MEDICAL EDUCATION
Theory and Practice

To Jane
Good reading!
Best wishes, John

Commissioning Editor: Laurence Hunter
Senior Development Editor: Ailsa Laing
Project Manager: Alan Nicholson
Designer: Kirsteen Wright
Illustration Manager: Gillian Richards

MEDICAL EDUCATION
Theory and Practice

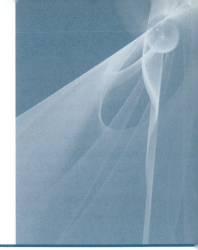

Edited by

Tim Dornan PhD DM FRCP MHPE
Professor, Maastricht University, the Netherlands, and Honorary Professor, University of Manchester, Manchester, UK

Karen Mann BN MSc PhD
Professor Emeritus, Division of Medical Education, Faculty of Medicine, Dalhousie University, Halifax, Nova Scotia, Canada, and Honorary Professor, University of Manchester, Manchester, UK

Albert Scherpbier MD PhD
Professor, Scientific Director of the Institute for Education and Associate Dean of Education, Faculty of Health, Medicine and Life Sciences, Maastricht University, the Netherlands

John Spencer MBChB FRCGP
Professor, and Sub-Dean for Primary and Community Care, School of Medical Sciences, Newcastle University Medical School, Newcastle-upon-Tyne, UK

Foreword by

Geoff Norman PhD
Canada Research Chair in Cognitive Dimensions of Clinical Expertise; Assistant Dean, Programme for Educational Research and Development (PERD), McMaster University; Professor, Department of Clinical Epidemiology & Biostatistics, McMaster University, Ontario, Canada

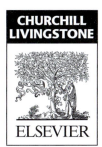

CHURCHILL LIVINGSTONE

ELSEVIER

Edinburgh   London   New York   Oxford   Philadelphia   St Louis   Sydney   Toronto 2011

CHURCHILL
LIVINGSTONE
ELSEVIER

© 2011 Elsevier Ltd. All rights reserved.

ISBN 978-0-7020-3522-7

British Library Cataloguing in Publication Data
A catalogue record for this book is available from the British Library

Library of Congress Cataloguing in Publication Data
A catalogue record for this book is available from the Library of Congress

Notices

Knowledge and best practice in this field are constantly changing. As new research and experience broaden our understanding, changes in research methods, professional practices, or medical treatment may become necessary.

Practitioners and researchers must always rely on their own experience and knowledge in evaluating and using any information, methods, compounds, or experiments described herein. In using such information or methods, they should be mindful of their own safety and the safety of others, including parties for whom they have a professional responsibility.

With respect to any drug or pharmaceutical products identified, readers are advised to check the most current information provided (i) on procedures featured or (ii) by the manufacturer of each product to be administered, to verify the recommended dose or formula, the method and duration of administration, and contraindications. It is the responsibility of practitioners, relying on their own experience and knowledge of their patients, to make diagnoses, to determine dosages and the best treatment for each individual patient, and to take all appropriate safety precautions.

To the fullest extent of the law, neither the Publisher nor the authors, contributors, or editors, assume any liability for any injury and/or damage to persons or property as a matter of products liability, negligence or otherwise, or from any use or operation of any methods, products, instructions, or ideas contained in the material herein.

your source for books,
journals and multimedia
in the health sciences
www.elsevierhealth.com

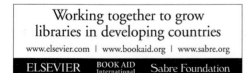
Working together to grow
libraries in developing countries
www.elsevier.com | www.bookaid.org | www.sabre.org

ELSEVIER   BOOK AID International   Sabre Foundation

The Publisher's policy is to use paper manufactured from sustainable forests

Printed in China

Contents

Foreword

The invitation to write a foreword for this book is a considerable honour, although I am first to admit that this small contribution hardly merits the appearance of my name in large font on the title page, alongside the editors who have contributed so many hundreds of hours toward the creation of this *magnum opus*.

Medical education is a growing field, with at least five peer-reviewed journals, (and likely many more, depending on how you count them), several hundreds of articles each year, and a regular presence in mainstream journals such as BMJ and JAMA. Somewhat paradoxically, however, there are few 'textbooks' to which one can refer. There is a real need – graduate degree programs in medical education are proliferating worldwide, and almost every medical school I visit has a number of faculty pursuing graduate training in medical education, either locally or as a student in one of the large international programs. Fellowship programs are becoming increasingly common. The FAIMER (Foundation for the Advancement of International Medical Education Research) Fellowship, sponsored by the Educational Commission for Foreign Medical Graduates in the United States, has graduated over 400 fellows.

All of these students need resources, but they are few and far between. While some groups like ASME and AMEE have produced monograph series, and review articles appear from time to time, neither can replace the systematic presentation of information provided by a textbook. Books do appear from time to time; the last comprehensive treatment I can recall is the *International Handbook for Research in Medical Education*, which I co-edited with Cees van der Vleuten and David Newble. It appeared in 2002 and disappeared soon after.

Why are books on the subject so rare? One explanation is that, unlike physiology or statistics, medical education, like all education, is not a discipline. As Shulman (1981) said many years ago:

A major reason why research methodology in education is such an exciting area is that education is not itself a discipline. Indeed, *education is a field of study*, a locus containing phenomena, events, institutions, problems, persons, and processes, which themselves constitute the raw material for inquiries of many kinds. The perspectives and procedures of many disciplines can be brought to bear on the questions arising from and inherent in education as a field of study. As each of these disciplinary perspectives is brought to bear on the field of education, it brings with it its own set of concepts, methods and procedures, often modify in them [sic] to fit the phenomena or problems of education. Such modifications, however, can rarely violate the principles defining these disciplines from which the methods were drawn.

Schulman LS 1981. Disciplines of inquiry in education: an overview. *Educational Researcher* 10(6):5–12.

Indeed, the editors of this book share a similar perspective. In the introductory chapter, they speak of medical education as a domain, with 'boundaries, a landscape, a colourful mix of inhabitants, social systems... and a role in the wider world.' A far cry from how a biochemistry book might begin. The consequence of this viewpoint is that it is well-nigh impossible to define precisely what medical education *is*. When we say that someone has a graduate degree in medical education, what new skills does she now possess? If we were to set a licensing examination for medical educators, what content should we cover? In a field like statistics, this is easy. Virtually every statistics book has the same chapters, and examination questions would show great commonality. In medical education, this is not the case. A few years ago, program chairs of degree programs in medical education met to discuss common standards. The discussion terminated without any attempt at consensus within an hour; all present agreed the task was impossible. A similar conclusion results from perusing the table of contents of our old *International Handbook* with its 31 chapters, and the 19 chapters of *Medical Education: Theory and Practice*. I counted 2 chapters that appeared to cover similar ground. However, such divergence is not simply a case of random variation. The three of us who drafted the outline of the *Handbook* were unabashedly quantitative in our orientation.

Medical Education: Theory and Practice has a different and unique perspective. Beginning with their 'domain' metaphor, the authors and the editors share a humanitarian viewpoint that is, I think, unique among the books in this field. Nowhere is this more evident than in the first chapter by Tan, Sutton and Dornan, which discusses medical education as a 'social good'. In a subsequent chapter on learning, they discuss four orientations – behaviourist, cognitivist, social and humanist, but as the story unfolds, the dominant orientation is clearly to the social and humanist. Their preoccupation is with the wellbeing of students, teachers and patients, a concern that is too frequently lost in the research literature, with its preoccupation with *p*-values and effect sizes.

Like all large edited books, *Medical Education: Theory and Practice* represents an enormous collective effort among many academics. While it may never be possible, or even desirable, to define precisely what the field of medical education represents in terms of specific knowledge or skills, one conclusion is clear from this volume – practitioners of medical education research share a commitment to scholarship that is second to none. I am proud to be associated, if only in a minor way, with such an authoritative treatise.

Geoff Norman
Ontario, 2011

This book is the product not so much of a collaboration as of an extended family. It started with a conversation between the nuclear family (Tim Dornan, Karen Mann, Albert Scherpbier, and John Spencer) and Laurence Hunter from Elsevier. Where, we wondered, would a Masters student, PhD student, or scholarly educator wanting to learn above the basic operational level find the underpinning principles of medical education clearly articulated, and linked to practice? There seemed a need to set educational method in a well-articulated theoretical context that was both scholarly and practical. Conversations with Laurence have an uncanny habit of turning into book proposals because he makes the perspiration of book-writing seem more like inspiration, at least in anticipation. After an over-long gestation period, a set of proposals emerged and the hunt for authors began. The specifications were ambitious. We wanted authors who would think and write outside the box while knowing the contents of the box very well. We wanted a geographical spread of authors, not exclusively anglophone. We wanted both well-established scholars and rising stars. And we wanted willingness to write to a brief against quite a tight timeline.

The nuclear family is quite diverse. Tim Dornan is a British internist and endocrinologist turned education researcher, who completed Masters and PhD degrees in medical education rather far on in his career. His main interest is now in education research, particularly methodological aspects and research into workplace learning. Karen Mann is Canadian and her background is in nursing, health education, and education. She is a medical educationalist with experience of undergraduate programme leadership, who has conducted research and published extensively in the field. She has held a number of lead roles in North American medical education. Albert Scherpbier is a Dutch doctor who, early in his career, was drawn from a career in surgery into the world of medical education. He has been the academic lead of a clinical skills laboratory, and then of an internationally renowned undergraduate medical programme. He has published extensively on a whole variety of medical education research topics. John

Spencer is an English general practitioner, who is a leader in community-oriented medical education. He has been very active in the teaching of communication skills and has latterly developed a strong interest in professionalism. He has also been a journal editor. His time is now delicately balanced between caring for patients, teaching, leading an undergraduate programme, writing, and research.

The extended family is certainly not linked by genetic inheritance, or even by 'nurture', because we sought out people from diverse disciplinary backgrounds. It is, however, linked by a common passion for what Chapter 1 describes as 'a good'-medical education. The extended family is also linked by a preference for well-reasoned argument and sound empirical evidence over tradition and dogma, and by having the courage to say unfamiliar, even unpopular things.

The book lays out some underpinning principles of medical education in the six chapters of Section 1, and then reviews the contexts, processes, and outcomes of medical education in the remaining 13 chapters that constitute Section 2.

Naomi Tan, a British medical student who went through the transition into early postgraduate life while working on Chapter 1, wrote it with Adrian Sutton, a psycho-analytically oriented British child psychiatrist with a keen interest in ethics, and Tim Dornan. They compare and contrast the *morality and philosophy of medicine and education*. They explore the rights and responsibilities of patients and then meld a perspective on human development with their expert knowledge of educational processes. They frame workplace medical education in a novel way as 'the participative emergence of form'.

Karen Mann was the principal author of Chapter 2, which she wrote with Pim Teunissen, a Dutch Obstetrics and Gynaecology resident who was awarded a PhD in medical education during the book's gestation, and Tim Dornan. This chapter presents and explores similarities and differences between an eclectic selection of theoretical *perspectives on learning*. It shows how good awareness of theory can inform practice – and help 'raise the game' of medical education.

Chapter 3 teams Ayelet Kuper, a Canadian internist with a doctoral background in literature, with Brian Hodges, a Canadian psychiatrist, qualitative researcher, and research group leader, to consider *medical education in its societal context*. They explore five different theoretical perspectives – a Foucauldian discourse perspective, a Bourdieuvian perspective on education as symbolic capital, a Neo-Marxist perspective, the perspective of a combined (feminist and anti-racist) equity agenda, and finally a post-colonial perspective. They show how each might be used to frame questions in medical education practice and research, and consider how they illuminate medical schools' social missions.

While there are important similarities between medical education and education for other knowledge-rich health professions, which include dentistry, veterinary medicine, and pharmacy, the central thrust of this book is uniprofessional. Chapter 4, however, places *medical education in an interprofessional context*. Scott Reeves, a British sociologist working in Canada whose research pedigree is in the ethnographic tradition, teamed up with Joanne Goldman, a health services researcher from Canada, to consider the theoretical background of interprofessional education (IPE), methods of delivering it, and evidence of its effectiveness.

Chapter 5 was written by Angela Towle and William Godolphin, two scholars from Vancouver, BC, Canada, who share a background in biomedical science and medical education and a long history of working together to ensure that patients' voices are clearly heard in the education of doctors. They write of how *patient involvement in health professional education* has changed from relatively passive involvement as 'teaching aids' to active participation. Their writing spans practical matters that must be attended to when involving patients through to matters of international policy and practice, ending with a look into the future.

One of just two with a single author, Chapter 6 was written by Colin Coles, a widely published British scholar of *curriculum development in learning medicine*. He reflects on the later consequences of the recommendations for curriculum reform Flexner made a century ago. He frames 'a curriculum' as 'something that exists, whether people know it or not, in any educational event or activity' and which may take the form of a curriculum on paper, a curriculum in action, or a curriculum as experienced by teachers and learners. Chapter 6 tells us that curriculum development must be based on sound educational principles and grounded in values, and that the true curriculum developers are the teachers and learners: they are the people who make education 'work'.

Section 2 begins with Chapter 7, which was written by two doctors still going through their own postgraduate education, both of whose PhD theses concerned *creating a learning environment*. Klarke Boor is a Dutch obstetrics and gynaecology resident, while Rachel Isba is a British physician with a background in paediatrics, who entered public health residency while the book was in preparation. In addition to the fruits of their research, they bring experiences of optimising medical students' learning environments in two different European countries to bear on the topic. They consider what (in material, social, and intra-psychological terms) a learning environment is, and why it is important. Chapter 7 shows how considering teaching as a feature of a learning environment shifts the emphasis from a traditional teacher-centred environment to a learner-centred one.

Chapter 8 was written by two US scholars of medical education, Casey White and Larry Gruppen, who share a research and practice interest in *identifying learners' needs and self-assessment*. The focus of the chapter is on how to help learners take responsibility for identifying and addressing their learning needs. The authors weave between theory – notably adult learning principles – and practice, considering how theory defines effective teaching behaviours. Like the previous chapter (and the next one), this chapter is a rich source of advice about how to be an effective teacher in a learner-centred environment.

Chapter 9 brings together Reg Dennick, a British educationalist with a background in biochemistry and an interest in *teaching and learning in small groups*, and John Spencer. They argue that small group interaction not only takes learners to higher levels of learning but also teaches them important (social) skills. They show how a wide range of theoretical perspectives on small group learning can inform the all-important skill of group facilitation and describe various stages in the developmental trajectory of small groups, including the group dynamics that characterise them. They bring us into the information age by describing virtual groups and the special facilitatory and participatory skills they call for.

Chapter 10 takes us from small groups to *teaching and learning in large groups*. Tim Dornan's perspective is supplemented by the expertise of Rachel Ellaway, a British educationalist who works in Canada, in applying education technology to medicine. The authors rise to the challenge of an authority in the field, who asked why the large group genre has not been scrapped, by considering the cognitive benefits of skilfully delivered lectures. This chapter is deliberately practical in its orientation, but draws on cognitive psychology to justify some of its suggestions. It ends by considering how new educational technologies can augment this time-honoured educational method and sustain its relevance in the hands of skilled educators.

Roger Kneebone and Debra Nestel wrote Chapter 11. Roger is a UK doctor, whose background includes surgery and general practice (GP) and who both researches *learning and teaching clinical procedures* and leads a Masters programme in Surgical Education. After completing a doctorate on clinical communication in Hong Kong, Debra worked for many years with Roger in the United Kingdom and is now Professor of Medical Education in Australia. They start the chapter by considering how traditional medical apprenticeship is coming under pressure in the modern age, survey a wide range of relevant theoretical perspectives, and then bring both real and simulated patients into the frame. They present some of the intricacies of simulation and end by presenting their concept of layered learning.

Chapter 12 spans not just the lifelong learning continuum but also the globe because it was written by Pim Teunissen from the Netherlands, who completed a PhD thesis on *learning and teaching in* (postgraduate) *workplaces* while the book was in preparation (see also notes on Chapter 2, earlier), and Tim Wilkinson, a geriatrician and Professor of Medical Education in New Zealand, whose research has included both undergraduate and postgraduate workplace learning. Such is the power of electronic communication that they had nearly finished the chapter before they met for the first time! Workplace learning, they tell us, can be serendipitous and messy, or planned and systematic. The triadic relationship between learner, patient, and expert physician lies at its core and the context in which it occurs is an important component of learning. Participation supported by effective feedback, the chapter tells us, is fundamental to workplace learning.

Erik Driessen is a Dutch educationalist, who has made the study of reflective, portfolio learning his major academic interest. He has done much research with Jan van Tartwijk, also Dutch and also a scholar of reflective, portfolio learning, but with a background in teacher education. In writing Chapter 13 about *learning from practice: routines, mentoring, feedback,*

and portfolios, they were joined by Karlijn Overeem, a resident in GP and PhD student. They revisit Chapter 8 to highlight the centrality of self-assessment in learning from practice and also highlight the importance of mentoring for learning. They explore, in tandem, the interrelated roles of teachers and learners.

Chapter 14 again straddles the lifelong learning continuum, having been jointly written by Val Wass, a general practitioner and Professor of Medical Education who is internationally eminent in the field of *assessing learners* and wrote her PhD thesis on the topic, and Julian Archer, a paediatric resident similarly with a PhD in assessment, who is co-developing his career in clinical medicine and education, and is a leader in the development of workplace-based assessment methods for learning. Having acknowledged that assessment drives learning, they take a forward-looking perspective on assessment as a developmentally formative process. They make complex concepts, including psychometric ones, accessible by introducing them in quite simple terms.

Chapter 15 is another Dutch team effort, having been written by Diana Dolmans, Renée Stalmeijer, Henk van Berkel, and Ineke Wolfhagen, all educational psychologists, who are well-established researchers and leaders in the field of *quality assurance of teaching and learning*. They are a team, not just in sharing expertise but in working together to bring it to bear on educational processes in their own institution. Starting from simple concepts, they build towards a vision of quality improvement as something which has to permeate the entire culture of any institution that aspires to excellence.

Rachel Ellaway, who was introduced in the note earlier about Chapter 10, is the book's other solitary author, for Chapter 16. She is solitary because her level of expertise in *developing learning resources* is at a premium in the medical education world – Scotland's loss of it became Canada's gain! She takes readers on a whirlwind tour of types of learning resources, ways of developing and using them, and economic considerations when adopting them, to which a vignette like this cannot do justice. Justice can, however, begin to be served by quoting her own warning against being seduced by the affordances of technology: 'Simply making learning resources available to learners will not guarantee any kind of result. At best … learning (can be) catalysed by the use of a learning resource'.

Harold Reiter and Kevin Eva, both from McMaster University in Canada, jointly collaborate in research into *selecting for medicine*, the topic of

Chapter 17. Harold is a radiation oncologist with a Masters of Education focusing on psychometry, and is a medical school admissions chair. Kevin, a cognitive scientist and education researcher, is also Editor-in-Chief of a leading medical education journal. With a timeline from Flexner on, they chart the topic of medical admissions. Selection for medicine at the start of the twentieth century, they tell us, fully deserved the criticism Flexner poured on it. They describe a process of progressive enlightenment, bringing us to the present time when social pressures again threaten to compromise the task of selecting the most suitable people for medicine.

Katherine Woolf, another British author who completed a PhD in medical education during the gestation of this book, wrote Chapter 18 with Chris McManus, a dual-qualified British scholar of medicine and psychology, who has conducted a large corpus of research into *predicting and guiding career success in medicine*. They plunge us straight into the apparent paradox that a good understanding of careers must pay equal attention to the way people are similar and the way they are different; in the authors' words, 'any understanding of careers has to acknowledge..(the).. three levels, of invariance, similarity and individuality'. Having illuminated their field from psychological, social cognitive, and sociological theoretical perspectives, they draw out sound practical guidance.

Chapter 19 is unique within the extended authorship family in having been written by a husband and wife partnership from the David Geffen School of Medicine at the University of California, Los Angeles, which has also been a very productive scholarly one. LuAnn Wilkerson (who has applied her doctorate in education to the study and improvement of medical education over the past 25 years) is widely recognised as an authority on *developing teachers* and her expertise is complemented by the scholarly and practical experience of Hy Doyle (known across the United States for his work in cultivating, recruiting, admitting, and supporting a broadly diverse medical student body) in *developing learners*. Every preceding chapter having framed education in terms of human relationships within social contexts, it is entirely fitting that the book rounds up with their complementary perspectives on how to make the best of the human capital in a medical curriculum – its teachers and students. The authors go to great lengths to place their wisdom within an international context, so it is both practically relevant to individual contexts, and generalisable enough to transcend them.

Professor Kieran Sweeney, whose interpretation of the 'Human Effect in Medicine' spanned philosophy, clinical medicine, and a compassionate understanding of the human condition, graciously turned down our invitation to write for the book because of a recently diagnosed disease. He sadly died before it appeared in print, but he is part of it insofar as he inspired some of its material, albeit expressed nowhere near so well as if he had written it.

We hope that readers of this book will regard the authors and their backgrounds as a very integral part of what lies between its covers. Our effort to recruit authors from across the globe, who we believed would have something fresh to say, ranged from medical student to senior professor, represented a spectrum of disciplines, and was perhaps our major contribution. We thank them for what they have taught us and for being, without exception, such fun to work with and so prompt and diligent in their efforts. We have already acknowledged Laurence Hunter's role in the conception of this book and thank him for his part in its gestation and delivery. Ailsa Laing, also from Elsevier, was a staunch supporter as our efforts began to pay fruit. A person who stands apart from all others in deserving our thanks is Kim Hunter, who kept the project on track throughout and came to be known as the member of the extended family who could be relied on for courteous, timely, and supportive communication. Her efforts, most particularly in pulling the book together at the end, were above price. In that, she was helped by Angee Khara, who put the references in order. A surprisingly large part of the extended family did not use reference management software, so that was no mean task and we thank Angee for accomplishing it in such a timely way. And two final comments. We thank three unwittingly honorary members of the extended family – Ceri, Ian, and Gail – whose support to Tim, Karen, and John was also a very integral part of our work. Albert invested himself in the other three of us in his characteristically unselfish way, so let us hope that we three provided some sort of support to his efforts – it was certainly fun working together!

Tim Dornan
Karen Mann
Albert Scherpbier
John Spencer

Contributors

Julian Archer MB ChB MRCPCH FHEA MEd PhD FAcadMed
Clinical Lecturer in Medical Education, National Institute for
Health Research Academic, Peninsula College of Medicine
& Dentistry, Plymouth, UK

Klarke Boor MD PhD
Specialist trainee in the field of Obstetrics and
Gynaecology, VU University Medical Centre, Amsterdam,
The Netherlands

Colin Coles BSc MA PhD
Professor, Faculty of Education, Health and Social Care,
University of Winchester, Winchester, UK

Reg Dennick BSc PhD MEd FHEA
Professor of Medical Education, and Assistant Director
of Medical Education, University of Nottingham,
Nottingham, UK

Diana Dolmans PhD
Associate Professor Faculty of Health, Medicine and Life
Sciences (FHML), University of Maastricht, Maastricht,
The Netherlands

Lawrence Hy Doyle Ed.D
Executive Director UCLA PRIME, David Geffen School of
Medicine, UCLA, Los Angeles, California, USA

Erik Driessen PhD
Assistant Professor in Medical Education, University of
Maastricht, Maastricht, The Netherlands

Rachel H. Ellaway PhD
Assistant Dean and Associate Professor Informatics,
Northern Ontario School of Medicine, Sudbury, Ontario,
Canada

Kevin W. Eva PhD
Associate Professor and Director of Education Research
and Scholarship, Department of Medicine; Senior Scientist,
Centre for Health Education Scholarship, University of
British Columbia, Vancouver, BC, Canada

William Godolphin PhD
Professor Emeritus, Department of Pathology & Laboratory
Medicine, Faculty of Medicine, The University of British
Columbia, and Co-director, Division of Health Care
Communication, College of Health Disciplines, The University
of British Columbia, Vancouver, British Columbia, Canada

Joanne Goldman MSc
Research Associate, Keenan Research Centre, Li Ka Shing
Knowledge Institute of St. Michael's Hospital and Office of
Continuing Education and Professional Development,
University of Toronto, Toronto, Ontario, Canada

Larry Gruppen PhD
Chair, Department of Medical Education; Josiah Macy, Jr.
Professor of Medical Education, University of Michigan
Medical School, Ann Arbor, MI, USA

Brian Hodges MD PhD FRCPC
Professor, Scientist and Director, Wilson Centre for Research in
Education; Richard and Elizabeth Currie Chair in Health
Professions Education Research, Faculty of Medicine/University
Health Network, University of Toronto, Toronto, Ontario, Canada

Rachel Isba BA MSc DLSHTM BM BCh MA DRCOG MAcadMed
PhD
Clinical Lecturer in Medical Education, Lancaster University,
and Specialty Registrar in Public Health, Mersey
Deanery, UK

Roger Kneebone PhD FRCS FRCGP
Reader in Surgical Education, Imperial College London,
London, UK

Ayelet Kuper MD DPhil FRCPC
Assistant Professor, Department of Medicine, and Scientist,
Wilson Centre for Research in Education, University of
Toronto, Toronto, Ontario, Canada

Chris McManus FRCP(Lond,Ed) FMedSci
Professor of Psychology and Medical Education, University
College London, London, UK

Debra Nestel PhD
Professor of Medical Education, Gippsland Medical School, Monash University, Victoria, Australia

Karlijn Overeem MD
PhD student in General Practice, and Researcher, Scientific Institute for Quality of Healthcare, Radboud University Nijmegen Medical Centre, Nijmegen, The Netherlands

Scott Reeves PhD
Director of Research, Centre for Faculty Development, and Scientist, Keenan Research Centre, Li Ka Shing Knowledge Institute, St Michael's Hospital; Scientist, Wilson Centre for Research in Education; Associate Professor, University of Toronto, Toronto, Ontario, Canada

Harold Reiter MD MEd FRCPC DABR
Professor, Department of Oncology, McMaster University, Hamilton, Ontario, Canada

Renée Stalmeijer MSc
Educationalist, Researcher, Faculty of Health, Medicine, and Life Sciences, Maastricht University, Maastricht, The Netherlands

Adrian Sutton BSc (Hons) MB BS FRCPsych
Senior Teaching Fellow & Curriculum Lead for Ethics and Law, Manchester Medical School, University of Manchester, Manchester, UK

Naomi Tan MBChB BSc (Hons)
F1 Doctor, Royal Free Hospital, London, UK

Pim W. Teunissen MD PhD
Medical Education Researcher, Maastricht University, Maastricht, The Netherlands, and Resident in Obstetrics and Gynaecology, VU University Medical Centre, Amsterdam, The Netherlands

Angela Towle PhD
Associate Professor, Department of Medicine, Faculty of Medicine, and Co-Director, Division of Health Care Communication, College of Health Disciplines, University of British Columbia, Vancouver, British Columbia, Canada

Henk van Berkel PhD
Associate Professor Faculty of Health, Medicine and Life Sciences (FHML) University of Maastricht, Maastricht, The Netherlands

Jan van Tartwijk PhD
Professor of Education, Faculty of Social and Behavioural Sciences, Utrecht University, Utrecht, The Netherlands

Valerie Wass BSc FRCGP FRCP MHPE PhD FHEA FCGP SL
Professor of Medical Education, Keele University, Keele, UK

Casey White PhD
Assistant Professor, and Assistant Dean for Medical Education, University of Michigan Medical School, Ann Arbor, MI, USA

LuAnn Wilkerson Ed.D
Professor of Medicine, and Senior Associate Dean for Medical Education, David Geffen School of Medicine at the University of California, Los Angeles, California, USA

Tim J. Wilkinson MB ChB M Clin Ed PhD MD FRACP
Professor of Medicine, and Associate Dean (medical education), University of Otago, Christchurch, New Zealand

Ineke Wolfhagen PhD
Associate Professor Faculty of Health, Medicine and Life Sciences (FHML) University of Maastricht, Maastricht, The Netherlands

Katherine Woolf BSc(Hons) PhD FHEA
Lecturer in Medical Education, UCL, London, UK

An introduction to the medical education domain

Tim Dornan   Karen Mann   Albert Scherpbier   John Spencer

Outline

This chapter starts by explaining why it is helpful to think of medical education as a 'domain'. Then, it describes the domain in enough detail to provide a meeting point between readers who have only recently arrived in it and others who are already familiar with it. The first section represents medical education as a lifelong learning continuum, explaining how learners enter the continuum and what they experience thereafter. It highlights nodal points along the way that can give learners a sense of discontinuity; in particular, the summative assessments that allow them to progress, and their experiences of transition when they do so. The next section explains a number of themes that are common to all stages of the continuum and therefore characterise the domain. The last section identifies some contemporary tensions in the scholarship of medical education, which is relatively young, restless, and forward-looking, seeking to define how medical practice can be made most useful to society. The aim of the chapter is to 'problematise' medical education – readers who are unfamiliar or uncomfortable with the term will find a very good illustration of it in the way Coles teases out 'the curriculum problem' in Chapter 6. Essentially, we set out to define the problems to which this book provides solutions. There are some matters on which most people agree. There are others on which people disagree. Indeed, one person's orthodoxy can be another's heresy. Even in those parts of the domain that are commonly regarded as orthodoxy, why are they orthodox and what are the dangers of leaving their orthodoxy

unchallenged? And why are there tensions in the domain? The word tension must not be regarded as a pejorative because it is along fault lines that progress is made. Perhaps we should even be more afraid of peace than struggle! This chapter draws its material almost exclusively from the other 19 chapters of the book. It leaves the fault lines gaping wide to motivate you to find resolution in the later chapters.

Introduction

The 'domain' metaphor is a fit one because medical education, like geographical domains, has boundaries, a landscape, a colourful mix of inhabitants, social systems that energise it and manage power within it, and a role in the wider world. Unlike geographical domains, however, this is a global one with more similarities than differences in its delivery around the world. There is a good chance its uniformity will change because, historically, North American and Western European thinking has had a hegemonic grasp over traditionally less powerful parts of the world, which it may have to relinquish. But that is over the horizon so, for now, there is more uniformity than variation.

Section 1: The medical lifelong learning continuum

Although it is truly a continuum, the domain divides easily along a timeline into undergraduate medical education, postgraduate medical education, and continuing medical education (CME). The latter is increasingly called continuing professional development (CPD) to emphasise that it concerns personal development but we term it CME throughout this chapter in line with the book's focus on medical education.

Undergraduate medical education

Admission

Entrants to medical education have typically been grounded in physical and perhaps biological science in high school, in an access course, or in a prior degree programme. They may arrive fresh from secondary school, from another degree course, or from another career. A prior degree is an entrance requirement in the United States and Canada. Programmes in other parts of the world are more typically non-graduate entry, although calls for widened participation have led to the development of graduate entry tracks, which make medical education attractive to older entrants. The age of medical school entrants ranges from 18 – completion of secondary school – to the early forties, after which age the number of years serving society is insufficient to offset the cost of educating a doctor. Everywhere in the world, undergraduate medical education (confusingly, the same term is used to include the education of both undergraduate and graduate entrants) is higher education (i.e. delivered by a university). The attributes of practising doctors are determined to an important degree by the attributes of the people who enter medical school, so the selection of learners for medicine is a very important feature of the domain. Becoming a doctor is a popular career choice and a demanding course of study, so academic thresholds for entry are very high. In addition to measures of academic performance, some programmes use aptitude and personality tests and/or admission interviews to select their entrants. In Chapter 17, Reiter and Eva chart how admissions procedures have come to be 'reliable' insofar as they select entrants with a particular set of measurable attributes with any precision. Reliability, however, comes at a cost because the humane qualities of a good doctor are so personal that they are hard to measure in a replicable way. For that reason, replicable testing can distract from the elusive goal of identifying the best future professionals. Reiter and Eva explain how the process of selection for medicine is further complicated by today's social trends such as equity in access to medical school.

Length of the programme

Graduate entry programmes typically last 4 years while undergraduate entry programmes last longer. The length of the programmes is determined, in part, by whether they include a period of internship at the end (performing as part of a clinical care team in the capacity of a junior apprentice). Medical schools on the European mainland and some parts of Australasia do so, while internship in the United Kingdom begins after qualification perhaps because UK society is very intolerant of people who have not yet passed an exit test of competence delivering health care. The global picture is very confused. Programmes in the United States and Canada are all graduate entry and last 4 years, the final two being delivered along apprenticeship lines (a pre-internship if not an internship). At the other extreme, some 7-year programmes in southern mainland Europe withhold any authentic clinical experience until very late, at which time students start a type of internship. UK programmes provide clinical experience early and throughout the programme but often not integrated into real-time patient care. To make matters more complicated, the UK General Medical Council (accrediting body) is, at the time of writing, reversing trends by reinstating a type of pre-internship in the final year. The length of time before students get authentic experience in some programmes and the unofficial involvement of unqualified learners in authentic patient care in others will surely not be tolerated indefinitely in the European Union, which is seeking to standardise educational processes. For now, it is only possible to say that undergraduate medicine around the world lasts 3–7 years with widely varying clinical exposure (both quantity and timing) and engagement in authentic practice.

Curriculum

The early years

The rather specific description that follows is intended to complement what Coles has written in Chapter 6 about 'curriculum' as a construct, and how that construct applies in the medical domain. Undergraduate medical curricula have a fairly standard structure, although more integrative approaches described later are beginning to change the mould. The first 2–3 years are spent more in classroom than clinical settings and devoted primarily to learning the underpinning sciences of medicine with some clinical and communication skills. Biomedical sciences include anatomy, physiology, biochemistry, and pharmacology. Behavioural sciences include psychology and sociology. Medical schools tend to have a much stronger leaning towards biomedical than behavioural sciences, reflected in the large number of biomedical scientists among their faculty and the lesser emphasis given to behavioural sciences. Humanities – including literature, graphic arts, and music – tend to have an even smaller but increasing place in medical programmes. Disciplines like medical ethics and law, pathology, radiology, and population health/epidemiology, which bridge 'pure science' and practice, have a variable presence in medical curricula. University-employed scientists predominate over practitioners in the early medical curriculum years. The amount of exposure to authentic workplace or community settings in the early years varies from none at all to extensive.

Transition to clinical learning

There is, typically, a point of transition when the focus switches markedly from theory to practice, the settings switch from classrooms to clinical workplaces, and faculty change from university scientists to practitioners. The timing of that transition ranges from 2 to 6 years after entry, typically 2–3 years. Undergraduate entry programmes may give students the opportunity to insert an extra year of study at that point to obtain a Bachelor's degree, typically in one of the foundation disciplines of medicine. One way or another, the experience of transition is a powerful one. Learners undergo an identity change from being a university student to being a student doctor. Norms of dress and behaviour change from student to professional ones. The subject matter switches from theory to practice. There are clinical skills to learn. Working days are long and tiring. The whole purpose of studying medicine – to be able to promote health and relieve suffering – comes into focus, which can be very motivating. But the possibility of doing harm and the distance between where students are now and the point they have to reach become uncomfortably obvious. Some practitioners provide inspiring role models in their humanistic behaviour towards patients and students, while others are arrogant and unfeeling. There are incidents of student belittlement and abuse. Emotional peaks are high, troughs are deep, and learners may move erratically from one to the other. Most settle into the new way of learning very quickly. Some accelerate their progress because there is a better outlet for their abilities and they feel more motivated. Others

spiral down into failure and even withdraw from their programmes. There is a general increase in anxiety and depression, which may reach clinical proportions. It is at this stage that one of its more worrying features of undergraduate medical education emerges – the growth of cynicism and consequent decline in empathy. Partly, cynicism is a protection against the emotional forces that are at play in clinical settings. Partly, it is a response to the gap between the altruistic ideals that brought students into medicine in the first place and what it is really possible for doctors to do on behalf of patients. Partly, it arises from negative role modelling, whereby practitioners' cynicism rubs off on learners.

Clerkships

Typically, the clerkship years start with an orientation to clinical settings coupled with intensive instruction in basic clinical skills when it has not been provided in earlier years. There follows a rotation through placements in the major specialities: internal medicine; surgery; obstetrics/gynaecology; paediatrics; psychiatry; and primary care. Whereas classroom instruction predominates in the early years, educational activities now centre on encounters with patients, observed, set up for instructional purposes, or arising out of students' participation in authentic patient care. There may also be formal 'off the job' education including, increasingly, learning in simulated settings. The faculty includes both trained and trainee practitioners, senior students, and peers. It also includes members of other health professions, notably nurses and midwives. It may include scientists as well as practitioners. The extent to which clinical staff are university-employed, affiliated, or even non-affiliated varies by programme and country.

A tension within undergraduate medical education arises from the already large and increasing number of specialities that can offer clerkships. A set of specialities that raises one particular tension includes dermatology, ophthalmology, and ear, nose and throat surgery. The diseases in question are very prevalent and cared for either by generalists or by a number of specialists that is too small to allow specialist instruction for every student. Clerkships in those specialities, therefore, are typically of short duration with the potential for various negative consequences. There is a lack of continuity, which prevents practitioners and students from developing the relationships on which clinical learning depends. Coverage of subject matter is limited. Practitioners are worn down by 'production line' educational pressures, often superimposed on the clinical pressures of delivering a minority speciality. Another set of disciplines – exemplified by neurological medicine and surgery, and by musculoskeletal medicine and surgery – exemplifies a rather different problem. There is not so much a shortage of experts as a question about how truly relevant their increasingly specialised practice is to generalist education. The question manifests itself in struggles for curriculum time and protagonists' perception that their disciplines are not being given the prominence they deserve, often coupled with a perception that poor performance by qualified generalists could have been prevented by a more favourable apportionment of curriculum time. A third type of speciality, whose inclusion in undergraduate medical curricula is problematic, is what might be called 'service specialities'. They are generously staffed and play important roles in clinical care but have not traditionally been accorded the same importance as other clinical disciplines. Practitioners in those specialities include the pathologists who process morbid specimens (from biopsy material to recently deceased bodies), blood, and other bodily fluids; radiologists, who image (and, increasingly, treat) the body's disordered workings; and anaesthetists who render sick people operable by the surgeons who are in the curriculum mainstream. Those large specialities are important career pathways, so is it right that they should not be regarded as foundational disciplines and, if they are, how can they best be represented in a curriculum?

A final problematic aspect of clerkship education concerns primary care. To start with, huge semantic difficulties are posed by different usages of the term in US and UK medical English. Primary care includes internal medicine, paediatrics, and obstetrics/gynaecology in US terminology, but not in UK terminology. Britain, which has a strong tradition of GP, or 'family practice' in US medical English, uses the terms GP and primary care to mean much the same thing. Canada, Australia, and New Zealand are more aligned with UK English usage. Much of a GP's practice involves paediatrics and women's health, but paediatricians, obstetricians/gynaecologists, and general internists in UK practice are in secondary care, not primary care. The problem goes deeper than semantics and highlights how differences in health care systems affect medical curricula. No matter how primary care is defined, however, the undue dominance of tertiary (super-specialist) and secondary care specialities is a global issue, given the generalist goals of undergraduate medical education. Primary care, it can be argued,

is too important a facet of medical practice to be just one of many specialities in a clerkship rotation. A good case can be made that a generalist basic education is needed more than ever, supported by convincing evidence that primary care education can support a wide range of outcomes, including ones that were traditionally attained in hospital settings. To put the case for primary care education in a broader context, countries with better established primary care systems tend to have better health outcomes. Finally, many countries have difficulty recruiting generalists, so one important role of undergraduate medical education is to make careers in primary care attractive to students.

Choice and integration

Resolving the tension between specialities competing for space in medical curricula must be a local or national matter, and the decisions that are made must reflect the needs of the health care system and availability of disciplines to resource medical education. There are, however, two generic solutions that are becoming increasingly common. One is to differentiate between core learning, which must be common to all students, and optional placements, which students (usually) choose for themselves, such that there are differences in different students' experiences within one programme. Those optional placements may support a single, shared set of intended learning outcomes (ILOs) or they may each have different ILOs. Even then, the motivation to provide placements may be common to the different specialities involved – to provide 'tasters' which give learners an appetite to choose the speciality of the placement for their subsequent careers. A prime example is offering experience of remote or aboriginal care in countries with large land masses to foster recruitment to remote health care – particularly among students who themselves came from remote regions and might otherwise be drawn into urban practice.

The second generic solution to competition between disciplines for curriculum space is a more radical one, with a strong educational rationale. That is not to base the curriculum on disciplines at all, but to integrate them. Two terms are used to describe integration. Horizontal integration is to merge the subject matter of different disciplines into curriculum blocks, which are themed according to the various structures or functions of the body. Vertical integration is to break down the pre-clinical–clinical divide and have continuous, parallel strands of theory and practice running through the length of the undergraduate programme. Vertical integration breaks down disciplinary boundaries by encouraging scientists and practitioners to coordinate, or even pool, their educational efforts. Horizontal integration breaks down boundaries by putting the subject matter first and regarding faculty as exponents of subject matter rather than exponents of their disciplines. Vertical and horizontal integration are popular solutions to the theory–practice divide discussed later in this chapter and the proliferation of disciplines explained earlier. Vertical integration is mandated by the UK General Medical Council, has been strongly advocated in the United States and Canada, and is being adopted quite widely simply because it makes sense to expose medical students to practise early. Vertical integration of a scientific emphasis into the later curriculum years is progressing slowly, partly because practitioners assume that students will have achieved fluency in science disciplines by the time they enter clerkships and respond to finding that they have not by expressing frustration rather than sharing their practical understanding of them. Abandonment of that rather rigid assumption (which too easily results in belittlement of students) and greater enthusiasm on the part of practitioners to help students obtain fluency in science through the medium of practice is an important area for future curriculum development.

Horizontal integration deserves special mention because it lies behind one of the most important of higher education's instructional design developments in recent decades, which medicine was very quick to adopt; problem-based learning (PBL). Dennick and Spencer discuss PBL in the context of small group learning in Chapter 9. Not only does it embody horizontal integration, it embodies a student-centred, active learning educational design. Students are given a narrative, video, or other instructional material, which represents a problem of some sort and acts as a trigger for inquiry. Their task is to define the problem, articulate what they already know that could explain the problem, identify what they do not know, articulate a set of learning goals, meet those goals, explain the problem to one another in the presence of a tutor, and identify what they have learnt. Over the past three decades, PBL has become a new educational orthodoxy of the early curriculum years, reframing scientific disciplines and faculty within them as resources of knowledge rather than the organisational structure of the curriculum. When, as is often the case, the problem is a clinical scenario,

sciences integrate to provide not just explanations but solutions to problems. Adventurous curriculum designers have extended PBL into the clinical years with at least moderate success. There are, however, two problems in adopting PBL in the later years. One is that the understandable desire to 'heal' turns PBL into problem-solving, which changes what is intended to be an integrative exploration of underpinning theory into a discipline-based heuristic exercise. The second problem is that medical practice is not integrated, so the integration of declarative knowledge in a seminar room is perpetually contradicted by the disciplinary nature of practical bedside knowledge. A more general problem, which bedevils research into its outcomes, is that different people interpret the term PBL differently. New medical schools, in particular, have tended to adopt a hybrid approach, so PBL is not one single, clearly defined entity.

Assessment

The unfitness for practice of medical graduates a century ago sparked off a determination to implement rigorous assessment processes, which dominate undergraduate medical education to this day. The tension between reliable selection of competent people and valid selection of humane ones is as apparent in the judgement about which students are fit to qualify as in their selection for medical school entry. What losses are there of humane people, we might ask, if nobody who falls below a reliably measurable threshold of competence is allowed to graduate from a medical school? The problem is accentuated by modern society's intolerance of unprofessional behaviour on the part of doctors. It is, of course, a shocking fact that the worst serial killer in modern history was not just a UK doctor, but one who was very popular with many of his patients. It is understandable that steps should be taken to qualify only truly humane people. But what is society losing when it reduces humanity to the reliably measurable attributes captured by the word 'professionalism' and assessing it? And how sure can we be that inhumane, devious individuals will lack the cunning to work such an assessment system to their advantage? Wass and Archer pick their way through those complex issues in Chapter 14, explaining the trade-off between reliability and validity. Acknowledging that assessment drives learning, they propose that competency assessment should move away from examinations alone to a more developmental, formative approach in which decisions about learners' progression are guided by information from multiple and diverse sources.

Postgraduate medical education

Postgraduate education differs fundamentally from undergraduate education because learners are not spectators or even *peripheral* participants in the clinical workforce. They are salaried, productive members of it, who contribute an important part of the skill mix, albeit the most junior one. Put simply, clinical services could not be provided without the contribution of postgraduate learners. As a result, most postgraduate learning is 'on the job' and informal, although formal events are making an increasingly important educational contribution. Teunissen and Wilkinson explain workplace learning in Chapter 12, reminding us from the outset that the main purpose of a workplace is to get a job done. Learning is, for much of the time, subordinate to provision of patient care, though Teunissen and Wilkinson highlight ways in which the routine activities of workplaces can be designed to optimise learning.

Transition

While the first part of this chapter has highlighted international variability in the responsibility taken by learners before qualification and variability in the degree of specialisation in their posts after qualification, there is general agreement that entering the workforce represents a second point of transition. Again, there is an important shift in a learner's sense of identity, now from student to practitioner. The task of writing prescriptions exemplifies that transition very clearly. Up to the moment a person's medical qualification legally comes into force, they may not write prescriptions, a complex and socially embedded task which it is difficult to learn without actually performing it. From the moment of qualification, learners are not just able to write prescriptions but are the members of the workforce to whom this potentially harmful task most often devolves and who must accept responsibility for its outcomes. Not surprisingly, the 'shock of practice' created by such an abrupt transition brings about much the same emotional reactions as medical students' entry to clinical environments.

Curriculum

It is harder to generalise about postgraduate than undergraduate curricula because there is considerable variation by speciality and country. Residency typically lasts 5 years. Entry to it may follow directly after qualification or may follow an internship of up to 2 years. Competition to be accepted may impose a time gap between qualification and entry to residency, typically filled by taking on a junior non-training position. Until recently, residency curricula were described in terms of the experiences that should be provided, typically a rotation between learning contexts and subspecialities. While the rotational design of residencies has not changed, programmes tend now to be specified more in terms of competencies that must be acquired and assessments that must be passed. As with undergraduate curricula, we urge you to note that what we are describing here is, according to Coles in Chapter 6, the 'curriculum on paper', which may be very different from the 'curriculum in action', and different again from the 'hidden curriculum'. Note also the contrast between the relative simplicity of this description and the complexity that, according to Coles, is characteristic of curricula. Finally, we draw your attention to Coles' warning that the contemporary move towards competency-based postgraduate curricula threatens to change medical education into a form of technical training.

Instructional methods

The instructional approach of residency can loosely be described as an apprenticeship. Learning results from participation in practice under expert supervision with formative feedback, reflection on experience, and appraisal. In Chapter 12, Teunissen and Wilkinson underscore the importance of feedback for effective apprenticeship learning while Driessen, Overeem, and van Tartwijk, in Chapter 13, explain how important it is that masters mentor the reflective learning of their apprentices. Increasingly, instructional activities during residency include skills instruction using one of the simulation techniques described by Nestel and Kneebone in Chapter 11. Progression depends on successful performance in summative assessments, overseen by a process of regular appraisal. Beyond that it is hard to generalise because educational methods are very speciality-specific.

Assessment

Concomitant with the shift to competency-based education, it has become usual to assess the competence of postgraduate learners using one or more of the workplace-based assessment techniques described by Wass and Archer in Chapter 14. Typically, clinical performance and procedural skills are assessed by fully trained practitioners observing learners directly, making summative judgements, and providing formative feedback. The diet of assessments may also include a chart review. Professional attributes are assessed by a variety of co-workers, using a multi-source feedback instrument. In some countries – notably the United States and Canada – fitness for certification as a specialist is assessed by a summative test of knowledge and skills.

CME

CME is the least developed part of the medical education continuum although systems in Canada, Australia, and the United States have been developed considerably further than ones in many European countries. There have been two main drivers behind the introduction of CME. One is a pedagogic one, seeking to sustain and develop the expertise of fully trained practitioners throughout their careers. The other is a regulatory one, politically driven, and seeking to demonstrate to society that the medical profession is 'policing' the continuing education of its practitioners. They pull in different directions because the pedagogic approach is emancipatory, while the regulatory approach is more restrictive. The problem is that specialist expertise is so individual, contextually bound, and tacit that any system seeking to apply reproducible, standard criteria of competence is doomed either to failure or to undermining rather than reinforcing expertise. That, perhaps, is why research to date has shown little impact of formal CME on practice. The uneasy situation pertaining at the time of writing in the United Kingdom, whose system is more regulatory than emancipatory, is that enrolment in a CME scheme is a criterion for continued licensure. The system is designed for its regulatory purpose, with rather scant attention to the pedagogy of sustaining and developing expertise. Credits are awarded for participation in educational activities. The scheme is conceived of in terms of individual learning, sometimes without considering how individual and corporate development can subserve one another. Beyond accumulating credit hours, assessment is not yet a consistent feature of CME schemes although moves towards periodic relicensure will doubtless strengthen the case for summative assessment as a criterion for continued practice.

Conclusion to Section 1

Despite the discontinuities we have identified, a medical lifetime is more than a sequence of educational experiences arranged along a timeline. Medical students and doctors are bound together by professional activities and values. They co-participate in the educational events described in the next section. The responsibility of doctors to be teachers is a clearly defined part of the ethic of medicine and peer-assisted learning is an increasingly common feature of the undergraduate medical landscape. Learners in the later part of the continuum teach those in the early part of it – and are, in due course, replaced by them. In that sense, medical education takes place within a closed community. From an individual point of view, the continuum is a 'career', as described by Woolf and McManus, who start Chapter 18 by making the simple point that 'people differ'. So do their careers, supported by colleagues further along the continuum.

Section 2: Educational themes that run through the continuum

History

It is perhaps unsurprising that a pedagogic discipline whose history dates back two millennia sees today's educational practice in a historical context. Nestel and Kneebone (Chapter 11) explain how the need for simulation education has arisen from the passing of an era when the whole pace of medicine was slower, educational relationships were stable over long periods of time, and skills could be acquired through performing routine duties. The year of writing this chapter – 2010 – is the centenary of arguably the most influential event in the history of medical education, the publication of Abraham Flexner's recommendations for undergraduate medical education in the United States and Canada. Reiter and Eva (Chapter 17) explain how today's system of selecting for medicine was shaped by forces unleashed by the report, while Coles (Chapter 6) charts the 'explosion of curriculum development in medical education' that resulted from it. Kuper and Hodges (Chapter 3) characterise the Flexner report as so influential that medical educators still tend to regard its precepts as 'normal' without acknowledging that Flexner articulated them at a moment in history far removed from the one in which they are now being applied. At the time of writing, the Carnegie Foundation (which employed Flexner) had just published recommendations for a second step change in US medical education. They were to: move from time served to competencies achieved as the focus for medical education; achieve greater horizontal integration between theory and practice across the lifelong learning continuum; foster interprofessional collaboration; supervise learners more effectively; orientate medical education more towards doctors' role in society; foster a spirit of inquiry and improvement; and select/develop faculty more intentionally for their educational roles.

The humanist orientation of medical education

A humanist orientation, which, in the words of Mann, Dornan, and Teunissen (Chapter 2), 'focuses on human potential for growth and the freedom of individuals to become what they are capable of becoming', is common to the practices of medicine and of medical education. Chapter 2 goes on to explain that adult learning principles, which have come to the fore in recent decades, are humanist insofar as they see adults as 'actively seeking out experiences that contribute to and reflect their ongoing development'. Dennick and Spencer (Chapter 9) argue that similar humanist principles underpin relationships between teachers and learners in small group activities. Carl Rogers, according to Chapter 9, conceived of education in terms of relationships of mutual trust between teachers and learners, which encourage students to be curious and motivate them to learn. Tan, Sutton, and Dornan (Chapter 1) note similarities between patient-centred practice and learner-centred education founded on 'kindness' – an 'ability to bear the vulnerability of others, and therefore of oneself'.

Medical education as 'a social good'

The value system that governs one-to-one relationships in medicine and medical education, coupled with medicine's ability to promote health and relieve suffering, makes medical education a potential 'social good', though Tan, Sutton, and Dornan's exploration of this issue (Chapter 1) warns of the ethical difficulties that arise when trying to decide exactly how

education should realise its virtuous potential. Kuper and Hodges (Chapter 3) examine the issue of medical schools' social responsibility, pointing out how differently that responsibility can be defined depending on the theoretical perspective from which it is viewed. Towle and Godolphin (Chapter 5) explain the moral imperative to give people other than doctors a voice in medical education and describe ways in which education can be enriched by doing so. Certainly, there could be no medical education without the participation of people from the community, who are generally very ready to acknowledge its importance and participate in it.

Experience and context

What lies at the heart of medical education, more than any one pedagogic approach, is *experience* in *context*. A defining characteristic of clinical practice, according to Nestel and Kneebone (Chapter 11), is its complexity. Coles frames practice as a 'complex system' and warns against seeing it as 'a machine that simply needs oiling'. The fact that the experiential world of medicine is so complex creates opportunities and poses problems; opportunities because it has great power to stimulate learning; problems because its complexity can be bewildering, particularly to novices. Essential elements of experience can, however, be abstracted into the relative simplicity and safety of a small group discussion centred on a PBL scenario (Chapter 9) or instruction in a simulation laboratory (Chapter 11).

Mann, Dornan, and Teunissen (Chapter 2) argue that, however it is presented, experience is pivotal to learners' development at all points along the lifelong learning continuum because it lies at the heart of participation, which is central to social and collaborative perspectives on learning. Experience may arise 'simply as a result of living' or be provided in a way that gives teachers more control over it (Chapter 11). Experience is, however, only one of the variables that influences learning. Chapter 2 conceptualises learning as a cyclical process, which creates knowledge through the transformation of experience; learning, from that perspective, begins and ends in the experiential world. It follows logically that the more experience a person has, the more they stand to learn (Chapter 2). Teunissen and Wilkinson (Chapter 12) distinguish physical and social aspects of learning contexts, both of which must be attended to when constructing or choosing learning environments (see the next paragraph) or quality assuring them (end of Section 2, this chapter). While acknowledging that the complexity of clinical contexts may force at least some learning activities to be conducted in non-clinical ones, we must remember that 'all competencies are context bound' (Chapter 14); learners are better able to recall and apply competencies in places that are similar to those where they learnt them (Chapter 12). The workplace is, therefore, a centrally important context for learning because it is the context in which learning must later be applied. In that sense, workplaces present learners with both their learning opportunities and their ILOs (Chapter 12).

Learning environments and social interaction

The concept of a learning environment is an important one in contemporary medical education. Of course, learning environments provide the context for learning discussed in the previous section but they do more than that; they serve as catalysts (or inhibitors) of learning and, from a social perspective, even represent the subject matter of learning. Boor and Isba (Chapter 7) distinguish material elements of learning environments – facilities, resources, and organisational aspects – from social elements – people and the way they interact. 'Perhaps the most valuable element of any learning environment', they suggest, 'remains the people within it – learners, teachers and patients. People can have profound impacts – either positive or negative – upon learners and play a large part in the process of learning'. Boor and Isba also distinguish between 'formal' (lecture theatre or skills laboratory) and 'informal' (clinical workplace) environments. Finally, they point out that learning environments exist at many different organisational levels. Boor and Isba argue that teaching is not the central activity of medical education it was once considered to be but a feature of learning environments that influences the quality of learning.

Material aspects of learning environments

The technologies that support skills education described by Nestel and Kneebone (Chapter 11) and the learning resources described by Ellaway (Chapter 16) are very important material features of contemporary learning environments. While emphasising their importance, Ellaway places learning resources in a contextual, rather than central, relationship with learners and their learning – in her words, 'simply making learning resources available to learners will not guarantee any kind of result'. Some types of learning resources have more agency and are, themselves, able to generate other learning resources. Still other types can simulate activities that take place within learning environments or contribute to those activities by scaffolding or supporting social interactions (see also Chapter 8) but material aspects tend to subserve social ones.

Social aspects of learning environments

One-to-one or several-to-one relationships

One of the strongest themes that runs through this book is that social relationships between individual teachers and learners underpin medical education (Chapters 1,2,5–9,12,13,18). Tan, Sutton, and Dornan (Chapter 1) write of teachers and learners committing themselves jointly to the service of learning. Mann, Dornan, and Teunissen (Chapter 2) consider how relationships support participation in practice. Dennick and Spencer (Chapter 9) frame the dialogue between teacher and learner as a 'conversational apprenticeship'. The relationship cannot be a truly equal one because learners are less competent but teachers can limit learners' experiences of failure and build relationships by showing humility and being sure not to humiliate (Chapter 1). An effective educational relationship is one of mutual trust which, when teachers and learners provide clinical care together, is in patients' interests. Teunissen and Wilkinson (Chapter 12) take patients' involvement in medical education a step further by regarding the clinical teaching relationship as a triadic (rather than dyadic) one in which patients are participants rather than passive onlookers. Towle and Godolphin (Chapter 5) take the logic a stage further again when they describe how patients can take on the officially sanctioned role of mentors to learners. Sensitivity towards learners' emotional reactions is an important facet of an educational relationship, which (according to Driessen, Overeem, and van Tartwijk; Chapter 13) must provide honest feedback without being judgemental. The relationship between a small group facilitator and learners, according to Dennick and Spencer (Chapter 9), should be one that engenders a climate of trust, and helps learners build confidence and self-esteem. A final type of relationship between teachers and learners is a 'vicarious' one (Chapter 9) in which teachers may even be unaware they are serving as role models. Teachers can make role modelling explicit by drawing attention to aspects of their practice, which might otherwise pass unnoticed, and thereby help learners acquire tacit knowledge (Chapter 12).

Relationships within communities of practice

Mann, Dornan, and Teunissen (Chapter 2) parse out perspectives on learning and development according to whether they focus on individuals or on practice in a society and culture. The latter, known as socio-cultural perspectives, locate teaching and learning between rather than within individuals and go beyond one-to-one relationships to locate learning within groups of people; so-called 'communities of practice'. A socio-cultural perspective is not at odds with the individual social perspective articulated in the previous paragraph, but considers teachers and learners in terms of the communities they belong to more than as individuals. It is a remarkable fact that ethnographic research conducted in West African tailors, Mexican midwives, quartermasters in the US Navy, and Alcoholics Anonymous reported by Jean Lave and Etienne Wenger in 1991 should resonate so strongly in the world of medical education that no fewer than nine chapters of this book refer to it directly (Chapters 1,2,6,7,9,11,12,14,19). Communities of practice theory is discussed at greatest length in Chapters 2 and 12. To avoid undue repetition, this chapter quotes or paraphrases how the theory is represented at various points in the book: learners gradually become part of a professional group and their learning takes place through gradual absorption into a shared activity with common goals (Chapter 11). Learning is an integral and inseparable aspect of social practice and participation is the key to understanding how learners develop within a community (Chapter 12). A community of practice is a set of relations among persons, activity, and world over time that is the result of collective learning in the pursuit of a shared enterprise (Chapter 12). Learning is located squarely in the processes of co-participation, not in the heads of individuals. It is distributed among co-participants not a one-person act (Chapter 2). The work of Lave and Wenger moved the notion of apprenticeship from a dyadic relationship between teacher and learner centred on the performance of tasks to a social relationship between learners and communities of practice, centred on the co-construction of meaning and identity (Chapter 2). There is a reciprocal dynamic between learners' individual development and the development of their communities such that, at the end of the lifelong learning continuum,

'old-timers' may be transformed by more junior participants or come into conflict with them (Chapter 2). Medical learners are in a constant process of defining and redefining their identities throughout the lifelong learning continuum (Chapter 2). Avidly though communities of practice theory has been taken up by the medical education community, it sets up tensions that have yet to be fully explored. If learning resides so squarely within communities, how is it possible for learners to transfer their learning to other communities? One must assume the 'inter-subjectivity' (Chapter 12) that exists within communities rubs off on individuals in ways that extend beyond the confines of any one community in both space and time.

The subject matter of medical education

Section 1 described the specialities that contribute to medical education at different points along its continuum. Apart from the early undergraduate years and, in some specialities, when postgraduate learners prepare for summative knowledge tests, the subject matter of medical education is dominated by practice, either as a perspective that gives theory relevance and meaning, or as a perspective that is sufficient unto itself and far removed from theory. If that is true of Coles' 'curriculum on paper' (Chapter 6), it is even truer of his 'curriculum in action' and 'hidden curriculum'. Trained practitioners who espouse the importance of understanding theory usually do so only insofar as it is relevant to their practice. One can only imagine what would happen if a medical student, chastised by a surgeon for his lack of 'pure science' knowledge of skeletal anatomy, were to ask his (tor)mentor detailed questions about the physiology of the kidney. And how much would a nephrologist, whose practice depends on good knowledge of renal physiology, know about the surgical anatomy of the patella (kneecap)? That is not to belittle the knowledge that is required to be an effective doctor, but it is of a more tacit, contextualised nature than official curricula and clinical teachers tend to acknowledge. Possessing practical skills (Chapter 11) is more characteristic of doctors than members of some other professions, as is the possession of a highly developed system of values that is applied through the medium of practice (Chapter 1). It is conventional to categorise competence into knowledge, skills, and attitudes, a categorisation that is too crude and dichotomous to capture the hidden curricula and curricula in action of medicine; the tensions created by framing curricula on paper in such terms are considered in Section 3 of this chapter. Suffice it to say that the skills of fully trained practitioners are imbued with a highly encapsulated and applied form of knowledge and, as our surgeon and nephrologist illustrated earlier, knowledge is useful only insofar as it supports practice. Finally, 'attitudes' are useless if they are just warm feelings. They must be informed by good practical knowledge of medical ethics and law and applied with good interpersonal communication skills and moral purpose. The subject matter of medical education is a nexus, teased out in curricula so that learners can enter into conversations with the practitioners they must, eventually, emulate.

The pedagogy of medical education

The large group tradition (Chapter 10) is very strong in medicine, particularly at the two ends of the continuum: the undergraduate years and CME. Small group learning (Chapter 9) is increasingly strong in the undergraduate years but only variably strong in the later years, given how much cheaper it is to educate one large group than multiple small ones, and how superficially attractive it is to stay within one's comfort zone in a lecture theatre when one is senior enough to choose. The development of clinical skills (simulation) centres, as described in Chapter 11 by Nestel and Kneebone, has been one of the most conspicuous changes in the medical education landscape over the last two decades and is set to continue given the practical nature of the domain and the increasingly technical nature of practice. Methods of assessment have, likewise, changed rapidly, partly because of the affordances of simulation technology. Objective structured clinical examinations (OSCEs; see Chapter 14) have become a standard way of testing practical competence in simulated settings during the undergraduate years and are becoming more apparent in early postgraduate education as well. Knowledge tests have changed from oral examinations to more reliable, standardised, impersonal formats over the same period of three decades. More recently, workplace-based assessments of knowledge, behaviour, and clinical performance have been very rapidly adopted across the postgraduate education domain and are beginning to penetrate CME as well. The sheer scale and relative affluence of medical education has positioned the domain well to adopt the education technologies described in Chapters 11 and 16, fuelled by society's understandable wish for doctors to demonstrate their competence in 'safe' ways before patients are exposed to them. A notable import, originally from the world of graphic arts, has been the learning portfolio (Chapter 13). There has been persuasive scholarly writing about reflective learning, so it is now an unusual undergraduate, residency, or CME/CPD programme (in more developed countries, at least) that does not have reflective learning, supported by a portfolio, as part of its pedagogy.

The pedagogies described in the previous paragraph support 'formal' medical education, but a characteristic of the domain, which has changed only superficially in recent years, is that most practical learning takes place informally in workplaces. So, the individual and social relationship described in the preceding paragraphs and workplace activities described in Chapter 12 are, above all others, defining and abiding characteristics of the domain. One of the most important tasks of medical educators is to keep the centrality of experiential learning within supportive relationships at the forefront of their minds whenever whim or fashion temporarily conceals its importance.

Developing the human capital

A main theme of this book, previewed in preceding paragraphs and further developed in the chapters that follow, is that the vitality of medical education resides in its teachers and learners. Wilkerson and Doyle consider how to develop the human capital of an educational institution in Chapter 19. They recount how there was a move in the second half of the twentieth century away from the belief that content expertise in the subject matter of medicine was all that was needed to prepare a doctor to be a teacher and that, beyond that, teachers were born not made. They explain that good education calls for 'an organisational structure to support the work of teaching and teachers, a variety of faculty development activities and resources targeted at the differing educational roles and individual needs of teachers, and a reward system that values excellence in the various educational roles needed in the institution'. So, it is now an expectation that medical education institutions will have mechanisms in place to develop doctors and other faculty members as teachers. A more recent change has been to recognise and address the development needs of learners as well as teachers, moving away from a 'survival of the fittest' culture. Alongside faculty development, learner development is thus an emerging feature of the medical education domain.

Quality assurance

Having now described all the component parts of a medical curriculum, this final paragraph of Section 2 previews the content of Chapter 15, in which Dolmans, Stalmeijer, van Berkel, and Wolfhagen describe the steps that have to be taken to enhance the quality culture of an educational institution. The incentive to introduce quality assurance systems to medical education has come from a new climate of accountability and a need to be efficient in order to educate increasing numbers of medical learners without parallel increases in funding. The prerequisites for quality assurance are remarkably consistent with the prerequisites for good education: a coherent community working to agreed goals, with a sense of mutual engagement and accountability. Dolmans and colleagues describe the scrutiny of inputs, processes, and outputs, and evaluative processes that go into a cyclical process of continuous improvement, which, they argue, should be at the heart of a medical education institution.

Conclusion to Section 2

Medical education is closely in touch with its history, which has seen an explosion of curriculum development over the last century. Despite that pace of change, medical education has maintained a humanistic orientation, which makes it a social good. At its core, the pedagogy of medical education is a simple one: learners gain experience in context within supportive relationships. The material aspects and social processes of the environments within which learning takes place, however, are anything but simple. While the centrality of the master–apprenticeship relationship has long been recognised, recent developments in educational theory have broadened out the concept of apprenticeship to one that is situated within the nexus of relationships that constitutes a community of practice. The subject matter of medical education is, ultimately, very practically oriented but richly imbued with knowledge and values. While relationships are prerequisite, the learning that takes place within them can be strengthened by large and small group events, supported by education technology. Despite technological advance, informal learning through practice remains the defining pedagogy of medical education. Medicine's power to do harm as well as good calls for a strong emphasis on summative assessment, though contemporary education theory and practice is placing greater emphasis on the formative role of assessment with feedback. Education has traditionally been so deeply embedded in practice that it was often invisible. Two important features of its increased visibility in recent years are faculty and student development, and quality assurance of its processes and outcomes.

Section 3: Tensions

Tensions in the domain of medical education are not so much between different people holding clearly opposed points of view as between what best scholarly opinion holds to be most appropriate and the forces of either conservatism or change, though contradictions inherent to education can set scholars against one another. The type of conservatism that sets up tensions is often apparent in what people tacitly hold to be 'normal' or worthy of defending. The type of change that sets up tensions is driven by fashion, politics, or some other social force. Sections 1 and 2 have identified some such tensions:

- Having abrupt points of transition in what is supposedly a continuum,
- Selecting learners on the basis of their academic ability for a practice that depends, at least partly, on their humanity,
- Learning a practice (as in the case of prescribing, discussed under 'transitions') that one can only participate in as an onlooker,
- Espousing biomedical science as the main foundation discipline of what is, in practice, a humane art,
- Exposing altruistically motivated novices of the humane art to a hidden curriculum that breeds cynicism,
- Exposing learners to an adequate range of clinical experiences while allowing sufficient time for immersion in each of them,
- Balancing an adequate primary care experience against the wealth of learning opportunities that reside in specialities,
- Obtaining a good balance between the summative and formative roles of assessment,

- Balancing work and learning in workplaces,
- Regulating learning for regulatory purposes while emancipating learners to 'be as good as they are'.

This section explores five other, important tensions.

What is truth and how do we learn it?

Mann, Dornan, and Teunissen (Chapter 2) contrast a positivist perspective, according to which knowledge is value and context-free and exists outside the learner, with a constructivist perspective, according to which learners actively construct their individual understandings of the world. They contrast acquisition and participation metaphors for learning, according to which truth either passes from teacher to pupil, or arises from teachers' and learners' mutual engagement in education activities. They contrast 'universalist' approaches, which are preoccupied with what is common to different individuals' learning processes, with socio-cultural approaches, which are preoccupied with the diversity of people's processes of learning and development. While medical education is avidly adopting constructivist pedagogies, what many teachers tacitly hold to be 'normal' or worthy of defending is firmly rooted in positivism, the acquisition metaphor, and universalism.

Competency (outcome)-based education

This chapter has highlighted the breadth, depth, and interconnectedness of medical education's subject matter, and the central place of relationships in developing expertise. In Chapter 11, however, Nestel and Kneebone note a move from an apprenticeship model of education (which is founded on relationships centred around complex problems) to a competency-based model. Nestel and Kneebone warn that the competency movement risks over-simplifying complexity, aspiring to adequacy rather than excellence, causing learners and teachers to lose sight of the bigger picture, and leaving learners to cope with the problem of transferring generic skills they have acquired to specific contexts. Wass and Archer (Chapter 14) note that 'some believe this approach' (competency-based education) 'undermines medical professionalism and fails to provide the appropriate learning platform for CPD. Instead, it fosters a "tick box," "can do" mentality'. 'Even more seriously, there is a risk of generating "incompetency" if learners

perceive prematurely that they have achieved "competency"'. Coles (Chapter 6) is forthright in warning that a competency-based approach 'may be changing contemporary medical education into a form of technical training'. Far beyond the 'competent' person, the 'man of practical wisdom sees the particularities of his practical situation in the light of their ethical significance and acts consistently on this basis'. Competency-based education, according to Coles, is based on a 'product' model of education, when a 'process model would be more appropriate if the curriculum intention is to help people understand what is being taught'. Without specifying that learning outcomes should be expressed as competencies, White and Gruppen (Chapter 8) raise the important counter-argument that learners need specified learning outcomes if they are to assess themselves and prepare for assessment by others.

Self-direction and self-assessment

The existence of a plethora of interrelated terms and concepts scattered throughout this book – self-direction, adult learning, self-regulation, self-actualisation, self-assessment, self-monitoring, self-guidance, student-centred learning – highlights a fact and number of tensions. The fact is that contemporary medical education puts the rights, responsibilities, tasks, and development trajectories of learners and their learning ahead of 'teaching'. The tensions arise from balancing that principle against the rights, responsibilities, tasks, and development trajectories of individual teachers and the communities of practice of which they and their learners are co-members. All those stakeholders are, of course, bound together by a shared commitment to the rights, responsibilities, tasks, and development trajectories of the people they care for, which can heighten the tension. The different perspectives of a number of chapters illuminate those issues in ways we now briefly overview.

Mann, Dornan, and Teunissen (Chapter 2) note that becoming a self-directed learner is widely regarded as the fundamental basis of self-regulation, in turn, a *sine qua non* of professional practice. They juxtapose their treatment of it with an explanation of adult learning principles, used also by White and Gruppen as a perspective to illuminate self-assessment in Chapter 8. Self-directed learning, according to Chapter 2, can be viewed in two different ways: as a personal attribute or a set of skills. It is perhaps best characterised as a humanist orientation, which sees learning as progression towards a fully developed 'self-actualised self', though Mann, Dornan, and Teunissen note that self-directed learning 'has not had an easy path as a guiding principle for curriculum design and as a perspective in its own right'. One reason is that a person's self-directedness is as much a product of the environment in which people find themselves as an individual attribute. Yet, 'self-direction remains a deeply valued goal and tenet of the profession and a critically important attribute to identify educational needs and keep up to date over a lifetime of practice'.

A major criticism of self-directed learning is that it depends on self-assessment, which Wass and Archer (Chapter 14) urge us to 'view with caution as an assessment tool' because unconscious, self-serving processes make us unreliable at making judgements of our competence that accord with external judgements. Teunissen and Wilkinson (Chapter 12) describe how individuals learning in workplaces use self-monitoring and self-guidance, which together contribute to self-regulation, to react and respond to events. Self-regulation, they explain, is receiving increased attention within medical education as an alternative way of conceptualising self-assessment. Driessen, Overeem, and van Tartwijk (Chapter 13) take the concept a step further when they write of effective learners creating 'internal feedback and cognitive routines while they are engaged in academic tasks', as opposed to less effective learners, who 'have minimal self-regulation strategies and ... depend more on external factors (such as the teacher or the task) for feedback'. Driessen, Overeem, and van Tartwijk neatly reconcile self-reliance with external support in their concept of 'self-assessment seeking behaviour'. Within their model of reflective learning, 'self-directed assessment seeking and reflection are critical and a mentor is of great importance'. Chapter 8 is wholly devoted to the concept of self-assessment, the educational principles and methods of which it analyses in great detail and relates to the concept of self-regulated learning. White and Gruppen make a very useful practical contribution by describing a rich set of tools 'for self-identifying and addressing gaps in knowledge and skills'. They describe how faculty can assume roles as effective facilitators of self-regulated learning. Continuing on the theme of supporting learners' autonomy, Woolf and McManus (Chapter 18) state that 'autonomous motivation is not inborn or static, but can be nurtured ... by clinical teachers'. In the context of career counselling, that is achieved by 'listening to the needs of students and trainees, understanding their points of view, encouraging them to make their own choices and giving them sufficient information to make those choices'. Dennick and Spencer (Chapter 9) give a small group learning perspective on teachers' relationships with autonomous learners, drawing on Rogers' view of trust as the ingredient that changes teaching to the facilitation of learning. A facilitator helps learners 'become as much as (they) possibly can' – that is, to self-actualise.

While this chapter can give only limited insights into the self-directed learning debate, which is far from over, we conclude our overview by turning to a perspective from which other ones gain much of their legitimacy; a moral and philosophical one. Sutton, Tan, and Dornan (Chapter 1) ask whether 'selfness' means 'self to the exclusion of others or self in relation to others'. They discuss the strengths and weaknesses of 'self-direction' in terms of where it places the responsibility for learning and how it makes relationships between learners and teachers more or less legitimate. They question whether the high level of autonomy some people infer from the term is realistic or desirable. They find resolution by locating autonomy within the arena of 'individual development, interpersonal relationships, and organisational structures rather than individual "selfness," which the term is often taken to mean'. They reword the point at issue as 'the learning-directed self' to reduce the danger of learners being left unsupported. Through the inherently social process of participation, they propose, the formed practitioner emerges. A good learning environment, we may conclude from their analysis, models good medical practice within 'a culture which places a high regard on both trustworthiness and a "kindness" which protects the most vulnerable'.

Uniprofessionalism or interprofessionalism?

The way this book has a uniprofessional title but speaks of learning taking place within communities of practice, whose members are drawn from many professions, highlights a tension that characterises the domain. It is noteworthy, also, how the topic of interprofessionalism is largely confined to Reeves and Goldman's consideration of it in Chapter 4, which was commissioned to be sure it was represented. A notable exception is Towle and Godolphin's description in Chapter 5 of how community educators, recruited from patient organisations and advertisements, lead interprofessional education workshops in which students of the various professions learn with, from, and about one another. A cynic might observe that this self-evidently valuable initiative is worthy of mention primarily because it is so much an exception to the uniprofessional rules of the domain, and might note the irony that specially recruited community leaders are needed to get health professionals working together. Against that is set Reeves and Goldman's treatment of the topic which, from beginning to end, makes interprofessionalism 'normal', or at least the way things could and should be. Reeves and Goldman, moreover, explain why it is in medicine's interests to be slow to adopt interprofessionalism; they explain how medicine ensured its dominant position over other health and social care professions by being the first to 'engage successfully in a professionalisation project', which secured for it 'the most highly prestigious areas of clinical work – the ability to diagnose and prescribe'.

Simulation or reality

The tradition, as was explained earlier in this chapter, was for most or all of a doctor's education to be gained through authentic experience of practice as a clinical apprentice. The last century saw an increased proportion of first undergraduate then postgraduate education shift to classrooms and laboratories. Over the last three decades, an explicit focus on clinical skills instruction led to the emergence of clinical skills laboratories, most of whose activities involve simulating reality. A typical PBL scenario, it should also be noted, simulates reality, albeit as a written narrative for discussion in a seminar room rather than a practical activity in a simulation laboratory. Replacement of reality and meaning with symbols and signs, such that 'experience' is of a simulation of reality rather than reality itself, was

named by Baudrillard a 'simulacrum'. Nestel and Kneebone, in Chapter 11, are very circumspect in their narrative of skills education and the use of simulation, seeking to 'bridge the gap between formulaic, impoverished model-based training and the richness and unpredictability of clinical practice'. They warn against a fragmentation of skills education 'into isolated components' which 'can lead to over-focusing on the technical elements of procedures'. Teachers do that because, amongst other reasons, they feel swamped with the large numbers of students they have to teach and because altered patterns of care and concerns about patient safety make reality hard to access. The preceding description of how context is a vital element of learning makes it clear that retreat into a simulacrum is, ultimately, counter-educational. Coupling best use of simulation with imaginative use of reality is a pressing challenge, to which Chapter 11 suggests innovative solutions.

Conclusion to Section 3, and of this chapter

To keep up momentum in the domain of medical education, we should be at least as interested in its unresolved problems as its successes. We have drawn on the rest of this book to highlight difficulties and contradictions in the selection of learners, in the philosophy, morality, and subject matter of medical education, in the instructional design of what is supposedly a lifelong continuum, in its pedagogic methods, in the balance between instruction and experiential learning and the balance between different experiential elements, and in the balance between developing individuals and the relationships between them while assuring their competence, and regulating the whole process. We promised to leave the 'fault lines' of the domain gaping wide, so this chapter, unlike the other nineteen, does not conclude with 'implications for practice'. We leave you to read on and find how the authors derive practical implications from their detailed consideration of principles overviewed earlier.

Section 1

Theoretical and social foundations

Morality and philosophy of medicine and education

1

Naomi Tan   Adrian Sutton   Tim Dornan

CHAPTER CONTENTS

ABC

Glossary

Autonomy; see also conditional autonomy and principled autonomy The ability to live one's own life, according to one's own motives and reason.

Complexity theory This theory concerns the interactivity of elements in open systems, where the magnitude of effects cannot be predicted in a linear fashion from the magnitude of the elements relative to each other.

Conditional autonomy The delineation by an authority of particular areas of activity as ones within which a subordinate may act autonomously.

Consequentialism Ethical theory in which the act that is morally right is determined by the consequences of the act rather than the act itself.

Defensible practice Activity that is carefully negotiated with a patient to take account of scientific knowledge and moral principles.

Defensive practice When fear of litigation encourages (unhelpfully) restricted professional activity.

Developmental resonance The re-emergence of unresolved personal conflicts around autonomy and authority which may then be re-enacted in the relationship between supervisor and supervisee.

Continued

© 2011, Elsevier Ltd.
DOI: 10.1016/B978-0-7020-3522-7.00001-2

"The point of philosophy is to start with something so simple as not to seem worth stating and to end with something so paradoxical that no one will believe it"

Bertrand Russell (1918) 'The philosophy of logical atomism'

Outline

This chapter describes some ethical and philosophical concepts that are key to medicine and medical education. It applies them to issues medical practitioners and educators are currently facing and suggests some core texts in the field. We use the phrase 'health and sickness care' because there can be different and even competing demands between the care of health and the care of sickness. In particular, the way 'health', 'sickness', 'health care', and 'sickness care' are defined depends on the value attached by the definer to the different experiences of life and the functions performed in living. We start by considering how such definitions are arrived at. Next, we describe a variety of schools of thought about the nature of human development and relationships. Having introduced the principles of ethics primarily from the perspective of health and sickness care, we turn our attention to medical education, analysing and differentiating the rights and responsibilities of learners, teachers, and patients, as both individuals and members of society.

Medicine and education as social goods

From whatever ethical or social standpoint they are viewed, the goals of both medicine and education are, in principle, 'good'. The practice of medicine aims to prevent suffering when it is avoidable and alleviate suffering when it is inevitable. Education strives to meet individual learners' and society's needs for enhanced knowledge and ability. What amounts to 'a good' and how education can achieve it are, however, debatable.

The chance to 'do good' and be 'useful' is motivating to those who seek to learn and teach medicine. In return for their altruistic motivation, health professionals are given intimate access to people's lives at times of vulnerability. However, medicine has limitations, so professionals can be faced with the feeling that they cannot be 'useful'. Worse than that, treatments can cause harm, so practising medicine means balancing the positive and negative effects of treatment. As if that were not difficult enough, one person's appraisal of an outcome as 'good' or 'bad' does not necessarily agree with another person's. Such value judgements are not the only factor at play; what is actually available to treat a patient may be determined by the need to allocate resources equitably. The basis on which such decisions are made cannot be divorced from the value that is placed on the benefits or harms that may accrue. Other value judgements are even more delicate – e.g. is treating someone in order that they can return to work a greater good than treating someone who will never be able to return to work? The ability to examine why treatments may or may not be available and why an outcome is described as 'good' or 'bad' is a fundamental component of both medical practice and medical education.

The ability to do something is not a sufficient basis for actually doing it and deciding what is useful to do can be complex. If medical practice is defined as prolonging life or improving health, there comes a time for every individual when there is no useful course of action. At such times, the art of medicine is to resist both the temptation to "strive officiously to keep alive" (in the words of the poet Arthur Hugh Clough) and the temptation to abandon the person to death or suffering. In the language of Winnicott (1971), the task of health and sickness care has elements of both 'doing [to] and being [with]'. Tolerating *feeling* useless or helpless – coping with one's patients being ill and not getting better – is an essential contribution of health and sickness care professionals.

The way in which medicine is practiced may influence individual and societal attitudes towards health and illness and be influenced in turn by those attitudes. The consequences of this interactivity – for example, the development of policies about how time and finance should be allocated – need to be part of public and professional discourse. Prioritising one treatment over another involves decisions not only about the *cost* but also about the *value* of the outcomes to individuals and to the whole community. Individual medical scientists and practitioners all contribute to this discourse alongside patients and experts in other relevant fields such as social policy and ethics. One final consideration in this overview of health and education as social goods is that health interventions can be at the level of whole populations rather than single identifiable individuals. Whilst a net increase in the health of a population must surely benefit individuals, that effect may not be recognisable in any specific person. Practitioners must have a balanced view of the interplay between collective and individual good and help learners to see the collective perspective when they are, as is inevitable, preoccupied with the needs of sick individuals.

The relationship between medical ethics and law

Laws tell us which activities are sanctioned and what will happen to people who engage in activities that are not sanctioned. The fact that laws can change in any one jurisdiction and are different in different jurisdictions emphasises that laws are not absolute. What is *legal* and what is *morally correct* are not necessarily the same. Ethical analysis plays an important part in the evolution of legal process by systematically and rigorously questioning what is 'good'.

Medicine exists within the bounds of what is legal in the country in which it is practiced. Learners, educators, and practitioners in any one country must know which activities are sanctioned and which ones are proscribed both in professional practice and lay life. However, the fact that a law exists does not mean that it should be accepted without question; neither should previous interpretations of a law nor the application of those interpretations be left unchallenged. Fear of litigation may encourage unhelpfully restricted professional activity (*defensive practice*) rather than activity that is carefully negotiated with an individual patient to take account of scientific knowledge and moral principles (*defensible practice*). An understanding of the principles of ethics is therefore fundamental to the everyday practice of medicine and medical education just as much as it is at the scientific and technological frontiers of practice.

Ethical and moral principles

While variation between individuals in what they find morally acceptable in their personal lives is inevitable, professional practice requires agreement on ethical and moral principles. Consensus in such matters is arrived at by ethics committees (usually at national level), which hear academic, lay, ethical, and legal opinion. They disseminate guidance in published documents; advise the bodies that regulate professional practice; and give opinions when new, difficult issues come to public attention. When differences of priority and opinion arise, it is right that there should be moral debate. Intuition and individualism have their place in such debates but rigorous philosophical enquiry is about starting from solid premises to develop arguments which lead to solid conclusions. The 'perfect argument' would result from a series of irrefutable premises. But, just as scientific truth is provisional rather than absolute, a particular ethical stance stands only until a more valid argument is put forward. It is the complexity of constructing and comparing well-reasoned arguments and deciding which actions are to be sanctioned or proscribed that makes it necessary to have ethics committees and professional ethicists. Their existence, however, does not obviate the need for informed ethical reflection and analysis in day-to-day practice and a willingness to question the *status quo*. We must always be open to new ethical questions since we will never know if we have formulated all the questions that could be asked.

Intuition, as the expression of an inherent sense of right and wrong, commonly alerts health care professionals to ethically questionable situations. It leads them to ask *why* something is morally uncomfortable and to seek an answer by a logical analysis of their own position and that of their colleagues. Arguments have to be examined for the quality of their reasoning. Rhetoric and emotion play little role in the final formulation and exposition of ethical arguments, but this does not mean that ethics is without feeling. Emotions are a fundamental component of the human condition, particularly when caring for people who are at their most vulnerable, so emotions are inseparable from ethics.

Current themes in medical ethics

In presenting this chapter, we have chosen to give an overview of various schools of thought about moral philosophy and the nature of human development and relationships. One of our goals has been to integrate ethics with developmental and dynamic processes of human relatedness. Another has been to encourage readers to take a discriminating approach to ethics and we provide tools to help them do so.

Principlism

Principlism (Beauchamp and Childress, 2001) has been a major influence on modern medicine. It has four central 'pillars': the principles of

- Beneficence
- Non-maleficence
- Respect for autonomy
- Justice

Beneficence and non-maleficence

At the start of the chapter, we said that doing good is a major pillar of medicine. Avoiding harm is at least as important. The aphorism "primum non nocere" – "first

do no harm" – emphasises the primacy of this principle. The benefits of treatment always interplay with concurrent risks so it is part of the day-to-day work of doctors to understand and balance those risks.

Autonomy

Individual autonomy is 'an idea that is generally understood to refer to the capacity to be one's own person, to live one's life according to reasons and motives that are taken as one's own... to be directed by considerations, desires, conditions, and characteristics that are not simply imposed externally upon one' (Stanford Encyclopedia of Philosophy [S.E.P.], 2009; http://plato.stanford.edu/entries/autonomy-moral/). Only in the past half century has medicine begun to leave behind the paternalism of 'doctor knows best' in favour of autonomy. Respecting autonomy means accepting a patient's right to make their own choices, regardless of whether those choices are in accord with the doctor's preferences and whether the reasoning is acceptable to the doctor.

Gillon (1985) subdivided autonomy into three components:

- Autonomy of thought: the ability to think and reason for oneself,
- Autonomy of will: the ability to form the wish and intent that something should be made to happen,
- Autonomy of action: to be equipped to act and be unrestrained from action.

Justice

The principle of justice is that decisions should be made on the relative usefulness of different actions and resources should be distributed equitably ('to each according to need' rather than 'to all equally'). The principle of justice applies to education just as it applies to health care. It demands that mechanisms be in place to distribute resources fairly, whether such resources are reliant on finance, suitably trained practitioners, equipment, or available time.

Beyond the primacy of individual autonomy

Principlism provides a useful framework to analyse clinical, research, and educational practice but the primacy it accords to individual autonomy has been a matter of recent debate. Campbell (1991) highlights how confusions may arise: "[If] 'autonomy' is to carry a high value, then what is its polar opposite which is to be equivalently disvalued?... [In] confusing autonomy with independence, the current political mood regards dependency as moral inadequacy. The weak and needy are increasingly being seen as an inconvenient burden which the strong and successful must only grudgingly bear." 'Maximal' autonomy, in which the individual has unlimited freedom to exercise self-rule, is more a theoretical concept than a reality because it is unattainable. Conversely, a more 'basic' level of autonomy, consisting of the ability to make reasoned judgements and freedom from explicit oppression (SEP, 2009), is far more inclusive.

Interconnectedness was encapsulated by the poet John Donne's phrase 'No man is an island, entire of itself; every man is a piece of the continent, a part of the main'. Simplistic adherence to the principle of autonomy is at odds with interconnectedness. Sennett (1998) argued that a political culture during the latter part of the twentieth century, which set 'independence' as a virtuous state for individuals, led to a 'corrosion of character'. O'Neill (2002a) believed that problems arise when autonomy and individual independence are viewed as synonymous, with the corollary that 'dependence' is an affront to autonomy. Sutton (2001), arguing from a psychoanalytic perspective, similarly challenged an absolutist view of individual autonomy; "Instead of a culture which sets dependence and independence as value-loaded polarities, what is required is one which accepts that what can be depended upon may lie within or outside an individual and that this is a dynamic state within and between individuals." Given that both clinical and educational processes rely on identifying where or within whom resources can be located, interconnectedness is an important perspective in medical practice and education.

Principled Autonomy

O'Neill (2002a) proposed a framework of 'Principled Autonomy', whose application to one person does not interfere with its simultaneous application to any other person. She identified three components that, unlike Principlism, reflect the dynamic interrelationship between an individual and the situation they are in:

* Relational (autonomy from someone/something),
* Selective (the matters in which autonomy is expressed),
* Graduated (the extent to which different people have autonomy).

Graduated autonomy is a developmental perspective, which acknowledges that capacity increases from childhood through to adulthood as a result of maturational processes. Hence, adolescents have 'conditional autonomy' (Sutton, 1997, 79); in other words, autonomy of action in areas negotiated with their parents. That process of negotiation (implicitly and explicitly) defines the limits of the responsible adult(s)' own autonomy. There may be psychosomatic and social dynamics to particular individuals' experiences of self-determination at different times; for example, the ability to perform at one's best is influenced by health and sickness. In comparison with their wider peer group, learners participating in professional education programmes such as medicine may have constraints placed upon their activities through the requirements of 'protoprofessionalism', a term proposed by Hilton and Slotnick (2005) to describe the undergraduate stage of professional development.

Principled Autonomy strives to balance the rights of individuals against benefits to the widest possible number of people (utilitarian arguments), contextualising ethics to relationships and community interactions. Clinical practice based on Principled Autonomy is the "...provision of sufficient and understandable information and space [to] patients, who [have] the capacity to make a settled choice about medical interventions on themselves, [and] to do so responsibly in a manner considerate to others" and "best fits the optimal patient–doctor relationship in which there is a mutual, unspoken agreement between the parties that recognises the duties and obligations each to the other." (Stirrat and Gill, 2005) This relationship between what individuals can reasonably expect *for* themselves and *of* others needs careful consideration. Since rights and obligations are inextricably entwined, a right cannot be fulfilled unless there is a clear duty on someone to fulfil it. That means that the person(s) on whom an obligation rests must be equipped to fulfil it; an attempt by professionals to present themselves as capable of providing a treatment they are not equipped to provide is dishonest. O'Neill (2002a) eloquently demonstrated the corollary of this in relation to a 'right to health': "...since it will never be possible to guarantee health for all, there can be no obligation so to do... there can therefore be no right to health." Similarly, learners and teachers have the right to expect their medical school to provide resources to support them, but patients and society have to authorise learning and teaching. Fulfilling an obligation, whether in clinical or educational terms, involves both *duty* and *ability*: a person's *right* is that there should be an aspiration for, and reasonable actions towards, an equitable approach.

Interdependence and trust in medical education

The preceding descriptions approached ethics primarily from the perspective of health and sickness care, sometimes showing how principles of clinical ethics apply to medical education. We now take a wholly educational perspective.

Respect for the task of learning

Patient–learner

The true risks and benefits of learner–patient interactions are unquantifiable because what the learner has learnt from any one encounter will become apparent only at a later date and the learning will not pertain solely to the patient involved. Any direct benefit or harm to the patient may be equally intangible. Learners and teachers must try to anticipate the significance of situations so patients can give truly informed consent. Unfolding processes of involvement should be negotiated in which patients are treated as full partners who understand their right to veto any action at any time.

Education in clinical settings relies on patients' altruism, optimism, and faith, which depend on the trustworthiness of learners and the medical profession. Baier (1986) describes trust as requiring "good grounds for [...] confidence in another's good will, or at least the absence of good grounds for expecting their ill will or indifference" and entailing "accepted vulnerability to another's possible but not expected ill will (or lack of good will) toward one." Patients, however, cannot always understand why they trust or mistrust a learner or doctor. Baier (1986) writes of *conscious (proper/reasonable)* and *unconscious* processes of trust. O'Neill (2002) considers that there has been a crisis of trust in the medical profession in the UK as a result of well-publicised breaches such as in Bristol and Liverpool and by Dr Harold Shipman. In Bristol, unfavourable surgical audit data were ignored, which resulted in further deaths. In Alder Hey Children's Hospital, Liverpool, a pathologist removed and retained organs at post-mortem examinations without informing or seeking the consent of parents. Over many years, Harold

Shipman systematically killed elderly patients by administering drugs and the death certification system failed to bring his misdeeds to light. O'Neill (2002) further emphasises that the problems that ensue from 'misplaced *mis*trust' can be as great as those that follow from 'misplaced trust'.

Learner–patient interactions rely, at least to some extent, on an extension of trust to learners in their role as (future) members of the medical profession. Patients must be confident about the value of learners being involved, the reasonableness of the proposed activity (particularly if a learner has not carried it out before), and that learners and teachers are competent judges of its reasonableness. The same professional standards apply to learners as to fully trained doctors; as emphasised by the UK General Medical Council (GMC, 2006), teachers and learners must enact their roles only if they are fit to "be honest and open and act with integrity – act without delay if you have good reason to believe that you or a colleague may be putting patients at risk." Of specific importance to both learner and patient is that the teacher can judge what can reasonably be expected of a learner.

Learner–teacher

A learning contract – a shared agreement to be interested in and extend understanding and abilities relating to health and sickness care – is what brings learner and teacher together, whether in the immediacy of caring for a patient or remote from it. All parties have to be able to put themselves in the service of learning, whilst simultaneously ensuring that whatever action is taken is in the best interests of the patient. Teachers play the important role of providing guidance and setting tasks that are within learners' 'zones of proximal development' (Vygotsky, 1978). By challenging learners, teachers help them expand their knowledge (including awareness of what they have yet to learn) and acquire new abilities. By doing so in a controlled and thoughtful manner, teachers limit the extent to which learners experience failure (Lave and Wenger, 1991). Learning requires humility but is undermined by humiliation, which demotivates learners, undermines relationships between learners and teachers, and can undermine doctor–patient relationships too. Attempting but not succeeding is not necessarily the same as failing. It may be only through trying to perform a skill that it becomes clear what elements of the skill learners have acquired and what elements they still need to acquire.

There are three key issues for clinical education: the safety of patients, the maintenance of a developmental trajectory towards enhanced professional capability, and judging whether the achieved standard is sufficient for continued progress. For that positive process to occur, there needs to be a particular form of trust between learners and teachers. Phillips and Taylor (2009) argue that kindness is derived from 'kin-ness' – similarities in experiences and/or aspirations – and calls for an 'ability to bear the vulnerability of others, and therefore of oneself'. Applying that concept to the learner–teacher relationship, the two parties need to show kindness in rather different ways, not least because of the different parts they play in safeguarding the welfare of patients. Learners and teachers will do that best if they feel confident in the support of their institution and society in general.

The particular relationship between learners and teachers can usefully be thought of in terms of what each is putting in the hands of the other, their engagement with developmental processes, and the unconscious dynamics that result. Chronological definitions of 'adolescence' vary, some authors suggesting that it continues into the early twenties, which includes most undergraduate entrants to medical education and even early postgraduate learners. In putting oneself forward for vocational education, there is an understanding that one is not 'equipped to act' in certain ways but an expectation that one will become so and that carrying out such actions will rely on appropriate authorisation by patients and a proper authority. Since adolescence is a stage of 'conditional autonomy' (see page 7), adolescents and adults have to "negotiate which of them can 'speak' with sufficient authority about a particular issue and therefore assume responsibility for what will or will not be done" (Sutton, 1997). Teachers and teaching institutions need to respect the developmental stages of their learners. Sutton (1997) further suggested that postgraduate training can be conceived of as a form of "professional adolescence" in which conditional autonomy applies to learners' professional responsibilities despite them having become fully autonomous in other aspects of their lives. Professional adolescence may be complicated by *developmental resonance* in which there is "re-emergence of unresolved conflicts around autonomy and authority, which may then be re-enacted in the relationship between supervisor and supervisee," something that must be taken into account in managing relationships.

Learner–teacher–patient

Safe and productive learner–patient interactions rely on teachers' guidance, learners' ability to recognise their own limits, and patients' trust that proper professional standards are being upheld. Even patients who do not understand statements such as 'I'm a third year medical learner' may at least appreciate that a professional apprentice will be carrying out tasks appropriate to their level of training. Patients' expectations of learners may, however, be unrealistic so the grounds for learners' participation need to be made clear; for example, whether they can carry out a procedure as a substitute for a doctor or only under a doctor's direct supervision. Committed teachers and patients can see that learners are an investment for the future, and may also benefit from a naive, 'fresh' perspective, for example, when a learner's need for clarification and correction exposes lay misunderstandings.

Why should patients be involved in medical education. . . a responsibility to future patients?

Principled Autonomy implies that there must be some basic mutuality of purpose if being involved with others is to be considered morally justifiable. If there is no mutuality, the relationship becomes an exploitative one. Learners in clinical environments may contribute much or little directly to patient care, but any educational situation involves an element of looking into the future because learners represent – as the GMC put it – "Tomorrow's Doctors" (http://www.gmc-uk.org/education/undergraduate/tomorrows_doctors_2003.asp). Learners who see patients without being able to help may be experienced as an intrusion, perhaps even as *voyeurs*. Being present, however, and actively observing without acting upon a patient, is both a key clinical skill and an expression of empathy, or 'kindness' (Philips and Taylor, 2009). Learners must experience authentic clinical encounters in order to be equipped for their later role; even a dying patient may sincerely wish to contribute to the future by allowing a learner to be present.

In the immediate situation, patients who see learners may not gain anything directly, so it is hard to regard mutual benefit as a reason for them to agree to such interactions. But, do present patients have a *responsibility* to future patients they will never meet, such that they should be expected to allow learners to examine them? Or, should they be *allowed* to reject any responsibility towards future patients? An approach grounded firmly in 'Individual Autonomy' would answer 'No' to the first question and regard the second question as irrelevant because patients do not need to be *granted permission* to refuse. 'Principled Autonomy' would argue that the answer should take into account the communities of which patients are part; since current treatments were made possible by the educational experiences of prior doctors, the continued availability of care relies on mutuality and reciprocity. Further, patients may also have a right to the *opportunity to participate* in building the bank of experience that helps doctors achieve competence. The application of the principle of equal opportunity relating to research involving human participants in the Declaration of Helsinki (1964) to education warrants further attention.

Does individual responsibility depend on health or sickness status?

In health and sickness care systems that require citizens to contribute financially through tax or insurance, there is a clear expectation that the fruits of paid work, made possible by sufficient health, will be used to ensure that care exists and will continue to exist. Should that expectation extend to contributing to medical education? It might be argued that medical learners have a 'right' to learn. They have entered into a contract to learn to be doctors and clinical learning requires access to patients. That argument could be seen to place an obligation on patients to serve as a resource for learning. There is acceptance, however, that ill people may be unable to fulfil their usual duties and that special allowance should be made to minimise hardship; this is manifest, for example in paid sickness leave. Illness may limit patients' autonomy across a wide range of their usual activities, from total incapacity because of pain, mechanical, or physiological impairment, through to constraints arising from fear. Impairment resulting from illness (or even fear of illness) places people in a different position in the relationships upon which they depend and it can be argued their rights and obligations change accordingly. The extent of patients' obligations to the health and sickness care system is clearly contingent upon their state of health. Learners' needs for learning opportunities cannot take absolute priority over sick people's needs and rights.

Promoting patients' sense of responsibility for learners' learning without obligation

The preceding argument might suggest that interacting with learners is perceived negatively or as a burden by patients. That is often not the case. Once the purpose of learner interaction – the promotion of learning and the possibility of helping future patients (including themselves next time) – has been explained, many patients feel they can turn their illness into something positive. Contributing to learners' learning counteracts emotional strains which result from dependence, so becoming educators, or at least active participants in educational processes, can be beneficial. 'Expert Patients', who give personal accounts of their chronic diseases and/or teach physical examination, contribute by building bridges between text books and the reality of living with disease. They mix personal with generalisable experience, though they may repeat lay misunderstandings as well as understandings of diseases. One way or another, patients are the ultimate truly authentic teaching resource – and giving them the opportunity to teach places their experiences in a pivotal position to be of value and valued. A respectful system recognises the mutual benefits of learner–patient interaction, encourages patients to be involved, supports them in being so, and avoids actions that are coercive or even subtly change the contribution from a voluntary one to a perceived obligation.

Professional autonomy, the patient, and teaching

Professionals do not simply exchange goods or services for remuneration, nor are they simply purveyors/distributors of goods produced by others. The exchange is one in which judgement must be exercised as to whether what is proposed is reasonable. Professionals must give their own informed consent to the process alongside patients and be prepared for potential disagreement about proposed courses of action. Stirrat and Gill (2005) summarise this as "the doctor fulfilling his or her duty to the patient by exercising his or her own autonomy and, as such, [this] may be entirely justified. Indeed, there will be some occasions in which acquiescence to a requested intervention against one's clinical or ethical judgement will be abrogation of one's duty as a doctor." Similarly patients cannot be viewed simply as recipients of goods from a third party (e.g. The UK National Health Service [NHS]). Neither can professionals be viewed simply as agents of a third party, acting without exercising professional judgement.

Arguments derived from Principled Autonomy, in line with Baier's formulation, highlight the central importance of the dynamics of trust, placing a reasonable expectation of mutual trustworthiness as a central pillar. This must also be understood in terms of human development, the dyad of patient/ professional, and the wider community in which the members of that dyad live and practice.

Becoming a doctor: the participative emergence of form

Evolution provides a useful analogy for developmental processes. Different constituents in an evolutionary system impact on each other, sometimes changing each other's form or function; there is a dynamic of compatibility and incompatibility, complementarity and non-complementarity. Changes may be irreversible. They may alter the integrity of one or more components. They may even bring about the destruction of other components. Although Darwin's model is often presented as 'the survival of the *fittest*', the issue is actually one of the survival of the *fit* between the needs, demands, and effects of biological systems in relationship to each other and their environment. The perpetuation of a particular system does not indicate anything about optimal functioning or desirability; only that equilibrium has been obtained. No *intent* to bring about the outcome is present, but the result can be ascribed *value* in terms of its potentially beneficial or detrimental influences.

When considering human actions, the possibility that they may have adverse effects on individuals or groups needs due consideration. Examining outcomes and reflecting on whether it is justifiable to continue the actions that lead to them is an essential component of practice. Evidence-Based Medicine supports such a process of examination by making available robust evidence about outcomes to support decision making. 'Values-Based Medicine' (Fulford, 2004) goes one stage further by evaluating the desirability (as opposed to likelihood) of different outcomes from different people's points of view.

Individual development can be considered as a person's 'evolution of form' under various internal and external influences. Future possibilities are defined by how those internal and external influences interact. Winnicott's (1965) book "The Maturational Processes and the Facilitating Environment" captures this evolution in terms of its developmental desirability ('maturity') and the contributions of both individuals themselves and the relational and physical environments in which their time is spent (the 'good-enough', facilitating environment). The title underlines the fact that human development arises from interaction between *possibilities* present in the human givens of genetic endowment and *possibilities* arising from physical and relational environments. The co-existence of genetic and environmental possibilities in particular forms at particular times means that the likelihood of any form continuing or being feasible again in the future can increase or decrease through the same operations. There is not an infinite number of possibilities but patterns arise, indicating that different outcomes or ranges of outcomes are more or less *probable* or *improbable*. Translated into our expectations of people admitted to undergraduate or postgraduate medical education, there is an acceptably high likelihood that they will be suitable for progression. This progression, which must be within an acceptable range of diversity, occurs through a dynamic interaction between developmental processes and environmental influences.

Complexity Theory uses the term *self-organisation* to describe the emergence of systems that are identified by their structures and functions but not by any intent that they should come into being or remain in being (see, e.g. Sweeney and Griffiths, 2002). In considering organisation and management, Shaw and colleagues propose the term 'participative self-organisation' to capture the fundamental influences of interactivity, whereby there occurs 'an inescapably self-organising process of participating in the spontaneous emergence of continuity and change' (Shaw, 2002). Philosophical and psychodynamic considerations, however, mean that even the inclusion of the word 'self' introduces further complexity. To what extent are we considering this process of change as fundamentally the experience and expression of *self as agent*? To what extent can the *experience* of self as agent be equated with the *fact* of oneself as having been 'an/the agent' of what occurs?

There is no doubt that self *and* others participate in medical education, so we need to consider the different contributions that are necessary and sufficient for individual evolutionary journeys of practitioners as they are influenced by and influence the system within which they are learning. All parties come under the influence of each other simultaneously and bear responsibility to consider the impact they may have on the primary task. Changes in pre-university education may alter medical schools' expectations of learners at entry; financial currents may influence the ability to study; or changes in employment law may alter the educational opportunities available for learners. Such processes call for an ability to consider intended and unintended outcomes, the part different factors have played in those outcomes, and whether the form that emerges truly serves the desired purpose of providing good practitioners. We suggest the term *participative emergence of form* to capture this process in which even subtle changes in one part of the system may have disproportionate effects on the whole, whether intended or not.

Self-directed learning?

In considering medical education, professionalism, and different expressions of personhood, ideas of 'self' related to living the *good life* (in philosophical rather than hedonistic terms) present further questions. 'Self-directed learning' (SDL) has been a powerful theme in medical education during the last two decades. In the context of this chapter, what does it mean in terms of *self-ness*? Does it mean 'self to the exclusion of others' or 'self in relation to others'? Could it suggest *selfish*, the idea of *self in the service of others*, or are both possible simultaneously?

My (AS) experience is that the term 'SDL' has strengths and weaknesses. The emphasis on 'self' promotes personal responsibility to learn (including learning how to learn) but may unintentionally deny the importance of learning relationships. It can leave some learners feeling alone and teachers feeling disqualified from teaching. Winnicott (1971) emphasises that, since autonomous individuals are never truly independent of their environments, 'Independence does not become absolute', although mature individuals 'may *feel* free and independent, at least so far as is necessary for happiness and a sense of personal identity'.

The formulation of education as a participative emergence of form is consistent with the tenets of Principled Autonomy. It places autonomy in the arena of individual development, interpersonal relationships, and organisational structures rather than

individual 'self-ness', which the term is often taken to mean. It also allows links with psychological theories of personal, relational, moral, and social development related to learning. Eriksen (1950), for example, described themes in personal and social development across the life-span, using a vocabulary shared with moral philosophy – for example, '*trust* versus *mistrust*' and '*autonomy* versus shame and doubt'.

Does *self*, however, exist as an entity that an individual experiences without it having externally recognisable features or must it be manifest in a form identifiable, by self and other, in actions? This issue of the experience and expression of self as acting and being acted upon leads psychological and educational theories, along with moral philosophy, to a shared interest in the concept of the 'self as agent'. This self as agent also needs to be integrated with an ability to appraise situations, recognising their similarities and differences, in order that further potentially beneficial actions can increase and detrimental ones decrease. It needs to take account of how relating with others may sequentially influence the perception of events and actions. An example would be where the wish to please someone influences activity in a way that overrides one's 'better' judgement. The ability to have 'a mind of one's own', know that one can be 'in two minds', and appreciate that one's autonomy of action may be limited is crucial in assimilating new experiences and being able to reflect on motivations and actions.

The picture presented is one of abilities changing and different facets of self emerging and being expressed in the course of development. We suggest that it is useful to think of a '*learning-directed self*' in conjunction with other aspects of self. This 'learning-directed self', which motivates people to learn, may have various roots: pleasure derived from novelty and learning; altruistic desires to make a difference; pleasure in participating and learning alongside others; and the wish, eventually, to earn a living. It may also have a variety of routes for expression: intellectual; artistic; physical; and philanthropic. The primary, shared focus of education is engagement with this learning-directed self in order to produce 'fit-for-purpose' health and sickness care practitioners. The framework should also provide practitioners with the experience of a *good life* in philosophical terms, or in Winnicott's terminology, a *good-enough* experience of life.

There is, therefore, an interlinking of necessary and sufficient components for this participative emergence of form at each stage of medical training from application to medical school through to retirement. In order to withstand ethical scrutiny, frameworks for education must provide for learning about what is necessary and sufficient for full and reasonable use to be made of these people as they live their lives trusting that expectations of them will be reasonable.

In terms of the psychodynamics of trust, a model of a necessary and sufficient sense of common purpose is pivotal. Misplaced trust can distort interactions through lack of scrutiny and accountability; misplaced mistrust can disrupt through fear of scrutiny and blame leading to unhelpful, defensive practice. Although patient safety cannot be left to the vagaries of learning by 'trial and error', the process of clinical practice and learning is inevitably one of 'trial and improvement'. Establishing and maintaining an environment for medical education in conjunction with good medical practice relies on a culture that places a high regard on both trustworthiness and a 'kindness' which protects the most vulnerable.

Selection for medical school... and beyond

It is plainly necessary to identify those who should or should not be admitted to medical school, awarded a degree, and allowed to practice. Active participation by learners and staff in selection, whether as selected or selector, is a moral imperative – certainly for the good of patients and perhaps also for the good of individuals who might otherwise be training or practicing when not fit. There are good arguments for involving patients and other members of the public in selection, not least to promote a sense of responsibility among members of the public to participate in medical education.

Trusting in development

Clearly, the aim of selection is to choose people who have a high probability of being 'a good' to society. Careers in medicine cover a wide range of work practices including direct clinical practice with patients, direct input to patient care without direct patient contact, education and training, research, and the planning and management of health and sickness care. All of these represent useful societal functions, which have particular developmental pathways, draw upon different qualities or abilities, and are hindered by different inabilities or disabilities. Articulating what such qualities are and identifying indicators of their potential development are areas of continuing exploration.

In order to make good use of the doctors they consult, patients must trust the quality of their *practice*, which is an admixture of the art and science of medicine; but how do they know if that trust is deserved? Being trustworthy is not the same as putting patients at their ease or agreeing to their requests. Circumstances may not allow the continuity of care which makes for a well-informed decision about *this* practitioner; yet the practice of medicine relies on trust developing in an often short timescale. Clinical situations are riddled with uncertainty, which has to be managed honestly, consciously, or unconsciously (see Jackson, 2001). Preparation for practice therefore requires *education for uncertainty coupled with a need for decisive action* (which may include 'watchful waiting' or deciding no action is required).

If articulating why we believe a doctor is trustworthy is not straightforward, identifying learners who have the potential to be trustworthy doctors is no less complex, yet an effort must be made. Sulmasy (2000) highlights an inherent dilemma of attempting to measure trust "...truly virtuous physicians are those who can be trusted to do what is right and good for patients even when no one is measuring." The way developmental and relational processes interweave makes it particularly challenging to articulate what makes somebody morally suitable for the practice of medicine. McMillan et al (2009) summarise the challenge posed by applicants who have a criminal conviction for which they have served their sentence. There is no uniform practice in UK medical schools; decisions range from the 'hard-nosed' (absolute rejection) to the 'contrition view' (consideration of a learner's application being based on whether they are felt able to let sound moral judgement govern their future behaviour). Will the more 'hard-nosed' approach ensure safer practitioners and maintain patients' confidence in the medical profession? Or can it exclude potentially useful doctors on a 'morally healthy' developmental trajectory, which has included antisocial activity? Decision-making must take into account whether aberrant behaviour is particularly relevant to future medical practice (see Colliver et al, 2007). Ziliak and McCloskey (2008) highlight the importance of differentiating between whether or not a finding of *statistical* significance is of real significance to the desired aims. Aberration in one aspect may or may not be a powerful influence on the desired outcome; they call this the difference between 'precision' and 'oomph'.

Selection for medical education must, in summary, have inclusion and exclusion criteria that command the confidence of patients, practitioners, and commissioners of services. A comparable confidence is needed for processes governing progress during undergraduate education, postgraduate education, and continuing professional development. This remains an area of extreme complexity given that individuals' life experiences (e.g. health and social adversity) affect their abilities in unpredictable ways, which only time can tell.

Does the range of doctors that are available need to conform to other societal characteristics?

A recurrent theme of this chapter is that the range of attributes needed to provide the workforce with appropriate medical practitioners is wide. Academic/intellectual ability, relational attributes, physical attributes such as manual dexterity, developmental potential, and trustworthiness are notoriously difficult to specify, particularly when they come to be synthesised to produce good-enough practitioners. Mechanisms to decide whom to offer places for training are required but there is a real dearth of evidence about reliability, validity, specificity, and sensitivity. Interviews, for example, are frequently used. But could they lead to bias because the conscious or unconscious manifestations of 'kin-ship' propagate a well-established, if not necessarily optimal, system? If there is no reasoned way of differentiating between applicants, is random allocation of people meeting a necessary minimum academic threshold a more just system? This was used in Holland but had to be modified because very able learners were not being selected (De Gruiter, N.M. (2006) cited in Stasz and van Stalk (2007)).

A policy of *Widening Participation* [W.P.] in higher education has been adopted in England "...to promote and provide the opportunity of successful participation in higher education to everyone who can benefit from it. This is [viewed as] vital for social justice and economic competitiveness...

[and is]... closely connected with broader issues of equity and social inclusion" (Higher Education Funding Council for England, 2009). Hilton and Lewis (2004) assert that "The need for widening participation in medicine is essential." There is a pragmatic argument in this for medical schools: there is an established government policy, so substantial institutional funding relies on compliance. However, the same authors also assert, "The underrepresented sectors of society that widening participation aims to include are also those same sectors with high health and social care needs. If the NHS is to understand and serve the community the make up of its workforce should reflect that community." Assertions of the value of social change like this contain an implicit view of how systems, relationships, and individuals can best operate in relation to policy aims. However, *thinking*, as a prerequisite for understanding, does not reside in a 'system' although the individuals involved may share ways of thinking and understanding. So, can a health service *understand* and can people *feel understood* by a health service? The answer to the former must be 'No' although the answer to the latter may be 'Yes'.

Furthermore, does equating 'similarity' with 'understanding better and serving better' withstand scrutiny? From a psychological point of view 'being-like/not-being-like' are not reasonable grounds to determine whether someone is capable of 'being of good service to/not-being-of-good-service-to'. Particular forms of prior experience may make a person better able to appreciate how others are affected by similar experiences and act as their advocates, though the judgment of *similarity* may obscure what is *different* in the other person's experience. It may lead to collusive over-generalisation, obscuring rather than enlightening, or a failure to recognise the individuality of the other. Is such political rhetoric any more defensible than a child's retort when insulted "It takes one to know one?"

The Dutch lottery system and WP initiative pose further questions relating to the place of medical education in meeting societal goals. Does the value gained fit sufficiently with those other qualities necessary for and the resources (personal, institutional, financial) available to produce the necessary range of doctors? Should medical schools be established to meet only the needs of a particular form of health service in a particular country at a particular time or is there a responsibility to the wider world, current and future? There needs to be further exploration of medicine's ability to bring about social change in an international context to identify medical education's core tasks and the impact of linking these with other societal aims.

Assessment

One theme of this chapter is that there has to be an on-going process of selection that determines progression through medical education and continued licensure once fully trained. Clinical work forces practitioners to examine their interactions, opinions, recommendations, and actions constantly. Thus practice, or more specifically, truly reflective practice, is an iterative, formative assessment. In common usage, however, the term *assessment* refers to mandatory punctuations which determine progress within training or confirm fitness to remain in specialist practice. It is vital that those assessments test what they set out to test, or at least act as suitable surrogates for the desired outcomes. From an ethical standpoint, the principles described in the first part of this chapter apply to assessment. Principled Autonomy, which underpins the learning contract between all parties in the service of medical education, provides a framework to define and enact rights and obligations.

Assessment influences learning, particularly in *strategic learners*, people adept at shaping their learning to assessment (well represented among medical learners). The contribution of assessment to shaping learning outcomes is not always positive. Newble and Jaeger (1983) described how an alteration in assessment could produce the opposite of an intended effect on learning through "distortion. . . [where] there is a mismatch between the Faculty's real objectives and the objectives expressed in the assessment scheme." I (AS) have experienced comparable concerns in undergraduate communication skills and post-graduate psychiatry examinations. The time-limited nature of formal tests and high stakes create a difficulty for candidates because preparing for assessments may have an undue effect on how they behave in everyday practice. Punctuating progress in that manner could unintentionally perpetuate inappropriate practice. Socrates' aphorism "The unexamined life is not worth living" may not win much favour with those in the process of being examined but an unexamined professional is certainly not worth entrusting one's life to! Assessments must not only stand practical and scientific scrutiny but also be based on enquiry about their own validity and humanity.

Implications for practice

Medical education is a complex interweaving of the sciences and arts of education and medicine. At its heart is the welfare of human beings. Those practicing and training for practice must be concerned with alleviating suffering, assisting adaptation to illness and disability, extending life, and contributing to a better death. Ultimately, there is no area of practice that can be regarded as value-free, so the ability to examine the values influencing action is an essential part of professional practice. If action is to be well reasoned and reasonable, the study of ethics is an essential, foundation component of medical education.

We have introduced some key areas of medical ethics and directed readers particularly towards the contribution we believe 'Principled Autonomy' can make because we believe it strikes a balance between the reasonable and unreasonable aspirations or expectations individuals may have of themselves and others. It also readily links to developmental and relational influences on learning and practice. Implicit in the presentation have been references to other schools of moral philosophy, for example, Consequentialism and Virtue Ethics; we encourage a deeper investigation into them. The goal is to be able to maintain personal integrity, remain sane whilst being in at least two minds (one's own doubts, in addition to one's own mind and that of a patient), and still achieve productive activity with others.

The educational process itself should help learners examine the moral basis of medical practice; it has to be a living model conducted on a morally sound basis. Implicit in our exposition is the need for research into the impact on patients, learners, teachers, and the wider community of the educational methods in common use. Further to this is the place of kindness in establishing and maintaining practitioners' usefulness and ability to respect and be worthy of trust.

"The real moral question is what kind of a self is being furthered and formed."

Dewey, J. (1932)

References

Baier A: Trust and antitrust, *Ethics* 96:231–260, 1986.

Beauchamp TL, Childress JF: *Principles of biomedical ethics*, ed 5, Oxford, 2001, Oxford University Press.

Campbell A: Dependency revisited. The limits of autonomy in medical ethics. In Brazier M, Lobjoit M, editors: *Protecting the vulnerable: autonomy and consent in health care*, ed 1, London, 1991, Routledge.

Colliver JA, Markwell SJ, Verhulst SJ, Robbs RS: The prognostic value of documented unprofessional behaviour in medical school records for predicting and preventing subsequent medical board disciplinary action: the Papadakis studies revisited, *Teaching Learning Med: An Int J* 19:3213–3215, 2007.

Eriksen E: *Childhood and society*, New York, 1950, Norton.

Gillon R: *Philosophical medical ethics*, Wiley, 1985, Chichester, pp. 61–62.

Fulford KWM: Ten principles of values-based medicine. Radden J, editor: *The philosophy of psychiatry: a companion*, New York, 2004, Oxford University Press, pp 205–234.

Higher Education Funding Council for England: *Widening participation* [Online]. Available at http://www.hefce.ac.uk/widen/ Accessed November 21, 2009.

Hilton S, Lewis K: Opening doors to medicine, *BMJ* 328 (7455):1508–1509, 2004.

Hilton SR, Slotnick HB: Proto-professionalism: how professionalization occurs across the continuum of medical education, *Med Educ* 39:58–65, 2005.

Jackson J: *Truth, trust and medicine*, London and New York, 2001, Routledge.

Lave J, Wenger E: *Situated learning: legitimate peripheral participation*, ed 1, Cambridge, 1991, Cambridge University Press.

McMillan J, Wright B, Davidson G, Bennett J: Criminal records and studying medicine, *BMJ Careers* 30 May:166–167, 2009.

Newble DI, Jaeger K: The effect of assessments and examinations on the learning of medical learners, *Med Educ* 17:165–171, 1983.

O'Neill O: *A question of trust*, 2002a [Online]. Available at http://www.bbc.co.uk/radio4/reith2002/ Accessed November 21, 2009.

O'Neill O, *Autonomy and trust in bioethics*, Cambridge, 2002b, Cambridge University Press.

Phillips A, Taylor B: *On kindness*, London, 2009, Hamish Hamilton.

Sennett R: *The corrosion of character: the personal consequences of work in the new capitalism*, New York and London, 1998, W.W. Norton & Co.

Shaw P: *Changing conversations in organisations: a complexity approach to change*, London and New York, 2002, Routledge.

Stanford encyclopedia of philosophy [Online]. Available at http://plato.stanford.edu. Accessed November 2009.

Stasz C, van Stalk C: *Working paper: the use of lottery systems in school admissions*, Rand Europe, 2009 [Online]. Available at http://www.rand.org/pubs/working_papers/2007/RAND_WR460.pdf Accessed November 21.

Stirrat GM, Gill R: Autonomy in medical ethics after O'Neill, *J Med Ethics* 31:127–130, 2005.

Sulmasy DP: Should medical schools be schools of virtue? *J Gen Int Med* 15(7):514–516, 2000.

Sutton A: Authority, autonomy, responsibility and authorisation: with specific reference to adolescent mental health practice, *J Med Ethics* 23(1):26–31, 1997.

Sutton A: Disrupted dependence and dependability: Winnicott in a culture of symptom intolerance, *Psychoanal Psychother* 15(1):1–19, 2001.

Sweeney K, Griffiths F: *Complexity and healthcare: an introduction*, Oxford, 2002, Radcliffe Medical Press.

Vygotsky LS: *Mind and society: the development of higher psychological processes*, Cambridge, MA, 1978, Harvard University Press.

Winnicott DW: *The maturational processes and the facilitating environment: studies in the theory of emotional development*, London, 1965, Hogarth Press and the Institute of Psychoanalysis.

Winnicott DW: Contemporary concepts of adolescent development and their implications for Higher Education. In Winnicott W, editor: *Playing and reality*, Harmondsworth, UK, 1971, Penguin Books, p 11.

World Medical Association: *World Medical Association Declaration of Helsinki: ethical principles of medical research involving human subjects*, 1964, World Medical Association. Available at http://www.wma.net/en/30publications/10policies/b3/17c.pdf.

Ziliak ST, McCloskey DN: *The cult of statistical significance: how the standard error costs us jobs, justice, and lives*, Ann Arbor, 2008, University of Michigan Press.

Further reading

General Medical Council [Online]. Available at: www.gmc-uk.org/ Accessed November 2009.

O'Neill O, *Autonomy and trust in bioethics*, Cambridge, 2002, Cambridge University Press.

Perspectives on learning

2

Karen Mann   Tim Dornan   Pim W. Teunissen

CHAPTER CONTENTS

ABC

Glossary

Adult learning; see also andragogy Describes a set of principles, originally described by Knowles in 1984, that differentiate how adult learners differ from children. They include the experience the adult has accumulated, motivation and self-direction, and the interest in solving problems that are relevant to their everyday lives.

Approaches to learning; see also deep learning and surface learning These describe how students approach learning tasks. *Surface* and *deep* learning represent two different approaches. A surface approach is characterised by accepting new facts and ideas uncritically and attempting to store them as isolated, unconnected, items (rote learning). Deep learning is characterised by examining new facts and ideas critically, tying them into existing cognitive structures and making numerous links between ideas.

Cognitivism A *cognitivist* orientation focuses on perception, memory, and meaning. The various cognitive perspectives share two important assumptions: (a) the memory system is an active processor of information and (b) knowledge plays an important role in learning. Learning is seen as reorganizing experience to increase meaning.

Continued

© 2011, Elsevier Ltd.
DOI: 10.1016/B978-0-7020-3522-7.00002-4

Glossary (continued)

Epistemology The theory or science of the method or grounds of knowledge.

Humanist orientation to learning Focuses on human potential for growth and the freedom of individuals to become "what they are capable of becoming." Theories of self-direction, transformative learning, and adult learning fall within the humanist category.

Lifelong learning An ongoing process through which individuals acquire the knowledge, skills, and values they will need through their life.

Practical theories of learning and teaching These are based on individuals' experiences, the combination of their formal and informal knowledge, and their values and beliefs. Practical theories strongly determine educational practice.

Self-directed learning Self-directed learning refers to an ongoing process through which individuals identify their learning needs, identify means to meet them, engage in relevant learning activities, and evaluate their progress and achievement in meeting their needs.

Socio-cultural theory Current conceptualisations of socio-cultural theory draw heavily on the work of Vygotsky (1978). A key feature of this emergent view of human development is that higher-order functions develop out of social interaction. Social relationships and culturally constructed artefacts – including language and tools – mediate learning and there is a two-way relationship between culture and individual learning. People learn meanings through activities that take place within individual, social, and institutional relationships.

Tacit learning; see also implicit learning The acquisition of knowledge independently of conscious attempts to learn, and without knowing exactly what has been learnt.

Outline

This chapter presents perspectives on learning selected for their ability to inform practice and research. We use 'perspectives' more or less interchangeably with 'theories' but prefer the term perspectives because it emphasises that any situation can be viewed from more than one angle; one perspective might be more informative for one purpose while a different perspective might be more informative for another purpose. After a brief overview of how perspectives might be grouped, we present them in the form of a map – far from any definitive 'truth', the map is intended to provoke discussion

about why a perspective might more appropriately be positioned in one place in the map than another and how it relates to other perspectives. The following perspectives are then presented: Cognitive psychological theory, Experiential learning, Reflective learning, Tacit learning, Adult learning, Self-directed learning (SDL), and Lifelong learning. Social perspectives including Social cognitive theory (SCT) and Socio-cultural theory are introduced, ending the overview with the two main 'neo-Vygotskian' socio-cultural perspectives: Activity theory, and Communities of Practice theory. We conclude the chapter by suggesting some implications for both educational practice and research.

Introduction

Medical education is located at the crossroads between medicine and education. Practitioners and scientists from both the biomedical and social science domains contribute to it in the joint pursuit of two goals: to develop and provide an education that effectively prepares medical professionals for their current and future tasks, and to develop an evidence base that can inform and be informed by practice. Understanding learning plays an important role in meeting both of those goals. If we have insight into how medical students, residents, and practising physicians develop the knowledge, skills, and behaviours that allow them to work as professionals, the development of programmes and assessments and the evaluation of their effects will benefit.

In ways that are both explicit and tacit, our understandings of and perspectives on learning inform our practice as educators. They inform the decisions we make about curricula and teaching, the ways we interpret the outcomes of teaching, the candidates we admit to educational programmes, and the questions we ask in research projects. Our perspectives on teaching also affect our views of learning. These perspectives arise from our experience as teachers as well as from formal study. Educators' deeply held values about teaching and learning translate into "practical theories" (Handal and Lauvas, 1987) that influence how they see their own roles and responsibilities and the roles and responsibilities of their learners.

An understanding of what learning entails contributes significantly to education research as well as practice. It informs the framing of research questions, design of interventions and experiments, and choice of outcome measures. To advance the field of medical education, researchers are encouraged to reflect on their practical theories and place them within a conceptual framework that can build a coherent body of evidence and, eventually, a better understanding of learning itself (Eva and Lingard, 2008; Prideaux and Bligh, 2002). Importantly, given that those involved in medical education range from busy clinicians to phenomenological researchers, there is a rich variety of perspectives on teaching and views on learning from which to choose.

The field of learning is complex and evolving. Beyond the personal and practical understandings discussed earlier, scholars have provided theoretical perspectives that illuminate learning more broadly, and reach far wider than the confines of medical education. Among these are behaviourist, cognitive, and social perspectives, as well as developmental and socio-cultural ones. Perspectives have arisen from the disciplines of psychology, education, sociology, and anthropology. Some overlap with others, which can be confusing but can also provide opportunities for deeper understanding. In this chapter, we discuss some key perspectives on learning. We also explore how such theories illuminate educational practice, and how they can complement each other in guiding understanding. Our two overarching goals are that, in reading and considering the subject matter of this chapter, you will

- acquire an up-to-date picture of the range of perspectives on learning that may inform your educational practice;
- be able to select from and use these perspectives as frameworks that can both guide the design of educational activities and help analyse and understand their effects.

Orientations to learning

People who come to education from a medical background may at first be perplexed by this emphasis on underpinning theory and even people who come from theory-rich disciplines may be surprised by the variety of theoretical perspectives they encounter in the world of medical education. Psychology is a rich source of educational theory so developments in education have been very closely linked to developments in psychology. Over the last century, psychology has moved first from a dominant behaviourist stance to a cognitive one and then to focus more on situated views of cognition, which accounts for some of the

breadth of perspectives. However, psychology is not the only social science that provides perspectives on learning. Wertsch (1991) wrote of the need for other perspectives – notably socio-cultural ones – because psychology has had 'very little to say about what it means to be human in the modern world (or any other world for that matter)'. No one perspective is inherently 'better' than any other, and certainly not just because it is newer, which is why this chapter discusses such a range of them. We do not by any means provide an exhaustive list of perspectives in use within (medical) education but aim to give the reader a broad overview of informative ones.

Behaviourist, cognivitist, social, and humanist orientations

We begin the chapter by outlining some very broad perspectives on learning, which we term 'orientations'. We have followed the categorisation of Merriam et al (2007), except that we regard constructivism as a broad philosophical position that underpins most contemporary ideas about learning; we devote the section following this one to it in preference to treating it as just one of five orientations to learning.

- A *behaviourist* orientation focuses on overt behaviour and the measurement of that behaviour. The assumptions of behavioural theorists about the nature of learning focus on the role of the environment in both stimulating and shaping behaviour. What happens within individuals is of less interest as it is unobservable. Learning equates to changes in behavioural responses to environmental stimuli. An individual's response, such as formulating a differential diagnosis or solving a clinical problem, produces a consequence. What an individual learns will depend on whether the response is rewarded or penalised. Proponents of this view were, for instance, Pavlov and Skinner. Skinner introduced "operant conditioning," acknowledging that individuals can instigate behaviour as well as respond to external stimuli. Behavioural approaches to learning are still very visible in educational practice today. Through the use of behavioural objectives, which emphasise that learners must demonstrate certain behaviour(s) under specific circumstances in response to specific stimuli, behaviourism still exerts a firm influence on curricula in professional education. Training approaches to simple skills like suturing and complex ones like advanced life support, where repeated practice and feedback are essential elements, have characteristics of behaviourism.

- A *cognitivist* orientation focuses on perception, memory, and meaning. The various cognitive perspectives share two important assumptions: (a) the memory system is an active processor of information and (b) knowledge plays an important role in learning. Learning is seen as reorganizing experience to increase meaning. In addition to responding to environmental influences, cognitive structures change as a result of maturation. Perspectives that fall within this orientation include information-processing, memory and meta-cognition, transfer of learning, and expertise. There are also theories of instruction that link instructional methods to the acquisition and processing of knowledge (Ausubel, 1963; Gagné, 1985). The two opposing concepts of meaningful and rote learning have their roots in the cognitive orientation. Meaningful learning is connected to learners' concepts and integrated into their existing knowledge structures, whereas rote learning is more superficial, not connected to other learning, and therefore not so 'durable'. The term 'deep learning' equates to the former, and 'surface learning' to the latter. The essential components of learning are organisation of the information to be learned, the learner's prior knowledge, and the processes of perceiving, comprehending, storing, and retrieving information.

- A *social* orientation takes as its assumption that learning is a social activity; it occurs in interaction between the learner and other people. Social perspectives take account of learners, their environments, and the interaction between the two. From a social perspective, learners are not just the products of their experiences, but also proactive producers of the environments they operate in. Social learning theorists believe that people learn from observing and acting alongside others from which skill, knowledge, rules, strategies, beliefs, and attitudes ensue. People also learn about the appropriateness of behaviours and do so by observing others whom they regard as models, and seeing the consequences of their actions. Two different social learning perspectives are recognisable, one with a primary focus on learning as an intra-individual process – SCT (Bandura, 1986) – and another focusing on

learning as an inter-individual process – socio-cultural theory (Tsui et al, 2009).

- A *humanist* orientation focuses on human potential for growth and the freedom of individuals to become "what they are capable of becoming." (Maslow, 1970) Perhaps the most familiar of these perspectives is Maslow's hierarchy of needs, according to which needs at the lower end of the hierarchy must be met before those above can be addressed. Basic needs, such as hunger and thirst, are physiological. Above those are safety needs, for example shelter. Above those are needs for belonging, love, and self-esteem. At the top comes the need for self-actualisation. Theories of self-direction, transformative learning, and adult learning fall within the humanist category.

Constructivism

To understand constructivism, it is necessary to go deeper into the philosophies of knowledge and learning. In the language of philosophy, perspectives on learning differ in their 'ontologies' and 'epistemologies'. As explained by Guba and Lincoln (2005), the study of *ontology* is concerned with the question 'What is the form and nature of reality?' According to them, 'If a "real" world is assumed, then what can be known about it is "how things really are" and "how things really work"'. 'Questions, such as those concerning matters of aesthetic or moral significance, fall outside the realm of legitimate scientific enquiry'. That would be described as a 'positivist' system of beliefs, which contrasts with a constructivist one. *Epistemological* questions concern 'What the nature of the relationship between the knower ... and what can be known is'. Guba and Lincoln (2005) go on to show how a positivist ontology leads logically to a positivist epistemology when they argue that 'If a real reality is assumed, then the posture of the knower must be one of objective detachment or value freedom in order to... discover "how things really are" and "how things really work"'.

Since this book concerns education, we can confine ourselves to epistemology and consider how the different perspectives we discuss view the relationship between the knower and the known. The positivist epistemological perspective in the aforementioned quotations of a "real" reality that can be apprehended through an 'objective detachment' is characterised by Guba and Lincoln (2005) as 'naive realism'. From a positivist standpoint, knowledge is outside the learner; it is value and context-free. In contrast, a constructivist system of beliefs does not see such a distinction between 'real' and 'experienced' realities because its epistemology is, according to Guba and Lincoln, 'transactional/ subjectivist'. So, the focus is not on knowledge as an absolute external reality, but on its construction by the knower: 'Realities are apprehensible in the form of multiple, intangible mental constructions, socially and experimentally based, local and specific in nature (although elements are often shared among many individuals and even across cultures), and dependent ... on the individual persons or groups holding the constructions' (Guba and Lincoln, 2005). The knower and the object of their knowing are 'assumed to be interactively linked' so their knowledge is 'literally created'. In an educational context, constructivism can be seen as a process whereby learners actively construct their understandings based on previous experience, knowledge, and their perceptions of the world. Constructivism also contrasts with positivism in attaching more importance to 'matters of moral and aesthetic significance'; in other words, values and beliefs. A progressive shift towards a more constructivist view of (medical) education explains many of the recent changes in the field and much of the subject matter of this chapter reflects the dominance of a constructivist epistemology of learning.

Two axes for mapping constructivist perspectives

Because it can be difficult to see how different perspectives relate to or differ from each other, we offer two organizing principles to group them. First, the extent to which they focus on individual versus societal/cultural processes; second, the extent to which they provide abstract conceptualisations (AC) versus principles that can be applied directly to practice.

Individual-social axis

Learning can be viewed more as an individual or a collaborative process. Within cognitive psychology, studies of perception, meaning, and memory have focused on the processes developed and used by individual learners. Early cognitivist thinkers focused on individuals' mental processes in order to understand

learning and behaviour. Later thinking stressed the importance of embodiment, according to which cognition depends not just on the brain but also on the body. Metaphors that are in common use reinforce the view of learning as an individual process, notably the *acquisition* metaphor, from which perspective learning involves the acquisition and accumulation of goods by individuals. In the case of medical education, those 'goods' include knowledge, skills, attitudes, values and (more recently) competence. We talk about a person attaining, developing, accruing, and 'getting a grasp' of an idea or skill. Once someone has accumulated one of those entities, they can transfer or apply it to a different context and share it with others. As Sfard (1998) pointed out, this metaphor has been so much a part of our thinking that we scarcely noticed it until another metaphor began to emerge. This was the *participation* metaphor, which represents the other end of the individual-collaborative spectrum. Participation centres on activities and doing. While the acquisition metaphor implies that we can reach the point where we have 'achieved' learning, participation is ongoing and continuous. Learning through participation can never be separated from the context in which it occurs. Learning theories from fields such as sociology and anthropology have helped us understand how participation is shaped by societies and cultures. The participation metaphor (also known as the embedding thesis) highlights how important it is that we understand learning and development as situated in a social and physical environment. This perspective opened up the possibility of "cognition extending beyond the boundaries of individual organisms" (Robbins and Aydede, 2009). Research into team functioning and learning, for instance, often incorporates this extension thesis.

Abstract-applied axis

The second organizing principle centres on the extent to which a theory is abstract or applied. Cognitivist or socio-cultural perspectives present quite abstract notions of how people behave, interact, or learn. Based on observation and study, theorists try deductively to identify principles that underlie learning. Other theoretical perspectives are less abstract and more readily applicable; for example, adult learning principles. Some perspectives seem to be so 'applied' that they bear hardly any relationship to developed bodies of knowledge and are open to the criticism that they lack a solid theoretical basis (Norman, 1999).

Mapping individual perspectives

Figure 2.1 maps the theoretical perspectives discussed in this chapter to where they sit on the continuum between learning being situated primarily within (parts of) individuals or situated within a society and culture, and on the abstract-applied continuum. Of course, those positions are not fixed. Different people will conceptualise the same perspective in different ways and argue for different positions on the map. Theoretical perspectives are 'alive' in the sense that they are continuously being researched, applied, further developed, and extended. The purpose of the map is to indicate that perspectives differ along at least two dimensions and each perspective can be characterised by the two organizing principles we discussed. We hope this insight will help readers understand differences between theoretical perspectives and stimulate them to reflect on their own practical theories of learning.

Individual perspectives on learning and development

Cognitive psychology

Cognitive psychology is the basis for many aspects of (medical) education and this perspective underlies much of the current emphasis on active learning,

reflective practice, problem-solving, diagnosis, clinical reasoning, and expertise. The relationship has been a reciprocal one because education research has also refined cognitive theory. As explained earlier, cognitive psychology is concerned with what goes on in learners' minds and views learning as an active constructive process. To illustrate how cognitive principles apply in practice, we now explain some underlying principles of problem-based learning (PBL), an educational method that has been widely adopted in recent years.

The importance of prior knowledge

Prior knowledge, which provides meaning, context, and a connection for new knowledge, is an important determinant of the new knowledge a learner can master at any moment.

Activation of prior knowledge

For prior knowledge to be used effectively to connect and integrate new knowledge, it must be activated. This activation is brought about by considering relevant aspects of the problem (case); importantly, prior knowledge is activated by the social process of discussion (see Chapter 9 for an explanation of PBL as a small-group learning process) which elicits what each student can draw on to help explain the problem. For example, students may have family members who have experienced a health problem

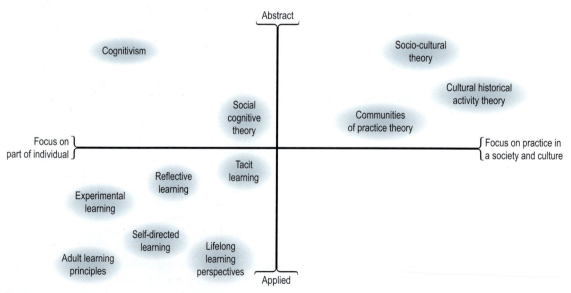

Figure 2.1 • Constructivist outlooks on learning and development.

similar to the one under discussion. Discussion draws in their individual experiences and analyses their relevance to the problem under consideration. Similarly, summarizing what has been learnt to date about the problem can activate knowledge.

Elaboration of knowledge

To be effective and available for use, rich knowledge structures need to be developed. Those structures contain knowledge that is connected to many other bits of knowledge. Having a richer network of interconnections creates alternative pathways to stored information such that knowledge is adaptable and flexible. Elaboration can happen in several ways including discussion of the case, sharing past experience, sharing what learners have learned, peer teaching, taking notes, and gaining additional real or simulated experience with patients.

Learning in context

Learning something in a meaningful context enhances a learner's ability to retrieve it for the solution of future problems. The closer the situation in which it is learnt is to the one in which it will be used, the more readily usable the information will be. So, the meaningful context of PBL problems and their relevance to the real problems of future practice are intended to enhance learning and memory.

Transfer of knowledge

To develop a usable, durable, flexible, and adaptable knowledge base, one must be able to transfer what is learnt in one problem or setting to another problem or setting. While it was once thought that transfer occurred quite readily, it is now clear that both teachers and learners have to encourage transfer actively. Two kinds of transfer have been described: low-road transfer, the product of exposure to and opportunities to practice on multiple examples of a problem, which can happen without explicit awareness; and high road transfer, a more deliberate process in which principles are extracted that can be applied to other relevant situations. Transfer can occur by looking backward, to see what from our previous experience and learning is helpful, or looking forwards, to identify which aspects of a problem may be useful in the future. Learners might need help to develop the habit of identifying salient aspects of problems, rather than just those that are on the

surface. Transfer of a concept can be improved by embedding it in a problem, as is the case in PBL, though conventional curricula can also accomplish transfer. The process of looking for underlying concepts and principles can be strengthened by effective tutoring; for example, by encouraging students to compare the current case with others in their experience or think of other examples that reveal similar concepts. Actively rehearsing concepts in the context of a case promotes transfer (Norman, 2009a).

Developing generic problem-solving skills?

While PBL was hailed initially as a means to develop generalised problem-solving skills, subsequent research showed convincingly that a person's ability to solve a problem is closely related to their knowledge in that specific area. So PBL may only enhance problem-solving skills in so far as it develops learners' knowledge and critical thinking skills, and their ability to work as part of a social group to accomplish a shared goal.

To round off this review of cognitive perspectives on learning, Box 2.1 lists what Simons et al (2000) label *new learning outcomes*, a set of desirable features of learning outcomes, which relate very well to the preceding description of cognitive processes.

Box 2.1

New learning outcomes

Durable: Learning endures over a period of time and is not just for today or tomorrow.

Flexible: Learning can be approached from different perspectives and angles – not tied to just one perspective. Learning should be adaptable to new contexts and changes in contexts. This requires deep learning and internal relational networks (elaborated knowledge).

Functional: Learning (knowledge and skills) should be available when needed (right time, right place)

Meaningful: Deep understanding of a few basic principles with far reaching significance is more important than superficial understanding of many facts that may become obsolete.

Generalisable: Learning is not restricted to one situation but reaches out to other situations.

Application-oriented: people should know the possible applications and conditions of their knowledge and skills.

Simons et al (2000).

Experiential learning

From a constructivist standpoint, experiences are pivotal in the development of undergraduate medical students, postgraduate learners, practicing physicians, and other health care professionals. Experiences lie at the heart of participation, and participation, as discussed in relation to Figure 2.1, is central to social and collaborative perspectives on learning. Experiential learning encompasses a range of concepts and has been influenced by educational theorists like Piaget, Lewin, Dewey, and Kolb. Experiential learning starts from the generally accepted notion that an individual's concepts and behaviours arise from and are adjusted through their life experiences. The work of Kolb offers a way of understanding the cognitive processes that underlie such learning. In his influential 1984 book entitled 'Experiential Learning: experience as the source of learning and development', he defines learning as "the process whereby knowledge is created through the transformation of experience" (Kolb, 1984, p. 41). He proposes a four-stage cyclical model of knowledge development that combines the grasping and transformation of experience by individuals. According to Kolb, the first stage of learning starts with a concrete experience (CE), followed by reflection on that experience, leading to the formation of abstract concepts and generalisations regarding the experience, and finally the testing of new or adjusted concepts through new experience. This leads again to CE, which closes the learning cycle. Honey and Mumford (1986) slightly adapted this learning cycle. According to them, learners move from having an experience to reviewing the experience, to drawing conclusions based on the experience, and to planning the next steps. Kolb acknowledged that learning does not necessarily start with an experience and that the cycle may be entered at other stages as well (Kolb, 1984). Subsequent developments of experiential learning theory have paid less attention to the cyclical aspect.

Meanwhile, Kolb and others focused more on the two opposed modes of grasping and transforming experience (Kolb et al, 2001). CE and AC were the two modes of grasping experience whilst reflective observation (RO) and active experimentation (AE) were the two modes of transforming experience. According to Kolb, learners have a preference for a certain approach to acquiring experience and transforming it, which he called their learning style. This underlies the Learning Style Inventory (LSI)

(Kolb, 2005). The LSI identifies four types of learners: convergers (AE-AC), accommodators (AE-CE), assimilators (RO-AC), and divergers (RO-CE). The LSI was designed to determine an individual's learning preference. It was one of the first learning style questionnaires developed, and is used widely, including in the medical domain (Curry, 1999). There is, however, considerable criticism of its use and value (Norman, 2009b). According to Coffield and colleagues, the reliability of the LSI has not been established and it has low validity as a predictive test. The implications for teaching have been drawn logically from the theory rather than from research findings and there is no evidence that 'matching' education with preferred learning styles improves performance (Coffield et al, 2004, https://crm.lsnlearning.org.uk/user/order.aspx?code=041543). Moreover, Kolb's underlying theory of the four-stage experiential learning model has received much criticism on very diverse grounds (see Greenaway, 2009, http://reviewing.co.uk/research/experiential.learning.htm#styles). The idea that learning takes the form of a neat four-stage cycle is challenged. For instance, Schlesinger argues that the separate elements of the cycle may be relevant, but that in practice learning is much more fragmented and chaotic (Cheetham and Chivers, 2005; Schlesinger, 1996). Bleakley pointed to the paradox of a model of 'experience' that neglects the social context of that experience and its influence on what is learnt from the experience (Bleakley, 2006). Nonetheless, researchers have found Kolb's experiential learning theory useful to explain a number of phenomena related to learning in medical workplaces (Chung et al, 2003; Smith et al, 2004; White and Anderson, 1995).

Reflective learning

Reflective learning is also based in and on experience. Reflection as a means of learning has been discussed by educators as early as 1933 (Dewey, 1991), when Dewey described learning as "active, persistent and careful consideration of any belief or supposed form of knowledge in the light of the grounds that support it and the further conclusion to which it tends" (p. 9). Reflection and reflective practice have moved into a more visible and central position in definitions of competence (Epstein and Hundert, 2002), and are clearly stated to be elements of learning in the activities of such bodies as the Royal College of Physicians and Surgeons of Canada and the General Medical Council of the United Kingdom, among others. Undergraduate pre-licensure medical education programmes require learners to keep portfolios to serve not only as evidence of their experiences but also as a basis for demonstrating the ability to reflect on and synthesise experience.

While reflective practice cannot strictly be said to be a discrete perspective, it incorporates a number of cognitive theoretical constructs and its potential effectiveness as a way of learning can be highlighted through exploration of these. Reflection, as defined by Boud et al (1985), is the process by which we examine our experiences in order to learn from them. This examination involves returning to experience in order to re-evaluate it and glean learning that may affect our predispositions and action in the future. Others describe it as the process of turning something over in our minds to frame a problem or shape a solution in an unstructured situation (Moon, 1999). Finally, reflection has been conceptualised as a process whereby new learning is assimilated into our cognitive structures through becoming part of our existing knowledge and skills, attitudes, beliefs, and values (Moon, 1999). Each of these definitions emphasises different aspects of reflection, which include critical thinking as well as personal reflection and integration of learning.

Generally, reflection as a method of learning is conceptualised as an interactive set of activities, whereby we are prompted, either deliberately or unexpectedly, to return to our experience to re-examine it and learn from it. Kolb (1984) described reflection as an integral part of a cycle of learning from experience. Following a study of several professions, Schön too described an interactive process, which he depicted as follows (Schön, 1987). He described professionals' 'knowing-in-action' as their accumulated body of knowledge and skills are gained through formal and informal learning and through experience, which they apply to framing, identifying, and addressing the problems of authentic practice. When professionals encounter a 'surprise' a process of 'reflection-in-action' ensues. In this period of 'thinking on one's feet', solutions may be considered and rejected which may lead to a slightly altered or new course of action. The final stage in the iterative process involves 'reflection-on-action' or returning to the experience to evaluate its outcomes and learn from it. New learning can then be incorporated into professional 'knowing in action' so that it is altered by each learning experience.

Theoretically, reflection has been proposed as an active approach to learning which can (a) add to one's knowing-in-action, (b) surface assumptions and biases that may influence one's perceptions, (c) promote deep learning of new concepts, (d) help in the framing of difficult complex problems, (e) assist in integration of effective experiences, (f) facilitate the acceptance of feedback, and (g) help connect one's work and learning to a broader context. Above all, it seems to hold potential for practitioners to become more self-aware, in order to better develop as balanced professionals, and to be able to think critically about both the scientific nature of their work and the nature and meaning of their experience. Such self-awareness can assist in self-regulation, and holds potential for professionals to uncover the tacit knowledge and understanding that applies in their practice and can be shared with others.

Although the evidence for its existence and any effects on learning is dispersed in the health professions education literature, a recent systematic review of the literature for the years 1994–2005 (Mann et al, 2009) confirmed its existence as a strategy employed by physicians, nurses, and other health professionals as well as students. Analyses of the structure of this activity (Mamede and Schmidt, 2004, 2005) revealed a five-factor structure consisting of openness to reflection, deliberate induction, and deliberate deduction, testing, and meta-reasoning. Reflection appears to be linked to learning and positively associated with deep learning across several studies. While it appears that some individuals are more naturally inclined to reflect than others, there is also evidence that the skills of reflection can be developed through practice, feedback, and supervision (Mann et al, 2009). It also seems that reflection can be encouraged in some contexts but discouraged in others. More recently, the literature has suggested that, at least in resident learners, a reflective approach may reduce diagnostic errors in complex problems (Mamede et al, 2008). Lastly, reflection seems to be an integral aspect of practice in high-performing physicians, and a critical process to enable acceptance and use of feedback on performance (Sargeant et al, 2006, 2009b).

The aspect of reflection to which Schön paid most attention was 'reflection on experience'. More recently, however, scholars have tried to theorise 'reflection-in-action', which represents the ongoing minute-to-minute monitoring of our performance; they have posited that it is a critical element of self-assessment and self-monitoring (Eva and Regehr, 2007; Moulton et al, 2007).

Attempts to assess the presence of reflective capability and reflective practice have been reported in the literature. These reports have taken two directions: (a) the development of quantitative, self-report questionnaires completed by learners and practitioners and (b) the development of methods to assess the products of reflection, such as journals and reflections on experience. Although several have been reported, two scales have emerged in medical education, for which information about development and psychometric properties are available. These are the Reflection in Learning Scale (RLS) (Sobral, 2005), and the Groningen Reflection Assessment Scale (GRAS) (Aukes et al, 2007).

The RLS is a 14-item scale, requiring responses on a Likert-type scale, designed to measure students' self-reported use of reflection in their learning. It has high internal consistency ($\alpha = 0.84$) and test–retest stability ($\alpha = 0.86$); it has also shown positive statistically significant relationships with measures of deep learning (Sobral, 2001). The GRAS is a 23-item scale, also using Likert Scale responses, developed to measure personal reflection ability in medical students. Developed from a theoretical and empirical base, the scale had satisfactory psychometric properties ($\alpha = 0.76$), and content validity. A factor analysis led the authors to conclude that the scale measures a single underlying construct, with three related aspects: self-reflection; empathetic reflection; and reflective communication. Both of these scales appear to be easy to administer and score and offer potential means of assessing students' level of and growth in reflective ability.

Measurement of reflective ability from writing, such as in journals or narrative accounts of experience, seems also to be possible. Reports of such assessments have generally come from the nursing and health professions literature; generally, they are based on criteria drawn from models of reflection, such as those by Boud et al (1985) or Mezirow (1991). These models categorise reflection in terms of both the processes involved and the depth of reflection achieved. Difficulties with inter-rater agreement and coding have been reported; nevertheless, it appears that acceptable consistency can be achieved.

Despite challenges in teaching and modelling reflection in the professional context, there is increasing support for its use to promote professional development, deepen learning, and encourage development of habits of mind for future practice. Reflective learning is not, however, without its critics, nor is it without its challenges within the professional context (Boud and Walker, 2002). Indeed, concerns

have been raised about the potential for creating a 'ritualised' form of reflection. Coulehan and Williams (2001) described a non-reflective professionalism in which individuals were unable to see gaps that existed between their espoused ways of behaving and their professional behaviour in action. Further, as the tendency to be reflective varies across individuals, there are some who find reflection an artificial and unhelpful process (Sargeant et al, 2009a,b). Others express concern about the burden of keeping reflective journals, some seeing reflective writing as redundant (Grant et al, 2006). Concerns are expressed about the assessment of reflection, particularly the validity of written reflective material submitted for assessment.

Tacit learning

In contrast to the 'formal learning' that is emphasised by official curricula, much important learning results from everyday activities. This 'informal learning' contributes 'tacit knowledge', which accumulates without awareness and tends to be regarded as things a practitioner "just knows" (Eraut, 2000). As practitioners develop expertise, tacit knowledge of how to do things and which actions to apply in which situations frees their cognitive resources to frame and solve problems. Their tacit knowledge, however, is difficult to articulate, which means that they are more likely to pass on explicit aspects of their knowledge when they 'teach'. That emphasis on the explicit rather than the tacit is strongly reinforced by outcome-based curricula, particularly ones that codify professional expertise as competencies (Chapter 6).

Constructivism's acknowledgement that we learn experientially from daily activities, in contrast to positivism's preoccupation with the codified knowledge that learners acquire as a result of teaching, has made it possible to give more prominence to tacit learning.

Tacit as it may be, this type of knowledge affects our expectations and the way we frame and perceive events, which has very important implications. Many would agree that professional education is in large part a process of socialisation, which means internalising the knowledge structures, routines, norms, expectations, attitudes, and values of the profession. Those matters may be explicitly taught, but much of what is learnt about them is tacit. Moreover, tacit learning may actually be in opposition to explicit teaching. Hafferty and Frank (1994) described how the "hidden curriculum" could directly oppose explicitly espoused values such as patient-centredness and ethical practice. Coulehan and Williams (2001), describing a conflict between tacit learning and stated values, elicited three types of response: detachment, in which affective aspects of activity become distanced and competence comes to be viewed as objective and technical; entitlement, in which students come to believe that, in return for their hard work, they are entitled to prestige, money, and power as well as respect for the value of their work; and finally, a non-reflective professionalism, where professionals become unaware of the gap between those values they espouse and those they enact in their practice. Coulehan and Williams went on to describe ways that learners might resolve the conflict experienced. The first is a conflating of values, in which individuals come to believe that the detachment and objectivity, which protects them, is actually best for their patients; deflating values, in which they may become cynical and lower their expectations of themselves and of others; and a positive one in which some people seem to have a natural immunity to these responses and hold on to their values. The latter response has been associated with being female, being older or more mature, and holding traditional religious or spiritual values.

Adult learning, self-directed learning, and lifelong learning

Perhaps the most strongly espoused perspectives on professional development and practice at the present time are (1) adult learning principles; (2) SDL; and (3) lifelong learning. In contrast to most perspectives discussed so far, these are 'principles' in that they are couched more in terms of how learning and teaching should be than how they actually are. So, adult learning principles, SDL, and lifelong learning are prescriptive rather than descriptive. We now examine how they relate to the perspectives discussed earlier.

Adult learning principles

At every level of the medical education continuum, the term "adult learners" is used to justify the design of educational experiences, expectations of learners, and the way learners are expected to approach their

education. In fact, the term is so embedded in our conversation that our tacit understandings of what we mean by it are rarely shared or examined.

Adult learning principles were first discussed in the educational literature by Knowles (1984), who elucidated them as a means of explaining why *andragogy*, or the science of teaching adults, was different from *pedagogy*, or teaching children. Knowles outlined the following principles to describe adult learners, which he saw as fundamental to programme design.

- Adults move from dependence to self-direction in their learning.
- Adult learners bring to any learning experience significant prior experience, which serves as a rich resource for their new learning.
- They are motivated by internal rather than external factors.
- They value learning which is relevant to the problems and questions that they must address in their everyday lives.
- Adult learners have a greater focus on problem-centred than on subject-centred learning.

Other writers have studied adult learners and described similar principles (Merriam, 2001), which have guided the design of curricula in many fields, including the education of health professionals other than doctors. The principles imply that adults come to learning experiences with a rich array of experiences and learning skills and can use those experiences to help them navigate new situations. Despite their widespread and continued incorporation into medical education curricula, adult learning principles have not proved as useful in explaining and predicting behaviour as was hoped. They apply, moreover, to teaching and learning in childhood as well as adulthood: an observation that Knowles ultimately acknowledged. The validity of individual tenets of this approach has been questioned both theoretically and empirically. Critics have noted that the model assumes education to be value-neutral and all learners to look the same. Although the relevance of learning related to individuals' daily lives and roles is included in the model, the relationships between individuals and the societal context of their learning is ignored. Lastly, critics have asserted that the model reproduces society's inequities. In the medical education literature, Norman (1999) described the adult learner as a "mythical species" and the assumptions as largely untested. Norman suggested the assumptions may be more a product of the environment in which adults find themselves than any fundamental difference in how adults and children learn. Relatively little empirical work has been conducted on the model and its assumptions, which therefore remain to be directly validated.

Criticisms notwithstanding, the principles of adult learning can be useful when planning learning, particularly because they focus on strengthening learners' agency in teacher–learner relationships. They align with a cognitive perspective, which sees learners' prior experiences as giving meaning to new information, and emphasises that prior learning becomes a powerful resource for new learning when it is activated. The adults who constitute, for example, a PBL group will collectively have accumulated very significant prior experience, both in the domain they are learning about and their learning skills. Relevance to authentic problems is another commonality between adult learning principles and a cognitive perspective. Practitioners participating in a continuing education programme, for example, will have an understanding of the problems of practice that helps them see some experiences as more relevant than others. Regarding learners as intrinsically motivated is also important, though learners respond to a mixture of intrinsic and extrinsic influences (Misch, 2002). Bandura describes extrinsic motivation as most powerful early in learning; intrinsic motivation increases once learners reach a level of knowledge and that makes an activity rewarding in its own right (Bandura, 1986).

In addition to the cognitive perspective, adult learning principles are grounded in the humanist perspective in that adults are seen as actively seeking out experiences that contribute to and reflect their ongoing development. Adult learning principles are underpinned by constructivism, in that they see experience as both a resource for and stimulus for learning, and imply that an adult's work is to understand the important meanings of their society.

Self-directed learning

Becoming a self-directed learner is widely regarded as fundamental to self-regulation, in turn a *sine qua non* of professional practice. So, SDL forms the basis for some widespread approaches to designing medical education. PBL as a teaching–learning method explicitly incorporates the goals of self-direction in encouraging learners to determine both 'what' and 'how' to learn. Those who classify SDL as a theoretical orientation (Merriam et al, 2007)

classify it as one of the humanist group; so it is a perspective that views learning as a process of human growth and development. Learning, therefore, is progression toward a fully developed 'self-actualised' self (Maslow, 1970). Transformational learning is central to SDL, requiring a capacity for critical reflection and knowing oneself as a prerequisite for autonomy (Mezirow, 1991).

Published literature has viewed SDL from two quite distinct points of view. The first sees self-directedness as a personal attribute, an attitudinal disposition that is reflected in observable behaviours. We describe as self-directed those individuals who recognise learning needs or interests, pursue them, access the requisite resources, and evaluate their progress. Those individuals strive for personal growth and autonomy. From that viewpoint, many different traits contribute to self-directedness. The second view is of self-direction as a set of skills that can be developed through experience and practice. These skills include the ability to identify one's learning needs, set goals for learning, undertake learning, and evaluate the outcomes. Notwithstanding the motivation to be self-directed, the skills are separate, not necessarily inherent, and needing to be learned and practiced. The two viewpoints imply somewhat different educational approaches, and have stimulated different research questions. The two approaches have been brought together in a model of 'self-direction in learning', according to which self-direction comprises both instructional processes and learner attributes, and is undergirded by personal responsibility for learning (Brockett and Hiemstra, 1991).

As a guiding principle for curriculum design and a perspective in its own right, SDL has not had an easy path. Many learning approaches of the past have employed a transmission approach to learning, which relies on two main means of teaching: the first is a formal, didactic approach, where the content of the discipline is transmitted to upcoming generations, and the second is an apprenticeship approach, where the learner is placed in an authentic clinical setting, to work with an experienced practitioner or 'master' and where learning has both formal and large informal components. Opportunities to be self-directed are limited by the sheer volume of knowledge and skill that are required, which drives learners and focuses their attention on what they must master. In addition to these constraints, we have also learnt that self-direction and the demonstration of requisite skills do not generalise consistently across fields. One may be very self-directed in a field where one has experience, yet require considerable guidance and support when encountering new learning challenges. This has been attributed both to misunderstanding what is actually meant by self-direction and to a lack of clarity about the processes and goals of teaching and learning, a difficulty described extremely well by Miflin et al (1999) in relation to pre-licensure medical students entering a PBL self-directed curriculum.

Measuring self-direction has proved difficult; however, two widely used scales with known psychometric properties have been developed: The Self-Directed Learning Readiness Scale (SDLRS) (Guglielmino, 1997) and the Oddi Continuing Learning Inventory (OCLI) (Oddi et al, 1990). The 54-item SDLRS was developed to assess the degree to which people perceived themselves as possessing skills and attitudes conventionally associated with SDL. The scale has several factors: self-concept as an effective learner; initiative and independence in learning; acceptance of responsibility for learning; love of learning; creativity; future orientation; and ability to use basic study and problem-solving skills. The OCLI is a 26-item scale, developed to identify clusters of personality characteristics that relate to initiative and persistence in learning over time. The four main clusters include self-confidence; the ability to work independently and through involvement with others; avid reading; and the ability to be self-regulating. It is of note that both scales include both predispositions to self-direction and the skills to put it into practice. Also, in measuring individuals' ability to be self-directing, these approaches tend to ignore the impact of social environments on self-directedness. As Norman suggested with respect to adult learning principles, a person's self-directedness may be a product of the environment in which people find themselves rather than any fundamental difference between individuals. Research in this area has been complicated by the co-existence of different perspectives and challenges in reaching common operational definitions. Yet self-direction remains a deeply valued goal and tenet of the profession and a critically important attribute to identify educational needs and keep up to date over a lifetime of practice.

Viewing SDL as a set of skills that must be learnt has several implications for learning: As with other skills, those that constitute effective SDL can be improved through repeated practice with feedback; the feedback must target not only content but also the SDL process the learner has employed; learners will exhibit less self-direction and need more direction and support when they engage in new educational experiences. It is also important to remember that SDL does not mean behaving completely independently; an important part of self-direction may be choosing a mix of learning methods including formal didactic sessions. In 1989, a landmark study in continuing education was published, entitled 'Change and Learning in the Lives of Physicians' (Fox et al, 1989). The 'Change Study' as it came to be known involved interviews with 336 physicians, who identified more than 770 changes they had made in their professional practice over the previous year. These changes and in-depth analysis of them generated a model of learning and change that has stimulated much subsequent research. At the core of the model is the physician's self-direction, a trigger that identifies the learning needs and the processes the individual uses to specify the need. The model also identified the processes of undertaking new learning and incorporating it into practice. SDL, however, is much more than a set of behaviours. To be effective, self-directed learners must have a well-developed reflective capacity and ability to assess or monitor themselves (Eva and Regehr, 2007).

Lifelong learning

Entering a profession where knowledge and skills expand and change at lightning speed impels a commitment to learning across one's entire professional lifetime. Not so many years ago, the belief was still held that medical education could impart to graduating physicians all there was to know about medicine, a store of knowledge and skills that would last them from their launch into professional practice until their retirement, at which time their fund of knowledge might also be no longer very useful. Who could have foreseen the gains that have revolutionised medicine and science and therefore required huge ongoing learning and change on the part of physicians?

Many examples of lifelong learning exist both inside and outside medical education. A particular example of lifelong, self-directed medical learning may be found in the Canadian Practice-Based Small Group Learning (PBSGL) programme (Premi et al, 1994), which began under the leadership of John Premi. PBSGL was first developed to mirror PBL but adapted to consider authentic practice situations rather than hypothetical scenarios. Members of a PBSGL group meet regularly, often for well over a decade, to work on cases and learning resources relating to a problem-oriented curriculum developed by The Foundation for Medical Practice. Each group selects modules that its members believe best meet their learning needs and learn around both those cases and patients under their individual care, sharing information and understanding through discussion. This group learning, which has been shown to improve patient outcomes (Herbert et al, 2004), is an exemplar of how a community of practice can incorporate both self-directed and lifelong learning.

While self-direction and lifelong learning are separate constructs, they often come together in such activities as noted above (Candy, 1991). Lifelong learning is a broader concept, of which self-direction is an important part. Longworth and Davies (1996) have defined it as follows: the development of human potential through a continuously supportive process which stimulates and empowers individuals to acquire the knowledge, values, and skills and understanding they will require throughout their lifetimes and apply them with confidence, creativity, and enjoyment in all roles, circumstances, and environments (p. 22). These authors have also described the skills required for lifelong learning; these skills, while not outlined with medicine in mind, describe well the skills required by practicing professionals (Box 2.2).

Researchers have reported the psychometric properties of a scale to measure lifelong learning (Hojat et al, 2009), which they define as: "A set of self initiated activities and information-seeking

skills with sustained motivation to learn and the ability to recognise one's own learning needs" (p. 1066). In a recent study to validate this Jefferson Scale of Physician Lifelong Learning, the authors found empirical support for lifelong learning as a multi-factorial trait. Three factors were identified in practicing physicians' and academic clinicians' responses: learning beliefs and motivation; attention to learning opportunities; and technical skills in seeking information. These three factors are conceptually congruent with those described by others. The scale itself was highly reliable and correlated positively with indicators of learning motivation. Ratings correlated positively with medical school rank and indicators of professional achievement.

Social perspectives

One of the strongest recent forces in learning theory has been the rise of social perspectives on learning. These include SCT and socio-cultural theory, including two 'neo-Vygotskian' socio-cultural perspectives: Activity theory and Communities of Practice theory.

Social cognitive theory

SCT, as described by Bandura (1986), was based on his earlier social learning theory. It unites two important theoretical perspectives: one that can be traced back to behaviourism and that emphasises the influence of the external environment on our learning and change; and cognitivism, which focuses on the processes of information gathering, processing, cognition and memory, and how they guide learning and function. Bandura labelled the theory as social, acknowledging the social origins of thought and action; the cognitive element acknowledges that thought processes mediate motivation, affect, and action.

SCT describes human behaviour and function as resulting from a dynamic, triadic, reciprocal *determinism*, a continuous relationship between and among the individual, the individual's actions, and the environment. Individuals bring their background, beliefs, skills, knowledge, and personal attributes to every interaction with the environment, and their behaviour is affected by factors in the environment, which influence and interact with their individual goals. The individual also acts on the environment, and thus both affects the environment and receives feedback from it. According to Bandura (1986, 2001)

Box 2.2

Lifelong learning skills

- Learning to learn
- Putting new knowledge into practice
- Questioning and reasoning
- Managing oneself and others
- Managing information
- Communication skills
- Team working
- Problem-solving skills
- Adaptability and flexibility
- Understanding the responsibility to update and upgrade one's own competence

Adapted from Longworth and Davies (1996)

individuals have basic capabilities, which have implications for both teaching and learning. These include

- *Symbolising capability:* Humans have a remarkable ability to use symbols to transform their experience so that it can be stored and used as a guide to future actions. This enables them to draw on stored experience when they encounter new situations in the future.
- *Capability to form intentions:* Individuals are proactive in shaping the outcomes of events and in creating their environment. Their behaviour is partly the results of intentions; cognitive representations of future courses of action to be performed. According to Bandura, intentions are "not simply an expectation or prediction of future actions but a proactive commitment to bringing them about" (Bandura, 2001).
- *Forethought capability:* Whereas intentions represent an individual's future actions, forethoughts are cognitive representations of anticipated outcomes. Based on the anticipated consequences of their actions, individuals "select and create courses of action likely to produce desired outcomes and avoid detrimental ones" (Bandura, 2001). Through the exercise of forethought, people motivate themselves and guide their actions in anticipation of future events.
- *Vicarious capability:* It is this capability that allows individuals to learn from observing the actions of others and the consequences of others' behaviour. If learning occurred only through personal experience, it would be an inefficient and lengthy process. Observational or vicarious learning is a very powerful means of learning behaviours through the process of modelling; often these are social behaviours such as interacting with others, for example with patients. Even if learning can occur in many other ways, vicarious learning can shorten the process and enhance it. Vicarious learning is not limited just to behaviours; others can observe and learn from our thinking, as well as the attitudes and values we convey.
- *Self-regulatory capability:* In SCT, a self-regulatory function is central to individual development. Much individual action is regulated by the internal standards people hold and by their evaluative reactions to their actions.
- *Self-reflective capability:* Bandura explains this capability as an ability to analyse experiences and

think about thought processes. This ability, which cognitive theorists call meta-cognition, allows people to understand themselves, their behaviour, and its context.

These six basic capabilities are profoundly important in guiding teaching and learning. They validate and align with the powerful assumptions that professionals have an ability to remain competent; learn from experience; and understand the context of their work, and the limits of their knowledge and skills. The ability to set goals for themselves and plan, implement, and evaluate progress towards those goals provides a basis for self-directed lifelong learning.

A central concept in SCT is self-efficacy. Perceived self-efficacy is people's belief in their abilities to arrive at certain attainments (Bandura, 1997). Self-efficacy is not a global trait; it is linked to distinct areas of function. For example, a surgeon might have a high sense of efficacy in relation to surgical abilities, but a low sense of efficacy with regard to sports ability. Efficacy beliefs have been shown to impact not only on behaviour but also on goals and aspirations, and the opportunities and barriers individuals see in their environments (Bandura, 2001). They influence (a) The courses and actions people choose to pursue; (b) the challenges and goals they see for themselves and their levels of commitment to them; (c) how much effort they put forth; (d) how long they persevere in the face of barriers; (e) their resilience to adversity; (f) the quality of their emotional life, particularly in response to challenging environment; (g) the life choices they make; and (h) what they can achieve.

Perceived self-efficacy arises from four major sources. They are (a) interactive mastery experiences that give strong indicators of capability; (b) vicarious experiences that are gained from observing others and making comparisons with oneself; (c) verbal persuasion and other social influences on how individuals see themselves; and (d) physiological and affective states that provide feedback on how vulnerable or capable individuals are. For these sources of information to affect efficacy perceptions, they must be integrated, interpreted, and influenced by many personal, social, and situational factors. Generally, the most powerful efficacy information comes from interactive experiences; the other sources of information tend to exert influence in descending order. With respect to vicarious learning, role-modelling is a powerful influence on efficacy beliefs.

Feedback is also central to Bandura's understanding of learning. According to Bandura, the provision of feedback both speeds up learning and increases accuracy. It also increases the level of goal that individuals set for themselves and their level of goal achievement. The provision of feedback has been a much discussed element of medical education's teaching and learning repertoire for a very long time. Originally it was understood through the behaviourist lens and was understood to affect behaviour through the rewards, reinforcements, or punishments, which followed learners' responses. Learners were understood to respond by improving or increasing certain behaviours and decreasing or stopping others. The same techniques were involved in shaping behaviour.

Not only does feedback as described by Bandura have a behaviourist element, but it is also mediated cognitively by learners who receive it under the influence of their prior experience, goals, attitudes, values, and perceptions. It is also affected by learners' contexts and interactions with those contexts. A recent definition follows: "Feedback is conceptualised as information provided by an agent (e.g. teacher, parent, book, parent, self, experience) regarding aspects of one's performance" (Hattie and Timperley, 2007). As noted, SCT views individuals as able to set goals and monitor their progress toward those goals. Key to being able to judge progress is receiving feedback about performance on a particular task – feedback that can help an individual reduce the gap between their current level of performance and their desired goal. Learners can benefit from feedback not only on their performance of a task but also on the processes they used in executing the task and they can develop improved strategies for self-monitoring and for error detection and error correction. Feedback is also integrally related to development of self-efficacy, which in turn improves learners' ability to seek out feedback and improve performance further. Clear goals and expectations are essential to guide learners in achieving desired levels of performance and achieving their own goals. Maximally effective feedback is related to the goals; in fact feedback that is unrelated to goals can readily be dismissed (Hattie and Timperly, 2007).

Socio-cultural theory

Socio-cultural theory had its origins in the first half of the twentieth century in the work of the Russian scholar Vygotsky, though it was considerably later that his work was translated into English and became more widely known (Wells, 1999). There are other terms to describe this theoretical orientation, which emphasise its historical dimension as well as its social and cultural ones. Wertsch (1991) characterised socio-cultural theory as concerning the diversity of different people's processes of learning and development, in contrast to the preoccupation of other theories of learning with 'universalism'. So, subject matter and educational processes are not uniform but as diverse as the people who learn. Social relationships and culturally constructed artefacts – including language and tools – mediate learning and there is a two-way relationship between culture and individual learning. People learn meanings through activities that take place within individual, social, and institutional relationships. People's understandings, their actions, and the artefacts they use are both shaped by, and shape, the contexts and cultures in which they learn (Lantolf and Thorne, 2006). Learning, from a socio-cultural perspective, is transactional. So, socio-cultural theory makes it possible to consider the development and functioning of the mind without divorcing it from its social context. Vygotsky's claim that higher mental functioning is rooted in social life is rooted in Marxist theory – so, both the origins of socio-cultural theory and the long delay in it impacting on western thinking can be attributed to Russian communism (Wertsch, 1991).

Wertsch (1991) distinguished a socio-cultural perspective, which puts learners' actions at the heart of learning, from a positivist/behaviourist system of beliefs, which treats individuals as passive recipients of information provided by their learning environments. In contrast to the latter perspective, socio-cultural theory treats knowledge as dependent on the knower and the cultural conditions under which it is developed and used. It is also to be distinguished from cognitive learning perspectives, linked to the metaphor of 'the mind as computer', which focus on the individual and treat the environment as a relatively inert source of material for the mind to work on. Socio-cultural theory differs from SCT (both, confusingly, can be abbreviated to SCT) in the extent to which it locates learning outside the individual mind in language usage, interpersonal interactions, institutions, cultures, and the legacy of history. Socio-cultural theory can be best understood by considering: mind, knowledge and meaning; mediation of learning; action; context; culture; and the dynamics of learning.

Mind, knowledge, and learning

From a socio-cultural perspective, the development and higher mental functioning of individuals is inseparable from the social milieu in which they take place and the activities that take place there. Relationships and culturally constructed artefacts (including language) play a central role in organising learning. Knowledge is not something fixed or autonomous, and it is not contained wholly within the minds of individual people; it is 'emergently constructed and reconstructed between participants in specific situated activities using the cultural activities at their disposal as they work towards the collaborative achievement of a goal' (Wells, 1999).

Mediation of learning

Vygotsky proposed that sign systems (notably language) and material artefacts (including works of art, legal codes, models, and theories that are created with the use of the primary artefacts) 'mediate' learning. Language and those artefacts both constitute, and are constituted by, culture.

Action

The actions of learners and other people in their social milieu, which are mediated by language and the artefacts mentioned above as well as culturally determined practices, have a central place in socio-cultural theory. Action can be conceived of as goal-directed, joint activity – which fits closely the participation metaphor introduced earlier (Sfard, 1998). Action is both moderated by, and moderates, the cultural, institutional, and historical context in which it is situated.

Context

Learning, from a socio-cultural perspective, is inseparably linked to the specific context in which it takes place. This attribute, called the 'situatedness' of learning, predicts that the way tasks are performed in any context determines what is learnt there.

Culture

This has been described as 'an objective force that infuses social relationships and the historically developed use of artefacts' (Lantolf and Thorne, 2006). Within a culture, values that are displayed in social practice are rooted in the history of that culture, and language usage is the most tangible characteristic of any particular culture.

The dynamics of learning

The preceding paragraphs illustrate the dynamic, interactional nature of learning according to socio-cultural theory. Each component of the theory is dynamically linked to each of the other components in a way that has been described as interdependent and mutually constitutive. Wells goes on to write of the 'triple transformation'; of the object or situation towards which an activity is directed; of the ability to participate and thus of the knowledgeable skills of those involved; and of the cultural artefacts and practices that are drawn upon to mediate the activity (Wells, 1999). For the learner, mastering ways of speaking, thinking, and acting in a particular practice are fundamental to cognitive development. Medical schools, postgraduate medical education institutions, and individual workplaces can be seen as places where interactions among people and between people and cultural artefacts must be systematically structured to promote learning.

Neo-Vygotskian perspectives

An individual in dynamic interaction with their social milieu is clearly seen in two socio-cultural perspectives that are influential in twenty-first century education theory. The first is cultural historical activity theory; the second is communities of practice theory.

Activity theory

Vygotsky's collaborator Leontiev developed socio-cultural theory's central focus on human action into activity theory. Now, activity theory is most closely associated with the name of Yrjö Engeström, a contemporary Finnish scholar, who expounds 'third generation' activity theory. This broadens and deepens the scope of previous writing to consider more complex activity systems and highly subjective issues such as emotion, embodiment, identity, and moral commitment (Engeström, 2009).

Activity theory locates the agency and learning of individuals or groups of individuals within social systems, operating within social contexts. Activity systems are collective and social in nature. Figure 2.2 shows the conventional representation of such a system and this description follows the account of Tsui et al (2009). Actions within activity systems are directed towards some specific object or goal. Those actions are performed by one or more subjects and mediated by cultural tools, language, behaviours,

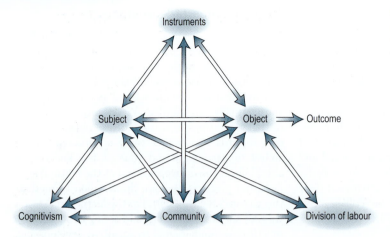

Figure 2.2 • Components of an activity system (from Tsui et al, 2009 with permission).

and physical artefacts. Activity systems are embedded within communities, whose rules and division of labour influence their outcomes. From a learning perspective, the human mind develops as a result of interactions between individual people and cultural tools. Activity is transformational because it mediates between individuals and their social worlds. Collective and individual learning are bound together by activity. 'Expansive learning', an important concept in activity theory, results from interactions and 'contradictions' between activity systems. According to this perspective, learning is open-ended, transformative, and innovative. Activity theory's strength is the way it locates individual agency within whole social systems, with a reciprocal dynamic between individual people and the systems of which they are part.

Communities of practice (situated learning) theory

If *similarities* between the various strands of socio-cultural theory reside in their common perspectives on mind, mediation, action, context, culture, and the dynamics of learning (p. 33), *differences* between them reside in their different 'units of analysis', which can range from individual peoples' utterances – as in discourse analysis – to the functioning of whole social communities. Much early socio-cultural scholarship, such as Vygotsky's interest in how social interaction could draw a learner into their 'zone of proximal development', took interactions at the level of teacher and pupil as the unit of analysis. More recent work has been at a more communal level, examining the relationship between cultural institutions, social practices, language, interpersonal relationships, and individual development (Tsui et al,

2009). The previous section described how Engeström's unit of analysis is activity systems, as characterised in Figure 2.2. Lave and Wenger's unit of analysis is the interaction between individual learners and 'communities of practice' in whose activities they participate. Their work was published in two books (Lave and Wenger, 1991; Wenger, 1998) and is concisely summarised by Tsui et al (2009). It has been enthusiastically adopted by the medical education community worldwide because it so well applies to medical work-based learning in ways we now describe. In his foreword to their first book, Hanks (p. 13) described how Lave and Wenger's writing excited him 'because it located learning squarely in the processes of co-participation, not in the heads of individuals'. According to them, 'Learning is distributed among co-participants not a one-person act'. Lave and Wenger originally set out to reconceptualise apprenticeship, an age-old tradition that is still strongly represented in the discourse of medical education. Their work moved the notion of apprenticeship from a dyadic relationship between teacher and learner centred on the performance of tasks, to a social relationship between learners and communities of practice, centred on the co-construction of meaning and identity. In Hanks' words (p. 15), 'while the apprentice may be the one transformed most dramatically by increased participation in a productive process, it is the wider process that is the crucial locus and precondition for this transformation'. Learning, from this new perspective, became 'a way of being in the social world, not a way of coming to know about it' (p. 24).

Chapter 11 revisits communities of practice theory in relation to acquiring team working skills and learning skills in the context of functioning clinical teams, while Chapter 12 views workplace learning from a communities of practice perspective, particularly in relationship to the growth of medical learners from novices to established physicians, and then to 'old-timers'. This description sets out to familiarise readers with some of the terminology and concepts of this perspective. The suffix to the title of Lave and Wenger's 1991 book was 'legitimate peripheral participation', a phrase that encapsulates important elements of their perspective. Learning is through participation in the activities of authentic workgroups, or communities of practice. For participation to be possible, the learner must be legitimate in the eyes of the community. Novices – such as medical students – enter such a community at its periphery because they are not yet equipped to be full participants. Through participation, for example as a senior medical student or foundation trainee, they move centripetally to become full members of the community. There is a reciprocal dynamic between their development and the development of the community such that, at the end of the lifelong learning continuum, 'old-timers' may be transformed by more junior participants or may come into conflict with them. Lave and Wenger see no distinction between work and learning – according to them, 'learning is an integral and inseparable aspect of social practice'. Through participation, members of a community of practice construct meaning and develop identity. The place of language in learning, meaning, and identity is nicely captured by their notion that learners learn both from talk and to talk. Importantly, Lave and Wenger decouple learning and instruction, because learning can take place without instruction, even when activities are conducted with no educational intent. So, learning is an inevitable part of everyday life.

For present purposes, the term 'community' can be taken more or less at face value but the term 'practice' is characterised by Wenger (1998) as having several important components: 'mutual engagement' between members of the community; relationships of mutual accountability; and 'shared repertoires' of routines, words, tools, ways of doing things, stories, gestures, symbols, genres, actions, and concepts. A communities of practice perspective places great weight on identity, which is neither individual nor abstractly social. Identity exists in the mutual engagement of person and community. Identity 'exists in the constant work of negotiating the self'. Medical learners, from this perspective, are in a constant process of defining and redefining their identities throughout the lifelong learning continuum.

Summary and conclusions

We have presented a range of perspectives on learning, selected because they are relevant to medical educators in their educational practice and scholarship, and researchers in their explorations of the field. We have framed them along two dimensions: the extent to which they are abstract or applied and the extent to which they emphasise learning as an individual or a collaborative process. We recognise that such distinctions cannot be absolute, as many perspectives encompass aspects of both ends of these dimensions; however, we hope this 'mapping' will help readers conceptualise them in ways that can support their practice. We have also introduced the idea of metaphors for learning, to highlight how they influence discourse and practice. We agree with others that the two metaphors of *acquisition* and *participation* are both necessary to develop maximally effective learning. In addition to presenting more abstract theoretical perspectives such as SCT and socio-cultural theory, we have presented more applied perspectives, such as adult learning, SDL, and lifelong learning. We have included them because we regard it as important to understand the origins and assumptions of perspectives that, whilst questionable in terms of their theoretical 'purity', are pervasive in the contemporary discourse of learning and teaching. Above all, our goal has been to provide perspectives that can guide practice and research and encourage educators to examine their own perspectives on teaching and learning.

Implications for practice

Kurt Lewin famously said 'there is nothing as practical as a good theory'. Educators wishing to do more than unquestioningly replicate previous practice will find that keeping the following questions at the forefront of their minds will lead to better practice:

Which theoretical perspectives guide my practice?

Does my practice actually reflect the perspectives I espouse?

How can I use these perspectives to:

- plan activities that support the attainment of the goals I want my learners to achieve
- align objectives, teaching and learning activities, and assessment
- frame hypotheses that lead to worthwhile research questions
- Interpret the results of research.

Adopting a constructivist view of learning makes it logical to place the learner at the centre of teaching and learning activity and see the teacher's role as facilitating learning. Shifting the emphasis from individual learning towards social and collaborative learning makes it logical to consider clinical learning environments as communities of practice where learners develop their professional identities through both explicit and implicit processes. A socio-cultural perspective leads teachers to encourage both individual and collective learning; take advantage of cultural tools and other mediators available; use other learners, both peers and more senior learners, to facilitate learning; and consider learning and teaching as a joint enterprise, for which teachers and learners together assume responsibility.

References

Aukes LC, Geertsma J, Cohen-Schotanus J, et al: The development of a scale to measure personal reflection in medical practice and education, *Med Teach* 29:177–182, 2007.

Ausubel D: *The psychology of meaningful verbal learning*, New York, 1963, Grune & Stratton.

Bandura A: *Self-efficacy: the exercise of control*, New York, NY, 1997, Freeman.

Bandura A: *Social foundations of thought and action. A Social Cognitive Theory*, Englewood Cliffs, NJ, 1986, Prentice Hall.

Bandura A: Social Cognitive Theory: an agentic perspective, *Ann Rev Psychol* 52:1–26, 2001.

Bleakley A: Broadening conceptions of learning in medical education: the message from teamworking, *Med Educ* 40:150–157, 2006.

Boud D, Walker D: Promoting reflection in professional courses: the challenge of context. In Harrison R, Reeve F, Hanson A, Clarke J, editors: *Supporting lifelong learning* (vol 1), London, UK, 2002, Routledge Farmer, pp 91–110.

Boud D, Keogh R, Walker D, editors: *Reflection:turning experience into learning*, London, 1985, Kogan Page.

Brockett PG, Hiemstra R: *Self-direction in adult learning: perspectives on theory, research and practice*, New York, NY, 1991, Routledge.

Candy P: *Self-direction for lifelong learning*, San Francisco, CA, 1991, Jossey Bass.

Cheetham G, Chivers G: *Professions, competence and informal learning*, Cheltenham, UK, 2005, Edward Elgar.

Chung PJ, Chung J, Shah MN, et al: How do residents learn? The development of practice styles in a residency program, *Ambul Pediat* 3:166–172, 2003.

Coffield F, Mosely D, Hall E, et al: *Learning styles and pedagogy in post-16 learning: a systematic and critical review*, London, 2004, Learning and Skills Research Centre.

Coulehan J: Today's professionalism: engaging the mind but not the heart, *Acad Med* 80:892–898, 2005.

Coulehan J, Williams PC: Vanquishing virtue: the Impact of Medical Education, *Acad Med* 76:598–605, 2001.

Curry L: Cognitive and learning styles in medical education, *Acad Med* 74:409–413, 1999.

Dewey J: *How we think*, Amherst, NY, 1991, Prometheus Books.

Engeström Y: The future of activity theory: a rough draft. In Sannino A, Daniels H, Gutierrez KD, editors: *Learning and expanding with activity theory*, Cambridge, 2009, Cambridge University Press.

Epstein RM, Hundert EM: Defining and assessing professional competence, *JAMA* 287:226–235, 2002.

Eraut M: Non-formal learning and tacit knowledge in professional work, *Brit J Educ Psychol* 70:113–136, 2000.

Eva K, Lingard L: What's next? A guiding question for educators engaged in educational research, *Med Educ* 42 (8):752–754, 2008.

Eva KN, Regehr G: Knowing when to look it up: a new concept of self assessment ability, *Acad Med* 82:581–584, 2007.

Fox RD, Mazmanian PE, Putnam RW, editors: *Change and learning in the lives of physicians*, New York, 1989, Praeger.

Gagné RM: *The conditions of learning and the theory of instruction*, New York, 1985, Holt, Rinehart and Winston.

Grant A, Kinnersley P, Metcalf E, et al: Students' views of reflective learning techniques: an efficacy study at a UK medical school, *Med Educ* 40:379–388, 2006.

Greenaway R: *Critiques of David Kolb's theory of experiential learning*, [internet] Available at: http://reviewing.co.uk/research/experiential.learning.htm#styles Accessed November 23, 2009.

Guba EG, Lincoln YS: Paradigmatic controversies, contradictions, and emerging confluences. In Denzin NK, Lincoln YC, editors: *The Sage handbook of qualitative research*, ed 3, Thousand Oaks, CA, 2005, Sage, pp 191–215.

Guglielmino LM: Contributions of the self-directed learning readiness scale (SDLRS) and the learning preference assessment (LPA) to the definition and assessment of self-direction in learning. In Paper presented at the First World Conference on Self-Directed Learning, Canada, 1997, Montreal.

Hafferty F, Frank R: The hidden curriculum, ethics teaching and the structure of medical education, *Acad Med* 69:861–871, 1994.

Handal G, Lauvas P: *Promoting reflective teaching: supervision in action*, Milton Keynes, UK, 1987, The Society for Research into Higher Education and Open University Press.

Hattie J, Timperley H: The power of feedback, *Rev Educ Res* 77:81–112, 2007.

Herbert CP, Wright JM, Maclure M, et al: Better Prescribing Project: a randomized controlled trial of the impact of case-based educational modules and personal prescribing feedback on prescribing for hypertension in primary care, *Fam Pract* 21(Oct):575–581, 2004.

Hojat M, Veloski JJ, Gonnella JS: Measurement and correlates of physicians' lifelong learning, *Acad Med* 84(8):1066–1074, 2009.

Honey P, Mumford A: *Manual of learning styles*, London, UK, 1986, Peter Honey Publications.

Knowles MS, et al: *Andragogy in action: applying modern principles of adult learning*, San Francisco, 1984, Jossey-Bass.

Kolb DA: *Experiential learning: experience as the source of learning and development*, Englewood Cliffs, NJ, 1984, Prentice Hall.

Kolb DA: *Learning Style Inventory. Version 3.1*, Boston, MA, 2005, Hay Group, Hay Resources Direct.

Kolb DA, Boyatzis RE, Mainemelis C: Experiential Learning Theory: previous research and new directions. In Sternberg RJ, Zhang LF, editors: *Perspectives on thinking, learning and cognitive styles*, New Jersey, 2001, Erlbaum.

Lantolf JP, Thorne SL: *Sociocultural theory and the genesis of second language development*, Oxford, 2006, Oxford University Press.

Lave J, Wenger E: *Situated learning. Legitimate peripheral participation*, Cambridge, 1991, Cambridge University Press.

Longworth N, Davies WK: *Lifelong learning*, London, 1996, Kogan Page.

Mamede S, Schmidt H: The structure of reflective practice in medicine, *Med Educ* 38:1302–1306, 2004.

Mamede S, Schmidt H: Correlates of reflective practice in medicine, *Adv Health Sci Educ Theory Pract* 10:327–337, 2005.

Mamede S, Schmidt H, Penaforte J: Effects of reflective practice on the accuracy of medical diagnoses, *Med Educ* 42:468–475, 2008.

Mann KV, Gordon JJ, MacLeod AM: Reflection and reflective practice in health professions education a systematic review of the literature in the health professions, *Adv Health Sci Educ Theory Pract* 14:595–621, 2009, DOI 10.1007/s10459-007-9090-2.

Maslow AH: *Motivation and personality*, ed 2, New York, NY, 1970, Harper Collins.

Merriam SB: Andragogy and self-directed learning: pillars of adult learning theory. In Merriam SB, editor: *The new update on adult learning theory: New directions for adult and continuing education* (vol 89), 2001, pp 3–14.

Merriam SB, Caffarella RS, Baumgartner LM: *Learning in adulthood. A comprehensive guide*, ed 3, San Francisco, CA, 2007, Jossey-Bass.

Mezirow J: *Transformative dimensions of adult learning*, San Francisco, 1991, Jossey-Bass.

Miflin B, Campbell CB, Price DA: A lesson from the introduction of a problem-based, graduate entry course: the effects of different views of self-direction, *Med Educ* 33:801–807, 1999.

Misch DA: Andragogy and medical education: are medical students internally motivated to learn? *Adv Health Sci Educ Theory Pract* 7:153–160, 2002.

Moon J: *Reflection in learning and professional development*, London, UK, 1999, Kogan Page.

Moulton CA, Regehr G, Mylopoulos M, et al: Slowing down when you should: a new model of expert judgement, *Acad Med* 82:S109–S116, 2007.

Norman G: Teaching basic science to optimize transfer, *Med Teacher* 31:807–811, 2009a.

Norman GR: The adult learner: a mythical species, *Acad Med* 74:886–889, 1999.

Norman GR: When will learning style go out of style? *Adv Health Sci Educ Theory Pract* 14:1–4, 2009b.

Oddi LF, Ellis AJ, Robertson JEA: Construct validation of the Oddi continuing learning inventory, *Adult Ed Quar* 40(3):139–145, 1990.

Premi J, Shannon S, Hartwick K, et al: Practice-based small-group CME, *Acad Med* 69(Oct):800–802, 1994.

Prideaux D, Bligh J: Research in medical education: asking the right questions, *Med Educ* 36:1114–1115, 2002.

Robbins P, Aydede M: A short primer on situated cognition. In Robbins P, Aydede M, editors: *The Cambridge handbook of situated cognition*, New York, 2009, Cambridge University Press, pp 3–10.

Sargeant J, Mann K, Sinclair D, et al: Learning in practice: experiences and perceptions of high-scoring physicians, *Acad Med* 81:655–670, 2006.

Sargeant J, Armson H, Chesluk B, et al: *The processes and dimensions of self-assessment*, Malaga, Spain, 2009a, AMEE, Research presentation.

Sargeant J, Mann K, van der Vleuten C, et al: Reflection: a link between receiving and using assessment feedback, *Adv Health Sci Educ Theory Pract* 14(3):399–410, 2009b.

Schlesinger E: Why learning is not a cycle, *Ind Commer Training* 28:30–35, 1996.

Schön D: *Educating the reflective practitioner: toward a new design for teaching and learning in the professions*, San Francisco, CA, 1987, Jossey-Bass.

Sfard A: On two metaphors for learning and the dangers of choosing just one, *Educ Res* 27:4–13, 1998.

Simons R-J, Vander Linden J, Duffy T: *New learning*, Dordecht, NL, 2000, Kluwer.

Smith CS, Morris M, Francovich C, et al: A qualitative study of resident learning in ambulatory clinic. The importance of exposure to 'breakdown' in settings that support effective response, *Adv Health Sci Educ Theory Pract* 9:93–105, 2004a.

Sobral DT: Medical students' mindset for reflective learning: a revalidation study and the reflection in learning scale, *Adv Health Sci Educ Theory Pract* 10:303–314, 2005b.

Sobral DT: Medical students' reflection-in-learning in relation to approaches to study and academic achievement, *Med Teach* 23:508–513, 2001.

Tsui ABM, Lopez-Real F, Edwards G: Sociocultural perspectives of learning. In Tsui ABM, Edwards G, Lopez-Real F, editors: *Learning in school-university partnership. Sociocultural perspectives*, New York, 2009, Routledge.

Vygotsky LS: *Mind in society: the development of higher psychological processes*, Cambridge, MA, 1978, Cambridge University Press.

Wells G: Language and education: reconceptualising education as dialogue, *Annu Rev Appl Linguist* 19:135–155, 1999.

Wenger E: *Communities of practice: learning, meaning and identity*, Cambridge, UK, 1998, Cambridge University Press.

Wertsch JV: *Voices of the mind: a sociocultural approach to mediated action*, Cambridge, MA, 1991, Harvard University Press.

White JA, Anderson P: Learning by internal medicine residents: differences and similarities of perceptions by residents and faculty, *J Gen Intern Med* 10:126–131, 1995.

Further reading

Bandura A: Social Cognitive Theory: an agentic perspective, *Ann Rev Psych* 52:1–26, 2001.

Guba EG, Lincoln YS: Paradigmatic controversies, contradictions, and emerging influences. In Denzin NK, Lincoln YS, editors: *The Sage handbook of qualitative research*, ed 3, Thousand Oaks, CA, 2005, Sage, pp 191–215. ISBN 0-7619-2757-3.

Kaufman DM, Mann KV: *Teaching and learning in medical education: how theory can inform practice*, Edinburgh, UK, 2007, Association for the Study of Medical Education.

Lave J, Wenger E: *Situated learning. Legitimate peripheral participation*, Cambridge, 1991, Cambridge University Press.

Sfard A: On two metaphors for learning and the dangers of choosing just one, *Educational Researcher* 27:4–13, 1998.

Medical education in its societal context

3

Ayelet Kuper   Brian Hodges

CHAPTER CONTENTS

ABC

Glossary

Constructivism Constructivism is a theory of knowledge (epistemology) whose philosophical roots can be traced back to Kant and whose psychological assumptions can be traced back to Piaget. It holds that the reality humans perceive is constructed by their social, historical, and individual contexts such that there can be no absolute shared truth. In an educational context, constructivism can be seen as a process whereby learners actively construct understandings based on their perceptions, previous experiences, and knowledge of the world. They assimilate new ideas and information by linking them to existing ideas and information. That is in contrast to a view of learning as having knowledge transmitted by a teacher. Constructivism is not a specific pedagogy, but it underlies many approaches to learning today. In small groups, those include ascertaining prior knowledge, challenging misconceptions, promoting active learning, and encouraging learners to take responsibility for their learning.

ABC

Glossary (continued)

Critical theory A theoretical framework that assumes an oppressive relation between the powerful and the powerless; critical theorists try to use their explanations of oppression to eliminate current inequities of power.

Discourse analysis A methodology that analyses language to understand its role in constructing the social world. Critical discourse analysis focuses on the macro-level features of oral and written texts in their social contexts (as opposed to 'linguistic discourse analysis', which includes the micro-level analysis of grammatical features).

Normalisation A process by which ways of thinking, statements of truth, roles for individuals to play, hierarchies, processes or institutions that are socially constructed and historically contingent come to appear obvious and immutable.

Social construct An organised perception of reality that is created, shared, and modified over time by the members of a social group.

Outline

Medical education takes place in socially constructed institutions. What medical education is and the role it plays in a society are specific to the historical period and socio-cultural place in which it arises. Social science theories can be used to explore how particular modes of medical education are constructed, examine unexplored assumptions about their nature and function, and make visible implications and adverse effects of the way they have come to be.

© 2011, Elsevier Ltd.
DOI: 10.1016/B978-0-7020-3522-7.00003-6

Examining medical education through this lens makes it possible to (re)construct, consciously and proactively, what medical education is and what it does *vis-à-vis* the societies in which particular educational institutions are located. While Chapter 2 introduced a variety of perspectives on individual learners, their learning, and the contexts in which they learn, this chapter brings a wider view to bear on the interaction between those learning contexts (specifically, institutions) and the societies within which they reside. We begin by introducing how a social scientist might view medical education, revisiting the notion introduced in Chapter 2 that reality is 'constructed'. We then turn to a brief exploration of five different theoretical perspectives, showing how each might be used to frame questions in medical education practice and research. They are a Foucauldian discourse perspective, a Bourdieuvian perspective on education as symbolic capital, a neo-Marxist perspective, the perspective of a combined (feminist and anti-racist) equity agenda, and finally a postcolonial perspective. While those five approaches represent just a small subset of many schools, traditions, and perspectives in the rich domain of social sciences, they can together help a novice reader appreciate how a slight change of perspective can shift practice and research questions and data collection appreciably. Following that overview, we consider some implications of bringing social science perspectives to bear on medical education. We finish with some key sources for people wanting to pursue further study of the concepts we introduce.

Introduction

Every medical educator has an idea in his or her own mind about what medical education should be. That idea is mediated by many things – for example, the individual's positive and negative experiences of particular institutions, their knowledge of pedagogy and curriculum design, and their own academic training. It is also mediated by larger forces: membership of a particular society, as part of a particular cultural group, at a particular point in history. Those small- and large-scale influences come together to inform a unique perspective on medical education.

The educators who run medical schools, postgraduate training programmes, continuing education courses, and national medical education organisations are each individually subject to these contexts and contingencies, which lead them to construct their ideas about, and ideals for, medical education. Collectively they create the idea of medical education. They decide what it should be and what it should do; they operationalise those decisions as actions, institutions, and statements of 'truth'. This shared construction of the idea of medical education may not be explicit, but it is a necessary precondition for working together towards a common goal.

The implicit, social construction of medical education leaves many preconceptions and preconditions unspoken. In North America, for example, nobody needs to say that basic sciences are important to medical education, that doctors should have good communication skills, or that health professionals should collaborate in teams. However, since such preconceptions are the product of individuals and, even more powerfully, of their socio-historical situations, they are not 'truths', nor are they unalterable. Indeed, they may not be as self-evident on close examination as they initially seemed.

Before going any further, it is useful to explore more fully this notion of medical education as a 'construction' by addressing more broadly the definition of a 'social construct'. As we have written elsewhere, and as has been considered in Chapter 2, constructivism is a 'belief about knowledge (epistemology) that asserts that the reality we perceive is constructed by our social, historical, and individual contexts, and so there can be no absolute shared truth' (Kuper et al, 2008). Each of the resultant organised perceptions of reality is called a 'construct'; when such constructs are created, shared, and modified over time by the members of a social group, they are called 'social constructs'. Examples of social constructs include not only medical schools and other training programmes but also such deceptively obvious terms as professions (and professionals), classrooms, hospitals, and universities. Perhaps the broadest implication of the idea that knowledge, processes, and objects are social constructions is that it may be possible (though sometimes very difficult) to change them if we do not like the way they are constructed. Thus, far from being ivory tower concepts debated by armchair theorists at great remove from 'real' clinical and educational settings, social constructivist theories are very useful ways to analyse the nature of medical schools and the roles people play within them, in the service of imagining and enacting anything from a minor change to a radical reform. It may be difficult to conceive of our everyday roles, processes, and institutions as social constructions because they have become so familiar in their current form that we cannot imagine any other. Re-examining our situation from the perspective of a different historical time or a different cultural context is an effective way of rendering strange that which is familiar in order to see it anew.

Lessons from history and culture

One of the easiest ways to bring into focus the impact of the social on the construction of a practice or of an institution is to look at its history. It is helpful, then, to examine medical education in its historical context. In North America, at least, it is impossible to think about this history without considering the impact of Abraham Flexner. Today North American medical educators almost uncritically accept that the Flexnerian model of undergraduate medical education – scientifically based, with years in the classroom and years on the wards, conducted within a research-intensive university – is the only way in which medical education could be constructed. This model has become 'normalised' to such an extent that scant attention is paid to its constructed nature. But of course, like everyone else who has written about medical education before and since, Flexner was a product of his time. In his case this was early twentieth-century North America, a time and place in which faith that science would bring about unabated progress was combined with admiration for traditional European models of medical education.

Flexner's reforms have since become 'the' canonical view of medical education in North America, where Flexner is seen as the founder of 'modern medical education'. However, his reforms were necessarily rooted in the society in which he had been educated and in his personal experiences within that society. Any claim on behalf of these reforms to neutrality (by appealing, perhaps, to 'academic standards' or 'medical necessity') must therefore be suspect, by virtue of their social construction. Indeed, seen through the lens of early twenty-first-century equity politics, some of Flexner's ideas seem quite reactionary, particularly when one considers both their intended and unintended consequences. Yet, like all who came before and those who came after him, he was trying to create a system of medical education that fitted his ideal of medical education as constructed in that place and at that time (Hodges, 2005).

It might come as a surprise that the Flexner report, much lauded as an heroic accomplishment

in a maturing scientific profession, is framed by some contemporary authors as an oppressive and discriminatory turning point that led to the closure of medical schools for Blacks and women, groups who would not achieve admission to medical schools again in significant numbers until several decades later (Strong-Boag, 1981). Other authors have argued that the Flexner reforms marked the beginning of the economic conflation of medical education with corporate capitalism, a shift that has subsequently led to ethical problems like the conflicted relations between physicians and the pharmaceutical industry (Brown, 1979). The Flexnerian reforms provide a clearly delineated example of the construction of particular medical education institutions (in this case medical schools) as products of the society and historical period in which they arose.

Just as taking an historical perspective helps illustrate the constructed nature of current practices, so too does examining institutions, processes, and roles from the vantage point of other cultures. A few simple examples illustrate that what is *taken for granted*, or even framed as 'universal' about medical education, in one place is actually strange or unimaginable in another (Hodges et al, 2009). For example, Scandinavian countries have a cultural value called 'Jantelov' (loosely, the idea of not considering oneself to be too important) that renders the idea of competitive examinations inappropriate. So Scandinavian countries have very few exams. Japan, meanwhile, has a strong value of respect for elders that renders student evaluation of teachers inappropriate. Finally, Germany has traditionally held that the purpose of medical education was to develop in-depth scientific knowledge so, until very recently, there was no clinical skills teaching during the first 6 years of medical school. Contrast these observations with the *taken for granted* nature of rigorous examinations, frequent teacher evaluations, and early clinical training in North American medical schools and it quickly becomes apparent that 'global' concepts of medical education or 'universal' standards are tenuous at best.

Because we are all constrained by our point in history and culture(s), it is inevitable that the institutions, processes, and roles that appear 'normal' to us disguise constructions that would be highly visible from the perspective of another time or place. The implications are not trivial. Indeed the choices that educators are making in every country of the world today will have both positive and adverse effects on graduates and on their societies, just as Flexner's did in his day. Given the likelihood of being blind to these effects, it is important to consider ways of rendering visible the social construction of medical education and its many effects. It is in this 'rendering visible' that the power of the social sciences lies.

The usefulness of theoretical perspectives

While the long view of history helps to 'make strange' assumptions and practices of past eras, it is more difficult to recognise how odd or even absurd some of our contemporary constructions are, or even recognise the implicit assumptions we currently make about medical education. While adverse effects of current approaches to medical education may not be fully visible to those who have not had 50 years to look back on them, there are means we can use to render visible what is tacit or implicit about medical education today. A powerful means of uncovering such preconceptions and elucidating some of the implications of particular constructions is to use social science theory (Reeves et al, 2008).

Many different theories can be used for this purpose. For example, Marxist theories illuminate the way institutions serve to channel power and privilege in societies. Feminist and anti-racist theories cast light on the ways institutions create inequities on the basis of gender or race, while anti-colonial theories examine the function of institutions in extending and maintaining the power of dominant countries and cultures. Foucauldian analysis draws attention to ways in which certain kinds of institutions are made possible by specifically sanctioned ways of thinking, of being, and of speaking, while a Bourdieuvian approach illustrates the ways in which institutions are implicated in the struggle for power, prestige, and dominance in professional fields. These five perspectives are summarised in Table 3.1.

Foucault and discourse

Michel Foucault's work is important for medical education in many ways. Foucauldian discourse theory draws attention to ways in which certain kinds of institutions are made possible by specifically sanctioned ways of thinking, speaking, and being. Working in France in the late twentieth-century, Foucault wrote a history of the birth of clinical medicine (Foucault, 1963/2003) and an analysis of the ways in which schools, hospitals, and other post-Enlightenment institutions shape and control the behaviour of individuals (Foucault, 1975/1977). He also wrote histories and case studies about ethics, the body, sexuality, identity, and many other topics that are pivotal to medical education. Among the many ways in which scholars of medical education can incorporate the work of Foucault, no concept is more useful than that of 'discourse'.

Foucault's work illustrates how particular discourses 'systematically construct versions of the social world' (McHoul and Grace, 1993). Discourses are involved in the way we see and understand the world; they act like lenses or filters and are 'productive' in that we use them to create 'reality'. Certain discourses make it possible for us to say some things but not others, act in certain ways, and have certain roles in our social worlds. The research approach associated with this perspective is called 'discourse analysis' and, while there are many different approaches that share this term (Hodges et al, 2008), Foucauldian discourse analysis involves both the examination of language and of the individuals and institutions that are made possible by, and make possible, particular ways of thinking and speaking. Foucault's study of madness, for example, uncovered three distinct discourses that have constructed what madness is in different historical periods and in different places: a discourse of 'madness as spiritual possession' that was dominant in the Middle Ages in western countries; a discourse of 'madness as deviancy' that was dominant in the Victorian era; and, more recently, a discourse of 'madness as medical illness' that has been prominent since the beginning of the twentieth-century (Foucault, 1965). These different discourses create very different possibilities for people and institutions. For example, a discourse of 'madness as spiritual possession' makes visible 'possessed individuals' and creates a role for spiritual healers and religious institutions, while a discourse of 'madness as deviancy' makes visible 'deviant individuals' and creates a role for judges and jailors working in courts and prisons. By contrast, a discourse of 'madness as medical illness' makes visible 'mentally ill individuals' and creates a role for psychiatrists and psychologists who work in clinics and hospitals. This approach is echoed in a more recent study of how the very different terms 'patient', 'consumer', and 'survivor' are each made possible by particular institutions and individuals who themselves are aligned with specific discourses (Speed, 2006).

Table 3.1 Five theoretical perspectives, assumptions, and possible adverse effects

Theorist or school	Assumptions made visible	Examples of adverse effects made visible
Foucault and discourse theory	Medical schools are institutions of social control and use many mechanisms and technologies to shape the behaviours and roles of those (faculty, students, patients) engaged with them.	Both overt and 'hidden' curricula, as well as systems of examination, can embed and reinforce problematic or undesirable behaviours and ways of being. Uncritical acceptance of concepts such as 'professional self-regulation' can disguise problematic power structures or ways of being.
Bourdieu and symbolic capital theory	Medical schools are ways for individuals and social groups with social, cultural, and economic capital (e. g. power, legitimacy, money, etc.) to maximise such capital.	Admissions processes and assessment of 'professionalism' may embed markers of social and cultural capital (e.g. ways of dressing, talking, carrying oneself) that are learnt at home by certain social groups but become important in selection processes (e.g. at interview).
Neo-Marxism	Medical schools function as means for privileged individuals and social groups to maximise their economic capital and exert dominance in society.	High tuition fees in many North American jurisdictions (and elsewhere) mean that only the wealthy (or those comfortable enough with risk to go into huge debt) can afford medical school, reproducing a monopoly on the wealth produced within the profession.
Feminist/Anti-racist theories and the combined equity agenda	Medical schools continually reproduce the power differentials visible elsewhere in society (e.g. those due to gender, race, religion, sexual orientation).	The 'pink-collarisation' of specialties such as Family Medicine and devaluing of medicine as a whole is linked to feminisation of the profession. Professional norms reflect white, male, heterosexual, Christian standards of behaviour.
Post-colonial theories	Medical schools activities in lower-income countries may be forces of Europeanisation/Americanisation that devalue indigenous, traditional cultures and practices and contribute to economic and human resource destitution (e.g. neo-liberal Westernisation).	Inappropriate importing of Western professional norms into a very different professional context leads to loss of traditional cultural practices. Brain drain of physicians to Europe and North America.

Discourse analysis can also be used to study medical education. For example, professional competence, like madness, has been defined in very different ways at different times. In the 1700s, a 'competent' doctor was a member of a guild who carried a blade for blood letting and emetics for purging, with the goal of balancing the humors of the body. In 1850, by contrast, a competent doctor was a gentleman (there were almost no women doctors) with a walking stick who diagnosed patients by looking at their tongue and smelling their urine. By 1950, a competent doctor, still most likely to be a man, wore a white coat rather than a suit and had at his disposition a host of physiological investigations and pharmacological treatments. Yet in the 1950s a 'professional' doctor was expected to discuss a woman's health with her husband and

withhold the true diagnosis from a dying patient so as not to provoke worry. In the twenty-first-century, blood letting, smelling urine, and withholding the truth from dying patients are all considered incompetent behaviours (Hodges, 2007).

So what is the interest of such an approach to medical education? It might occur to the reader that most of these changes to the associated discourses of competence simply reflect the advancement of science. Certainly, the urine-sniffing doctor of the nineteenth-century did not have the benefit of modern laboratory analysis. Similarly, the bloodletting eighteenth-century physician would have been unfamiliar with twentieth-century patho-physiological explanations of fever and inflammation. These changes in practice did indeed correspond to developments in science. But what of talking to a woman's husband about her illness? This aspect of professional competence reflected a set of cultural expectations that have since shifted. Indeed, it would be quite imaginable today to hold a debate with doctors from different countries of the world as to whether talking to a woman's husband about her health is 'competent' behaviour or not, and what regional, national, cultural or other variations might underpin the answer. There are other issues with little explanation in science. For example, why did it become important to wear a white coat rather than a 3-piece suit? Or, what is the reason that women, once thought to be too 'feeble-minded' to pursue studies in science, now represent more than half of medical students? Discourse analysis, in the tradition of Foucault, allows us to see many elements that are uncritically considered to be 'normal' aspects of medical education. It challenges us to rethink not just such notions as 'appropriate communication skills', 'professional behaviours', and dress, but also things that are more overtly 'scientific' like physical examination technique, history taking, laboratory investigation, and diagnostic classification. All are made possible at some level by the specific ways in which we talk, think, and act. These, in turn, are conditioned by, and particular to, our place in the world and our period of history. When we realise that such fundamental things can be constructed so easily by time, place, and discourse, it becomes obvious that the construction of dominant ways of thinking and being can potentially be harnessed for both helpful and harmful purposes and that, given enough attention, we can change them.

Bourdieu and symbolic capital

The work of French sociologist Pierre Bourdieu focuses on struggles for power, prestige, and dominance in various 'fields'. Within Bourdieu's theory, a 'field' refers to two things simultaneously: an arena for the production, circulation, and acquisition of goods, services, knowledge, or status that are centred on a particular issue (e.g. art, science, opera, medicine); and also the configuration of historical relations of power between the positions held by individuals, groups, or institutions who interact within this field (Bourdieu and Wacquant, 1992). Each field is characterised by a particular 'game', the focus of which is the legitimate definition of what is 'good' within that field as well as the measures used

within that field for the assessment of 'quality'. "In each field the competition for predominance of one definition over competing definitions as the recognised model of excellence in the field results in a struggle between players as each tries to promote a definition that places value on their own products and their own ways of doing things. The ultimate currency in this struggle is the acquisition of prestige, the power to influence activities within the field itself." (Albert et al, 2007)

There are many forms in which power can be active within a field. To account for this, Bourdieu developed the concept of 'species of capital', whereby capital can be thought of as being, for example, cultural, economic, social, or symbolic (Bourdieu, 1986). The concept of 'symbolic capital' is often the most difficult to understand. It refers to those aspects of being (whether belongings, degrees, job titles, or family linkages) that endow someone with elevated status and give them a certain amount of power within a given field. Studying any field therefore requires analysis of elements that are valued within that field (Bourdieu, 1980). Thus, the focus of competition between 'players' in a field is the accumulation of specific symbolic capital; the amount of such capital amassed by each player determines his or her power to influence the field. This approach to understanding the game being played in individual fields has been used successfully in a number of medical education-related domains such as the field of medical education research (Albert, 2004) and the field of university academia (Bourdieu, 1988). It has also been used within medical education (along with a related Bourdieuvian concept, the 'habitus') to study the socialisation of individual medical students as they become physicians (Luke, 2003; Brosnan, 2009).

The field of medical education can therefore, according to Bourdieu, be conceptualised as a field in which players struggle for various forms of capital (e.g. power, legitimacy, money) in order to maximise such capital for themselves. Players compete to establish the legitimate definition of the 'good' doctor, painting it in their own disparate images. They naturally include in their definitions things that support and reproduce the legitimacy of their own social and cultural capital, such as legitimising certain ways of dressing and speaking as more 'professional' than others. For Bourdieu, medical education is (and will always be) a struggle both to attain the capital associated with being a physician (including a conservative reproduction of current norms) and to control the legitimate definition of 'physician-ness'. An understanding of the nature of this struggle may help medical educators shift this definition in a more acceptable, and more equitable, direction in the future.

Marxist theory

In the late nineteenth-century, Marx and Engels (1844/1970) argued that a sector of society was not profiting from economic expansion of the industrial revolution and drew attention to the negative effects of separating labour from capital. Marxist analysis focuses on the oppression of the working classes by the middle and upper classes and the unequal division of capital in society. In medical education, 'neo-Marxists' have explored the ways in which the medical profession and its institutions are implicated. For example, in *Rockefeller Medical Men*, Brown (1979) documented the rise of the medical profession 'from ignominy and frustrated ambition to prestige, power and considerable wealth' by harnessing the momentum of capitalist society. In a radically different version of a familiar story, Brown recounted how Abraham Flexner, whose career was made possible by funds derived from the powerful petroleum and steel industries (Rockefeller and Carnegie Foundations) wrote a report on medical education (Flexner, 1910) that ultimately resulted in the closure of all but the elite medical schools in the United States and Canada.

Other neo-Marxists such as Johnson (1972), Larson (1977), and Larkin (1983) further explored the links between professional power and the capitalist system, analysed medicine's occupational dominance, and explored ways in which diagnostic categories could be modified in the service of economic goals. Larson argued that medical education, specifically, is a process that channels privilege and capital to a very select group of students:

> I see professionalization as the process by which producers of special services [seek] to constitute and control a market for their expertise. Because marketable expertise is a crucial element in the structure of modern inequality, professionalization appears also as a collective assertion of special status and as a collective process of upward social mobility (Larson, 1977, p. xvi)

More recently, authors working with this paradigm have noted that, one by one, western governments are adopting 'neo-liberal' arguments to disassemble systems of wealth redistribution, privatise national assets, and transfer power and resources to the profit-oriented sector. Neo-liberalism, they argue, also entails giving priority to the reduction of costs and efficiency of production (Teeple, 2000). The implication for universities in general, and medical education in particular, is the restructuring of curricula, of pedagogic methods, and of governance and administration to support neo-liberal ideology and objectives (Magnusson, 2000). The objective of scholars working with this paradigm is to raise consciousness among oppressed groups and re-centre education as a vehicle of emancipation rather than a tool to enrich the privileged yet further (Freire, 1970).

Feminist and anti-racist theories

The past 60 years have seen the rise of a multitude of theories that explore the systemic inequities in society perpetuated on the basis of gender, race, religion, class, sexuality, and/or physical ability. Feminist and anti-racist theories cast light on the ways in which institutions create inequities on the basis of gender or race. These perspectives have two functions: to generate understanding and to create change in order to improve the conditions of those who are subjugated by inequity. What these theories all have in common, besides their interest in inequity, is that they are 'critical' – that is, their mandate is to enable and foment social change.

For many years each of the 'equity' theories was taken up separately – written about by different authors, in different places, and addressed to different communities. More recently, however, there has been an effort to embrace commonalities between the agendas of different groups who are attempting to address inequities. This is sometimes referred to as the 'combined equity agenda'. Exploring the intersection of inequities acknowledges that one person might simultaneously embody a multiplicity of identities (Haraway, 1991). The rapprochement of theories that address gender, race, sexuality, ability, and other dimensions of human identity through an equity lens has resulted in a body of critical equity-based theories that are sometimes referred to as 'critical theory'. Critical perspectives are widely used within the broader education literature (Ng et al, 1995) and have been used to critique the medical profession and health care system generally (see, e.g. Witz's, 1992; *Professions and Patriarchy*). More recently, a critical approach has been used to address various aspects of medical education. Wear and

Aultman (2005) and Wear and Kuczewski (2004), for example, employed a number of equity-related critical perspectives to address both curricular and pedagogical aspects of undergraduate medical education, while Martimianakis (2008) addressed structural effects of equity and diversity policies in a Faculty of Medicine. Phillips (1995) has shown how decades of research conducted almost exclusively on white, middle-aged, Euro-American men means that the solid ground of 'evidence-based medicine' taught by medical schools is built on highly selective evidence.

An understanding of the impact of inequities on society enables us, at the simplest level, to make them visible to our students. However, we must not assume that patients suffer inequities and physicians do not. Structural inequities exist inevitably at all levels of medical education because it takes place in an inequitable society. Consistent with the critical paradigm, scholars working from this standpoint argue that, in order to address such issues as equitable access to medical education and leadership roles within the discipline, it is necessary to focus on the gendered, cultured, and racialised hierarchical nature of the profession itself and make efforts to (re)invent a more equitable society.

Post-colonial theories

One of the major historical shifts of the twentieth-century was the end of the Eurocentric colonial systems that had ruled much of the non-European world for hundreds of years. This enormous political change and the accompanying economic and social upheaval have been written about from many different cultural and disciplinary perspectives. Post-colonial theories give voice to the oppressions and disparities that are the legacy of old and continuing colonial power relations. This broad school of thought has emerged from the analysis of global changes and their aftermath, as well as the colonial conditions that preceded them. Although this group of theories interacts with, and often draws on, other theoretical groupings (including Foucauldian discourse analysis, feminism, and neo-Marxism), it makes visible certain assumptions and problems that other theories do not clearly address.

For example, although neo-Marxism problematises economic exploitation of the 'third world', post-colonial theorists have emphasised that cultural and social dimensions of such interactions are equally important. Theorists working from a post-colonial perspective have also argued against accepting a unified discourse of colonialism in order to expose the specificity of effects on different colonies and colonisers. In addition, post-colonial theorists have focused attention on the difficulties of translating western feminist ideals (and other aspects of the combined equity agenda) into the post-colonial realm, where nationalist struggles have often taken precedence over inequities and where western notions of equality can themselves be seen as 'colonising' ideas. Finally, a post-colonial movement known as 'subaltern studies' has struggled to give voice to those who are too culturally and socio-economically marginalised even to take part in such debates.

Although there has been research into the effects of colonial dominance in medicine generally, and into the effects on diverse cultures specifically, linkage of medical education and post-colonial theory is relatively new. Such theories have, however, been taken up in an emerging discussion of globalisation in medical education. Recent papers have problematised the straightforward export of copies of European and North American medical education curricula and institutions to other parts of the world. They argue that such exportation includes not only curricula but also, more problematically, the social and cultural assumptions embedded within them (Bleakley et al, 2008). Uncritical export of medical education models, products, and institutions is particularly troubling as it is being done with an implicit acceptance that there are globally appropriate professional values (Hodges et al, 2009) – values that most often stem directly from western professional ideals.

While post-colonial thought helps explain problems of globalisation in medical education, it is also a useful theoretical tool to understand complex problems at a more local level. Analysing medical education problems based on local histories and specific cultural norms can counter some of the negative effects and artificial disjunctions that are born of uncritically adhering to sweeping position statements about 'global standards' and 'best practices', which masquerade as universally validated constructs, but which often disguise very particular socio-cultural constructions. Other strands of post-colonial theory such as subaltern studies offer intriguing possibilities to teach our students to hear and represent appropriately the perspectives of the voiceless among our patients: elderly, homeless, and mentally ill people, immigrants, refugees, and other marginalised groups.

Implications for practice

While dramatic shifts in the nature of medical education (such as Flexner's reforms) are rare, medical education and its institutions are continually being (re)shaped. This process is often passive, resulting from circumstance rather than deep reflection on the nature of medical education and its relationship to societies. Currently, neo-liberalism, market economics, and the globalisation of medical education are reshaping many aspects of medical education. Yet their profound impact on issues like access to medical education institutions, the financing of medical education, and the role that its graduates play in different societies has not been actively studied or proactively influenced to any great degree. Their implications are worthy of study.

Understanding and harnessing the forces of social construction offer the possibility of re-imagining medical education and its institutions in a more active fashion. Educators and students need not be swept along passively in the currents of their socio-political environments. Rather, medical education institutions and medical educators hold a great deal of power and influence in their societies. While there are significant constraints on the degree to which individuals can shape what is possible to think, say, or be, collective reflection and concerted effort could make it possible to exert influence.

In this vein, the social science perspectives that have been considered in this chapter, while theoretically bound, can be used to inform practical changes in the nature, governance, and/or management of medical education institutions. To illustrate this point, it may be helpful to consider social responsibility, a notion of central concern to medical educators and students. At the risk of cross-cultural generalisation, social responsibility implies that medical education institutions, in various parts of the world, exist through a tacit understanding with the societies in which they are located. That is, there is an unwritten agreement that, in exchange for significant financial resources, a high degree of prestige, protection for education and research activities, a set of legal, financial, and other structures that allow for self-regulation, and a relative monopoly for the professional services of their graduates, each medical school will give back in some meaningful way to the society that supports it. This 'giving back' is usually framed as 'social responsibility' or even 'social accountability' and its nature varies tremendously.

However, were a faculty of medicine, its teachers, and its students to try to articulate the nature of their social responsibility, the various theoretical 'lenses' we presented in this chapter would prove most useful:

- A Foucauldian approach would draw attention to the ways in which medical institutions powerfully shape and control the beliefs, behaviours, and ways of being of their faculty and students. Since, as Foucault himself argued, power is always 'productive', medical schools could choose to shape the values and behaviours of their students in various ways. One could, for example, analyse the ways in which performance-based examinations with standardised patients (such as Objective Structured Clinical Examinations (OSCEs)) embed particular ways of 'being' for students, patients, and other health professionals. That might highlight problematic constructions and behaviours that run counter to the institution's avowedly socially responsible values.

- A Bourdieuvian perspective would focus on making visible any struggles for power and prestige. This approach could be used to understand how an admissions system reinforces the social power and privilege of particular socio-cultural groups. What might appear as a neutral interview process might be discovered to embed subtle and particular values related to communicating, dressing, or behaving 'appropriately' that function as social or symbolic capital because some groups of individuals can 'decode' them better than others. Such research could explain unsettling disparities between the demographics of medical students admitted and the demographics of the societies from which they come.

- A Marxist approach would examine the reproduction of economic inequality. The goal would be to render visible contradictions that arise between the avowed medical ethos of public service and social responsibility and the ways in which a medical school serves to advance the socio-economic standing of its small, elite graduating classes. The changing demographics of medical students in countries with deregulated and rising tuitions and the narrowing social stratum from which these students come, for instance, could be examined through a neo-Marxist analysis of governance, finance, and admissions policies.

- Feminist and anti-racist lenses would bring dimensions of gender and race (and, more broadly, of sexual orientation, physical ability, etc.) to the fore in critiquing medical education. Such approaches could be employed to illuminate the ways in which the hierarchy of various medical school constituencies (faculty, administration, students, patients, specialty groups, etc.) is related to power, remuneration, prestige, or legitimacy on the one hand and gender, race, culture, sexuality, and the intersection of these identities on the other. In response, an activist approach might then be taken to address the under-representation of certain groups at various ranks of the medical school.

- Post-colonial theory would be particularly useful for addressing the impact of socio-economic and cultural oppression in former colonies, but equally in the new hierarchies created by globalisation. The current movement of curricula, people, and ideas around the world could be studied from this perspective. For example, a post-colonial approach might analyse the degree to which imports and exports of medical curricula, medical students, or fully trained doctors are adapted to local cultural needs and contexts or, conversely, the degree to which they disguise a system of poaching resources from less powerful to more powerful cultures or countries.

These are brief examples of what each of the five theoretical perspectives could bring to the study of medical education in one domain: social responsibility. There are many other questions that lend themselves to the rich analytic frameworks of social science theory. Each of these frameworks, and many others that are beyond the scope of this chapter, force us to question the basic assumptions of our everyday educational practice and research. This questioning is, in turn, the first step towards actively shaping medical education to respond to the needs of the societies of which we are members.

References

Albert M: Understanding the debate on medical education research: a sociological perspective, *Acad Med* 79(10):948–954, 2004.

Albert M, Hodges B, Regehr G: Research in medical education: balancing service and science, *Adv Health Sci Educ Theory Pract* 12(1):103–115, 2007.

Bleakley A, Brice J, Bligh J: Thinking the post-colonial in medical education, *Med Educ* 42(3):266–270, 2008.

Bourdieu P: Quelques propriétés du champ. In Bourdieu P, editor: *Questions de sociologi*, Paris, 1980, Éditions de Minuit, pp 113–120.

Bourdieu P: The forms of capital. In Richardson JG, editor: *Handbook of theory and research for the sociology of education*, New York, 1986, Greenwood Press, pp 241–258.

Bourdieu P: *Homo Academicus* (Collier P, translator), Stanford, CA, 1988, Stanford University Press.

Bourdieu P, Wacquant JD: *An invitation to reflexive sociology*, Chicago, 1992, The University of Chicago Press.

Brosnan C: Pierre Bourdieu and the theory of medical education: thinking 'relationally' about medical students and medical curricula. In Brosnan C, Turner BS, editors: *Handbook of the sociology of medical education*, New York, 2009, Routledge.

Brown RE: *Rockefeller medicine men: medicine and capitalism in America*, Berkeley, 1979, University of California Press.

Flexner A: *Medical education in the United States and Canada: a report to the Carnegie Foundation for the Advancement of Teaching*, New York, 1910, The Carnegie Foundation.

Foucault M: *The birth of the clinic (Naissance de la clinique)* (Sheridan AM, translator), London, 1963/2003, Routledge (original work published 2003).

Foucault M: *Madness and civilization: a history of insanity in the age of reason*, New York, 1965, Random House.

Foucault M: *Discipline and punish: the birth of the prison (Surveiller et Punir: Naissance de la prison)* (Sheridan AM, translator), New York, 1975/1977, Vintage Books.

Freire P: *Pedagogy of the oppressed (Pedagogía del oprimido)* (Ramos MB, translator), New York, 1970, Continuum.

Haraway DJ: *Simians, cyborgs, and women: the reinvention of nature*, New York, 1991, Routledge.

Hodges BD: The many and conflicting histories of medical education in Canada and the United States: an introduction to the paradigm wars, *Med Educ* 39(6):613–621, 2005.

Hodges BD: Medical education and the maintenance of incompetence, *Med Teach* 28(8):690–696, 2007.

Hodges BD, Kuper A, Reeves S: Qualitative methodology: discourse analysis, *BMJ* 337:a879, 2008.

Hodges BD, Maniate JM, Martimianakis MA, Alsuwaiden M, Segouin C: Cracks and crevices: globalization discourse and medical education, *Med Teach* 31 (10):910–917, 2009.

Johnson T: *Professions and power*, London, 1972, Routledge.

Kuper A, Reeves S, Levinson W: An introduction to reading and appraising qualitative research, *BMJ* 337:a288, 2008. doi: 10.1136/bmj.a288.

Larkin G: *Occupational monopoly and modern medicine*, London, 1983, Tavistock.

Larson M: *The rise of professionalism: a sociological analysis*, Berkeley, 1977, University of California Press.

Luke H: *Medical education and sociology of medical habitus: it's not about the stethoscope!*, Dordrecht, 2003, Kluwer Academic Publishers.

McHoul A, Grace W: *A Foucault primer: discourse, power and the subject*, New York, 1993, New York University Press.

Magnusson J: Canadian higher education and citizenship in the context of state restructuring and globalization, *Encounters Educ* 1(Fall):107–123, 2000.

Martimianakis MA: Reconciling competing discourses: the University of Toronto's equity and diversity framework. In Wagner A, Acker S,

Mayuzumi K, editors: *Whose university is it, anyway? Power and privilege on gendered terrain*, Toronto, 2008, Sumach Press, pp 44–60.

Marx K, Engels P: *The German ideology*, New York, 1844/1970, International Publications.

Ng R, Staton P, Scane J: *Anti-racism, feminism, and critical approaches to education*, Westport, CT, 1995, Bergin & Garvey.

Phillips S: The social context of women's health: goals and objectives for medical education. *Can Med Assoc J* 152(4):507–511, 1995.

Reeves S, Albert M, Kuper A, Hodges BD: Why use theories in qualitative research? *BMJ* 337:a949, 2008. doi: 10.1136/bmj.a949.

Speed E: Patients, consumers and survivors: a case study of mental

health service user discourses. *Soc Sci Med* 62(1):28–38, 2006.

Strong-Boag V: Canada's women doctors: feminism constrained. In Shortt SED, editor: *Medicine in Canadian society: historical perspectives*, Montreal, 1981, McGill-Queen's University Press.

Teeple G: *Globalization and the decline of social reform: into the twenty-first century*, Amherst, NY, 2000, Humanity Books.

Wear D, Aultman JM: The limits of narrative: medical student resistance to confronting inequality and oppression in literature and beyond, *Med Educ* 39(10):1056–1065, 2005.

Wear D, Kuczewski MG: The professionalism movement: can we pause? *Am J Bioethics* 4(2):1–10, 2004.

Witz A: *Professions and patriarchy*, London, 1992, Routledge.

Further reading

Brosnan C, Turner BS: *Handbook of the sociology of medical education*, New York, 2009, Routledge.

Eagleton M: *A concise companion to feminist theory*, Oxford, 2003, Blackwell.

Johnson T: *Professions and power*, London, 1972, Routledge.

Loomba A: *Colonialism/Post-colonialism*, ed 2, London, 2005, Routledge.

Mills S: *Michel Foucault*, London, 2003, Routledge.

Swartz D: *Culture & power: the sociology of Pierre Bourdieu*, Chicago, 1997, University of Chicago Press.

Medical education in an interprofessional context

Scott Reeves   Joanne Goldman

4

ABC

Glossary

Before-and-after study A research design in which data are collected before and after an 'intervention' such as interprofessional education.

Before-during-and-after study Similar design to a before-and-after study except it entails collecting data at some point during the intervention.

Collaborative practice Collaborative practice in health and social care occurs when multiple professions provide comprehensive services by working with patients, their families, carers, and communities to deliver the highest quality of care across settings.

Continuous Quality Improvement; see *Quality improvement*

Curriculum (without a pronoun) This is used as an overarching term for all those aspects of education that contribute to the experience of learning, including aims, content, mode of delivery and assessment.

Evaluation The systematic gathering of evidence to enable judgement of effectiveness and value, often to promote improvement.

Interprofessional education Where groups of learners from different professions learn about, from, and with each other to enable effective collaboration and improve health outcomes.

Intervention A consciously developed and implemented activity, such as interprofessional education, that attempts to improve or change outcomes of some form such as interprofessional collaboration.

Continued

© 2011, Elsevier Ltd.
DOI: 10.1016/B978-0-7020-3522-7.00004-8

Glossary (continued)

Knowledge translation Knowledge translation is a dynamic and iterative process that includes synthesis, dissemination, exchange, and ethically sound application of knowledge to improve health, provide more effective health services and products, and to strengthen the health care system.

Multiprofessional education Members of different professions learning alongside each other without interaction between them.

Practice Includes both clinical and non-clinical health-related work such as diagnosis, treatment, surveillance, health communications, management, and sanitation engineering.

Professional An all-encompassing term that includes anyone with knowledge and/or skills to contribute to the delivery of care.

Quality Improvement An approach that is based on a manufacturing philosophy and set of methods for reducing time from customer order to product delivery, costing less, taking less space, and improving quality. Common forms of QI activities include Continuous Quality Improvement and Total Quality Management.

Review Literature reviews are collections of previously conducted research or evaluation studies. Reviews may be exploratory, narrative, critical, or systematic.

Scoping review An exploratory type of review that aims to undertake a broad scope of a particular field before more extensive review work can be undertaken.

Total Quality Management; see *Quality Improvement* A culture within an organisation that is aimed at continuous improvement of educational quality.

Uniprofessional education When members (or students) of a single profession learn together.

Outline

Traditional ways of delivering medical education to students and qualified practitioners are being questioned. In addition to clinical knowledge, both pre- and post-qualification learners need other attributes to work effectively within the health care system and provide high-quality care. Those attributes include strategies for communicating and working with non-medical professional groups involved in the delivery of care. Interprofessional education (IPE) gives learners opportunities to develop the attributes and skills needed to work collaboratively with other professions. This chapter has five sections exploring issues pertinent to IPE, which include its emergence and aims; different learning and teaching approaches; organisational elements needed for effective IPE; evidence of its effectiveness; and the application of social science theory to IPE. The implications of IPE for medical education are integrated throughout the chapter. The concluding section highlights some future directions for interprofessionalism.

Part 1 The emergence and aims of IPE

This first part outlines why IPE has emerged within medical and health professions education (e.g. nursing, occupational therapy, social work), and what it sets out to achieve. Globally for over three decades, health policy makers have identified IPE as having a key role in improving health care systems and outcomes (e.g. World Health Organisation, 1976), but it is over the past ten years in particular that IPE has come to the forefront of research, policy, and regulatory activity on an international level. IPE, whether before or after qualification, is defined as

> 'When two or more professions learn with, from, and about each other to improve collaboration and the quality of care' (Centre for the Advancement of IPE – www.caipe.org.uk/about-us/defining-ipe).

This definition applies to learners before and after qualification. The promotion of this type of education stems from the complexity and multifaceted nature of patients' health care needs and the health care system, and research demonstrating that effective collaboration amongst multiple health care providers is essential for the provision of effective and comprehensive health care.

Problems with communication and collaboration amongst different health care professionals have been well documented and continue to be a concern. For example, failures of collaboration were at the centre of well-publicised health and social care enquiries in the UK, such as the excessively high mortality of children undergoing cardiac surgery in Bristol and the death of Victoria Climbié, a child whose repeated physical abuse continued despite the involvement of various social agencies. A study of interprofessional (IP) teams in Sweden found that poor collaboration between health care professionals impacts on patient care and service (e.g. Kvarnstrom, 2008). Studies in the USA and Canada demonstrated the impact of communication problems on work processes and patient safety in surgical settings (e.g. Williams et al, 2007). In a US sentinel event alert of infant death and injury during delivery, communication issues were identified as a root cause in 72 per cent of the 47 cases identified (The Joint Commission, 2004).

The collective picture emerging from the literature is that doctors, along with other health and social professionals, need to develop attitudes, knowledge, and skills, which equip them to work effectively together if they are to deliver safe, high-quality patient care. It has been argued that a traditionally isolated approach to health professions education in both the pre-qualification (medical school) and post-qualification (from graduate to continuing medical education) stages fails to promote IP collaboration; hence the need for IPE.

Policy documents in various countries have delineated a role for IPE. For example, policy makers in the UK re-emphasised their commitment to it in the white paper *A Health Service of all the Talents* published in 2000. This outlined the future of education for the health and social care professions to support team working, flexible working, streamlined workforce planning and development, a maximum contribution from all staff towards patient care, and the development of new, more flexible carers (Department of Health, 2000). A number of health policy documents have been produced in Canada outlining the role of IPE within a Pan-Canadian Health Human Resources Strategy (see Box 4.1).

A sign of the emergence of IPE has been the creation of courses, programmes, and offices in higher education institutions in the United Kingdom, Canada, United States, continental Europe, and

Australia (Barr et al, 2005). The Royal College of Physicians and Surgeons of Canada CanMEDS framework outlines competencies needed for medical education and specialty practice organised around seven roles: Collaborator; Medical Expert; Communicator; Health Advocate; Manager; Scholar; and Professional (see: http://rcpsc.medical.org/canmeds/index.php). Similar frameworks are being adopted in other countries. In the UK, for example, the government's *Modernising Medical Careers* lists the following requirement of the curriculum for postgraduate education and training:

> 'The requirement for trainee doctors to learn a range of skills including communication, the undertaking and use of research, time management, team-working, leadership, quality and safety improvements, and use of evidence and data'.

Likewise, teamworking and communication skills are advocated for inclusion in patient safety education (see: www.dh.gov.uk/en/Aboutus/Ministersand-DepartmentLeaders/ChiefMedicalOfficer/Archive/FeaturesArchive/DH_4107830).

Health care organisations are also supporting IPE initiatives. For example, Barr et al (2005) report on programmes in the United Kingdom and United States, where primary care practices and medical centres have made a commitment to support health care improvements through initiatives that include IPE. Involvement of the medical profession in IPE programmes is essential, given the key role physicians play in IP collaboration. Furthermore, leadership from the medical community is critical, given the complexity of implementing such initiatives. In response, medical schools, associations, councils, practices, and organisations are recognising and supporting IPE for their students and practicing physicians. In a study comparing medical student learning about patient safety uniprofessionally versus interprofessionally, all students increased their knowledge, but those who participated in IPE gained added value and were better able to position their learning within safe IP team-working (Anderson et al, 2009).

 ## Box 4.1

Health Canada's statement on IPE

"Changing the way we educate health providers is key to achieving system change and to ensuring that health providers have the necessary knowledge and training to work effectively on interprofessional teams within the evolving health care system."

Available at: http://www.hc-sc.gc.ca/hcs-sss/hhr-rhs/strateg/interprof/index-eng.php

Part 2 Learning and teaching approaches

Building on Part 1, we probe in more depth a range of pertinent learning and teaching approaches. Specifically, we explore when to deliver IPE, the need for an interactive approach, initial activities, informal learning, IP group composition, programme focus and status, and facilitation.

When to deliver IPE to students

There is an ongoing debate about when is the most effective time to implement IPE. It has been found that students entering their first year of a prequalification programme already have established and consistent stereotypes about other health and social care professional groups (Barr et al, 2005). It may seem logical, therefore to deliver IPE at this early stage if negative effects of professional socialisation, such as hostile stereotyping, are to be prevented. Others, in contrast, have suggested that post-qualification IPE is more effective because participants have a firmer professional identity and understanding of their role. In a recent survey of pre-registration students from eight health care groups, including medicine, from three higher education institutions in the UK, the strength of professional identity in all professional groups was high on university entry but declined significantly over time in some disciplines. Students' readiness for IPE was also high at entry but declined significantly over time in all groups except nursing (Coster et al, 2008). Students' readiness and the existence of professional identities relatively early in their education argue for early and ongoing IPE.

It has been suggested that IPE should be part of an individual's ongoing professional development, starting pre-qualification and continuing throughout their career (Barr et al, 2005). Given that the objectives and nature of IPE differ according to the stage of learning, this seems appropriate; it could be used initially to prepare students for collaborative practice while, delivered at a later stage, it could reinforce early learning experiences and further support IP collaboration in practice.

The need for an interactive learning approach

The definition of IPE outlined previously stresses the need for interaction between participants as this interactivity is believed to promote development of the competencies required for effective collaboration (Barr et al, 2005). Educational strategies that enable

Box 4.2

Different IP interactive learning methods

- Exchange-based learning (e.g. seminar-based discussions);
- Observation-based learning (e.g. joint visits to patients/clients);
- Action-based learning (e.g. problem-based learning);
- Simulation-based learning (e.g. simulating clinical practice);
- Practice-based learning (e.g. IP clinical placements);
- E-learning (e.g. online discussions).

interactivity are therefore a requirement. Barr et al (2005) outline different types of interactive learning methods (Box 4.2).

The literature contains numerous examples of such learning activities. For example, Freeth et al (2009) in the UK report a one-day simulation-based course for obstetricians, obstetric anaesthetists, and midwives to improve IP working in obstetric care. The focus of the course is on non-technical aspects of care and their influence on patient safety. The course involves an initial orientation to the environment, simulation scenarios, and facilitated debriefings.

Combining different interactive learning methods can make IPE more stimulating and interesting and contribute to a deeper level of learning. For instance, the Seamless Care IPE programme in Canada, which aimed to develop IP patient-centred collaborative skills of students from medicine, dental hygiene, dentistry, nursing, and pharmacy, involved an orientation workshop, ongoing educational sessions, and an 8-week clinical placement with an IP student team (Mann et al, 2009). In an evaluation of IP clinical placements for teams of medical, nursing, occupational therapy, and physiotherapy students, it was reported that leaving the clinical learning environment to spend time reflecting upon experiences in interactive classroom activities deepened students' understanding of issues and processes related to IP teamwork (Reeves, 2008). The particular learning methods used depend on the objectives of the education initiative, the participants, and the resources available. Different students may be more or less familiar and experienced with particular learning methods, such as online learning or simulation, which can be challenging in an IPE programme.

Initial activities

When a group comes together for the first time to undertake IP learning, attention should be paid to the initial interactive processes of group formation. The use of an 'ice-breaking' session may help facilitate group cohesion. Ice-breaker sessions allow learners to focus interactively on professional stereotyping or professional assumptions they bring. For example, one study reported that students entering medical school considered nurses to be more caring and doctors more arrogant, and considered nurses to have lower academic ability, competence, and status, although comparable life experience (Rudland and Mires, 2005). Ice-breaker sessions are particularly helpful in unpacking and exploring issues of professionalism (e.g. boundary protectionism) that are central to any collaborative venture. They are also helpful in team-building, especially when a group of learners has not worked together before. These sessions can be useful in allowing established IP teams to unpack issues linked to hierarchy and power differentials that surround their daily practice. Existing problems within established teams, however, can make IPE programmes less effective.

Informal learning

Opportunities for informal learning – when learners meet socially and discuss aspects of their formal education – are a useful part of IPE. Informal learning can allow individuals to exchange ideas and obtain guidance from their peers, work colleagues, or managers. Informal learning activities can be explicitly built into an IP programme by including, for example, opportunities to discuss educational experiences informally during breaks. Informal learning can also occur as an 'unplanned' outcome of an IP initiative. In the evaluation of a community-based module (Reeves, 2008), medical, nursing, and dental students used pubs and cafes after their formal learning sessions to discuss informally and reflect upon their IPE; they saw this informal learning as a valuable part of their shared experience.

There are important differences in informal IP clinical placement learning. Informal learning opportunities in clinical contexts can be influenced by individual professional and organisational cultures as well as by students' confidence levels (Pollard, 2009). Informal learning opportunities and mentorship during them play large roles in students' learning and development.

Interprofessional group composition

Arguably, effective IP interaction requires a balance of professions. An equal mix of members from each profession is ideal because a group skewed too heavily in favor of one profession may inhibit interaction as the larger professional group can dominate. For programmes of longer duration, interaction is enhanced if learners work together within a stable group, with few established members leaving and/or new people joining the group. Furthermore, at the post-qualification level, the participation of all relevant professions is likely essential if the IPE is to have an impact on practice.

Ensuring this balance of professions can be challenging. For learners in full-time pre-qualification education, effective timetabling across profession-specific education programmes can be key to creating group stability. Wright and Lindqvist (2008), for example, discussed challenges coordinating IPE for students from eight different professions, including medicine, and the inevitability that students from some professions could only attend two of the three workshops because of conflicts with clinical placements. They noted that this caused friction as some students viewed incomplete attendance as a lack of commitment.

Some studies have noted the challenges of physician participation in IPE programmes and the need to ensure their presence given their key role in supporting changes in IP collaboration (Goldman et al, 2010). In post-qualification initiatives, learning activities can be affected by the demands of clinical work, especially if sessions are held near learners' clinical areas or the programmes occur over a number of weeks. One way of overcoming this difficulty is to offer IPE off-site. This may provide a more conducive learning environment and opportunities for important processes of informal learning; it is an expensive option, however, especially as one needs to secure clinical cover for the team. A recent study of an IP programme within maternity care revealed that sufficient representation from each of the professions was important for discussions concerning IP working and team processes yet there was sometimes only one physician, and participants were disappointed not to hear the physician perspective (Freeth et al, 2009).

For effective interactive learning to occur, the group size should not be too large because it is harder for larger groups to have high-quality interactions. IPE programmes generally report group sizes of between five and ten learners (Reeves, 2008). Fiscal restraints, nevertheless, may cause difficulties in creating such small group learning formats. As will be discussed later in this chapter, organisational support is critical to scheduling students from different professional groups and enabling health providers to attend IPE programmes.

Programme focus and status

There is evidence that IPE is more effective when principles of adult learning are used (e.g. problem-based learning, action learning sets), learning reflects real-world practice experiences (Barr et al, 2005), and interaction occurs between participants. With other research, health professions education, and policymaking colleagues, we are currently conducting a scoping review of IPE programmes, which has found a range in the focus of programmes. Some focus mostly on generic IP skills while others focus on IP skills within the context of particular clinical topics and/or settings.

Combining learning activities designed to promote *collaborative* outcomes with activities designed to promote more *profession-specific* outcomes can be problematic as learners experience uncertainty regarding the overall aim of the IPE. This issue emerged during work on an IP placement for medical, nursing, occupational therapy, and physiotherapy students (Reeves, 2008). In order to offer students a holistic insight into the clinical environment, students were offered both collaborative interactive learning activities such as team problem-solving and profession-specific activities such as drug administration – a task that only nursing students undertook. For students on this placement, the inclusion of both collaborative and profession-specific learning activities produced tension as it was found difficult to participate actively in both types of activity. After feeding this finding back to the group responsible for developing the placement, it was agreed to review this part of the placement in order to reduce the tension.

Making participation in IPE voluntary can give the message that it has a low status in relation to profession-specific learning, which may in turn reduce learners' commitment to it. In addition, if IPE is not assessed in a way that gives it equal weight to profession-specific education, its status can again be diminished. Eliciting public support from professional leaders and recruiting high-quality educators may help improve its status. Making attendance compulsory and scheduling flexibly can prevent logistic challenges from

becoming a barrier to effective IPE. For physicians, continuing medical education credits may also provide the needed status, and therefore incentive, to encourage participation. Nevertheless, practitioners undertake IPE on a voluntary basis, so the incentive is to further their own professional development and/or enhance the coordination and delivery of patient/client care.

Facilitating IPE

Facilitating IPE calls for skill, experience, and preparation to deal with the various responsibilities and demands involved. It is ideal to train facilitators from the diverse faculty involved, and the number of facilitators required can be large, particularly in a pre-qualification context, depending on the number of students. There are various attributes required for this type of work, some of which are outlined in Box 4.3.

In line with other forms of small group education, facilitators need to focus on team formation and maintenance, create a non-threatening environment, and help all members participate equally, but these aims are more challenging in an IP context given the history of social and economic inequalities, and friction that exists between the different health and social care professions. Friedson's (1970) work provides an understanding of those imbalances. He argued that all occupational groups actively engage in a process of professionalisation through engagement in a 'closure' project. The aim of this project is straightforward – to secure and then protect exclusive ownership of specific areas of knowledge and expertise to secure economic reward and status enhancement effectively. As medicine was the first of the occupations to engage successfully in a professionalisation project, participants claimed the most highly prestigious areas of clinical work – the ability to diagnose and prescribe – which ensured their

Box 4.3

Attributes of facilitators of IPE

- Experience of IP work (to draw upon when facilitating);
- In-depth understanding of interactive learning methods;
- Knowledge of group dynamics;
- Confidence in working with IP groups;
- Flexibility (to use professional differences within groups creatively).

dominant position over other health and social care professions. Exploring this theme more recently, Pecukonis et al (2008) argue that different professional cultures shape different definitions of health, wellness, and treatment success, as well as power differences. They argue that IPE is limited by profession-centrism, which must be addressed through a curriculum that promotes IP cultural competence.

Part 3 Organisational elements

This section aims to explore how organisational elements interplay with the development and implementation of IPE within medical education, and the need for faculty development.

Organisational support

Organisational support is crucial to the success of an IPE programme. To instill a positive attitude in students, the organisation and its faculty have to demonstrate their support (Wilhelmsson et al, 2009). The leadership must have interest, knowledge, and experience. Given the resources required to develop and implement IPE, institutional policies and managerial commitment are also crucial. Such leadership and 'buy-in' are needed from all participating departments within an organisation.

The particular type of organisational support required depends on the stage of education. Large numbers of students, professional accreditation requirements, and inflexible curricula are challenging aspects of pre-qualification IPE. Most pre-qualification programmes for medicine and nursing have cohorts of between 100 and 200 students, though occupational therapy and physiotherapy programmes typically have cohorts of just 20–60 students. Large numbers create the logistic difficulty of finding a suitable location. Differences in course timing create further problems. Obtaining approval from each of the participating professions' regulatory bodies and resolving issues of accountability add further complications.

Planning post-qualification IPE tends to be less problematic because there are fewer institutional barriers, though institutional support is required to foster a positive attitude and give staff the time and resources to attend. Organisational support is also critical if any knowledge gains are to be successfully translated into practice.

In addition, finance needs to be carefully considered during the planning of any IP initiative. Because it tends to span a number of different departmental budgets (Reeves, 2008), agreement over financial arrangements can be a major hurdle.

Planning the IP learning

Developing IP curricula is a complex process, which involves health care workers and educators from different faculties, work settings, and locations. Involving faculty from the different programmes is crucial so that all have a sense of ownership. Equal representation ensures that no one group dominates the planning and skews the initiative in any one direction; it is challenging, however, to ensure adequate representation from smaller faculties. As developing IPE takes considerable time and energy, group members need to have dedication and enthusiasm. When programme development depends on the input of a few key enthusiasts, however, the long-term sustainability of a programme is at risk because key individuals may move to other organisations. In the evaluation of an IP clinical placement for nursing, medical, occupational therapy, and physiotherapy students, it was found that sustained enthusiasm of steering group members was critical to overcoming practical issues such as joint validation and the establishment of pilot placements. Without group effort of that sort, IPE cannot be developed and implemented (Reeves, 2008).

The election of a project leader to coordinate group activities and ensure progress is important. Organisers must have IP skills and they need to arrange regular meetings that consider all perspectives (Reeves, 2008; Wilhelmsson et al, 2009). Group members need to share their aims and assumptions about the initiative to ensure that they all work towards a common goal. When differences are identified, they need to be discussed and resolved. Regular planning meetings allow group members to update one another and jointly solve problems.

Sustaining IPE can be equally complex and requires good communication among participants, enthusiasm for the work being done, and a shared vision and understanding of the benefits of introducing a new curriculum. Organisations need constantly to evaluate, revise, and discuss IPE in the organisation and remind all members that the general goal of IPE is to foster IP practice (Wilhelmsson et al, 2009).

The need for faculty development

Faculty development is needed for those involved in developing, delivering, and evaluating IPE. For most educators, teaching students how to learn about, from, and with each other is a new and challenging experience. Like students, faculty may also feel a tension between IP and uni-professional issues, which may challenge their professional identities. Faculty development may reduce feelings of isolation, develop a more collaborative approach, and provide opportunities for faculty to share knowledge, experiences, and ideas (Rees and Johnson, 2007).

The growing number of faculty development programmes offer similar preparatory activities, such as understanding the roles and responsibilities of the different professions, exploring issues of professionalism, and planning learning strategies for IP groups. IPE faculty development programmes must enable individuals to promote change at the individual and organisational level, and must therefore target diverse stakeholders and address leadership and organisational change (Steinert, 2005). To ensure that faculty maintain their facilitation skills, faculty development must be ongoing. Team teaching with more experienced colleagues can help develop facilitation skills, coupled with regular opportunities for discussion and reflection. When it is impossible for a person to be formally trained, it is advisable for them to seek informal input from a colleague more experienced in this type of work. For IPE to be successfully embedded in curricula and training packages, the early experiences of staff must be positive, which will ensure continued involvement and receptiveness to student feedback.

Part 4 The evidence

During the past decade, a number of systematic reviews have examined evidence for the effectiveness of IPE. They had different inclusion criteria and therefore examined different studies although there was overlap. We recently conducted a critical appraisal and synthesis of the evidence base (Reeves et al, 2008), which included six systematic reviews identified by an electronic search for published and unpublished reviews. The following section reports on this synthesis.

The six reviews reported the effects of over 200 studies spanning the period 1974–2005, differing in methodological quality and reporting a range of

Box 4.4

Barr et al modified Kirkpatrick typology

- Level 1: reaction (learners' views on the learning experience and its IP nature);
- Level 2a: modification of attitudes/perceptions (changes in reciprocal attitudes or perceptions between participant groups);
- Level 2b: acquisition of knowledge/skills (gains of knowledge and skills linked to IP collaboration);
- Level 3: behavioural change (individuals' transfer of IP learning to their practice setting and their changed professional practice);
- Level 4a: change in organisational practice (wider changes in the organisation and delivery of care);
- Level 4b: benefits to patients/clients (improvements in health or well-being of patients/clients).

outcomes, but sharing a common definition of IPE ('two or more professions learning with, from, and about each other to improve collaboration and the quality of care'). Five were undertaken by similar review teams and five shared similar (methodologically inclusive) inclusion criteria (Reeves et al, 2008). Five employed a similar approach to recording outcomes. Barr et al (2005) modified Kirkpatrick's four-point typology (learners' reactions, acquisition of knowledge/skills/attitudes, changes in behaviour, and changes in organisational practice), to the six-point typology shown in Box 4.4.

Given the broad range of types of evidence (quantitative, mixed methods, and qualitative studies), we adopted an interpretive approach to synthesising the evidence-base. This allowed a variety of methodologies to be synthesised to illuminate different elements of the social world.

Table 4.1 outlines the types of studies included and outcomes examined in each review; below, we summarise the main points in relation to the programmes, quality of studies, and outcomes of the six reviews.

Nature of the IP programmes

The synthesis shows that IPE was delivered in a variety of acute, primary, and community care settings and addressed a range of chronic (e.g. asthma, arthritis) or acute (e.g. cardiac care) clinical conditions. While different combinations of professional groups participated in the programmes, medicine

Table 4.1 Key details relating to the findings and quality of evidence in IPE reviews

Review	Types of studies	Reported outcomes
Barr et al	19 studies (7 pre-qualification, 12 post-qualification) based in a range of practice settings	Reactions and attitudes; handful of studies reporting changes to organisational practice/patient care
Cooper et al	30 studies (all pre-qualification) based in a variety of practice settings	Short-term self-reported changes to attitudes, beliefs, knowledge, skills
Reeves	19 studies (all post-qualification), range of different IPE programmes based in mental health settings	Short-term changes to individual knowledge/skills and organisational practice
Barr et al	107 studies (20 pre-qualification, 85 post-qualification, 2 mixed) based in a variety of practice settings	Changes to individual knowledge, and skills some reporting changes to organisational practice and delivery of patient care
Hammick et al	21 studies (14 pre-qualification, 6 post-qualification, 1 mixed) based in a variety of practice settings	Changes in learner reaction, knowledge, and skills acquisition
Reeves et al	6 studies (all post-qualification) based in a range of settings	Changes in professional practice and patient satisfaction

and nursing were most often involved. IPE was generally delivered as a voluntary (i.e. elective) learning experience to participants and few programmes included any form of formal academic accreditation. Duration varied from 1–2 hour sessions to programmes delivered over a period of months; most lasted between one and five days. Programmes were more commonly delivered to post-qualification learners (typically physicians and nurses) in their workplaces, although IPE is increasingly being delivered to pre-qualification learners as a classroom or practice-based activity. IPE programmes used a variety of different combinations of interactive learning methods but seminar-based discussions, group problem-solving, and/or role play activities were the most common.

Quality improvement principles were often drawn upon within post-qualification IPE programmes. In general, IPE programmes assessed learning formatively, typically using individual written assignments and/or joint/team presentations, which provided a collective account of learners' IP experiences. Most programmes drew, implicitly, upon adult learning principles developed by authors such as Knowles, Schön, and Kolb (Reeves et al, 2008).

Quality of the evidence

The majority of studies provided little discussion of methodological limitations associated with their research. As a result, it was difficult to discern

their biases. In addition, a number of studies offered only limited descriptions of the interventions, which made it difficult to detect whether reported changes were actually attributable to the programme delivered.

Most studies paid little or no attention to sampling techniques or study attrition. There was a tendency to report short-term effects of IPE on learners' attitudes and knowledge. As a result, there is only limited information about the longer-term impact of IPE, particularly on organisational change, patient care, and educational processes.

There was widespread use of non-validated instruments to detect the impact of IPE on learner and/or patient satisfaction. While such tools can support local quality assurance, they are of limited research value. Measures to detect changes in individual behaviour were particularly poor, often relying on simple self-reported descriptive accounts. Self-report is of limited value because it describes only a person's *perception of change*. Most studies were undertaken in single sites.

Despite weaknesses in the evidence, there were some encouraging aspects too. Most notably, there was use of quasi-experimental research designs (e.g. before-and-after studies; before-during-and-after studies); most studies gathered two or more forms of data (typically survey and interviews); and there was growing use of longitudinal designs, which could establish the longer-term impact of IPE on organisations and patient care (Reeves et al, 2008).

Reported outcomes

Most studies found that learners enjoyed their IP experiences. Such studies also reported positive changes in learners' perceptions of changes in their views of other professional groups, views of IP collaboration, and/or changes in the value attached to working collaboratively with other professions. In addition, they reported positive changes in learners' knowledge and skills of IP collaboration, usually related to an enhanced understanding of roles and responsibilities of other professional groups, improved knowledge of the nature of IP collaboration, and/or the development of collaboration/communication skills.

Few studies reported changes in individual behaviour, usually reported as practitioners working more collaboratively with colleagues from other professional groups. Of studies which did provide evidence at this level, positive changes in individual practitioners' interactions were usually cited. A number of studies reported positive changes to organisational practice, usually changes to IP referral practices/working patterns or improved documentation (i.e. guidelines, protocols, use of shared records) related to the organisation of care. A small number of studies reported changes to the delivery of care to patients/clients. They typically reported positive changes to clinical outcomes (e.g. infection rates, clinical error rates), patient satisfaction scores, and/or length of patient stay.

In general, studies of pre-qualification IPE reported changes in attitudes, beliefs, knowledge, and collaborative skills. Post-qualification studies report learner-oriented changes but they also reported changes in organisational practice and patient care. Box 4.5 summarises the findings of the synthesis:

As the synthesis indicates, evidence for the efficacy of IPE rests upon a variety of different programmes (in terms of duration, professional participation, etc.), methodologies, and methods (from experimental research studies to mixed methods and qualitative studies) of variable quality, as well as a range of outcomes (e.g. reports of learner satisfaction to changes in the delivery of care). While the quality of evidence for IPE is currently limited, higher-quality studies are increasingly being published (Reeves et al, 2008).

Part 5 Theories

Social science theory can inform the development and evaluation of IPE initiatives, yet there has been minimal explicit use of it to date, apart from the

Box 4.5

Summary of findings from IPE evidence synthesis

- IPE is generally well received by participants;
- IPE can enable students and practitioners to learn the knowledge and skills necessary for collaborative working;
- IPE can enhance practice, improve the delivery of services, and make a positive impact on care;
- The use of quality improvement approaches such as Continuous Quality Improvement or Total Quality Management can support IPE in enhancing practice, delivery of services, and patient care;
- IPE can be effectively delivered in a variety of clinical settings.

implicit use of adult learning principles noted above. Barr et al (2005) identified three foci at which social science theories could be situated:

- Preparing individuals for collaborative practice;
- Cultivating collaboration in groups and teams;
- Improving services and the quality of care.

This section describes and discusses social science theories that are relevant to each of these foci.

Preparing individuals for collaborative practice

The three theories discussed in this section – contact theory, social exchange theory, and negotiation theory – provide ways of supporting effective interaction between different groups.

Contact theory is based on Allport's (1979) studies of prejudice between different social groups, and his conclusion that contact between their members is the most effective way of reducing tension between them. Experience demonstrated, though, that simply bringing individuals from different groups together was insufficient to effect change. Allport identified three conditions that had to be addressed for prejudice to be reduced: equality of status between the groups; group members working towards common goals; and cooperation during the contact. More recent work added three other conditions in the context of IPE: positive expectations by participants; successful experience of joint working; and a focus on understanding differences as well as similarities between themselves.

Social exchange theory (Challis et al, 1988) explains social change and stability as a process of negotiated exchanges between parties. According to it, all human relationships are formed according to a subjective cost–benefit analysis and comparison of alternatives. This theory can provide insight into the nature of relationships amongst different professionals during an IPE programme and help develop individuals' understandings of their relationships with others in work settings (Barr et al, 2005).

Negotiation theory was developed by Strauss (1978) to help explain how formal roles are transgressed by informal trade-offs between individuals' own goals and those of others. This theory can be used to explain how negotiations shape the nature of IP relations between health providers and also how negotiations affect the development and delivery of IPE. This theory becomes more complex within the context of IPE when negotiations are IP and/or inter-organisational as well as interpersonal.

Cultivating group/team collaboration

Workgroup mentality and team learning theories are presented to help understand how they can support IP team learning.

Workgroup mentality theory (Bion, 1961) is based in a psychodynamic perspective, which aims to explain unconscious processes in a group unable to deal with its 'primary task'. According to this theory, groups avoid making decisions to save members having to address potentially divisive issues. Stokes (1994) and others have extended this theory to IP relations. Stokes suggested that IP team meetings can frequently be unproductive as a false sense of collaboration prevents members from dealing with potentially difficult issues. IPE programmes with a group dynamic format can enable participants to reflect on unconscious forces that shape IP relations within the group, with the aim of increasing their understanding of such forces in their workplace.

The concept of a learning team developed from the concept of a learning organisation (Senge, 1990); the team learning concept aimed to help high-performance teams develop. Typically, members of a team do not wholly trust one another and share collective goals, but members of a learning team develop a shared commitment, have mutually agreed goals, and share a concern for the well-being of the team. In relation to IPE, team learning can help transform a loosely affiliated work 'group' of health care professionals into a more effective IP 'team', whose members trust one another and share a commitment to collective goals and the welfare of their colleagues (Barr et al, 2005).

Improving services and the quality of care

This section discusses theories that can be used in the context of IPE to improve services and the quality of care. The theories described are systems theory, activity theory, and discourse theory.

Von Bertalanffy (1971) developed the concept of 'system' as a response to the limitations of specialist disciplines in addressing complex problems. It could be applied across all disciplines, from physics and biology to the social and behavioural sciences, seeing wholes as more than the sum of their parts, interactions between parties as purposeful, boundaries between them as permeable, and cause and effect as interdependent, not linear. The underlying philosophy of *systems theory* is the unity of nature governed by the same fundamental laws in all its realms. An intervention by one profession at one point in the system affects the whole in ways that can only be anticipated from multiple professional perspectives.

Systems theory has multiple applications in IPE. It offers a unifying and dynamic framework within which all participant professions can relate person, family, community, and environment, one or more of which may be points of intervention, interacting with the whole. It can also be used to understand relationships within and between professions, between service agencies, between education and practice, and between stakeholders planning, and managing programmes.

Activity theory provides a means to understand and intervene in relations at micro and macro levels in order to effect change in interpersonal, IP, and inter-agency relations (Engestrom et al, 1999). An analysis of activity involves an understanding of individual relationships and how they relate to the macro level of collective and community.

An important component of an activity theory approach is the notion of 'knotworking' – a concept that helps describe the nature of collaborative work in which individuals connect – through tying, untying, and retying separate threads of activity during their interactions.

According to Foucault (1972), discourse helps to define a particular culture, its language, and the

Table 4.2 Summary of theories and key authors

IP foci	Theory	Author(s)
Preparing individuals for collaborative practice	Contact theory Social exchange theory Negotiation theory	Allport (1979) Challis et al (1988) Strauss (1978)
Cultivating group/team collaboration	Workgroup mentality theory Team learning theory	Bion (1961) Senge (1990)
Improving services and the quality of care	Systems theory Activity theory Discourse theory	Von Bertalanffy (1971) Engestrom et al (1999) Foucault (1972)

behaviour of individuals who belong to it. Lessa (2006) helpfully summarises Foucault's approach, as he states that discourses are knowledge systems made up of ideas, attitudes, actions, beliefs, and practices that influence how individuals think, see, and speak. Koppel (2003) used this approach to uncover prevalent discourses in continuing professional development and IPE. Koppel demonstrated how three main discourses shaped the thinking and behaviour of the main parties in the education field, namely the discourses of management, professions, and education.

Table 4.2 provides a summary of the theories presented above.

As illustrated above, the use of theory can give more in-depth insights into the nature of IPE. Theory can be used to inform the format and curriculum of a programme and can also be used to interpret findings. Further research with an explicit use of such theories would provide insight into their value for IPE.

Conclusions

Accumulating evidence of problems with communication and collaboration amongst different health care providers, and the resulting impact on the quality of health care, has stimulated decision makers in education, health care, policy, and research, to invest in IPE. The premise is that IPE will give health care providers the skills and knowledge required to work effectively with other health care providers in the health care system. As a result, IPE initiatives for pre and post-qualification learners, including medical students and physicians, are being developed and implemented across the globe.

Investment in IPE must be based on rigorous evidence of effectiveness, which is gradually accumulating. Systematic reviews show that IPE can have positive effects on participants' reactions, attitudes, knowledge/skills, behaviours, and practice, as well as patient outcomes, yet many studies have methodological limitations. As the number of studies increases and their methodological quality improves, it is to be hoped the evidence supporting IPE will become increasingly robust. In addition to better methodologies, future research needs to explore more fully the application of social science theories to IPE. As noted, we are conducting a scoping review to map out the IP field at the time of writing, which has delineated three types of IP interventions, which we have termed IPE, IP practice, and IP organisation interventions. Further research will show when it is most effective to use which intervention or combinations of them, in relation to learners' stage of development, the context, the outcomes desired, and other important factors.

While research has shown how IPE can improve IP collaboration and health care, it is but one factor amongst many. As our synthesis of systematic reviews showed, medical students and physicians are participants whose involvement is essential if knowledge gained from IPE is to be translated into practice. Policy makers in various countries are emphasising that physicians need to be effective collaborators and communicators; IPE is a key strategy to developing those characteristics. As evidence accumulates, we will know better how IPE can most effectively be implemented, and how its implementation influences physicians' behaviours and clinical outcomes.

Implications for practice

Over three decades' research and experience have shown the value of IPE at both the pre- and post-qualification learning stages. Medical students can benefit from a pre-qualification perspective on the roles of different health care professionals in relation to a particular topic being studied in a classroom and/or placement, while a post-qualification initiative for physicians can address communication issues with other health professionals with whom they work, and support changes in practice. We also have knowledge about different interactive learning methods that can be used in IPE, and about how new technologies can widen the options available. Interactivity is an essential element, but the particular method used must depend on the objectives of the programme and available resources. Attention must be given to the composition and size of IP learning groups and good facilitation is needed. Organisational support and leadership are critical to address the extensive logistic and resource issues associated with IPE, to support faculty development, and to develop a culture that endorses IPE, and facilitates knowledge translation into health care settings. Leadership from medical schools, associations, and organisations is essential to encourage and support medical students and practitioners to engage fully in IPE programmes.

References

Allport G: *The nature of prejudice,* Reading, MA, 1979, Addison-Wesley.

Anderson E, Thorpe L, Heney D, et al: Medical students benefit from learning about patient safety in an interprofessional team, *Med Educ* 43(6):542–552, 2009.

Barr H, Koppel I, Reeves S, et al: *Effective interprofessional education: argument, assumption and evidence,* Oxford, 2005, Blackwell.

Bion WR: *Experiences in groups and other papers,* London, 1961, Tavistock Publications.

Challis L, Fuller S, Henwood M, et al: *Joint approaches to social policy,* Cambridge, 1988, Cambridge University.

Coster S, Norman I, Murrells T, et al: Interprofessional attitudes amongst undergraduate students in the health professions: a longitudinal questionnaire survey, *Int J Nurs Stud* 45(11):1667–1681, 2008.

Department of Health : *A health service of all the talents: developing the NHS workforce,* London, 2000, HMSO.

Engeström Y, Engeström R, Vahaaho T: When the center does not hold: the importance of knotworking. In Chaklin S, Hedegaard M, Jensen UJ, editors: *Activity theory and social practice,* Aarhus, 1999, Aarhus University Press.

Foucault M: *The archeology of knowledge,* London, 1972, Tavistock.

Freeth D, Ayida G, Berridge EJ, et al: Multidisciplinary obstetric simulated emergency scenarios (MOSES): promoting patient safety in obstetrics with teamwork-focused interprofessional simulations, *J Contin Educ Health Prof* 29(2): 98–104, 2009.

Friedson E: *Professional dominance: the social structure of medical care,* New York, 1970, Aldine.

Goldman J, Meuser J, Lawrie L, et-al: Development and implementation of primary care interprofessional protocols, *J Interprof Care* 24(6), 2010.

Koppel I: *Autonomy eroded? Changing discourses in the education of health and community care professionals,* University of London, 2003, Unpublished PhD Thesis.

Kvarnstrom S: Difficulties in collaboration: a critical incident study of interprofessional healthcare teamwork, *J Interprof Care* 22(2): 191–203, 2008.

Lessa I: Discursive struggles within social welfare: restaging teen motherhood, *Br J Social Work* 36(2): 283–298, 2006.

Mann KV, Mcfetridge-Durdle J, Martin-Misener R, et al: Interprofessional education for students of the health professions: the "Seamless Care" model, *J Interprof Care* 23:224–233, 2009.

Pecukonis E, Doyle O, Bliss DL: Reducing barriers to interprofessional training: promoting interprofessional cultural competence, *J Interprof Care* 22:417–428, 2008.

Pollard K: Student engagement in interprofessional working in practice placement settings, *J Clin Nurs* 18(20):2846–2856, 2009.

Rees D, Johnson R: All together now? Staff views and experiences of a pre-qualifying interprofessional curriculum, *J Interprof Care* 21(5): 543–555, 2007.

Reeves S: *Developing and delivering practice-based interprofessional education,* Munich, 2008, VDM publications.

Reeves S, Goldman J, Burton A, et al: Knowledge transfer and exchange in interprofessional education: synthesizing the evidence to foster evidence-based decision-making, [online] Available at www.cihc.ca Accessed July 6, 2009, 2008.

Rudland J, Mires G: Characteristics of doctors and nurses as perceived by students entering medical school: implications for shared teaching, *Med Educ* 39(5):448–455, 2005.

Senge PM: *The fifth discipline the art and practice of the learning organization,* ed 1, New York, NY, 1990, Doubleday/Currency.

Steinert Y: Learning together to teach together: interprofessional education and faculty development, *J Interprof Care* 19(Suppl 1):60–75, 2005.

Stokes J: Problems in multidisciplinary teams: the unconscious at work, *J Social Work Practice* http://www.informaworld.com/smpp/title~db=all~content=t713436417~tab=issueslist~branches=8-v8; 8(2): 161–167, 1994.

Strauss A: *Negotiations: varieties, contexts, processes and social order,* San Francisco, 1978, Jossey-Bass.

The Joint Commission: Sentinel Event Alert: Preventing infant death and injury during delivery, [online] Available at: www.aap.org/nrp/simulation/JCAHOSentinelEvent.pdf [Accessed July 6, 2009], 2004.

Von Bertalanffy L: *General systems theory*, London, 1971, Allen Lane/Penguin.

Wilhelmsson M, Pelling S, Ludvigsson J, et al: Twenty years experience of interprofessional education in Linköping – ground-breaking and sustainable, *J Interprof Care* 23(2): 121–133, 2009.

Williams RG, Silverman R, Schwind C, et al: Surgeon information transfer and communication: factors affecting quality and efficiency of inpatient care, *Ann Surg* 245:159–169, 2007.

World Health Organisation : *Continuing education of health personnel*, Copenhagen, 1976, WHO Regional Office for Europe.

Wright A, Lindqvist S: The development, outline and evaluation of the second level of an interprofessional learning programme-listening to the students, *J Interprof Care* 22:475–487, 2008.

Further reading

American Interprofessional Health Collaborative (AIHC): The AIHC offers a venue for health and social professions based in the USA to share information, mentor and support one another as they provide the leadership to influence system change with the implementation of interprofessional education and practice at their individual institutions and organisations. Available at: http://blog.lib.umn.edu/cipe/aihc/ [Accessed November 2009].

Australasian Interprofessional Practice and Education Network (AIPPEN): AIPPEN aims to provide a forum for sharing of information, networks, and experiences in the area of interprofessional practice and education in health and social care contexts across Australia and New Zealand. Available at: http://www.aippen.net/ [Accessed November 2009].

Canadian Interprofessional Health Collaborative (CIHC): The CIHC is a Canadian national organisation that provides health providers, teams, and organisations with the resources and tools needed to apply an interprofessional, patient-centred, and collaborative approach to health care. CIHC's core activities are designed to make them the 'go to' resource for these organisations when they require expert advice, knowledge or information on interprofessional collaboration. Available at: www.cihc.ca [Accessed November 2009].

Centre For The Advancement Of Interprofessional Education (CAIPE): CAIPE, based in the UK, is dedicated to the promotion and development of interprofessional education with and through its individual and corporate members, in collaboration with like-minded organisations in the UK and overseas. It provides information and advice through its website, bulletins, papers, and outlets provided by others, and has a close association with the *Journal of Interprofessional Care*. Available at: www.caipe.org.uk [Accessed November 2009].

European IPE Network (EIPEN): EIPEN aims to develop and sustain a network in the European Union to share and develop effective interprofessional vocational training curricula, methods, and materials for improving collaborative practice and multi-agency working in health and social care. Available at: www.eipen.org [Accessed November 2009].

Journal of Interprofessional Care: The *Journal of Interprofessional Care* is the vehicle for worldwide dissemination of experience, policy, research evidence, and theoretical and value perspectives informing collaboration in education, practice, and research between medicine, nursing, veterinary science, allied health, public health, social care, and related professions to improve health status and quality of care for individuals, families, and communities. Available at: http://informahealthcare.com/jic [Accessed November 2009].

Patient involvement in health professional education

5

Angela Towle   William Godolphin

CHAPTER CONTENTS

ABC

Glossary

Cooperative enquiry (also known as collaborative inquiry) Research 'with' rather than 'on' people, which emphasises that all active participants are fully involved in research decisions as co-researchers.

Continuous professional development (CPD) The continuing education of fully trained and accredited practitioners.

Expert patient A person with a chronic disease who has the confidence, skills, information, and knowledge to play a central role in the management of his/her health concern and to teach others.

Identity construction Social processes in the training of medical and other health professions students whereby they develop a coherent image of self that distinguishes them from other professionals and lay persons.

Kirkpatrick levels A commonly used framework for the evaluation of educational programmes comprising four levels: Reaction, Learning, Behaviour, and Results.

Senior mentor Older adults in the community who provide medical students with long-term mentorship related to ageing and geriatrics.

Social accountability Defined by the World Health Organisation as the obligation of medical schools 'to direct their education, research, and service activities towards addressing the priority health concerns of the community, region, and/or nation they have a mandate to serve'.

© 2011, Elsevier Ltd.
DOI: 10.1016/B978-0-7020-3522-7.00005-X

Outline

Patients have always been the 'clinical material' for learning medicine, but the role of the patient as teacher has more recently been developed beyond a teaching aid towards more formalised and active participation in the educational process. Many and diverse initiatives have been described in government pronouncements and scholarly activity in the field, including reviews of patient involvement in medical education (Jha et al, 2009; Morgan and Jones, 2009; Wykurz and Kelly, 2002), nurse education (Repper and Breeze, 2007; Warne and McAndrew, 2005), mental health training (Livingston and Cooper, 2004), and social work (Cairney et al, 2006). There has also been an international conference (Farrell et al, 2006).

This chapter explores why that change has occurred and what the benefits and outcomes of active patient involvement are. We identify the factors that need to be considered when involving patients in education and provide examples to illustrate a range of approaches to patient involvement that are being tried in different health professional programmes in different countries, focusing particularly on government policy directives, social accountability, and the role of expert patients. Finally, we identify future directions for educational development and research in this field. The chapter starts by clarifying two major sources of controversy and confusion for anyone who wishes to gain an understanding of the topic: terminology and language, and the spectrum of possible involvement.

Terminology and language

We use the term 'patient', for the sake of brevity, to include people with health problems (service users, clients, consumers, survivors, etc.), their care givers (including carers, parents, and families), and healthy people (community members, citizens, lay people, well women, etc.). We have chosen to use the term 'patient' as our umbrella term because it is the most commonly recognised word, though the choice is a controversial one. 'Patients' are associated with passivity and many people do not like to be labelled in that way. It also defines the person as being ill; in the context of health professions education, there are many healthy people who contribute important experiences, such as parents of children with disabilities, seniors,

refugees, and people from different ethnic groups. The term 'lay' may be more inclusive but, when contrasted with its opposite – 'professional' – it dismisses the expertise of non-professionals, defines them by what they are *not* (i.e. professionals), and, in our experience, is universally unpopular, even among people who cannot agree on any other term.

The most commonly accepted term in the United Kingdom is 'user' or more specifically 'service user', especially in professions other than medicine. However, a health practitioner in North America is more likely to connect the term with illicit drug use. There are even those in the United Kingdom who consider the term 'service user' as passive and not inclusive of people who cannot or do not access services. It also follows that the counterpart to a service user is a 'service provider', which implies a technical kind of interaction that detracts from the provision of more holistic, relationship-centred care. As many of the service users involved in education in the United Kingdom also have carers who play an important role, the collective term 'service user and carer' is frequently used. 'Carer' is a less controversial term though it is not familiar in North America, where the term 'caregiver' is used.

Other words that appear in the literature include 'consumer' or 'client', but these have overtones of health care as a market and, although favoured in some countries and professions, these terms are generally not used in medical education. The words people use to think of themselves in relation to the health care system vary according to the type of practitioner they are consulting, their condition, and the stage of their illness. Some people who have battled against cancer or mental illness, for example, prefer to call themselves 'survivors'. The lack of agreed terminology is important on several levels: strong emotions generated by language and labels can create barriers to communication and partnership; the plethora of terms complicates scholarly activity by making it difficult to search the literature; and it makes writing and talking about the topic cumbersome.

The other source of confusion in the area of terminology is the large number of names used to refer to those patients who are actively involved in health professions education. Patients may be involved as teachers, educators, instructors, teaching associates, professional patients, mentors, or partners. When we reviewed the titles used to describe well women who are trained to teach intimate examinations (pelvic and/or breast), we found a total of 18 different titles used in 41 different papers in the literature. The meanings of terms are not always consistent: at one institution they may be called 'standardised patients' because they teach in a standardised way but the same role may be designated 'teaching associate' at another institution. This makes good literature search difficult and is one reason why reviews of the literature using similar but not identical inclusion criteria may miss many relevant papers.

Spectrum of involvement

Patient involvement occurs throughout the continuum from undergraduate education (pre-registration), postgraduate or specialist education, continuous professional development (CPD), and in-service training, although the majority of reported initiatives occur in undergraduate courses or in the postgraduate training of mental health professionals (predominantly non-psychiatrists such as nurses and counselling psychologists). Patients can actively contribute to different aspects of the educational process. Direct involvement in curriculum delivery is the commonest role; students may learn from people who come into the classroom to talk about their experiences of, say, living with an addiction, HIV/AIDS, or a disabled child. They may also learn from patient educators, who teach clinical skills. Health professionals at all stages learn informally from patients in clinical settings (see below). Patient organisations may contribute to, or lead, CPD activities on specialised topics such as fetal alcohol syndrome and there may be public members on committees that plan CPD (British Medical Association, 2008). The most comprehensive list of potential roles is provided by Tew et al (2004), who give examples of patient involvement in

- direct delivery of teaching and learning
- curriculum and course planning
- programme management
- recruitment and selection of students
- practice learning
- student assessment
- course evaluation
- patients joining courses as participants.

The diversity of educational initiatives in which patients are actively involved demands a classification scheme. Without such a framework there is no agreed way in which authors can characterise the role of patients in their initiatives, which makes scholarly communication difficult and comparative evaluation or systematic reviews impossible. It is often difficult to find out from published work exactly what the patient's role was in the educational programme described, especially the degree to which patients were *actively* involved and the degree to which they participated in decision making. For example, early patient or community contact in medical school often consists of an attachment to a patient with a chronic illness, a pregnant woman, a family, or a community agency; in some cases the patient, family, or community agency may be explicitly identified as a teacher or mentor, whereas in other cases their role is simply to be interviewed. The expected learning outcomes would be quite different for those two different roles.

There are two useful classification schemes: the Cambridge framework developed by Spencer et al (2000), which describes the attributes of educational settings that shape learner–patient encounters, including Who? (the patient's culture), How? (a passive vs. an active role), What? (a general vs. a specific problem), and Where? (community vs. hospital); and the Ladder of Involvement described by Tew et al (2004), which identifies five levels of involvement – Level 1: No involvement, Level 2: Limited involvement, Level 3: Growing involvement, Level 4: Collaboration, and Level 5: Partnership. More recently, we combined both of these models into a Spectrum of Involvement tool (Towle et al, 2010). Our proposed taxonomy includes six main attributes:

- The degree to which the patient is actively involved in the learning encounter;
- The duration of contact with the learner;
- The degree of autonomy the patient has during the encounter;
- The extent of training the patient has had;
- The degree to which the patient is involved in planning the encounter and overall curriculum;
- The extent of institutional commitment to patient involvement in education.

We recognise that these categories, rather than being discrete entities, overlap, and the taxonomy represents a continuum of involvement.

Why involve patients?

Depending on the health profession, country, and time, there are many reasons why health professional educators choose to involve patients actively. We have chosen three different clusters of reasons to discuss in detail. These clusters are not mutually exclusive but each is rooted in a different discourse (see Chapter 3). It is important to know that the movement to involve patients actively in the education of health professionals is based more on the power of these rationales than on robust evidence of beneficial educational outcomes at the time of writing.

Public and patient involvement in health care: government and professional policy directives

The importance of public and patient involvement in health care is recognised in many countries. Members of the public are frequently consulted about health care services, health policy, and research as part of a growing consumerist model of health care. UK government policy has placed public and individual patients at the centre of health care over the past 20 years. Successive policy documents have emphasised a patient-led National Health Service based on choice, participation, and partnerships. It is within this context that the government has also made clear its expectations that service users will be involved in all publicly funded health and social care research and, more recently, that service users and carers should be involved in the education and training of health professionals.

This policy directive has been taken up by accrediting bodies in the United Kingdom. 'Skills for Health', the body that is responsible for the quality assurance of all health professional programmes in the United Kingdom, except medicine, requires evidence of patient involvement in education. The Nursing and Midwifery Council requires universities to involve a service user as a panel member during the approval process for pre-registration nursing programmes. The General Medical Council does not have the same explicit requirements for patient–public involvement, although it requires data on the quality of medical education programmes to include feedback from patients (GMC, 2009).

The most significant activity has been in the field of mental health, originally in mental health nursing, extended more recently to social work, psychiatry, and clinical psychology. The National Service Framework for Mental Health published by the UK Department of Health in 1999 proposed that 'service users should be involved in planning, providing, and evaluating education and training' (a recommendation that

had been made in relation to mental health nursing in a 1994 Department of Health review). In 2006, the Department of Health stated that higher education institutions should 'involve service users and carers in every aspect of education including recruitment, curriculum planning, teaching, and student assessment'. In some training programmes such as mental health or social work, practitioners have specific courses on 'user involvement' that include users in curriculum development or as teachers.

The 'user' discourse raises interesting questions about ideology, articulated mainly in the areas of health and social care, but also in research (Cowden and Singh, 2007). The user movement has given service users a voice in decision making, particularly in the areas of disability and mental health; recognition of the importance of their lived experiences has given them roles as educators, researchers, and consultants. Government policy, however, has framed user involvement within a consumerist model of improving the product through market testing and consumer feedback (manager-led/users as consultants) rather than a user-led, liberational model, where users are empowered to develop new kinds of services, research, or education. Health professionals are urged to consult about the quality of services but find that service users' views vary between individual patients, patient groups, and patient representatives, and also between those with radical and non-radical views. Under those circumstances, it is difficult to select the 'right' patients (Williamson, 2007). These groups bring different knowledge and expertise, so finding representatives from each of them is as relevant to health professions education as to health services.

UK policy directives have resulted in a large number of initiatives such that the United Kingdom leads in institutionalising patient involvement in education. No other country has embedded service user involvement in health and social care so deeply into its policies and structures and, by extension, the education of health professionals.

Irrespective of national government policy, however, almost all health professions espouse a version of patient-centred care in their particular good practice model, which involves patients in decision making, with a focus on individual people's preferences, life circumstances, and experience of illness. There is at least a theoretical link between patient involvement in education, patient involvement in care, and improved health outcomes; Figure 5.1 shows how the model might apply in an interprofessional context (see Chapter 4). Bleakley and Bligh (2008),

Figure 5.1 • The interprofessional continuum: education and service delivery systems.

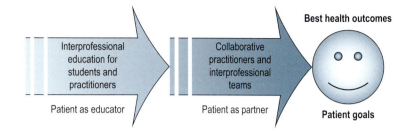

however, have pointed out that patient-centredness is still typically framed as a set of values and virtues learnt from doctors as role models, reinforced through structured educational input from medical educators, and, paradoxically, not from patients.

Social accountability of higher education institutions: the moral imperative

The World Health Organisation (WHO) has defined the social accountability of medical schools as 'The obligation to direct their education, research, and service activities towards addressing the priority health concerns of the community, region, and/or nation they have a mandate to serve. The priority health concerns are to be identified jointly by governments, health care organisations, health professionals, and the public'.

Social accountability is important because good education for health does not necessarily provide a nation with good health; there are many other factors involved such as the career choices of graduates, incentives and rewards for primary health care, and health policy. Translation of good education into good health requires the collaboration of key stakeholder groups. The framework for social accountability developed by the WHO, illustrated by the partnership pentagram (see Figure 5.2), has a central core reflecting a health system that meets human needs. Five partners have to respond to those needs – policy makers, health managers, health professions, communities, and academic institutions – and complex relationships between the stakeholders who serve and are served by the health care system must be managed for health needs to be met.

The Association of Faculties of Medicine of Canada (AFMC), influential in setting the direction for Canadian medical education, has adopted the

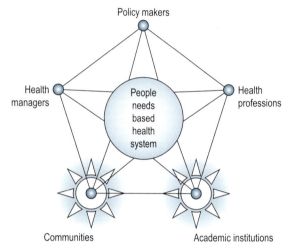

Figure 5.2 • Partnership pentagram for social responsibility (from Boelen, 2000, with permission).

WHO definition as its mandate for social accountability and the focus for its unifying vision for academic medicine in the country. Central to the AFMC vision was the creation of a 'Partners Forum' with representatives of key stakeholder groups, including the public. The concept of community engagement signals recognition by academic institutions of the importance of partnerships with the communities they serve. The Community Campus Partnerships for Health (CCPH), primarily a US organisation originating from a campaign to improve health care for those who need it most, has as its mission the promotion of health (broadly defined) through partnerships between communities and higher educational institutions. Many of the community engagement initiatives in the United States come from the moral imperative to address health disparities, especially by engaging large sectors of the population who do not have access to good health care. One of the major educational activities fostered by CCPH has been community-based service learning. Although active patient or community involvement is not in itself a prerequisite for service learning activities, people in the community play a variety of roles along the spectrum of involvement, from passive recipients of care (the classic provider–patient relationship), to facilitators of reflection seminars, mentors, and assessors of students. The provision of opportunities for service learning has recently been adopted as an accreditation standard for North American medical schools. Other patient involvement initiatives in the United States (e.g. the senior mentor programmes described below) have their origin in the need to improve health care for the underserved (in this case elderly people) through promoting more positive attitudes towards these populations among medical students.

The expert patient: enrichment of education

In the first published review of patients as active teachers in medical education, Wykurz and Kelly (2002) identified 23 studies that demonstrated the diversity of expertise patients brought to their teaching roles. The recognition of patients as experts comes in part from the concept of encounters between professionals and patients as 'meetings of experts', first elaborated by Tuckett et al (1985). From that point of view, not only do health professionals bring (biomedical) expertise but also patients bring expertise of their personal and cultural background and their experiences of living with illness or disability. Over the last two decades, educators have tapped into the expertise of patients in order to enrich student education in a variety of ways, providing learning experiences that could not otherwise occur, and broadening curricula from the biomedical model. In some disciplines, the expertise of patients has been used to augment a scarce pool of clinical teachers. Patient–teachers have been shown to create safe learning environments for students to practice clinical skills, especially intimate examinations, and they have been able to provide more in-depth feedback to students than could usually be provided by busy preceptors.

The extent of the expertise patients could offer has not yet been fully explored. At the University of British Columbia, we have worked with patients with mental health problems, arthritis, and epilepsy, and their caregivers, to develop patient-led workshops about a range of diverse topics, including

- living with chronic disease day to day and over time;
- the diversity of illness experiences;
- effects on partners and families;
- physical examination skills;
- diagnostic challenges;
- stigma and stereotyping;
- peer support;
- practical aids to daily living;
- advice about what health professionals can do;
- information about support groups in the community.

Outcomes of patient involvement

The diversity of motivations for involving patients predicts an equally diverse range of outcomes. Many reports in the mental health and social work education literature, for example, focus on service users' and carers' experiences of interacting with institutions of higher education, the outcomes of interest being more to do with user empowerment than student learning. The literature on patient involvement in general is marked by a lack of clear and measurable outcomes; most studies have been descriptive and few interventions rigorously evaluated. Most descriptions provide insufficient detail about what was done and few use rich, qualitative or mixed methodologies. Experimental studies give inadequate information about the interventions and research designs; initiatives are usually described only once in the literature, soon after implementation (often of a pilot project) along with preliminary evaluation data, usually student satisfaction and patient views. Typically, evaluation of short-term outcomes for a small subset of initiatives is reported (primarily in clinical skills teaching), but few such studies have had rigorous experimental designs.

A review by Morgan and Jones (2009), although limited to studies from the United Kingdom, provides a good summary of the state of the art. Most of the 41 papers they reviewed included some formal evaluation except for those that described patient involvement in curriculum design; in these studies, there were no attempts to demonstrate an impact on students who subsequently took the courses in question. Studies that included an evaluation generally captured the views of students and patients but not of the professional teachers. Using Kirkpatrick's four-level model of evaluation (Kirkpatrick, 1996), four papers reported evaluation data at Level 2 (changes in measured attitudes, skills, and knowledge), one at Level 3 (change in behaviour), and one at Level 4 (benefit to service users). With respect to Level 1 outcomes (reaction), overall student perceptions of patient involvement were generally positive; concerns that were expressed related largely to interaction with patients who had mental illnesses. Overall benefits for patients were reported, with no negative effects. Morgan and Jones (2009) conclude that 'despite a limited and weak traditional evidence base for impact on students' knowledge and practice, both students and service users identify benefits from engagement'.

Approaches to involving patients in education

Several 'good practice' guides that provide useful information have been produced in the United Kingdom for education in mental health care (Tew et al, 2004); clinical psychology (British Psychological Society, 2008); and social work (Ager et al, 2005; Levin, 2004). The INVOLVE guides, designed to promote patient involvement in health research, have information relevant to higher education (http://www.invo.org.uk). No such 'how to' resources yet exist for medical education but the British Medical Association (2008) has published some useful guidelines, especially on the important topic of ethics, including confidentiality and consent.

Each of these guides organises the key tasks slightly differently but all identify a core set of issues as critical. These include leadership (requires a champion); dedicated funding; recruitment of patients (diversity and representativeness); infrastructure for support, training, and supervision of patients; employment and contracting; payment and expenses; capacity building; and evaluation. They are a good resource for those needing advice about initiating and sustaining involvement. For example, Tew et al (2004) suggest that these activities may be more effectively facilitated by designated support and development workers, as teaching staff are not necessarily the best people to do outreach and capacity building work or to provide support to service users and carers. A network of development workers has been established in the United Kingdom

(the Ducie network), which has published guidelines for higher education institutions (Developers of User and Carers in Education, 2009). This liaison role, also referred to as being a 'culture broker' or 'boundary spanner', is one that many academic institutions have found essential to facilitate partnerships with community-based organisations.

A guide produced by the Social Care Institute for Excellence (Levin, 2004) articulates key practical considerations in 'preparing for participation', paraphrased as follows:

- Everyone who is involved benefits from working on and agreeing with the values and principles of involvement as early as possible in the process of developing partnerships;
- A comprehensive strategy for overall involvement makes it easier to include later new roles where progress may be slower or more complicated;
- Effective participation involves patients, academic staff, administrators, students, and others working together in new ways – an opportunity for development;
- Resources (people, time, money, and support) are needed to make it work;
- Actively promoting and sustaining participation is a process, not a one-off event. It takes time to build respectful and purposeful relationships and give attention to practicalities.
- Enthusiasm and goodwill are required to make it work; at the start only a small number of participants may be available and willing. Widening participation is a key task.

Often the words involvement, collaboration, and partnership are used interchangeably. Working in true partnership with people from the community, however, brings challenges for health professional educators: there is a large power imbalance; there may be tensions over decisions (e.g. whose objectives); and there may be barriers to communication. Recognising the difficulty of achieving authentic partnerships between academia and the community, the CCPH has developed a set of partnership principles that have been recognised and applied internationally (see Box 5.1).

Approaches to some of these issues are illustrated in the following four examples: three diverse initiatives at one institution that engage service users at different levels of involvement; patient educators who teach clinical skills (musculoskeletal examination), using expert knowledge of their own body; programmes developed to meet a national educational

> ### Box 5.1
>
> ### CCPH core principles of good community-campus partnerships (http://www.ccph.info/)
>
> - Partnerships form to serve a specific purpose and may take on new goals over time;
> - Partners have an agreed-upon mission, values, goals, measurable outcomes, and accountability for the partnership;
> - The relationship between partners is characterised by mutual trust, respect, genuineness, and commitment;
> - The partnership builds on identified strengths and assets but also works to address needs and increase capacity of all partners;
> - The partnership balances power among partners and enables resources among partners to be shared;
> - Partners make clear and open communication on ongoing priority by striving to understand each others'
> - needs and self-interests, and developing a common language;
> - Principles and processes for the partnership are established with the input and agreement of all partners, especially for decision making and conflict resolution;
> - There is feedback among all stakeholders, with the goal of continuously improving the partnership and its outcomes;
> - Partners share the benefits of the partnership's accomplishments;
> - Partnerships can dissolve and need to plan a process for closure.

need (better geriatrics curriculum) in order to meet a health care need (better care for an underserved population); and how to develop a new educational initiative that involves faculty and students from different health programmes and community organisations, and individual patients, as community educators.

Service user and carer participation in education of mental health practitioners

The University of Southampton School of Nursing and Midwifery, United Kingdom, has tried different 'socially inclusive' approaches to engaging service users and, in some cases, carers more fully in the education of mental health practitioners (Lathlean et al, 2006; Simons et al, 2007). The purpose of each project is to develop and evaluate different aspects of 'good practice' in which participants are active agents of change in processes of research and education. Each initiative represents movement on a continuum of participation from service users as passive recipients to service users as collaborators and co-researchers, and is grounded in theory.

The first initiative was a service user and carer reference group (i.e. users' role is collaborative and consultative). In existence for over 5 years, its aim was to share a range of views and knowledge of mental health matters and provide advice to guide the university in the development of its programmes. Challenges included the need to nurture participation, which requires energy, enthusiasm, commitment,

and sufficient funding. The benefits were the value of having established members with different contributions to make, including service users, carers, and students. They identified the group as a 'culture carrier', that is a shared belief in the value of participation as an essential contributing factor to organisational change towards more user-centred services.

The second was the service user academic initiative: the establishment of a position ('User Academic') in the university, modeled on the consumer academic concept from Australia (i.e. user integrated into the academic institution). The holder of the position was a person with experience of mental illness and mental health services, who was employed as a member of an academic team. An evaluation of the development and practice of the position revealed tangible benefits for students and the wider academic community; most importantly, the User Academic provided a powerful role model for students and challenged elitist attitudes by confronting notions of expertise. However, because of mixed expectations of the position and unintended discriminatory behaviour, the role did not become integrated into the team and key sources of support were unavailable.

The third initiative was the participation of mental health service users in the clinical practice decisions of mental health students in training, based on the theories of anti-oppressive practice, contact theory, and moral development. An emancipatory research design, co-operative inquiry, was used to study how service users could be more effectively engaged in students' clinical decision making (Tee et al, 2005). One of the most significant outcomes was to reveal how detached current concepts and theories of mental health, including the language used, could be from the day-to-day experience of people using services.

Arthritis educators

With the exception of clinical teaching associate programmes (teaching intimate examinations), the arthritis educator programme is unique as a long-lasting programme (the first paper was published in 1982), which has become institutionalised and widespread. It started in the United States as a development of the simulated patient concept but involved 'real' patient instructors with arthritis who were trained to teach the musculoskeletal examination through an intensive structured and standardised training programme (Gruppen et al, 1996). It spread through a cascade model to other schools in the United States and to Canada and Australia, thence to several other countries, as well as more recently appearing, apparently independently, in Switzerland and the United Kingdom. Long-term stable funding for the programme has come largely from pharmaceutical companies.

The patients are variously referred to as patient instructors, patient partners, patient educators, and arthritis educators. They are trained by physicians within the biomedical model; there is a strong emphasis on anatomy and the reliable assessment of the performance of the joint examination using a standardised checklist. The autonomy of the patient as educator is limited but patients also teach about psychosocial issues and the experience of living with arthritis in some programmes (Gruppen et al, 1996). The learners are generally medical students in the pre-clinical years, but some programmes teach clinical-level students or postgraduates and in some programmes the arthritis educators teach students from multiple programmes including physical therapy.

Because of differences in programme design and evaluation methods, it is difficult to draw strong conclusions about the outcomes of such programmes. In general, student satisfaction is high, although in comparative studies students tend to prefer being taught by specialists rather than by patients. Some programmes employ arthritis educators because of a shortage of specialists (rheumatologists). Students taught by patients generally have been shown to have examination skills equivalent to those of students taught by specialist physicians. Patient satisfaction is high and no adverse effects of being a patient teacher have been noted.

Senior mentor programmes

Senior mentor programmes (SMPs) have been developed by a number of medical schools in the United States (see e.g. Stewart and Alford, 2006) to meet the need for a better curriculum in geriatrics, including knowledge, skills, and attitudes (to counter ageism).

There are many different models but all have elements in common. Most SMPs are connected with an established 'doctoring' course that typically includes practical experience such as learning communication skills, sessions on professionalism (including ethics), and clinical reasoning, as well as contact with individual patients or populations. SMPs use older adults either directly as teachers or as 'sensitisers' to particular issues of importance to the medical care of elderly people. The relationship between student and senior is modelled on a learning relationship with mentors as teachers, rather than on a provider–patient relationship model. The programmes are therefore linked to the wider 'expert patient' movement in medical education; in this case the mentors' expertise is in ageing.

The programmes have been integrated into medical school curricula, which recruit seniors who are basically well, living in the community, and without cognitive problems; in this way, students interact with people who are 'ageing well' physically and mentally. Seniors are recruited through medical practices or community agencies, but recruitment of a diverse ethnic and socio-economic pool is a challenge.

The relationship that develops between student and mentor is at the heart of the programme and may include social events beyond academic activities. As both students and mentors are placed in new roles, programme staff may need to assist both parties to clarify and redefine their changing roles over time: students' roles change as they progress through the programme from being a friend to, for example, being asked to conduct a physical examination; mentors may develop health problems during the course of their relationship with students. In the SMPs that span several years, the relationship that develops can be very strong and a closing ceremony of some kind is important.

Community partnerships for interprofessional education

Our initiative at the University of British Columbia, 'Community Partnerships for Health Professional Education', aims to create sustainable partnerships with patient organisations that result in community-led educational initiatives for health professional students (Towle et al, 2009). Using a participatory design approach, community members, faculty, and students collaboratively develop, pilot, and evaluate interprofessional workshops led by community educators. Student and faculty collaborators come from medicine, nursing, pharmacy, occupational therapy, physical therapy, social work, human kinetics, and speech–language pathology. Community educators have been recruited through patient organisations, advertisements, and word of mouth.

The direction and evaluation of the project is overseen by an advisory board of students, faculty, and community members (representatives from patient support and advocacy organisations as well as individual patients). The advisory board has defined the mission, vision and goals, membership of the board, evaluation framework for the workshops, and policies for presentation and dissemination of the work. Evaluation methods include pre-workshop survey (student expectations); post-workshop survey (student learning); follow-up interviews, and focus groups with faculty, community educators, and students; and reflective journals maintained by students.

Reported student learning includes

- increased understanding of the effects of disease on quality of life and day-to-day living (new perspectives not based on pathology alone);
- improved knowledge of impact on families and significant others;
- importance of community resources and services reinforced.

With respect to interprofessional education (IPE), students learnt *with* each other and *about* each other by listening to each other's questions at all workshops. There were specific IPE activities at three workshops so students could learn *from* and *about* each other during small breakout groups and through working on a case study together. Although students were keen to learn about interprofessional care, this was not a high priority for the community teachers.

Community teachers found the experience to be positive:

- They were empowered through participation in the education of future health care providers;
- Participation resulted in positive health outcomes;

- They learnt from fellow community educators and from students.

Learning from patients in clinical settings

Although the formal 'patient as educator' roles described above are increasing in number, the majority of health professional contacts with patients still occur in clinical settings (hospital wards, clinics, family physician offices), where patients' main focus is on receiving health care. In those situations, patients may be too ill, disempowered, or focused on health care procedures to be willing or able to take on the additional role of a teacher in any formal way. The dynamics are most often between the student(s) and the clinical teacher, with the patient only peripherally involved. As Bleakley and Bligh (2008) point out, 'the main focus of the educational process, even where it is ostensibly based "around" the patient, tends to gain meaning and legitimacy only in the interaction between the student and the doctor (as educator)'. They call for a reorientation of the relationship between patient, student, and teacher to enhance collaboration between the student and the patient (for 'collaborative knowledge production') with the expert doctor as a resource. The work by Ashley et al (2008) provides some practical ways of achieving this 'patient-based curriculum' through a series of recommendations for supervising a medical student in an outpatient clinic or surgery.

The perceptions of patients about their role in student education in the clinical setting are more varied than in the studies in which patients are clearly recruited to be educators. Stockhausen's (2009) patients were 'experience brokers', who mediated and observed teaching and learning to care between nursing students and experienced preceptors, while also becoming participants in learning to care. Ashley et al (2008) found that the dynamics between student and patient were characterised by two themes, identification and participation; patients identified with students and students wanted to participate in the care of patients. McLachlan et al (2009) found that involvement in students' education was usually described by patients as 'ordinary', having little effect on them. There are also negative experiences. Although less commonly reported now, there are still official and anecdotal reports of patients who were uninformed or unwilling participants in the educational process and were unaware that an invasive procedure would be done by a novice student or that students would be performing pelvic examinations while they were anaesthetised for surgery. We have found, through interviews with faculty, health professional students, and patient educators, the following challenges to patient participation in student learning in the clinical setting:

Faculty

- Unpredictability of teaching encounters
- Balancing learning objectives with patient needs and safety
- Getting informed consent

Students

- Getting informed consent
- Faking it – students feeling under pressure to fake their level of experience when examining a patient or doing a procedure

- Theory and practice disjoint – what students are taught in class is not always modelled for them in practice

Patients

- Disrespectful teachers
- Physical and emotional discomfort

Working with the same groups, we have developed a set of guidelines for engaging patients as active teachers in the clinical setting (see Box 5.2).

Implications for practice

Theory

Very little of the literature about patients' involvement in education is informed by explanatory theory. Two exceptions are papers by Katz et al (2000) and Rees et al (2007), which take a social science

---

 ### Box 5.2

Guidelines for engaging patients as teachers

Identify patient's expertise
- Establish patient's prior experience;
- Identify patient's area(s) of knowledge/expertise (e.g. knowledge about procedure, condition, or lived experience);
- Determine which expertise fits with the student's learning objectives.

Informed consent
- Ensure patient's consent before student enters room;
- Give patient the option to say: 'Not today';
- Give patient options for level of involvement in teaching.

Prepare patient for teaching role
- Help patient to see how they can contribute (e.g. note their expertise);
- Tell patient about student's level of experience;
- Describe student's learning objectives;
- Ask patient to give feedback to student.

Prepare student
- Review case with student before entering the room;
- Assess student's level of experience with the problem and comfort with leading the interaction;
- Have student explain steps of the procedure to patient as it is done;

- Instruct student to get input from patient.

Connect student and patient
- Agree on student's level of involvement in the encounter;
- Facilitate interaction between student and patient to enhance their rapport and communication (e.g. patient and student face each other).

Facilitate feedback
- Demonstrate how to give feedback (then invite patient to give feedback);
- Ask patient to tell the student what they are feeling;
- Ask patient to describe to student what has worked or not worked for them in the past and this time;
- Provide options for giving feedback (e.g. verbal, written, suggestion box).

Closure
- Thank patient and validate their contribution to the student's learning;
- Validate patient's experience;
- Ask student to give feedback on the interaction and validate that experience;
- Acknowledge individual preferences of patient.

perspective to explore issues on how students learn 'with' rather than just 'about' patients. Bleakley and Bligh (2008) have proposed a theoretical model of collaborative knowledge production based on theories of text, identity construction, and work-based learning in which the prime locus for knowledge production is the student's reading of the patient's condition in collaboration with the patient. These examples provide glimpses of how the active involvement of patients could provide a new educational paradigm in which students, teachers, and patients can create new knowledge and novel solutions to health care problems by learning together.

research foci – antecedent variables, structures, processes, and outcomes – and given examples of needed enquiry in each category. For example, what are the drivers of patient involvement in health professional education, including external, institutional, faculty, and patient factors? (antecedent variables); what effect does the setting (e.g. patient's home, classroom, or clinic) have on learning? (structural elements); what are the meanings that involvement has for patients and how do these change? (processes); finally, what factors result in sustainable 'patient as educator' programmes and what are the successful models that can be replicated? (outcomes).

Research

There is a need for good-quality outcome studies with rigorous experimental designs, especially ones that investigate long-term outcomes. Most initiatives are described only once in the literature, usually at the end of a small-scale pilot or an early implementation phase. There are no studies of long-term outcomes or sustainability. Many initiatives do not last but the reasons why some become embedded within an institution while others fade away are not understood. Towle et al (2010) have identified four

Practice

There is a need for coordinated and sustainable programmes of patient involvement. Most initiatives described in the literature are single educational experiences for a specific group of learners. If education is to be patient-centred, we must move from these one-off experiences to coordinated and sustained programmes of development of a patient involvement curriculum and authentic partnerships at an institutional level.

References

Ager W, Dow J, Ferguson I, et al: *Service user and carer involvement in social work education: good practice guidelines*, 2005, Scottish Institute for Excellence in Social Work Education (now the Institute for Research and Innovation in Social Services, Glasgow, Scotland).

Ashley P, Rhodes N, Sari-Kouzel H, et al: 'They've all got to learn'. Medical students' learning from patients in ambulatory (outpatient and general practice) consultations, *Med Teach* 31:e24–e31, 2008.

Bleakley A, Bligh J: Students learning from patients: let's get real in medical education, *Adv Health Sci Educ* 13:89–107, 2008.

Boelen C: *Towards unity for health*, Geneva, 2000, Challenges and Opportunities for Partnership in Health Development, World Health Organization.

British Medical Association, Medical Education Subcommittee: *Role of the patient in medical education*, 2008. Available at: www.bma.org.uk. Accessed November 29, 2009.

British Psychological Society Division of Clinical Psychology: *Good practice guidelines: service user and carer involvement within clinical psychology training*, 2008. Available at: www.bps.org.uk. Accessed November 29, 2009.

Cairney J, Chettle K, Clark M, et al: Theme issue on involvement of service users in social work education, *Social Work Educ* 25(4):315–430, 2006.

Cowden S, Singh G: The 'user': friend, foe or fetish? a critical exploration of user involvement in health and social care, *Crit Soc Policy* 27:5–23, 2007.

Developers of User and Carer Involvement in Education: *Involving service users and carers in education: the development worker role*, United Kingdom, 2009, Higher Education Academy/Mental Health in Higher Education. Available at: http://www.mhhe.heacademy.ac.uk/silo/files/ducie-guidelines.pdf. Accessed November 29, 2009.

Farrell C, Towle A, Godolphin W: *Where's the patient's voice in health professional education?* Vancouver, Canada, 2006, Division of Health Care Communication, University of British Columbia.

General Medical Council : *Tomorrow's doctors*, London, 2009, GMC.

Gruppen LD, Branch VK, Laing TJ: The use of trained patient educators with rheumatoid arthritis to teach medical students, *Arthritis Care Res* 9:302–308, 1996.

Jha V, Quinton ND, Bekker HL, et al: Strategies and interventions for the involvement of real patients in medical education: a systematic review, *Med Educ* 43:10–20, 2009.

Katz AM, Conant JL, Inui TS, et al: A council of elders: creating a multi-voiced dialogue in a community of care, *Soc Sci Med* 50:851–860, 2000.

Kirkpatrick D: Revisiting Kirkpatrick's four-level model, *Train Dev* 50(1): 54–59, 1996.

Lathlean J, Burgess A, Coldham T, et al: Experiences of service user and carer participation in health care education, *Nurse Educ Today* 26:732–737, 2006.

Levin E: *Involving service users and carers in social work education*, 2004, Social Care Institute for Excellence, London, UK. Resource Guide No 2. Available at: www.scie.org.uk. Accessed November 29, 2009.

Livingston G, Cooper C: "User and carer involvement in mental health training, *Adv Psychiatr Treat* 10(2):85–92, 2004.

McLachlan E, Wenger E, King N, et al: *Patients' sense of identity in medical education, Phenomenological analysis,* 2009, Poster presentation at Association for Medical Education in Europe (AMEE), Barcelano, Viguera Editors SL, *Educacíon Médica* 12(suppl 2):S132, 2009.

Morgan A, Jones D: Perceptions of service user and carer involvement in healthcare education and impact on students' knowledge and practice: a literature review, *Med Teach* 31:82–95, 2009.

Rees CE, Knight LV, Wilkinson CE: "User involvement is a sine qua non, almost, in medical education": learning with rather than just about health and social care service users, *Adv Health Sci Educ* 12:359–390, 2007.

Repper J, Breeze J: User and carer involvement in the training and education of health professionals: a review of the literature, *Int J Nurs Stud* 44:511–519, 2007.

Simons L, Tee S, Lathlean J, et al: A socially inclusive approach to user participation in higher education, *J Adv Nurs* 58:246–255, 2007.

Spencer J, Blackmore D, Heard S, et al: Patient-oriented learning: a review of the role of the patient in the education of medical students, *Med Educ* 34:851–857, 2000.

Stewart T, Alford CL: Older adults in medical education – senior mentor programmes in US medical schools, *Gerontol Geriatr Educ* 27:3–10, 2006.

Stockhausen LJ: The patient as experience broker in clinical learning, *Nurse Educ Pract* 9:184–189, 2009.

Tee S, Coldham T: with Student Nurses: *Students and service users learning together: co-operative inquiry and its implications for curriculum development*, United Kingdom, 2005, Mental Health in Higher Education, UK Case Study. Available at: http://www.mhhe.heacademy.ac.uk/resources/-case-study-14/. Accessed November 29, 2009.

Tew J, Gell C, Foster S: *Learning from experience. Involving service users and carers in mental health education and training*, United Kingdom, 2004, Higher Education Academy/National Institute for Mental Health in England/Trent Workforce Development Confederation.

Towle A, Creak S, Kline C, et al: Community partnerships for interprofessional education, Abstracts of the Canadian Conference on Medical Education, Edmonton, Alberta, Canada, May 2–6, 2009, *Med Educ* 43(suppl 1):11–12, 2009.

Towle A, Bainbridge L, Godolphin W, et al: Active patient involvement in the education of health professionals, *Med Educ* 44:64–74, 2010.

Tuckett D, Boulton M, Olson C, et al: *Meetings between experts. An approach to sharing ideas in medical consultations*, London, UK, 1985, Tavistock Publications Ltd.

Warne T, McAndrew S: *Using patient experience in nurse education*, Basingstoke, 2005, Palgrave Macmillan.

Williamson C: 'How do we find the right patients to consult?', *Qual Prim Care* 15:195–199, 2007.

Wykurz G, Kelly D: Developing the role of patients as teachers: literature review, *Br Med J* 325:818–821, 2002.

Further reading

Towle A, Godolphin W: *Patient involvement in health professional education: a bibliography 1975–2009.*

Division of Health Care Communication, The University of British Columbia Available at: http://www.chd.ubc.ca/dhcc/node/67. Accessed November 29, 2009.

Curriculum development in learning medicine

6

Colin Coles

CHAPTER CONTENTS

ABC

Glossary

Assessment; formal That which occurs intentionally when someone comes to a view about someone's (possibly that person's own) learning, irrespective of

---

ABC

Glossary (continued)

what use (formative or summative) is to be made of that assessment.

Assessment; formative Assessment designed to help individuals develop by giving them information on their performance, usually in a non-judgemental and low-stakes environment (has no consequences in terms of the learner's progress). Often termed 'assessment for learning' or simply feedback.

Assessment; informal That which occurs naturally and often unrecognised when someone, somehow, comes to a view about someone's (possibly that person's own) learning, irrespective of what use (formative or summative) is to be made of that assessment.

Curriculum (without a pronoun) That which underpins any learning and may be seen in the actions of teachers and learners *in situ*.

Curriculum development The commonly used term to convey the work of people (curriculum developers) engaged in creating a curriculum plan. Together, often informally, and perhaps unrecognised by them, they determine learners' emergent educational needs.

Curriculum implementation The translation of a curriculum proposal into practice, involving people locally appreciating the contextual nature of the particular location of the curriculum.

Curriculum initiators A preferred term to 'curriculum developers' (see curriculum development above) which is used here to refer to people who initiate the formal development of a curriculum. Understood as such, their role is to enable curriculum development to occur locally (see curriculum development above).

Curriculum: the (or a) curriculum (i.e. with a pronoun) A plan or set of intentions, usually presented in a written

Continued

© 2011, Elsevier Ltd.
DOI: 10.1016/B978-0-7020-3522-7.00006-1

Glossary (continued)

form, often prepared as a document in order to guide teachers' and learners' actions.

Formal education That which occurs intentionally when some formal (and probably also some informal) learning happens.

Formal learning Learning that occurs within an organisation and context (formal education) that is designed for learning. Formal learning is intentional from the learner's perspective.

Formal teaching Teaching that occurs intentionally when someone (a 'teacher') seeks to help another person learn something.

Informal education/learning Learning resulting from unplanned activities within an educational programme and/or daily life activities related to work, family, or leisure. It is not structured in terms of learning objectives or teaching. Informal learning may be intentional but in most cases it occurs incidentally.

Informal teaching That which occurs naturally and often unrecognised when someone (a 'teacher') helps another person learn something worthwhile.

Professional practice The actions and underpinning thoughts of someone intentionally engaged in helping another in some morally determined capacity, involving making judgements in that person's best interests.

Summative assessment Coming to a view of someone's learning for the purpose of regulating the progression of that person and/or for some form of certification.

Syllabus The content of a curriculum.

Outline

The hundred years since the publication of Flexner's (1910) report, particularly the last 50 years, have seen an explosion of curriculum development in medical education. In this chapter, I look critically at those changes, make some observations of my own, and end with a vision for the future. In the course of those critical observations, I offer what I see as some essential educational principles on which curriculum development should be based. The chapter is not, however, entirely theoretical. I give examples at key points in the argument. Nevertheless, I hold that medical education generally, and curriculum development in particular, needs to be based on educationally supportable principles. Quite fundamentally, any curriculum for professional practice (since this applies not just to medicine) must begin

with a clear understanding of the nature of that practice. This means looking rigorously at the practice in question – researching it in ways that I describe here – from the perspective of the people most closely associated with it: practitioners themselves. Generally, this has not happened in medical education, which is the greatest weakness of many of the curricula that have emerged in recent years.

Background

A curriculum is usually thought of as an educational policy, which is often (though not necessarily) presented as a document, in

> ... an attempt to communicate the essential principles and features of an educational proposal in such a form that it is open to critical scrutiny and capable of effective translation into practice.
>
> Stenhouse (1975, p 4)

Thus, a curriculum is more than a syllabus – which is merely a list of 'content'. A curriculum exists, whether people know it or not, in any educational event or activity. In this sense, everyday teaching, learning, and assessment are founded on there being 'curriculum' present.

> The term 'curriculum'... refers to all the activities, all the experiences and all the learning opportunities for which an institution, or a teacher, or a learner, takes responsibility – either deliberately or by default. This includes: the formal and the informal, the overt and the covert, the recognised and the overlooked, the intentional and the unintentional.
>
> Fish and Coles (2005, pp 29/30)

This leads to the notion that, in any educational enterprise, there will be various forms of a curriculum. These can include

- The curriculum 'on paper' – the intentions or aspirations
- The curriculum 'in action' – what happens in practice, the 'enactment' of the intensions
- The curriculum that is experienced – how the teachers and especially the learners interpret what is required of them, sometimes called 'the hidden curriculum' (Snyder, 1971).

And these 'incarnations' of a curriculum may look very different, not just to outside observers but also to those engaged in and with it. In other words, people perceive a curriculum from different viewpoints, and their viewpoint is greatly influenced by how they see education more generally. Put another way, people's 'mindset' – their assumptions, expectations, beliefs and values about education – determines how they see, and then how they act in relation to, any curriculum. Generally, most people consider 'the curriculum' to be what is written down – the intentions. However, it is almost always more educationally useful to consider 'curriculum' as people's reactions and responses to those intentions in their educational practice, that is through the teaching, learning, and assessing that actually happen.

These are some of the challenges that curriculum developers face. Curricula are complex – nothing about them is straightforward – which has huge implications for learning medicine. The notion that there is a simple, one-way relationship between designing a curriculum and its educational effects is, to say the least, naïve, and, at worst, dangerous. One implication is this: the traditional view of the curriculum developer (or more usually a group of people) is 'a man with a mission' (Stenhouse, 1975, p 120); someone who offers 'a solution', with a stake (often their reputation) in having found 'the right answer'. That might not be helpful. On the hundredth anniversary of the Flexner report, have his ideas achieved fruition? Or was he simply 'a man with a mission'?

What is the curriculum problem?

So what *is* the problem? In this section I offer a broad critique of both undergraduate and postgraduate medical education, particularly in the United Kingdom (UK) and North America, to establish some key implications regarding curriculum development generally.

Undergraduate medical education

Factual overload

In the UK, by the time Flexner was writing his report, a regulatory body – the General Council for Medicine (later renamed The General Medical Council or GMC for short) – had been in existence for over 50 years, and was addressing what it saw as the educational concerns of the day. In 1863 it noted:

> ... an overcrowding of the curriculum of education, whether as to the number of courses, or of lectures in particular courses ... followed by results injurious to the student.
>
> GMC (1957, p 5)

Adding 6 years later:

> ... some limit must be assigned to the amount of knowledge that can be fitly exacted.
>
> GMC (1957, p 5)

Thomas Huxley made the point even more forcibly in 1876:

> The burden we place on the medical student is far too heavy, and it takes some doing to keep from breaking his intellectual back. A system of medical education that is actually calculated to obstruct the acquisition of sound knowledge and to heavily favour the crammer and the grinder is a disgrace.
>
> GMC (1957, p 5)

Yet little changed, and by 1918 Newman commented that, in the United Kingdom:

> The medical course [is] seriously overburdened ... and too fully occupied to permit a healthy assimilation of much which the student is taught.
>
> Newman (1918)

By the mid-1940s, a UK government report recommended 'a ruthless pruning' of the content, suggesting that the GMC review the curriculum. In 1947, the GMC wryly commented that they 'could not fail to share [this] anxiety' but regretted that they had very limited powers to effect any change, merely urging medical schools not to retain in their curricula 'anything which it is unnecessary or premature for students to learn' (GMC, 1947). By 1957, the GMC was becoming more assertive, challenging medical schools 'to teach less and to educate more', warning that

> ... students have tended to concentrate their attention unduly on memorising factual data. The Council feel no doubt that an effort should be made to reduce the congestion.

Yet, by the 1980s it was still saying:

> We ... reiterate ... that the student's factual load should be reduced as far as possible, to ensure that the memorising and reproduction of factual data should not be allowed to interfere with the primary need for fostering the critical study of principles and the development of independent thought.
>
> in GMC (1993, p 5)

And by 1993:

> Notwithstanding these repeated exhortations, there remains gross overcrowding of most undergraduate curricula, acknowledged by teachers as deplored by

students. The scarcely tolerable burden of information that is imposed taxes the memory but not the intellect. The emphasis is on the passive acquisition of knowledge, much of it to become outdated or forgotten, rather than on its discovery through curiosity and experiment. The result is a regrettable tendency to under-provide those components of the course that are truly educational, that pertain to the proper function of a university and that are the hallmark of scholarship.

GMC (1993, p 5)

Inappropriate educational processes

The same observations were being made of under-graduate medical education in North America. Becker (Becker et al, 1961), in what is now recognised as a classic study, noted increasing cynicism amongst students, who responded to the amount they had to learn by 'playing the system'; that is, finding what was immediately required of them and focusing their learning on just that. Flexner (1910, pp 60/1), though, had seen the problem not so much as *overload* to be *reduced* but as an inappropriate teaching *process*:

Out and out didactic treatment is hopelessly antiquated; it belongs to an age of accepted dogma ... when the professor "knew" and the students "learnt."

Rather, he argued:

The student throughout is to be kept on his mettle. He does not have to be a passive learner.

Flexner (1910, p 57)

His vision was that:

From the standpoint of the young student, the [medical] school ... seeks to evoke the attitude, and to carry him through the processes, of the thinker and not of the parrot.

Flexner (1910, p 54)

... advocating an education where:

The student no longer merely watches, listens, memorizes: His own activities...are the main factors in his instruction and discipline. An education [that] involves both learning and learning how; the student cannot effectively know, unless he knows how.

Flexner (1910, p 53)

Lack of structure

Flexner saw the medical curriculum as requiring two closely related phases, which shared the same educational goal. During the first, students would learn 'science', though not necessarily through lectures or from books but in what Flexner (1910, p 92) referred to as 'the laboratory'.

... a place constructed for the express purpose of facilitating the collection of data bearing on definite problems and the initiation of practical measures looking to their solution.

The second period was to be spent in the clinic – which he also saw as a kind of laboratory:

... the hospital and the dispensary are laboratories in the strictest sense of the term.

Flexner (1910, p 92)

He commented:

Certain conclusions as to clinical teaching follow. The student is to collect and evaluate facts. The facts are locked up in the patient. To the patient, therefore, he must go ... That method of clinical teaching will be excellent which brings the student into close and active relation with the patient: close, by removing all hindrance to immediate investigation; active, in the sense, not merely of offering opportunities, but of imposing responsibilities.

Flexner (1910, pp 92/3)

Lack of integration

In the United Kingdom, however, the GMC became more and more critical of what it called 'the pre-clinical/clinical divide', with:

... each part of the course proliferating without the moderating influence of the other and without a co-ordinated examination of the overall aims of the course.

GMC (1993, p 5)

Indeed, the second half of the century saw two broad attempts in both the United Kingdom and North America to solve what was now being seen as the *relevance* problem. Both involved a form of integration – horizontal and vertical. *Horizontal* integration focused on the study of bodily systems rather than separate 'pre-clinical' disciplines; for example at Case Western Reserve medical school in the United States of America. This initiative 'shook the world of medical education for some years to come' (Williams, 1980):

In the struggle for faculty receptivity. there were times when brave men of goodwill and high hope felt like sitting down and crying ... Experience in the pursuit of integrated systems teaching ... would appear to be less a confirmation of the practicability of using the total human organism as a unifying concept of a system of education than of its value as a means of stimulating a faculty to raise its sights from the service of professional self interest to the service of students in their education.

Williams (1980)

Indeed, integrating the content in this way had little effect on how students approached their learning:

> The first two years of the curriculum remain a largely passive learning experience, keyed to the lecture method of instruction. The advent of the 'new' curriculum ... with its apparent increase in 'free time' concomitant with a 50% reduction in planned exercises, in fact largely resulted in the elimination of the laboratory ... leaving the absolute number of hours devoted to lectures unchanged.

Williams (1980)

Similar problems were experienced at a horizontally integrated medical school in the United Kingdom (Coles, 1985) – the content was changed but not the educational process.

Lack of relevance; the advent of PBL

The second innovation, again an attempt to address the *relevance* problem, started in the mid 1960s at McMaster Medical School in Canada by relating theoretical teaching more closely to clinical experience, through an educational process called 'problem-based learning' (PBL):

> [The doctor] is never told ... "there is a patient out there with liver disease. You had better read up on it before the patient comes in." He must deal with the problem always initially as an unknown, as a stimulus for developing his problem solving skills and as a focus to determine what is the relevant learning in the basic sciences and the clinical sciences in medicine.

Barrows (1976).

PBL typically presents learners, particularly in the pre-clinical years, with a paper-based clinical problem, and provides opportunities for them to explore what they need to learn in order to understand the problem. Students generally work in small groups (with or without a faculty member acting as a facilitator to help their discussions), supported in their learning by resource materials and other educational facilities such as libraries and laboratories. Where PBL has been introduced, there are few lectures or time-tabled large-group activities.

Perhaps ironically, the educational processes introduced through PBL reflect many of the views of Flexner and his contemporaries in the early part of the

twentieth century such as Dewey in North America and Whitehead in the United Kingdom (see Doll, 1993, Chapter 6), with their emphasis on problem-solving, reflection, small group teaching, and the use of teachers as facilitators of learning (rather than transmitters of information), and encouraging in learners, as Flexner put it, *'the attitude...of the thinker and not of the parrot'*. Was PBL, then, a reincarnation of Flexner's notion of the patient – what he called 'the case' – being the 'laboratory' for medical student learning? He had, after all, noted in 1910 that:

> Some ingenious Harvard men, profiting by the experience of the Harvard law school, have evolved an effective discipline in the art of inference ... "Let us assume such and such a data: what do they mean? What would you do?" This is the essence of the case method, a method ... calculated there to develop the friction, competition, and interest which are powerful pedagogical stimulants.

(pp 98/9)

Criticisms of PBL

PBL has shown many gains, for example, in how students approach their studying (Coles, 1985), but it has not been without its critics in its 50-year history. A study of graduates entering clinical practice questioned whether they had sufficient 'basic knowledge', recommending that this should be given 'more attention in the curriculum' (Woodward and Ferrier, 1983). Another found that students in a problem-based curriculum covered up their inadequacies in an attempt to deceive others that they were competent, as at conventional medical schools (Haas and Shaffir, 1982). Gale (1980) noted that problem-based learning:

> ... leaves the question of structure open. The organising agents ... are not identified, thus no conclusions may be drawn about the structural properties of knowledge acquired through such learning.

A similar criticism saw little fundamental difference between what was called 'traditional' PBL and conventional programmes, which:

> ... are structurally similar, both following a knowledge first, application second view.

Margetson (1999)

In short, traditional PBL fails to address the *relevance* problem because it retains the conventional curricular separation of the pre-clinical and clinical phases – a discredited view of learning as 'preparation' for later practice, in that it isolates 'understanding' from 'action' (Fish and Coles, 2005, p 155). Margetson (1999, pp 362 and 363) added that the 'problems' – the 'cases' in PBL – that form the basis for students' learning are no more than what he called 'convenient pegs on which to hang the coat of basic science knowledge which students [are deemed to] need to acquire'. This, he argued, perpetuates an atomistic view of medical education in three ways:

- The pre-clinical and clinical phases of the curriculum are held structurally distinct from one another through the notion of the 'application' of knowledge learnt early on to later clinical experience,
- The two phases are quite separate in nature, the one being seen as 'theoretical' the other 'practical',
- The pre-clinical phase is seen as 'an absolutely secure foundation on which clinical practice rests'.

For Margetson, the weakness of problem-based learning curricula of this 'traditional' kind is that it fails to recognise that:

> Human action … makes no sense apart from understanding: rather, action raises questions of the extent of understanding and its soundness.
>
> (p 361)

As Schön put it, effective education requires:

> … a transaction with the situation in which knowing and doing are inseparable.
>
> Schön (1987, p 78)

Others make the same criticism that solving paper-based cases involves 'a significantly different process from that involved in diagnosing and managing real patients' (Rikers et al, 2004, p 1041). Margetson's solution – what he called a 'rigorously problem based' curriculum – requires a 'thorough integration of understanding (in the widest sense), knowledge and skill' (Margetson, 1999, pp 363 and 364), which he argued could occur only in clinical practice. PBL has some merits that are sufficiently appealing to contemporary curriculum developers to make it an attractive option for undergraduate medical education. However, it may 'work' for other reasons – for example, 'integration' has been shown to occur under those curricular circumstances where learners see more clearly why they need to know what they are being taught – that is, when their 'understanding' and their 'action' are brought together (Coles, 1985).

In short, PBL may not be the only way to achieve integration (Coles, 1990).

Postgraduate medical education

Preparedness for practice

In one sense, the 'curriculum problem' in undergraduate medical education was, by the end of the century following the publication of the Flexner report, appearing not to be the consequence of content overload, nor of relevance, nor resolved by making the educational processes more 'learner centred', nor by students learning the basic sciences through a 'case study' approach. The question curriculum developers were now being posed was more pragmatic: does the undergraduate curriculum prepare students well enough for clinical practice? In the United Kingdom these concerns, still the subject of the GMC's current review of the medical school curriculum (GMC, 2009), were being voiced over 40 years ago:

> The undergraduate medical course does not provide sufficient training for the immediate practice of medicine.
>
> Todd Report (1968) in GMC (1993, p 5)

A 100 years ago, Flexner reported that graduating doctors in North America generally had poor levels of understanding, which required:

> … an effort to mend a machine that was pre-destined to break down…to do what the medical school had failed to accomplish.
>
> (p 174)

Adding:

> … the young physician already involved in responsibility should acquire the practical technique which the medical school had failed to impart … aimed pre-eminently to teach the young doctor what to "do."
>
> (p 174)

In the United Kingdom, the tradition was that medicine was learnt chiefly through what was called 'an apprenticeship':

> … learning to be the professional by practising the profession under conditions of supervision and careful selection of appropriate levels of independent responsibility to meet them.
>
> Open University (2001, p 15)

Dangers were seen in this, however, and by the middle of the twentieth century, it was noted in the United Kingdom that:

Some [newly qualified doctors] undertook posts as resident house officers where they carried out surgical operations and gave anaesthetics without supervision. Although many made it their business to acquire a sound training in the specialty of their choice, postgraduate education was unstructured and ... there was no certification of its satisfactory completion.

GMC (1993, p 5)

Structuring postgraduate education

A first step towards structuring postgraduate education came in 1953 with the introduction in the United Kingdom of the 'pre-registration year' following graduation from medical school (see GMC, 1993, p 5). Even so, 20 years later a Royal Commission reported:

... all too often the graduate is treated as a much needed extra pair of hands rather than a probationer doctor still requiring supervision and training at a significant point in his career. Some young doctors find themselves burdened with responsibilities they are not yet in a position to assume; others are given duties not necessarily relevant to their training needs.

Merrison (1975)

It was then established that, following the pre-registration year ...

... all doctors entering the National Health Service are now required to undergo specialty training ... before they may practise independently.

GMC (1993, p 6)

Competency-based education

Recently, a further reorganisation was introduced under the title *Modernising Medical Careers* (Department of Health, 2004) or MMC for short. This marked a highly significant shift in postgraduate medical education in the United Kingdom:

Reform had been long overdue ... The apprenticeship model ... now needs to be set within efficiently managed, quality assured training Programmes.

MMC (2004, p 1)

Programmes need to achieve a set of pre-defined, published competencies and outcome

(2004, p 3)

Progress [as a doctor in training] will be achieved through the acquisition of competencies and the knowledge underpinning them'.

(2004, p 8)

What was being promoted, however, was (perhaps unwittingly) a particular form of education:

Modernising Medical Careers [has] signalled a move to competency-based training throughout the medical continuum.

(2004, p 12)

We will support and encourage ... the Royal Colleges to develop competency-based training and assessment.

(2004, p 7)

What, then, is 'competency-based training'? It is an educational movement that was strong in the United States of America in the 1970s and 1980s, though it never caught on in the United Kingdom at that time. Its major claim was (and still is) in relation to vocational (i.e. sub-degree) programmes that lead to technical qualifications. Educationists argue, however, that the competency-based approach is reductionist and instrumental, an attempt:

... to reduce educational practice to a kind of 'making action' through which some raw material can be moulded into a pre-specifiable shape.

Carr (1995, p 73)

Whereas, educationists agree that:

... the sum of what professionals do is far greater than any parts that can be described in competen[cy] terms.

ten Cate (2006, p 749)

Since:

A list of competencies cannot do justice to the quality and depth of thinking associated with the 'educated person', namely, the serious engagement with ideas, the struggle to make sense, the entry into a tradition of thinking and criticism.

Pring (2000, p 26)

Flexner held the same view, arguing that the technician:

... deals mainly with measurable factors ... Uncertainty is within fairly narrow limits. [Whereas] the reasoning of the [doctor] is much more complex. He handles at one and the same time elements belonging to vastly different categories: physical, biological, psychological elements are involved in each other ... Between the young graduate in medicine and his ultimate responsibility – human life – nothing interposes ... The training of the doctor is therefore more complex and more directly momentous than that of the technician.

(p 23/4)

More seriously, by pursuing a competency-based approach MMC may be changing contemporary medical education into a form of technical training:

> [This] new way of thinking about the relation of teacher and learner … employs different metaphors, different ways of describing and evaluating educational activities. In doing so, it changes those activities into something else … Once the teacher 'delivers' someone else's curriculum with its precisely defined 'product', there is little room for that transaction in which the teacher … responds to the needs of the learner. When the learner becomes a 'client' or 'customer', there is no room for the traditional apprenticeship into the community of learners. When the 'product' is measurable 'targets' on which 'performance' is 'audited', then little significance is attached to the 'struggle to make sense'.
>
> Pring (2000, pp 24–26)

What is the purpose of a medical curriculum?

This shift towards seeing medicine as a technical matter has been counterbalanced by others who suggest it is:

> … esoteric, complex and discretionary in character: It requires theoretical knowledge, skill, and judgement that ordinary people do not possess, may not wholly comprehend and cannot readily evaluate. Furthermore, the kind of work they do is believed to be especially important for the well-being of individuals or of society at large … It is the capacity to perform that special kind of work which distinguishes those who are professional from most other workers.
>
> Freidson (1994)

Wilfred Carr (1995, pp 68/9), an educationist, captures the same point:

> To 'practise' … is always to act within a tradition, and it is only by submitting to its authority that practitioners can begin to acquire the practical knowledge and standards of excellence by means of which their own practical competence can be judged.

Though he adds, hinting at a fundamental principle in professional education:

> … the authoritative nature of a tradition does not make it immune to criticism. The practical knowledge made available through tradition is not mechanically or passively reproduced: it is constantly being reinterpreted and revised through dialogue and discussion about how to pursue … the tradition. It is precisely because it embodies

this process of critical reconstruction that a tradition evolves and changes rather than remains static or fixed.

> Carr (1995, p 69)

Golby and Parrott (1999, pp 3 and 9) similarly comment:

> A practice exists whenever a more or less settled body of activities is carried out to some distinctive end … What people do within a practice, the activities they engage upon, are … intelligible only by reference to … the tradition of conduct of which they are part.

Adding that a 'tradition of conduct' is …

> … made up of contemporary practitioners who are in turn related to predecessors who have bequeathed their practice. When we engage in the characteristic activities of a practice, therefore, we are disciplined by its standards as represented by our peers and our predecessors. These standards are both technical and moral; they concern both the 'how to' and the 'why' of practice.
>
> Golby and Parrott (1999, p 9)

Gawande (2002, p 4) says this:

> Medicine is … a strange and in many ways disturbing business … What you find … is how messy, uncertain and surprising [it] turns out to be … These are the moments in which medicine actually happens.

Medicine (like education) is a complex professional practice. Doctors (and teachers) must deal appropriately not just with routine situations but more particularly with the situations of uncertainty that occur unpredictably. In short, they must learn to exercise judgement:

> … that form of wise and prudent judgement which takes account of what would be morally appropriate and fitting in a particular situation … not 'right' action in the sense that it has been proved to be correct [but] 'right' action justified as morally appropriate to the particular circumstances in which it was taken.
>
> Carr (1995, pp 71/2)

Professionals, then, must learn to decide what is 'best' for individuals in the circumstances in which they are found, rather than what is 'right' in some absolute sense (Tyreman, 2000). What knowledge does this require? Looked at from an educational perspective, the knowledge base is highly diverse:

> Medical decision making … is often presented only as the conscious application to the patient's problem of explicitly defined rules and objectively verifiable data … Seasoned practitioners also apply to their practice a large body of knowledge, skills, values and experiences that

are not explicitly stated by or known to them. This knowledge may constitute a different kind of evidence, which also has a strong influence on medical decisions.

Epstein (1999, p 834)

As Gawande (2002, pp 4 and 7) puts it:

We look for medicine to be an orderly field of knowledge and procedure. But it is not. It is an imperfect science, an enterprise of constantly changing knowledge, uncertain information, fallible individuals, and at the same time lives on the line. There is science in what we do, yes, but also habit, intuition and sometimes plain old guessing.

Fish and de Cossart (2005, 2007) argue that the doctor first determines what is the right thing to do generally – such as arriving at a differential diagnosis – largely based on bio-medical knowledge, which can be relatively easily taught, learnt, and assessed. The doctor then moves (often imperceptibly and very quickly) towards deciding what the best thing to do is in the particular instance:

Good [practice] is entirely dependent on what Aristotle calls *phronesis*, which we would translate as 'practical wisdom'. *Phronesis* is the virtue of knowing which general ethical principle to apply in a particular circumstance. For Aristotle, *phronesis* is the supreme intellectual virtue and an indispensible feature of practice. The *phronimos* – the man of practical wisdom – is the man who sees the particularities of his practical situation in the light of their ethical significance and acts consistently on this basis. Without practical wisdom … 'good practice' becomes indistinguishable from instrumental cleverness.

Carr (1995, p 71)

A 100 years ago Flexner argued that the practice of medicine – its 'doing' – was underpinned by two quite different kinds of knowledge:

The practitioner deals with facts in two categories. [The sciences] enable him to apprehend one set; [but] he needs a different apperceptive and appreciative apparatus to deal with the other, more subtle elements … The physician's function is fast becoming social and preventative, rather than individual and curative. Upon him society relies to ascertain, and through measures essentially educational to enforce, the conditions that prevent disease and make positively for physical and moral well-being.

(p 26)

Flexner's ideas were based, then, not on the 'facts' of science but its approaches:

A professional habit definitely formed upon scientific method … It goes without saying that this type of doctor is first of all an educated man.

(pp 26 and 56)

What educational models cultivate the educated practitioner?

How then might this 'type of doctor' become 'educated'? Stenhouse described three possible educational models, which he termed 'product', 'process', and 'research' (Table 6.1).

Experienced medical teachers at all levels will be familiar with these approaches. On occasions, the 'product' approach seems appropriate – when one needs to instruct someone about something. On another occasion, directly 'telling' people things would be inappropriate (and probably ineffectual). Then teachers help learners to work things out themselves. This is Stenhouse's notion of 'process'. In yet another setting, the teacher's role would be to supervise a learner's enquiry. This is the essence of the 'research' approach. Similarities will be apparent between the product versus process/research distinction and the contrast drawn between acquisition versus participation metaphors for learning in Chapter 2. The significance of Table 6.1, however, goes beyond this. It represents not simply 'teaching approaches' but 'educational models' – coherent views of education that are not just practically but logically distinct from one another. As the Table shows, the three models indicate not only what teachers do but define their relationship with learners and indicate the nature of other elements of the educational process such as how planning and assessment differ depending on the model chosen. The wise teacher works imperceptibly in all three models, drawing on each for particular educational purposes. The concepts contained within a particular model reflect a way of looking at education, an educational 'mindset'. Indeed, they can be thought of as the basis of curriculum models, as shown in Table 6.2.

An example of where a 'product' model could be appropriate as a basis for a curriculum is in 'trauma' courses, where it is vital that all those involved in patient care know precisely what is expected of them and of everyone else. The 'product' model is appropriate for 'training' – in situations where, if something happens, there is the 'right' (i.e. an agreed) thing to do. However, such forms of practice are rare in medicine. Even 'trauma' requires 'triage', which involves 'judgement'. Indeed, a curriculum based on the 'product' model was the kind of teaching and assessing that Flexner found abhorrent, and probably led to the problems of 'overload' and lack of 'relevance'. Current approaches to postgraduate

Table 6.1 Three educational models after Stenhouse (1975)

Educational issues	Three models		
	Product	Process	Research
	The term 'product' is used to characterise education as a technical or mechanical act involving 'transmission' of some sort	The term 'process' is used to mean education where the learner is an active participant	The term 'research' is used to mean 'any systematic, critical and self-critical enquiry which aims to contribute to the advancement of knowledge' (Pring, 2000, p 7)
Planning via . . .	Aims, objectives, detailed programme of all activities	Aims, intentions, principles of procedure, planned activities but flexible, may need to be changed as course proceeds following observations of and feedback by learners and their learning	Aims, intentions, negotiated agenda, statements of what the learner might explore, how they might explore it, and what might be the results of this
Intention	Teacher explains and tells	Teacher promotes learning	Learners explore to understand
Locus of knowledge	Teacher	Teachers and learners	Learners individually and as a group
Learners' role	Passive	Active	Seekers of knowledge and negotiators of learning activities
Learners' motivation	Comes from the teacher, but aware of a 'need to know'	Desire to learn, sees (appreciates) the need	Desire to discover, thirst for knowledge
Teachers' role	Instructor, lecturer, demonstrator, grades assessments	Facilitator of learning, sets up learning situations, a critic rather than a grader of assessments	Supervisor, enabler, facilitator, learns alongside the learner
Assessment	System: summative (or if intended to be formative, often seen as summative by learners), teacher assesses student, usually quantitative	System: part of teaching and learning, formative as well as summative, usually qualitative but can be quantitative, sometimes called 'feedback'	System: self-assessment, peer assessment, essentially formative can be summative, may be discursive
	Example: MCQs	Example: Case report	Examples: Reflective account, dissertation, thesis, portfolio

medical education in the United Kingdom, namely those based on a 'competency-based' formulation, also reflect a 'product' curriculum. A process model would be appropriate where the curricular intention is to help people understand what is being taught. That is the educational basis of 'learner-centred' and problem-solving approaches. What Margetson characterised as 'traditional PBL' reflects this model, as does an 'apprenticeship' approach to postgraduate medical education, where, although in both cases the teacher acts as a facilitator of the learner's learning, the teacher can remain the primary focus (and often the determiner) of what is taught, learnt, and

assessed. Whilst this may appear 'learner centred', it might constrain learners and their learning.

The research approach is harder to depict, yet is probably the most appropriate curriculum model for learning medicine at any level. It does not mean that learners undertake research projects. What Stenhouse had in mind was, as Pring (2000, p 7) more recently put it:

> . . . any systematic, critical and self-critical enquiry which aims to contribute to the advancement of knowledge.

In a curricular context, it is the learner's knowledge that is to advance. A medical curriculum based on

Table 6.2 A basis for choosing an appropriate model

Educational issues and questions	Three curriculum models		
	Product	Process	Research
Problem(s), what is (or are) the educational problem(s) for which one of these models might be the solution?	Clear to all those involved, self-evident, can easily be explained or demonstrated	Clear to some (especially the teachers), not always easily explained or demonstrated but not too difficult to understand	Unclear or understood by only a few, difficult to explain or demonstrate, must be experienced first hand
What do we want to achieve, what do we want to do educationally, what 'outcomes' ('ends') can we expect?	Agreed, can be easily explained or demonstrated, examples can be shown	Clear to some, can fairly easily be explained or understood, demonstration may help	Unclear, lack of consensus, several possibilities, different perspectives, difficult to explain or demonstrate, few (or no) relevant examples to refer to
How can we achieve these outcomes, what 'means' do we have at our disposal, what methods shall we use?	Agreed, limited choice, self-evident (or assumed to be without much thought or consultation)	Several possibilities become evident when people think this through, try them out, or have them demonstrated	Many possibilities, lack of consensus as to way forward, unclear, unknown, must be tested out in practice, few or no examples to refer to
Timescale, how long will it take to develop a curriculum based on a particular model?	Short	Takes time	Work in progress, continuous, never concluded
How do we know if it's working, how might we evaluate the curriculum?	Performance measures, objective outcomes, meets targets, mostly quantitative, often used as summative assessment of the course or programme	Self-report, observations of others, 'free text' comments most useful for course/programme development, some aspects can be quantified	Enlightened practice/practitioners, increased clarity of problems and purpose of curriculum, 'ends' and 'means' constantly reviewed, cannot be measured quantitatively and described only with difficulty
Example	Trauma course	Problem-based learning	Flexner's vision?

a research model, then, is one that engages learners in 'researching' their clinical practice. The 'knowledge' bound up in that practice is unearthed by the learners, not 'taught' prior to engaging in practice. Some of this 'unearthed knowledge' will be bio/psycho/social 'facts'. More will be 'discovered' through the action of practising and reflecting on that action. This will include 'professional judgement', 'practical wisdom', and 'the traditions of practice' – those higher-order forms of knowledge noted earlier to underpin professional practice. Indeed, 'practice' has its own inherent curriculum (Fleming, 2010), lying dormant (its nature and potential often under-recognised) in every practice encounter yet capable of being rendered 'known' in some form through appropriate forms of deliberation (Fish and de Cossart, 2007).

A research view of a medical curriculum is entirely consistent with Flexner's vision:

We may fairly describe modern medicine as characterised by a severely critical handling of experience ... [It] deals ... not only with certainties, but also with probabilities, surmises, theory ... It knows ... where certainties stop and risks begin. Now it acts confidently, because it has facts; again cautiously because it merely surmises; then tentatively, because it hardly more than hopes ... Scientific medicine, therefore, has its eyes open; it takes risks consciously.

(p 53)

He added, very significantly for the discussion here:

The main intellectual tool of the [scientific] investigator is the working hypothesis, or theory, as it is more commonly called ... Upon this he acts, and the practical outcome of his procedure refutes, confirms or modifies his theory ... This is essentially the technique of research: wherein is it irrelevant to beside practice? ... The progress of science and the ... intelligent practice of medicine employ, therefore, exactly the same technique. To use it ... the student must be trained to the positive exercise of his faculties; and if so trained, the medical school begins rather than completes his medical education.

(p 54)

Flexner, then, likened the thinking processes underpinning effective medical practice to 'research', meaning not 'the findings' of enquiries but 'the ways of finding' that researchers employ – professional practice as a form of thinking action. Carr (1995, p 71), following Aristotle, called this kind of action 'deliberation' or 'deliberative reasoning':

> ... in deliberative reasoning, it is always conceded that there may be more than one ethical principle ... and that there is no formula for methodically determining which one should be involved in a particular practical situation ... It is for this reason ... that deliberation is entirely dependent on the possession of what Aristotle calls *phronesis* ... 'Practical wisdom' is manifest in a knowledge of what is required in a particular moral situation, and a willingness to act so that this knowledge can take a concrete form.

He added, perhaps as a muted criticism of the current obsession with accountability:

> The man who lacks *phronesis* may be technically accountable, but can never be morally answerable.

(1995, p 71)

Perhaps that is what Flexner had in mind when he urged medical schools:

> ... to evoke the attitude ... of the thinker and not of the parrot.

(p 54)

The implementation problem

Any review of medical education over the past 100 years must inevitably conclude that a lot has been said, countless exhortations made, many recommendations formulated, innovations attempted, and radical change made; if there was 'an answer' – a 'solution' to the curriculum 'problem' – it would surely have been found. It is clear, however, that problems identified have not been satisfactorily resolved. Either there has been strong resistance to change or the changes introduced have not addressed the problems effectively. In short, implementation has not happened. The aspirations have not been fulfilled. Why not?

Problems with the implementation of medical curricula occur partly because developers fail to consider implementation as their task. The Flexner report, for example, says a lot about 'what might happen' but very little about 'how it might happen'. Curriculum proposals largely deal with educational 'ends' but often omit the 'means' for achieving those ends. The implementation problem is also bound up, in part, with our understanding of change – and in particular, how practices change. Schön, writing in 1971, characterised the most common approach to change as what he called 'centre-periphery' (popularly known as 'top-down'). This approach sees 'implementation' as a process of 'diffusion':

- The innovation to be diffused exists, fully realised in its essentials, prior to its diffusion
- Diffusion is the movement of an innovation from a centre out to its ultimate users
- Directed diffusion is a centrally managed process of dissemination, training, and provision of resources and incentives (Schön, 1971, p 81)

The success of this:

> ... depends first upon the level of resources and energy at the centre, then upon the number of points at the periphery, the length of the radii or spokes through which the diffusion takes place, and the energy required to gain a new adoption.

Schön (1971, p 81)

This fundamentally depends on:

> ... the level of technology governing the flow of men, materials, money and information ... [and the centre's] capacity for generating and managing feedback. Because the process of diffusion is originally regulated by the centre, the effectiveness of the process depends upon the ways in which information moves from periphery back to the centre.

(1971, p 82)

However:

> When the ... system exceeds the resources or the energy at the centre, overloads the capacity of the radii, or mishandles feedback from the periphery, it fails. Failure takes the form of simple ineffectiveness in diffusion, distortion of the message, or disintegration of the system as a whole ... Once new centres [at the periphery] are established, for better or worse, they pursue their disparate paths.

(1971, pp 83 and 84)

Examples of such failures abound in attempts to develop curricula in medical education.

More particularly, the implementation problem is a consequence of the very conceptualisation of the problem itself – as one of implementation. The word means 'to put a plan into action'. It invites a 'centre-periphery' approach. Looking again at Stenhouse's definition of curriculum with which I began this chapter, however, gives a clue to a different way forward. He speaks of the need for a curriculum proposal to be presented:

> . . . in such a form that it is . . . capable of effective translation into practice.

> (1975, p 4)

The first implication is that Stenhouse clearly puts the 'means' for change, not just the 'ends' of change, firmly on the curriculum development agenda. But also, and very significantly, he uses the term 'translation' – a term that carries a very different meaning from 'implementation'. It signals a particular way of going about this, and suggests two considerations:

- Any curriculum proposal may need to be modified to suit local circumstances
- Particular situations have their own characteristics that need to be appreciated and understood.

The message is this: because something works in one situation does not automatically mean that it will work in another. A medical analogy might help. Transplantation of an otherwise healthy organ can result in 'rejection' because of the effects of the recipient's 'immune response'. Curriculum change that is approached as 'a plan to be implemented', to be 'diffused' in a 'centre-periphery manner' (Schön, 1971), is like the use of immunosuppressant drugs in organ transplantation – medication is used to 'knock out' (suppress) the recipient's immune defence system. Rather, curriculum planners need to understand 'the immune system' of the people who they hope will take up their curriculum. Instead of 'suppressing' the recipient's immune system, they must understand it.

Pinar et al (1995) recommended not seeing the problem of curriculum change as deciding 'what' to do but an attempt to understand 'why' the problem exists:

> '. . . problems do not just require knee-jerk, commonsensical responses, but careful, thoughtful, disciplined understanding'.

> Pinar et al (1995, p 8)

It is for this reason that Stenhouse recommends that curriculum development should be seen as a form of educational research. Any curriculum proposal, he said, should be transformed:

> . . . into a hypothesis testable in practice. It [should invite] critical testing rather than acceptance.

> (p 142)

These views are well supported by recent observations that both education and medical practice are examples of 'complex systems' (Plsek and Greenhalgh, 2001, pp 635–638), where approaches that see them as 'machines' that simply need 'oiling' are liable to fail. Such mechanistic thinking:

> . . . is built largely on the assumption that plans for progress must provide 'the best' way, completely specified in great detail, and consistently implemented in that same level of detail across the board.

> Plsek and Wilson (2001, p 747)

Detailed specifications fail in complex systems because they do not:

> . . . take advantage of the natural creativity embedded in the organisation, [or] allow for the inevitable unpredictability of events.

> Plsek and Wilson (2001, p 747)

In the context of 'curriculum', Stenhouse (1975, p 143) argued that:

> . . . all well-founded curriculum . . . development . . . rests on the work of teachers. It is not enough that teachers' work should be studied: they need to study it themselves.

In other words, the teacher should be the focus of curriculum development. Seen in this way, curriculum development begins with an appreciation of what teachers and learners actually do, when they do it, how they do it, and why they do it that way. It is undoubtedly true that medical teachers (at all levels) teach well and highly appropriately, when they are committed to this work and adequately resourced to undertake it. Similarly, learners learn well where the curriculum allows them to (Coles, 1985). None of this requires 'detailed specification', and is more likely to occur naturally without it.

What then is curriculum development?

So where does this leave curriculum development? It is clear that:

The fundamental relationship between a trainee ... and the supervising consultant is critical for professional development ... There is no better way of realising the full potential of the trainee and passing on the wisdom of clinical experience.

Baldwin and Dodd (1999, p 28)

'Curriculum', then, is best seen not as a plan for action but rather as what underpins education (Fleming, 2010). It is the unseen (and often unrecognised) foundation of effective teaching and learning. Learning occurs in and through this relationship – the interactions and transactions – between a teacher and a learner. In that sense, teachers and learners together 'develop' what is to be learnt, how it is to be learnt, and how the effects of that learning are to be recognised, that is how it is best assessed and for what purpose that assessment is undertaken (AMRC, 2009). Curriculum development, then, actually (and naturally) occurs in and through that relationship between teachers and learners – a relationship that reflects that of researcher and supervisor – in the setting of authentic practice. The true curriculum developers are the teachers and the learners. They are the people who make education 'work', if the conditions are conducive to that happening. In the past, people have seen 'a curriculum' as a 'proposal' – usually a document that sets out educational intentions *for many contexts*. This contrasts with a second view of curriculum as an educational concept which defines the essential educational relationship between teacher and learner *in a particular context*.

Where does this leave those who up to now have been called 'curriculum developers'? If the role of curriculum developer is now to be given to (perhaps even given back to) teachers and learners, what is the function of people, frequently at national level, who are often the initiators of educational change? Quite fundamentally, the role of these 'curriculum initiators' is to help teachers and learners develop an appropriate curriculum for learning *in situ* – in their own setting – and certainly not to include anything in their curriculum plans that might constrain that development.

Some conclusions

A vision of learning medicine

What, then, ought a curriculum plan to entail that aspires to create the conditions for 'learning medicine'? What might a medical curriculum proposal look like from the perspective of my general conclusions about curriculum and curriculum development? My vision is speculative. It challenges some entrenched shibboleths. It is iconoclastic. It is (inevitably) a sketch, an outline, an overview. But it is not 'sketchy'; it is based on sound educational principles. Above all, it reflects the uneven history of curriculum development over the past 150 years. It rests on the concept of curriculum that I have drawn from my discussion in this chapter: moving from seeing curriculum as 'an educational plan', to curriculum in terms of the 'educational action' itself, that is *in situ*. The concept of curriculum I believe we now need to adopt is of something which underpins what teachers and learners do in practice. It is the basis for their educational actions. Strangely enough, Flexner might approve. His writing showed that he understood education, and he understood medical practice. He knew what teachers and learners did and why they did it, and then what they needed to do for their teaching and learning to be as appropriate as possible. Many curriculum developers since, for the reasons I have given, have lost that vision.

A vision for curriculum initiators

Those who initiate a curriculum plan must recognise that 'curriculum development' actually happens in and through the interactions of teachers and learners when they grapple, together, with their teaching and learning. Any curriculum plan must make this explicit – and make it possible for that 'grappling' to happen (Pring, 2000).

Any curriculum plan must show how:

– Teachers and learners will be well prepared for their role (this is likely to involve initial and ongoing 'professional development').

– Resources (in the widest sense of the word) are to be made available for teachers and learners to engage in effective education (that is the development of the curriculum *in situ*), including recognising the time needed to do this.

– This 'resourcing' will address how the education that is proposed will affect (and be affected by) developments in the clinical service and workforce (Tooke, 2008).

– Evaluation of the curriculum plans can support the on-going professional development of teachers and learners in their role as curriculum developers. (It should be seen as a 'formative' endeavour.)

A vision for teachers and learners

Teachers and learners are central to the effectiveness of any curriculum proposal. Their role needs to be fully recognised. Without them, there is no curriculum.

- Teachers and learners will need to recognise (and be helped to recognise through the curriculum plans and resources that are provided) that they are the true 'curriculum developers'.
- They will need to develop (and be helped and enabled to develop) the abilities and capacities to take on this role.
- They may, though, need to recognise that, in reality, curriculum plans might not always be as helpful to them as they could be (many are not!). In those circumstances, teachers and learners need to find ways to 'enrich' (Fish and de Cossart, 2007) what might be an otherwise 'impoverished' curriculum plan, which, sadly, is the situation facing many people today who are engaged in learning medicine.

Coda

I began this chapter by exploring thoughts that Flexner published a 100 years ago. Throughout, I have used his writings to critique what has happened in medical education since then. In sketching out my educational vision, I suggest that he might have approved of it. Flexner was a man both *of* his time and *before* his time. He saw the need for radical reform of medical education in North America. In doing so, he raised challenges that are as true today as they were then. However, despite considerable 'curriculum development' (a term I now use with some caution), little *educational* development has occurred. Indeed, some of it has been palpably 'counter-educational'. I have offered in this chapter some educational perspectives to account for that failure. The challenge now is to question models and structures of the past and to start afresh, though now equipped with an appreciation of sound educational principles. Medical educators can learn much from Flexner and from the curriculum failures of the 100 years since the publication of his report. Perhaps doing so brings us 'full circle', and helps us recognise the true contribution of his thinking. TS Eliot (1965) summed this up well:

We shall not cease from exploration
And the end of all our exploring

Will be to arrive where we started
And to know the place for the first time.

(section v of 'Little Gidding', Four Quartets)

Implications for practice

What conclusions can we draw from this account of curriculum development? The main educational principles emerging from this chapter are as follows:

- Understanding the principles of curriculum development is a crucial concern for all involved in the challenges of learning medicine, whether as students, trainees, teachers, planners, administrators, or policy makers; not just theoretically but in terms of what it means for them personally in their educational practice,
- History bequeaths some important lessons. Despite wise words, high ideals, and lofty intentions, curriculum plans generally have not always (perhaps not often) worked out in practice,
- Most curriculum development has been 'top down' and (increasingly) over-specified,
- Authentic medical practice (not some proxy for it such as 'problem cases' or even simulation) ought to be the primary focus for learning medicine, recognising through this its complexity, uncertainty, and unpredictability, and the centrality of 'judgement',
- The forms of knowledge that underpin professional judgment are highly complex and go well beyond knowing the so-called 'basic' facts. Learning to practise medicine effectively requires 'practical wisdom', acquiring 'traditions of conduct', and becoming a member of a community of practitioners (Lave and Wenger, 1991; Wenger, 1999),
- Acquiring factual knowledge prior to engaging in authentic practice is largely ineffectual. Facts still need to be reinterpreted in practice, and practice knowledge (practical wisdom) can be learnt only in practice,
- A 'research model' of education is most appropriate for learning to practise medicine, with learners researching medical practice (particularly their own), and with their teachers acting as 'supervisors' of that research,
- Learning medicine, then, occurs best in and through the relationship between the teacher and the learner,

- Such a 'minimum specification' is entirely appropriate for such a complex matter as learning medicine,
- 'Curriculum' is best conceived as that which underpins – conceptually it is the basis for – effective teaching and learning,
- 'Curriculum development', then, is best conceived as occurring within the educational transactions of teachers and learners,
- The curriculum development work of teachers and learners may be facilitated (enhanced) by 'curriculum initiators', and it should certainly not be hindered by them,
- Curriculum initiators (those people, often located nationally or regionally, who initiate curriculum development locally) must see their role as supporters and facilitators of, and providers of resources for, the curriculum development that is to be carried out by teachers and learners.

Paradoxically, perhaps, I return to what has been the situation for millennia in pursuing the curriculum problem – reinstating that educative relationship between the teacher and the learner as the locus for its solution. Maybe now, through a greater understanding of what is involved, those concerned with the curriculum problem can more confidently defend the central need for some form of 'professional apprenticeship' for learning medicine against a tide appearing to sweep them towards technical training.

References

AMRC: *Improving assessment*, London, 2009, Academy of Medical Royal Colleges.

Baldwin P, Dodd M: *Higher specialist training – early experience in Scotland*, Edinburgh, 1999, Scottish Council for Postgraduate Medical and Dental Education.

Barrows HS: Problem-based learning in medicine. In Clarke J, Leedham J, editors: *Aspects of educational technology 10: individual learning*, London, 1976, Kogan Page.

Becker HS, Geer B, Hughes EC, et al: *Boys in white*, Chicago, 1961, University of Chicago Press.

Carr W: *For education: towards critical educational inquiry*, Buckingham, 1995, Open University Press.

Coles C: *A study of the relationships between curriculum and learning in undergraduate medical education*, PhD thesis (unpublished). University of Southampton, 1985, Faculty of Educational Studies.

Coles C: Is problem based learning the only way? In Boud D, Feletti G, editors: *The challenge of problem based learning*, London, 1990, Kogan Page.

de Cossart L, Fish D: *Cultivating the thinking surgeon: new perspectives on clinical teaching, learning and assessment*, Harley, UK, 2005, TFM Publishing Ltd.

Department of Health: *Modernising medical careers; the next steps*, Leeds, 2004, UK Health Departments.

Doll WE: *A post-modern perspective on curriculum*, London, 1993, Teachers College Press.

Eliot TS: *Collected poems*, London, 1965, Faber & Faber.

Epstein RM: Mindful practice, *J Am Med Assoc* 282(9):833–839, 1999.

Fish D, Coles C: *Medical education developing a curriculum for practice*, Maidenhead, 2005, Open University Press.

Fish D, de Cossart L: *Developing the wise doctor: a resource for trainers and trainees in MMC*, London, 2007, The Royal Society of Medicine Press Ltd.

Fleming WF: *The curricular nature of practice*, United Kingdom, 2010, University of Winchester. PhD Thesis.

Flexner A: *Medical education in the United States and Canada: a report to the Carnegie Foundation for the Advancement of Teaching*, New York, 1910, Carnegie Foundation.

Freidson E: *Professionalism reborn: theory, prophecy and policy*, Oxford, 1994, Polity Press.

Gale J: *The diagnostic thinking process in medical education and clinical practice: a study of medical students, House Officers and Registrars with special reference to endocrinology and neurology*, PhD thesis. London, UK, 1980, University of London.

Gawande A: *Complications; A surgeon's notes on an imperfect science*, London, 2002, Profile Books Ltd.

GMC: *Recommendations as to the Medical Curriculum*, London, 1947, General Medical Council.

GMC: *Recommendations as to the Medical Curriculum*, London, 1957, General Medical Council.

GMC: *Recommendations on basic medical education*, London, 1980, General Medical Council.

GMC: *Tomorrow's doctors: recommendations on undergraduate medical education*, London, 1993, General Medical Council.

GMC: *Tomorrow's doctors 2009: a draft for consultation*. Available at: http://www.gmcuk.org/education/undergraduate/news_and_projects. Accessed November, 2009.

Golby M, Parrott A: *Educational research and educational practice*, Exeter, 1999, Fair Way Publications.

Haas J, Shaffir W: Ritual evaluation of competence: the hidden curriculum of professionalization in an innovative medical school program, *Work Occup* 9(2):131–154, 1982.

Haines A, Jones R: Implementing findings of research, *Br Med J* 308:1488–1492, 1994.

Lave J, Wenger E: *Situated learning: legitimate peripheral participation*, Cambridge, 1991, Cambridge University Press.

Margetson DB: The relation between understanding and practice in problem-based medical education, *Med Educ* 33:359–364, 1999.

Merrison AW: Report of the inquiry into the regulation of the medical profession, *Br Med J*, 25th June 1975.

MMC: *Modernising medical careers: the next steps. The future shape of foundation, specialist and general practice training programmes*, London, 2004, Department of Health.

Newman G: *Some notes on Medical Education in England*, London, 1918, HMSO.

Open University: *Evaluation of the reforms to higher specialist training 1996–1999: executive summary*, Milton Keynes, 2001, The Open University Centre for Education in Medicine.

Pinar WR, Reynolds WM, Slattery P, et al: *Understanding curriculum: an introduction to historical and contemporary curriculum discourses*, New York, 1995, Peter Lang.

Plsek PE, Greenhalgh T: The challenge of complexity in health care, *Br Med J* 323:625–628, 2001.

Plsek PR, Wilson T: Complexity, leadership and management in healthcare organisations, *Br Med J* 323:746–749, 2001.

Pring R: *Philosophy of educational research*, London, 2000, Continuum Books.

Rikers RM, Loyens SM, Schmidt HG: The role of encapsulated knowledge in clinical case representations of medical students and family doctors, *Med Educ* 38:1044–1052, 2004.

Schön D: *Beyond the Stable State: public and private learning in a changing society*, London, 1971, Temple Smith.

Schön D: *Educating the reflective practitioner*, London, 1987, Jossey-Bass.

Snyder BR: *The hidden curriculum*, New York, 1971, Knopf.

Stenhouse L: *An introduction to curriculum research and development*, London, 1975, Heinemann.

ten Cate O: Trust, competence, and the supervisor's role in postgraduate training, *Br Med J* 333:748–751, 2006.

Tooke J: *Aspiring to excellence: final report of the independent inquiry into modernising medical careers*, London, 2008, Department of Health.

Tyreman S: Promoting critical thinking in health care: *phronesis* and criticality, *Med Health Care Philos* 3:117–124, 2000.

Wenger E: *Communities of practice: learning, meaning and identity*, Cambridge, 1999, Cambridge University Press.

Williams G: *Western reserve's experiment in medical education and its outcome*, New York, 1999, Oxford University Press.

Woodward CA, Ferrier BM: The content of the Medical Curriculum at McMaster University: graduates' evaluation of their preparation for postgraduate training, *Med Educ* 17:54–60, 1983.

Section 2

Educational processes

Creating a learning environment

7

Rachel Isba   Klarke Boor

CHAPTER CONTENTS

ABC

Glossary

Approaches to participation: expansive approach
Fuller and Unwin describe a continuum of approaches to participation. At one end of the spectrum is an expansive approach. This approach has the following characteristics: departments offer their learners broad access to multiple communities of practice and stimulate boundary crossing; learners receive enough time for reflection and off-the-job time; departments aim to help learners become rounded experts and strive to align the development of learners' and organisational capabilities; a named individual is present to support learners; the status of learner is explicitly recognised.

Approaches to participation: restrictive approach
A restrictive approach represents the other end of the continuum from an expansive one. This approach has the following characteristics: departments offer their learners narrow access to learning in terms of tasks, knowledge, and different locations; there is limited boundary crossing; learners have practically no opportunities to reflect; departments aim to help learners become partial experts, tailored to organisational needs. *Ad hoc* support is offered to learners and there is ambivalent recognition of their status as learners.

Dundee Ready Educational Environment Measure (DREEM) An instrument widely used to measure undergraduate learning environments.

Dutch Residency Educational Climate Test (D-RECT)
An instrument to measure the postgraduate learning climate.

Herzberg's motivation-hygiene theory Herzberg developed his motivation-hygiene theory in 1959 according to which 'hygiene factors' (like working conditions or physical surroundings) prevent

Continued

© 2011, Elsevier Ltd.
DOI: 10.1016/B978-0-7020-3522-7.00007-3

ABC

Glossary (continued)

dissatisfaction, while 'motivation factors' (like recognition of achievement or the work itself) induce satisfaction. Dissatisfaction and satisfaction are, thus, not two ends of a continuum; they are separate entities. His work implies that some interventions will reduce dissatisfaction, but not necessarily generate satisfaction.

Learning environment See main Glossary, p 341
Maslow's Hierarchy of needs See main Glossary, p 341

Outline

Imagine that you are a medical student on your first day in hospital. You are feeling excited but also anxious. You are keen to get started but, when you arrive on the ward, you find it busier than you ever imagined. Your consultant does not expect you (in fact, he is not even on the ward yet), there is nowhere safe for you to put your bag, and the nurses tell you to stop getting in the way. You are put in an office and asked to wait until the consultant finishes the ward round. How would that influence your subsequent learning experience?

This is an example of a learning environment that is poorly organised at a number of levels, but probably all too familiar to many of our students. It shows how such an environment can have a negative impact on the learners within it. To be able to learn effectively, students need to be welcomed and supported. They need to feel that they belong to their place of learning and are not simply 'spare parts' getting in the way of other people. Learning environments are increasingly identified as having an influence on those within them – just as 'good' or 'bad' teachers can affect learners' experiences, so too can learning environments. This chapter explores learning environments in undergraduate and postgraduate medical education. It describes why they are important and what factors combine to make up one. It then explores some of those factors in detail before considering how learning environments can be measured. Towards the end of the chapter, we emphasise how important it is for organisations to invest in optimal learning environments, and offer some suggestions as to how organisations may optimise them. By aiming to develop learning environments that are positive, welcoming, and supportive to learners, institutions, organisations, and departments may avoid replicating the situation described above.

Why are we interested in learning environments?

From as early as primary school, learning environments have been identified as an important influence on the learners within them (DfES, 2006). Just as children's environments are vital to their development, so too are the environments in which our students and junior doctors learn. By gaining a better understanding of them and the particular influence they may exert upon students, it might be possible to alter them to improve learning experiences. Equally, by looking at the outcomes of individual ones, it may be possible to identify relationships between outcomes and the environments that produced them. If such a relationship can be shown, then it is reasonably to postulate that, by adjusting one, we may influence the other.

Many medical schools, specialty boards, and governments expect, and progressively, inspect the quality of their medical education. Policy makers want insight into the educational functioning of medical schools and teaching hospitals. Using those insights, institutions become aware of their strengths and weaknesses and are able to do something about them. Often, quality improvement efforts are doomed to fail because it is an arduous task to change daily routines. Evaluation of the current situation, however, is an important first step on the way towards better medical education. Of course, institutions should see to it that succeeding steps follow; they should make plans to improve the assessed shortcomings, and actually make the improvements and evaluate again to see whether the situation has really improved. That is, in fact, a description of the famous Plan-Do-Check-Act cycle, which Deming designed in the 1950s to promote quality improvements (Tague, 2004, pp 390–392). So, in conclusion, learning environments are important because they influence the learners working within them (and vice versa) and because measuring their climates shows how institutions are functioning educationally.

What makes a learning environment?

Meanings of the terms 'learning' and 'environment'

There are many published descriptions of the importance of learning environments (often interchangeably referred to as educational climates, educational environments, or learning climates) within the curricula of institutions but fewer publications explore what makes up a learning environment. The word 'environment' can mean physical space (with synonyms like surroundings, terrain, settings) and it can also mean atmosphere or ambiance. The term learning environments has several connotations, which include physical space and settings, teacher–learner relationships, and feelings. A big criticism of the term, however, is its all-embracing nature. People use it to describe purely material facilities such as the number of available computers or the architecture of a building or – at completely the opposite end of the spectrum – everything that happens on a campus or in a department (Genn, 2001; Hutchinson, 2003). For the purpose of this chapter, we must therefore be explicit about what we mean by learning environments.

First, it is important to dwell on our understanding of learning. As discussed in Chapters 2 and 12, Sfard describes two major outlooks on learning using two metaphors (Sfard, 1998). The first, traditional, metaphor is 'acquisition', which implies acquiring and possessing knowledge. The last few decades have seen a new metaphor of learning grow apace in medical education: the 'participation' metaphor. This term refers to learning by doing and becoming part of a greater whole. In this chapter, we have deliberately chosen not to use one metaphor because we agree with Sfard that both metaphors have value in understanding learning.

Formal and informal environments

Roughly, two types of environment exist within medical education. The first environment exists within universities and is predominantly designed for learning. Students attend classes, learn in small and large group formats, and are regularly assessed on their competence. The first and foremost aim of the students is to learn. The second environment is in (teaching) hospitals and community health facilities, where the focus is on working. Medical students in the clinical phase of their training and residents learn their craft through participating in daily practice. Their predominant aim is to work. Although most learners acknowledge the importance of learning by doing, there is always a tension between service delivery and education. Formal learning environments may have different characteristics from informal ones, but in our opinion non-clinical and clinical environments show many similarities when it comes to considering them as learning environments. In this chapter, therefore, we describe several general aspects that are equally applicable to both environments. In the section that considers how to measure learning environments, we list measures that are applicable to undergraduate and postgraduate environments.

Four aspects of learning environments

As was explained earlier, you can consider several aspects of learning environments. First, their *material* aspects: What kind of facilities exist to support learners? What aspects should be addressed in order to improve them? What are the organisational arrangements to facilitate learning? Second, the *social* world is an important facet of learning environments. During the last decade, interest in sociocultural perspectives on learning has grown apace, as discussed in Chapter 2. Those understandings draw heavily on the work of Vygotsky, who stated that all learning is social (Vygotski, 1962). For example, Vygotsky described children pointing their fingers. First, this is an accidental movement, but when they see the reaction of others, they start using it purposefully. Vygotsky's work led on to Lave and Wenger's conceptualisations of situated learning (Lave and Wenger, 1991; Wenger, 1998). Their theory stressed (even more) the importance of local contexts (i.e. learning environments). They stated that all learning is situated and that knowledge is intimately connected to participation in activities. The importance of 'experience-based learning' has been replicated in recent studies among medical students (Dornan et al, 2007) and residents (Teunissen et al, 2007). People learn from other human beings and together construct new understandings of the world. Third, it is important to look at learning environments' influence on learners' behaviour, emotions, and practical competences. As learners grow and develop in social worlds, learning environments have an impact on the *intra-psychological* 'worlds' of individual learners, which are evident in their behaviour, emotions, and practical competences, such as skills, knowing how to learn, and applied knowledge. Fourth, you can get an indication of the educational functioning of departments or medical schools through *measuring* learning environments. These four aspects will be described in further detail below.

Learning environments at different organisational levels

Finally, learning environments exist at a number of different organisational levels ranging from large national institutions to small groups of students in a single department. Each of those levels is subject to different pressures and influences and able to exert different degrees of influence on other organisational levels. Learning environments may encompass variable numbers of people – from single learners to entire universities or hospitals. They come in all shapes and sizes. Whilst general impressions or overviews of learning environments exist, individual students will experience their own unique personal versions of them. This presents a challenge for those who seek to measure and alter learning environments, as any one institution or department may be made up of multiple smaller learning environments that combine to make the whole.

Organisational levels

Material facilities

Learning environments are shaped by organisational arrangements that facilitate or impede learners' participation and learners' perceptions of the quality of those arrangements may not accord with faculty's perceptions of them. By arranging teaching sessions off the ward when it is very busy, for example, students may be pulled away from valuable 'informal' activities to attend 'formal' activities that they perceive (rightly or wrongly) to be less valuable. Papers referring to learning environments and how they should be improved often suggest focusing on material aspects; for instance, the need to buy more

computers. This section describes the importance of material contexts.

The influence of material context has been studied by researchers interested in satisfaction and motivation. Two psychologists, Maslow and Herzberg, have been highly influential in this regard. In 1943, Maslow described a hierarchy of needs for reaching 'self-actualisation' (see also Chapter 9, Maslow, 1943) and the need for each level to be fulfilled before it is possible to progress to the next level. The first level consists of 'basic physiological needs' such as getting enough food, sleep, and shelter. After those needs are fulfilled, one can move up to the next level and attain 'feelings of security and justice'. Only if these needs are satisfied, can one attain 'belongingness needs', such as having a partner, a family, and good relationships with friends or peers. Having fulfilled these needs, a person 'strives for achievement' and a reasonable amount of status. And only after fulfilment of those last needs does one reach 'self-actualisation'. This influential theory is used in many management courses. Few studies have, however, confirmed the strict hierarchy as originally proposed; for example, people can be motivated without basic needs being met.

Herzberg proposed his motivation-hygiene theory in 1959 (Herzberg, 1968; Herzberg et al, 1959). He claimed that job satisfaction is the consequence of motivation factors, whereas job dissatisfaction is the consequence of hygiene factors. According to his theory, job satisfaction and job dissatisfaction are not two ends of a continuum – they are separate entities. Hygiene factors are, for instance, salary, working conditions, and physical environment. If those factors are improved, they have no structural influence on job satisfaction but they prevent dissatisfaction. Motivation factors are, for instance, achievement, recognition of achievement, the work itself, and responsibility. They lead to increased job satisfaction. This theory implies that many interventions aimed at improving job satisfaction (like salary rises or improvements in physical surroundings) lead only to dissolving job dissatisfaction. To improve job satisfaction, Herzberg proposes *enriching* jobs by offering more responsibility, accountability, and acknowledgement of work delivered. The theory is based on data collected using the critical incident technique, where people are asked to recount vivid examples of situations under study. A diverse group of people – engineers, accountants, hospital maintenance personnel, nurses, and others – contributed. The distinction between job dissatisfaction and job satisfaction has been criticised and may be a result of the research technique used, although other studies have seemed to confirm the distinction. Also, many authors criticise the assumption that more satisfied workers get more work done, which is prevalent in the work of both Maslow and Herzberg.

The work of those two researchers sheds light on material components of educational environments. It is clear that the physiological needs of learners have to be fulfilled for a learning environment to stand any chance of being optimal. If medical students have not slept for days or are feeling hungry or cold, they will be less inclined to learn. Also, so-called hygiene factors are important to prevent dissatisfaction with the material context of learning environments. Learning environments can be enhanced by good facilities, although they are not a *sine qua non*. Institutions aiming to improve their learning environments often begin by investing in physical surroundings (relatively easy to change, 'just' costing time and money), while they fail to make long-lasting investments in the organisational and social context (which are much harder to change). Those relatively superficial changes may not lead to an improved perception of the learning environments (think back to Herzberg's hygiene factors).

To sum up, the material context is an important determinant of learning environments, which influences (at least) motivation. Departments should support learners' basic needs and offer amenities to facilitate learning. Efforts to improve learning environments should not, however, be restricted to investing in material aspects alone and should include attention for participation and interaction as well.

Organisational priority for education

Organisations exert a strong influence on the learning environments within them. An organisation that values teachers and teaching activities highly will provide its students with learning environments that reflect those values and will differ from other organisations where teaching is valued less. If learners see teachers being rewarded – for example by promotion – this may encourage them to strive to become good teachers themselves. Equally, showing that poor-quality teaching or unprofessional behaviour on the part of teachers is not tolerated is a positive feature of learning environments. Still, academic promotion is often awarded to researchers rather than teachers (Chandran et al, 2009). That

is partly because educators' contributions are not so visible (Simpson et al, 2007), which has led to the development of analytic tools to help evaluators see educators' achievements (Chandran et al, 2009; Simpson et al, 2007).

As stated earlier, learning environments exist at different organisational levels; for example at institutional and departmental levels, each of which is subject to different internal and external influences and potential conflict between them. The pressures on a medical school dean will be very different from those on first year medical students and the learning environments that surround them will reflect this. It is also true that the influence exerted by people in one learning environment on the development of others will be affected by their different hierarchical levels. Medical students will be able to shape their own learning environments and exert influence on their peers but will struggle to make major changes at an institutional level. Deans can influence learning environments around and downstream from them, but will find it harder to influence learning environments at a national level. Students themselves clearly have a role to play in this 'regulation' of learning environments. By asking them to complete a learning environment measurement tool and become more discerning about positive and negative elements of their learning environments, they will be better placed to shape their own microlearning environments, whilst also having a greater impact on the holistic learning environments within their institution.

Social processes

Participation

Lave and Wenger firmly put participation on the map by writing their landmark book, *Situated learning: legitimate peripheral participation* (Lave and Wenger, 1991). They described five case studies among midwives, Vai Gola tailors, quartermasters, butchers, and reformed alcoholics, showing how newcomers gradually became involved in daily practice and learned their craft 'just' through situated participation. Their work, also reviewed in Chapters 2 and 12, has had a strong influence on conceptions of learning today. Regarding learning environments, Fuller and Unwin (2003) built on Lave and Wenger's work to propose a continuum of approaches adopted by institutions offering apprenticeships in the United Kingdom. At one end of their continuum lies an *expansive approach*, which includes broad access to activities (boundary crossing), explicit acknowledgement of students' status as learners, and the aim of becoming a full participant. At the other end lies a *restrictive approach*, with access to a more limited range of activities, a greater focus on the benefits of work to the institution than on students' learning needs, and lack of explicit recognition of students' status as learners (see Table 7.1 for a complete oversight). Both approaches imply learning through participation. The expansive approach, however, offers a richer learning environment that is more focused on learners' growth than the restrictive approach. Recent work in the undergraduate medical setting by Dornan and colleagues showed the importance of supported participation, which resembles the expansive approach above (Dornan et al, 2007).

In summary, the availability of diverse opportunities for participation is an important property of learning environments. Newcomers should be able to move from the periphery to a more central position in a community of practice and, eventually, become full participants. All activities should be oriented towards reaching this status. For example, a resident in specialist training should be involved in the whole diversity of patient care and, in addition, the managerial and supervisory tasks of a specialist.

Table 7.1 Characteristics of approaches to participation

Expansive approach	Restrictive approach
Participation in multiple communities of practice in and outside the workplace	Restricted participation in multiple communities of practice
Primary community of practice has shared 'participatory memory': cultural inheritance of apprenticeship	Primary community of practice has little or no 'participatory memory': little or no tradition of apprenticeship
Breadth: access to learning fostered by cross-company experiences built into the programme	Narrowness: access to learning restricted in terms of tasks/knowledge/location
Access to range of qualifications including knowledge-based vocational qualifications	Access to competence-based qualification only
Planned time off the job including attending college and for reflection	Virtually all on job: limited opportunities for reflection
Gradual transition to full participation	Fast transition
Apprenticeship aim: rounded expert – full participant	Apprenticeship aim: partial expert - full participant
Post-apprenticeship vision: progression of career	Post-apprenticeship vision: static
Explicit institutional recognition of, and support for, apprentice's status as learner	Ambivalent institutional recognition of, and support for, apprentice's status as learner
Named individual acting as dedicated support to apprentices	No dedicated individual; *ad hoc* support
Apprenticeship used as a vehicle for aligning the development of individual and organisational capability	Apprenticeship used to tailor individual capability to organisational need
Apprenticeship design fosters opportunities to extend identity through boundary crossing	Apprenticeship design limits opportunities to extend identity: little boundary crossing
Reification of apprenticeship highly developed (e.g. through documents, symbols, language, tools) and assessable to apprentices	Limited reification of apprenticeship, patchy access to reificatory aspects of practice

After Fuller and Unwin (2003).

Teacher–learner relationships

Within learning environments, innumerable interactions take place every day. Interactions in medical education are between teachers and learners, teachers and patients, and learners and patients. Those interactions are complex and multi-faceted, and can contribute either positively or negatively to learners' experiences of their learning environments. Relationships between learners and teachers are a particularly influential aspect of any learning environment. The importance of those relationships was acknowledged by Hippocrates, who began his famous oath with the statement that one should "…hold him who has taught me this art as equal to my parents…" and, later on, one should "…give a share of precepts and oral instruction and all the other learning to my sons and to the sons of him who has instructed me and to pupils who have signed the covenant and have taken the oath according to medical law, but to no one else" (North, 2002). Those statements show that learning and teaching have been central to the medical profession from at least ancient Grecian times and they remain a powerful influence on learning to this day.

Tiberius et al (2002) describe changes in our understanding of teacher–learner relationships over the last half century. First, there was acceptance of the notion that teachers could be trained; rather than believing that 'good teachers are born, not made', people started to believe that didactic skills were trainable. In the 1960s and 1970s, objectivist models using metaphors like *transfer* and *malleability* became popular views of teaching and learning. Teachers possessed knowledge, which they could transfer to learners as if they were vessels waiting to be filled. Moreover, learners were seen as raw material that teachers could mould into any preferred form or shape. If learners did not learn enough, flaws in the material were to blame ('a leak in the vessel'). Those metaphors show similarities to the 'acquisition metaphor' described earlier in this chapter and Chapter 2. At the end of the 1970s and 1980s, interactionist and constructivist metaphors like *growth* and *conversation* came increasingly to the fore. According to this line of thought, the social context is pivotal to learning. Learners construct meaning through interaction with others in social settings. Teachers should arrange learning material in such a way that it engages learners' interest and helps them connect it to their earlier experiences. Teachers must interact with learners to find out how to incite their interest and, so, induce growth. The final understandings of teaching and learning Tiberius et al describe are relational models using the *inclusion* and *transformation* metaphors. Like good patient–doctor relationships, good teacher–learner relationships are the vehicle of learning. The difference between these last two understandings is the focus on individual relationships between learners and teachers in the latter and the roles of groups and community in the former. Both, however, have similarities to the earlier described participation metaphor.

Teaching as a feature of learning environments

Research on teachers predominantly focuses on clinical as opposed to science teaching. There have been many studies describing the roles of ideal clinical teachers. Ullian et al (1994) published a categorisation of four roles: the supervisor; physician; teacher; and person. A recent qualitative study among obstetric-gynaecologic residents showed the importance of the person role; almost half of all remarks related to this role. Apparently, residents value direct and personal interaction (Boor et al, 2008b).

Lyon's (2003, 2004) research on interactions between teachers and learners in the operating room (OR) has been very informative. She performed an extensive qualitative study including in-depth interviews, periods of observation in the OR, and student surveys. One important finding was that students had "…to negotiate the social relations of work, to find a legitimate role to play in order to participate in the 'community of practice', constituted by the operating theatre and its personnel." In further exploring this theme, she found that trust, legitimacy, involvement, and participation were factors facilitating positive learning experiences. In addition, she described the process of 'sizing up', where learners and surgeons continuously re-evaluated one another. Students sought out student-friendly surgeons, and procedures that offered possibilities for them to participate. Moreover, they presented themselves as pro-active, motivated students who deserved attention and teaching. Surgeons, for their part, observed students' motivation, interest, and professional conduct and then decided how to distribute valuable teaching time and participation opportunities (Lyon, 2003, 2004). Other authors have also stressed the importance of students trying to show 'good' behaviour in order to be rewarded with more opportunities to participate (Boor et al, 2008a; Sheehan et al, 2005).

It is important to realise that not only do learning environments influence learners but also learners influence learning environments. Moran and Volkwein (1992) have given a historical overview of understandings of organisational climates over the last few decades. First, organisational climates were seen to exist apart from the participants working in them. Then, organisational climates were seen as products of participants' perceptions of the climates. Third came an interactive view, where participants and organisations together formed emerging organisational climates. We favour this last view, which has also been replicated in qualitative studies among medical students (Boor et al, 2008a) and residents (Boor, 2009). A learning environment changes through its 'inhabitants'.

How teachers interact with their patients is an important influence on learning environments, which may have a direct impact on how learners then treat patients. By acting as role models (either implicitly or explicitly), teachers impart information to students about how they themselves should treat patients. Bandura has performed groundbreaking research on modelling. In his studies of aggressive behaviour, he showed how people could impart their behaviour to young children observing them (Bandura et al, 1961). This research from the 1960s has had a major impact on discussions about aggressive television shows and computer games as well as aggressive behaviour within families (for instance, children who witness abuse within their family have higher chances of becoming abusive themselves). Often, unintended behaviour is imitated; think of smoking or swearing. That has implications for teacher–learner relationships in medical education; teachers have to be aware of their position as role models *all the time*. They can *say* that it is important to take time to listen to patients but if they do not *show* that behaviour, students will copy their actual behaviour rather than follow their directions. In addition, Bandura suggested four steps in learning through modelling:

1. Learners must pay attention to certain behaviour before they can imitate it. A teacher can arouse this attention by 'cuing' (for instance explaining that a case is particularly helpful or interesting).
2. Learners must have the ability to *retain* what they have seen by imagination or language (by making a visual representation or verbal description of the behaviour).
3. Learners must have the (motor) ability to *reproduce* the behaviour.
4. Learners must be *motivated* to perform a behaviour. Possible incentives are past reinforcements, promised reinforcements, or vicarious reinforcements.

This work has clear implications for learning environments. Teachers and learners must be aware of the central role their interactions (not only with each other but also with patients and colleagues) play in the development of medical learning environments. If teachers want to serve as role models, they must be constantly aware of their behaviour and give learners opportunities to learn the behaviour by facilitating the above-described four steps. In turn, learners need to be aware of their own behaviour, as well as that of their teachers, and be pro-active in recognising those who may act as positive (and negative) role models. Ultimately, these learners will become teachers, and it is therefore important that they develop the attributes of positive role models.

Behaviour, emotions, and practical competences

Learning environments influence learners' behaviour and emotional well-being (Seabrook, 2004). Recent research that included in-depth exploration of undergraduate medical students' and staff's narratives suggests that learning environments have an important emotional element. Many students described learning environments using emotional language such as 'feel' and 'safe', and staff felt that it was important to make students 'feel welcome' (Isba, 2009). It is possible, therefore, that emotion represents a common final pathway between other elements. That is unlikely to be a static relationship, and the learning environment may then 'feed back'. It appears that emotional aspects of learning environments are more prominent in the perceptions of students than was previously been thought, and this fits with work emerging from other areas of medical education research on the value of emotions in learning (Isba, 2009). Observations relating to the role played by emotions in learning environments have huge implications for those responsible for delivering medical education, and may mean that a radical re-think of the 'How, why, and where' of teaching is on the horizon.

Another qualitative study amongst medical students clearly showed how learning environments affect learners' behaviour, emotions, and practical competences (Boor et al, 2008a). Students described, for instance, how they lost their motivation and enthusiasm in a department with a *restrictive* approach towards participation (Boor et al, 2008a). They felt discouraged from taking any initiatives. In addition, they described how they lacked practical skills (in this case obstetric and gynaecologic abilities). Another study showed how 'participation was influenced by, and influenced, respondents' emotions, which reached high peaks and low troughs': another example of learning environments' influencing students' emotions (Dornan et al, 2007). Organisational psychology also suggests a relation between environments and intra-psychological changes. Research shows a slight relationship between organisational climate and job performance (DeCotiis and Summers, 1987; Pritchard and Karasick, 1973), as well as a manifest influence on motivation (DeCotiis and Summers, 1987) and job satisfaction (DeCotiis and Summers, 1987; Pritchard and Karasick, 1973). It may, however, be difficult to prove a relationship between organisational culture and performance, since the former is such a multi-faceted construct (Scott et al, 2003).

Measuring medical learning environments

It is important to those involved in the delivery of undergraduate and postgraduate medical education to be able to quantify learning environments within their institutions for a number of reasons. By measuring them, it may be possible to identify strengths, weaknesses, and priority areas for improvement or resource allocation. Measuring learning environments can therefore act as a powerful curriculum evaluation and development tool, collecting data from those on the receiving end of a curriculum. By asking learners what they think about their learning environment, you are indicating that you value their opinion, and that is an important part of learner–institution interactions. An additional benefit of measuring learning environments is that their quantification allows comparison with other institutes. In addition, as stated in the introduction, measuring learning environments is the *beginning* of

a quality cycle that should then be followed by interventions and new evaluations.

Having said earlier that learning environments are many things to many different people, and operate at so many different levels, is it even possible to measure them? Research in the area of learning environments has, like many areas of medical education research, benefited from the duality of 'mixed methods'. By using qualitative approaches such as focus groups alongside quantitative methods, it has been possible to get a more detailed impression of learning environments than would have been possible from a single methodological approach alone (Boor, 2009; Isba, 2009). For the purpose of this chapter, however, we focus on quantitative instruments currently available for measuring learning environments. When considering an instrument, it is vital they not only measure what they set out to measure, but do so in a valid and reliable way. The American Psychological and Education Research Associations have published standards identifying five sources to support validity (American Education Research Association and American Psychological Association, 1999), summarised in Table 7.2. Reliability coefficients are used to estimate measurement error and are a means of quantifying an instrument's measurement consistency. The most commonly used measures of reliability are Cronbach's α (based on test–retest characteristics, and indicating internal consistency), the Kappa statistic (a correlation coefficient that indicates inter-rater reliability), ANOVA (also indicating inter-rater reliability), and generalisability theory (an estimate of the concurrent effects of multiple sources on reliability).

A number of instruments have been developed to quantify learning environments from the perspective of those learning within them – be they students, residents, or specialists. Each of those instruments has had its own set of strengths and weaknesses, both with regard to their design and also reliability and validity. A summary of survey instruments that have been developed to measure learning environments (all but one in medical education) over the last half century appears in Table 7.3.

Whilst some of the measurement instruments that appear in Table 7.3 are no longer widely used, some remain in extensive use across the world, despite not having the most robust psychometric qualities. Arguably, the most widely used instrument for measuring undergraduate medical learning environments at the current time is the Dundee Ready Educational Environment Measure (DREEM).

Table 7.2 Five sources of validity evidence

Validity evidence source	Definition
Content	The relationship between a test's content and the construct it is intended to measure. Refers to themes and wording of items. Includes experts' input. Also includes development strategies to ensure appropriate content representation
Response process	Analyses of responses, including the strategies and thought processes of individual respondents. Differences in response processes may reveal sources of variance that are irrelevant to the construct being measured. Also includes instrument security, scoring, and reporting of results
Internal structure	The degree to which items fit the underlying construct. Most often reported as measures of internal consistency and factor analysis
Relation to other variables	The relationship between scores and other variables relevant to the construct being measured. Relationships may be positive (convergent or predictive) or negative (divergent or discriminant)
Consequences	Surveys are intended to have some desired effect, but they also have unintended effects. Evaluating such consequences can support or challenge the validity or score interpretations

After Beckman et al (2005).

Table 7.3 Properties of surveys measuring the medical educational learning climate

Name	Authors	No. items, No. subcales	Study population	Validity evidence sources[a]		Reliability estimates
College Characteristics Index (CCI)[b]	Pace and Stern (1958)	300 items, 30 subscales	423 students, 71 faculty members	Content	Minimal	Inter-rater Reliability Item discrimination test
				Response process	No	
				Internal structure	Minimal	
				Relat. other variables	Minimal	
				Consequences	No	
Medical School Environment Inventory	Hutchins (1961)	180 items, 18 subscales	1901 medical school graduates	Content	Minimal	-
				Response process	No	
				Internal structure	No	
				Relat. other variables	No	
				Consequences	No	
Learning Environment Questionnaire	Rothman and Ayoade (1970, 1971)	65 items, 7 subscales	145 first year medical students	Content	Minimal	Internal consistency
				Response process	No	

Table 7.3 Properties of surveys measuring the medical educational learning climate—cont'd

Name	Authors	No. items, No. subcales	Study population	Validity evidence sources[a]		Reliability estimates
				Internal structure	Minimal	
				Relat. other variables	No	
				Consequences	No	
Medical School Learning Environment	Feletti and Clarke (1981), Marshall (1978)	50 items, 7 subscales	93 first year medical students	Content	Yes	Cronbach's α Other test–retest measures
				Response process	Minimal	
				Internal structure	Minimal	
				Relat. other variables	Minimal	
				Consequences	No	
	Rotem et al (1995)	46 items, 8 subscales (1 other section: No. of items not described)	209 first year residents	Content	Minimal	Cronbach's α
				Response process	No	
				Internal structure	Minimal	
				Relat. other variables	No	
				Consequences	No	
Dundee Ready Educational Environment Measure (DREEM)	Roff et al (1997)	50 items, 5 subscales	490 medical students, 256 nursing students	Content	Minimal	Cronbach's α
				Response process	No	
				Internal structure	Minimal	
				Relat. other variables	No	
				Consequences	No	
	Pololi and Price (2000)	31 (or 15) items, 3 subscales	619 non-clinical medical students	Content	Minimal	Cronbach's α
				Response process	No	
				Internal structure	Minimal	

Continued

Table 7.3 Properties of surveys measuring the medical educational learning climate—cont'd

Name	Authors	No. items, No. subcales	Study population	Validity evidence sources[a]		Reliability estimates
				Relat. other variables	No	
				Consequences	No	
Anaesthetic Theatre Educational Environment Measure (ATEEM)	Holt and Roff (2004)	40 items, 5 subscales	218 anaesthetical residents	Content	Minimal	–
				Response process	No	
				Internal structure	No	
				Relat. other variables	No	
				Consequences	No	
Surgical Theatre Educational Environment Measure (STEEM)	Cassar (2004)	40 items, 4 subscales	25 surgical residents	Content	Minimal	Cronbach's α
				Response process	No	
				Internal structure	Minimal	
				Relat. other variables	No	
				Consequences	No	
Practice-based Educational Environment Measure	Mulrooney (2005)	37 items, 4 subscales	48 GPs in training	Content	Minimal	–
				Response process	No	
				Internal structure	No	
				Relat. other variables	No	
				Consequences	No	
Postgraduate Hospital Educational Environment Measure (PHEEM)	Roff et al (2005)	40 items, 3 subscales	97 residents	Content	Minimal	Cronbach's α
				Response process	No	
				Internal structure	Minimal	

Table 7.3 Properties of surveys measuring the medical educational learning climate—cont'd

Name	Authors	No. items, No. subcales	Study population	Validity evidence sources[a]		Reliability estimates
				Relat. other variables	No	
				Consequences	No	
DREEM for residents	Oliveira Filho et al (2005)	50 items, 5 subscales		Content	Minimal	Cronbach's α Other test–retest measures
				Response process	No	
				Internal structure	Minimal	
				Relat. other variables	Minimal	
				Consequences	No	
Operating Room Educational Environment Measure (OREEM)	Kanashiro et al (2006)	40 items, 4 subscales	22 surgical residents	Content	Minimal	Cronbach's α
				Response process	No	
				Internal structure	Minimal	
				Relat. other variables	No	
				Consequences	No	
Mini-STEEM	Nagraj et al (2007)	14 items	83 final year medical students	Content	Minimal	Cronbach's α
				Response process	No	
				Internal structure	Minimal	
				Relat. other variables	No	
				Consequences	No	
Dutch Residency Educational Climate Test (D-RECT)	Boor (2009)	50 items, 11 subscales	38 experts, 1278 residents	Content	Yes	Cronbach's α Generalisability analysis
				Response process	No	
				Internal structure	Yes	
				Relat. other variables	No	
				Consequences	No	

[a]'No' indicates no data regarding this category; 'Minimal' indicates minimal data regarding this category; 'Yes' indicates sound and multiple data sources supporting the category.
[b]This is not a *medical educational* climate survey, but since it serves as a basis for many later developed surveys it is included in this list.

DREEM has spawned multiple other questionnaires like PHEEM (Roff et al, 2005), ATEEM (Holt and Roff, 2004), and STEEM (Cassar, 2004) (see Table 7.3) mostly developed by researchers working in Dundee, Scotland, United Kingdom. DREEM will now be explored in detail as an example of a tool to measure learning environments. There are, in addition, a number of newer learning environment measurement tools, which have set out to include rigorous testing of reliability and validity as part of their development; one will be described in more detail.

Undergraduate learning environments: DREEM

Undergraduate medical education takes place before qualifying as a doctor under the auspices of a medical school within a parent university. DREEM was developed in 1997 by a team of medical education researchers based in Dundee, Scotland, along with more than 80 collaborators around the world (Roff et al, 1997). Since then, it has been widely translated and remains the cornerstone of quantitative learning environment research in undergraduate medical education. It was developed as a generic tool for measuring learning environments in any country and was reported to be 'culture-free' and therefore transferable between any culture or curricular style. It uses a five-point Likert scale format, with 50 items each being assigned a score between 0 and 4. Combining those scores gives a total score out of a possible 200. The items can also be subgrouped into five headings – perceptions of learning, perceptions of teachers, academic self-perceptions, perceptions of atmosphere, and social self-perception – each containing a different number of items. However, recent work has shown these subscales are not reproducible across study cohorts (Isba, 2009).

Like any other instrument, DREEM has strengths and weaknesses. Whilst it is relatively easy to understand, there are some ambiguous items. It allows easy comparison with curricular outcomes like exam results, although reports of its reliability have not been uniformly positive. It has the potential to drive curriculum development because it represents student feedback but it may provide only a very broad overview of a learning environment. In sum, there is only minimal (and equivocal) evidence for its validity and reliability (Oliveira Filho et al, 2005).

Postgraduate learning environment: D-RECT

In 2008, a Dutch Residency Educational Climate Test (D-RECT) was developed with the specific aim of overcoming some of the above-mentioned psychometric shortcomings of existing scales (Boor, 2009). First, D-RECT built on earlier qualitative research among residents from various specialties and with different levels of experience. This research showed that an ideal learning climate integrated work and training while attuning to residents' personal needs. Those themes provided a basis for the preliminary D-RECT (75 items). Two complementary approaches safeguarded the psychometric quality of the instrument: in multiple anonymous rounds, a Delphi panel consisting of 38 experts (residents, specialists, educationalists, policy makers) (dis)approved of items to be included in it; at the same time, 1278 residents from 26 specialties filled out the preliminary questionnaire. Six hundred randomly selected questionnaires were used for an exploratory factor analysis. The outcomes from this combined with input from the Delphi panel led to a 50-item questionnaire, consisting of 11 subscales whose Cronbach's α coefficients varied from 0.64 to 0.85. The remaining surveys were used for a confirmatory factor analysis to confirm the subscale structure. This analysis showed a good fit. Generalisablity analyses showed D-RECT to be reliable with a number of 11 participating residents (although most scales could be interpreted reliably with the input of only eight residents). The 11 subscales cover subjects such as 'supervision', 'coaching and assessment', 'teamwork', and 'professional relations between consultants'. D-RECT's aim is formative, which means that departments can get information on the strengths and weaknesses of their clinical learning environments as a basis for improvement efforts. Two sources of validity evidence (content and internal structure) seem well accounted for and D-RECT's reliability has been carefully established.

Summary

Learning environments are of interest to those with responsibility for delivering medical education at all levels because they influence the ongoing development of medical students and qualified doctors and may have an impact upon curricular or programme outcomes. Learning environments are made up of, and influenced by, many things. Certain aspects of learning environments may be grouped into themes – preconditions, processes, and outcomes. Perhaps the most valuable element of any learning environment, however, remains the people within it – learners, teachers, and patients. People can have profound impacts – either positive or negative – upon learners and play a large part in the process of learning. Other elements of learning environments include physical space, opportunities, resources, and experiences.

Learning environments lend themselves to exploration in a number of different ways, both quantitative and qualitative. Whilst there are a number of quantitative instruments available to measure learning environments in postgraduate and undergraduate medical education, no one tool in current use is supported by the robust evidence and rigorous psychometric testing now expected in medical education research. However, new measurement tools are being developed. By measuring learning environments, it is possible to identify their strengths and weaknesses, which can lead on to improvement efforts. This is of particular importance as it offers institutions the opportunity to target their (often limited) resources on areas that learners have identified as important.

Much research remains to be done, particularly the further development of measurement instruments. Exploratory work also needs to be done to examine relationships between learning environments and learning outcomes. If such relationships exist, there is potential for harnessing learning environments to improve outcomes. Whilst learning environments are complex and hitherto poorly understood, they offer considerable potential for future development in medical education.

Implications for practice

Optimising learning environments

Each aspect of learning environments explored earlier in the chapter can, potentially, be improved. We now consider them in turn, suggesting how it might be possible to improve them to the benefit of the learning environment as a whole. Material aspects are the most easily optimised, though budgetary constraints will determine how close it is possible to get to the ideal. Learning environments need to be conducive to legitimate participation. Learners must feel they 'belong' and their learning is supported. Thinking back to the poor learning environment described at the start of this chapter, it is quite easy to see ways in which they could be improved. Learners need to be expected and welcomed, and supported emotionally as well as intellectually. They need to have positive role models and see how the environment encourages professional, ethical behaviour, and good clinical practice.

The evolution of learning environments is shaped by the multiple, complex interactions that occur within them, which opens the way to improving them by optimising teacher–learner relationships. 'Teach the teacher' courses and mentoring schemes that allow learners to align themselves with teachers for whom they feel a professional affinity have a clear role to play. Teaching and learning activities offered to learners, including supervision and feedback, may also be optimised. Finally, if it is possible to differentiate one learning environment from another and quantify their different strengths and weaknesses, then it should be positive for positive elements of one learning environment to be emulated by another.

References

American Education Research Association and American Psychological Association: *Standards for educational and psychological testing*, Washington, DC, 1999, American Education Research Association.

Bandura A, Ross D, Ross SA: Transmission of aggression through imitation of aggressive models, *J Abnorm Soc Psychol* 63:575–582, 1961.

Beckman TJ, Cook DA, Mandrekar JN: What is the validity evidence for assessments of clinical teaching?

J Gen Intern Med 20(12):1159–1164, 2005.

Boor K: *The clinical learning climate*, Amsterdam, 2009, VU Medical Center.

Boor K, Scheele F, van der Vleuten CPM, et al: How undergraduate clinical learning climates differ: a multi-method case study, *Med Educ* 42(10):1029–1036, 2008a.

Boor K, Teunissen PW, Scherpbier AJ, et al: Residents' perceptions of the ideal clinical teacher – a qualitative

study, *Eur J Obstet Gynecol Reprod Biol* 140(2):152–157, 2008b.

Cassar K: Development of an instrument to measure the surgical operating theatre learning environment as perceived by basic surgical trainees, *Med Teach* 26(3):260–264, 2004.

Chandran L, Gusic M, Baldwin C, et al: Evaluating the performance of medical educators: a novel analysis tool to demonstrate the quality and impact of educational activities, *Acad Med* 84(1):58–66, 2009.

DeCotiis TA, Summers TP: A path analysis of a model of the antecedents and consequences of organizational commitment, *Hum Relat* 40(7): 445–470, 1987.

DfES : *Early years foundation stage consultation document*, Nottingham, 2006, DfES.

Dornan T, Boshuizen H, King N, et al: Experience-based learning: a model linking the processes and outcomes of medical students' workplace learning, *Med Educ* 41(1):84–91, 2007.

Feletti GI, Clarke RM: Construct validity of a learning environment survey for medical schools, *Educ Psychol Meas* 41:875–882, 1981.

Fuller A, Unwin L: Learning as apprentices in the contemporary UK workplace: creating and managing expansive and restrictive participation, *J Educ Work* 16(4): 407–426, 2003.

Genn JM: AMEE Medical Education Guide No. 23 (Part 2): curriculum, environment, climate, quality and change in medical education – a unifying perspective, *Med Teach* 23(5):445–454, 2001.

Herzberg F: One more time: how do you motivate employees? *Harv Bus Rev* 46(1):53–62, 1968.

Herzberg F, Mausner B, Snyderman BB: *The motivation to work*, New York, 1959, Wiley.

Holt MC, Roff S: Development and validation of the Anaesthetic Theatre Educational Environment Measure (ATEEM), *Med Teach* 26(6): 553–558, 2004.

Hutchins EB: The 1960 medical school graduate: his perception of his faculty, peers, and environment, *J Med Educ* 36:322–329, 1961.

Hutchinson L: Educational environment, *BMJ* 326(7393):810–812, 2003.

Isba R: *DREEMs, myths and realities: learning environments within the University of Manchester Medical School*, Manchester, 2009, University of Manchester.

Kanashiro J, McAleer S, Roff S: Assessing the educational environment in the operating room – a measure of resident perception at one Canadian institution, *Surgery* 139(2):150–158, 2006.

Lave J, Wenger E: *Situated learning: legitimate peripheral participation*, Cambridge, 1991, Cambridge University Press.

Lyon P: A model of teaching and learning in the operating theatre, *Med Educ* 38(12):1278–1287, 2004.

Lyon PM: Making the most of learning in the operating theatre: student strategies and curricular initiatives, *Med Educ* 37(8):680–688, 2003.

Marshall RE: Measuring the medical school learning environment, *J Med Educ* 53(2):98–104, 1978.

Maslow AH: A theory of human motivation, *Psychological Review* 50:370–396, 1943.

Moran ET, Volkwein JF: The cultural approach to the formation of organizational climate, *Hum Relat* 45(1):19–47, 1992.

Mulrooney A: Development of an instrument to measure the Practice Vocational Training Environment in Ireland, *Med Teach* 27(4):338–342, 2005.

Nagraj S, Wall D, Jones E: The development and validation of the mini-surgical theatre educational environment measure, *Med Teach* 29(6):e192–197, 2007.

North, M: *Hippocratic oath*, Bethesda, 2002, National Library of Medicine.

Oliveira Filho GR, Vieira JE, Schonhorst L: Psychometric properties of the Dundee Ready Educational Environment Measure (DREEM) applied to medical residents, *Med Teach* 27(4):343–347, 2005.

Pace CR, Stern GG: An approach to the measurement of the psychological characteristics of college environments, *J Educ Psychol* 49(5):269–277, 1958.

Pololi L, Price J: Validation and use of an instrument to measure the learning environment as perceived by medical students, *Teach Learn Med* 12(4): 201–207, 2000.

Pritchard RD, Karasick BW: The effects of organizational climate on managerial job performance and job satisfaction, *Organ Behav Hum Perform* 9:126–146, 1973.

Roff S, McAleer S, Harden RM, et al: Development and validation of the Dundee Ready Education Environment Measure (DREEM), *Med Teach* 19:295–299, 1997.

Roff S, McAleer S, Skinner A: Development and validation of an instrument to measure the postgraduate clinical learning and teaching educational environment for hospital-based junior doctors in the UK, *Med Teach* 27(4):326–331, 2005.

Rotem A, Godwin P, Du J: Learning in hospital settings, *Teach Learn Med* 7:211–217, 1995.

Rothman AI, Ayoade F: The development of a learning environment: a questionnaire for use in curriculum evaluation, *J Med Educ* 45:754–759, 1970.

Scott T, Mannion R, Marshall M, et al: Does organisational culture influence health care performance? A review of the evidence, *J Health Serv Res Policy* 8(2):105–117, 2003.

Seabrook MA: Clinical students' initial reports of the educational climate in a single medical school, *Med Educ* 38(6):659–669, 2004.

Sfard A: On two metaphors for learning and the dangers of choosing just one, *Educ Res* 27(2):4–13, 1998.

Sheehan D, Wilkinson TJ, Billett S: Interns' participation and learning in clinical environments in a New Zealand hospital, *Acad Med* 80(3):302–308, 2005.

Simpson D, Fincher RM, Hafler JP, et al: Advancing educators and education by defining the components and evidence associated with educational scholarship, *Med Educ* 41(10): 1002–1009, 2007.

Tague RN: *The quality toolbox*, ed 2, Milwaukee, 2004, ASQ Quality Press.

Teunissen PW, Scheele F, Scherpbier AJJA, et al: How residents learn: qualitative evidence for the pivotal role of clinical activities, *Med Educ* 41(8):763–770, 2007.

Tiberius RG, Sinai J, Flak EA: The role of teacher-learner relationships in medical education. In Norman GR, van der Vleuten CP, Newble DI, editors: *International handbook of research in medical education*, Dordrecht, 2002, Kluwer Academic Publishers, pp 462–498.

Ullian JA, Bland CJ, Simpson DE: An alternative approach to defining the role of the clinical teacher, *Acad Med* 69(10):832–838, 1994.

Vygotski LS: *Thought and language*, Cambridge, MA, 1962, MIT Press.

Wenger E: *Communities of practice. Learning, meaning, and identity*, Cambridge, 1998, Cambridge University Press.

Identifying learners' needs and self-assessment

Casey White Larry Gruppen

8

CHAPTER CONTENTS

ABC

Glossary

Constructivism See main Glossary, p 338.

Learning agreements See personal learning plans

Learning Management Systems Systems that support and assist learners to plan, manage, customise, share, regulate, and evaluate their learning. These resources might include learning tools and guides, study guides, course management systems, and portfolios, among others. Currently, most learning management systems are computer-based and increasingly robust.

Learning Strategies See main Glossary, p 339.

Minute paper See main Glossary, p 339.

Personal learning plans These plans are formulated by learners, often in collaboration with teachers, and outline learners' goals, learning activities, and strategies they plan to use to reach the goals, resources they will use, and how they will monitor their progress and evaluate their learning. They are also called learning contracts or learning agreements in some settings.

Self-efficacy See main Glossary, p 340.

Self-regulated learning See main Glossary, p 340.

Outline

This chapter considers how educators can help learners take responsibility for identifying and addressing their learning needs. It considers the topic from

© 2011, Elsevier Ltd.
DOI: 10.1016/B978-0-7020-3522-7.00008-5

theoretical and empirical research perspectives as well as giving practical insights. Physicians must possess the skills we describe here if they are to be effective lifelong self-regulated learners. To help them discharge their responsibilities towards their own and others' learning, we describe tools for self-identifying and addressing gaps in knowledge and skills, educational principles, and methods that support self-regulated learning, tips, and principles for helping faculty assume roles as effective facilitators in more active and small-group methodologies, and information on electronic tools that can help learners manage and enhance their learning. Finally, we present some conclusions and a consideration of the chapter's implications.

Identifying and addressing learning needs

One of the major responsibilities of medical practitioners is to maintain knowledge and skills through continuous learning. A physician's motivation to learn should be driven by needs identified in the course of clinical practice; that is, day-to-day professional work including collaborations on teams and encounters with patients and colleagues. These provide an informal, opportunistic context for identifying personal learning needs (Grant, 2002). Despite its importance, there is evidence that physicians are not very effective at self-assessing their own learning needs (i.e. identifying 'blind spots' and gaps) (Bandara and Calvert, 2002; Davis et al, 2006; Eva and Regehr, 2005). Likewise, students enter medical school lacking skills to self-assess learning needs (Fitzgerald et al, 2003). By virtue of being in a learning phase, they lack the competence or knowledge to assess their own performance accurately within the domain of what they are learning (i.e. 'How can I know what I do not know when I do not know what I do not know?') (Eva and Cunningham, 2004).

As medical education becomes more learner-centred, approaches that shift responsibility for learning to students, including responsibility to identify and address learning needs, become more important. There is growing evidence that personal learning plans (PLPs) and portfolios – coupled with guidance, reflection, and feedback – can be effective tools for identifying (i.e. self-assessing) and addressing learning needs (Challis, 2000; Mathers et al, 1999). As a result, PLPs are becoming more common in medical education. Portfolios in particular have been under academic investigation as lifelong learning tools in medical practice for some

time, particularly in the United Kingdom. Given changes in certification for physicians in the United States, they will likely become more common there as well in the near future. Tools like portfolios provide a structure for recording, reflecting on, and assessing learning needs. Thus, it makes sense to introduce them as early as possible so students become increasingly facile by the time they are autonomous medical practitioners.

Personal learning plans

Personal learning plans (PLPs), also called learning contracts or learning agreements, have been linked with 'deep' learning (Marton et al, 1984), adult learning principles (Knowles, 1986), self-assessment, self-regulated learning, and lifelong learning (Knowles, 1975; see Box 8.1).

As with all learning, guidance and feedback from a mentor are key to developing a PLP and its ongoing implementation and adaptation. It is important to gauge and encourage motivation and self-confidence, particularly for learners who are accustomed to having their learning needs dictated and assessed by faculty (Challis, 1997). A critical underlying philosophy is that a PLP challenges students to assume responsibility for learning – including identifying learning needs or gaps, setting learning objectives, choosing resources, and self-assessing. This responsibility can be increased over time, as skills become sharper. Ultimately, the PLP should be designed to help students develop into motivated and skilled self-regulating learners throughout their professional lives (Anderson et al, 1996).

Portfolios

Portfolios, which are considered at greater length in Chapter 13, have become an increasingly popular tool in the context of student-centred learning. They

Box 8.1

How learning plans help learners (Challis, 2000)

Learning plans help learners identify:
- What needs to be learnt
- Why it needs to be learnt
- How it will be learnt
- How learners will know when they have learnt it
- A timeframe for learning
- Links to past and future learning

are similar to PLPs in that they challenge students to take more responsibility for their own learning but they often also involve writing and reflection combined with collection and assessment of learning goals, resources, events, and outcomes. Portfolio-based learning has been shown to improve acquisition of factual knowledge (Elango et al, 2005) but, as important, its use fosters autonomy and self-assessment (Challis, 2000). Again, continuous guidance and feedback by a mentor are key. In assessing a portfolio, mentors should see evidence of completion of the self-regulated learning cycle: learning needs identified; strategies to meet needs customised to learning styles and activities; structured self-assessment and reflection on experience; and use of feedback and critical events to modify or reformulate learning objectives (Mathers et al, 1999). Principles of reflective learning are presented in Chapter 2.

Reflection

The notion of being a reflective practitioner is not new – in fact there is a wealth of literature on the topic dating back to the early twentieth century (Dewey, 1933). Effective methods to help students become more reflective, however, have been more elusive; in part, that is due to a lack of appropriate skills on the part of instructors (McGrath and Higgins, 2005). While concrete, purposefully worded learning outcomes and time set aside specifically for reflection are a good start, these can be insufficient. Learners need to know how they will achieve their intended outcomes. Without facilitation and an appropriate environment, time set aside to reflect might lead to diffuse and disparate outcomes (Boud and Walker, 2001). Thoughtful writing with individualised feedback (Wald et al, 2009) and other forms of structured reflection such as reflective practice groups (Platzer et al, 1997) and critical incident analysis (Ghaye and Lillyman, 1997) have been shown to yield deep (as opposed to surface) learning (Mathers et al, 1999) and foster insight into personal accountability and responsibility.

There is relatively less attention in the literature to what instructors need to know in order to help learners acquire reflective skills. These include synthesis and evaluation (high-order skills on Bloom's taxonomy of the cognitive domain) (Bloom, 1956), clinical reasoning, problem solving, and self-awareness (McGrath and Higgins, 2005). Boud and Walker (2001) argue that ritualised processes or pre-written sets of questions to be pondered and answered are more comfortable for facilitators but do not allow learners to construct their own meanings. Reflection is not solely a cognitive process – feelings are key elements of reflection and unique to individuals so learners must be able to express themselves intellectually and emotionally. Effective environments to promote reflection require respect, trust, boundaries, and appropriate understanding of the learning milieu (context), which influences instructors and learners in different ways (Boud and Walker, 2001).

Self-regulated learning and self-assessment

The need for self-regulated learning

Although there are established links between self-regulated, continuous medical education and the quality of care provided by physicians (Lowenthal, 1981; Westberg and Jason, 1994), there is evidence that physicians are not particularly effective at identifying gaps in their own knowledge and skills (Davis et al, 2006; Eva and Regehr, 2005). We know that good self-regulated learning (SRL) habits can be taught (Pintrich, 1995) and it therefore seems logical to help students develop such behaviours when they enter medical school. To achieve successful outcomes, however, SRL has to be intentionally integrated into a curriculum – meaning that it will require additional time and resources in the curriculum in order to ensure appropriate mentoring, monitoring, and feedback.

Integrating SRL into curricula has shorter-term benefits as well. Research has suggested that learners who are proactive tend to learn more and learn better than learners who expect instructors to transmit knowledge (Knowles, 1975); proactive learners are more persistent, resourceful, motivated, and confident (Pintrich, 1995; Zimmerman and Schunk, 2001). Developing SRL in learners can be fostered by creating learning environments that make learning processes explicit, offer opportunities for practicing self-regulation (Schunk and Zimmerman, 1994), set clear expectations for goal-setting, self-monitoring, and reflection, and provide specific and comprehensive feedback linked with learner self-assessment and achievement of learner-set goals (White and Gruppen, 2007).

The student's role

A self-regulating learner takes initiative for diagnosing learning needs, formulating goals, identifying resources, implementing appropriate learning/studying activities and strategies, and evaluating progress and outcomes (Spencer and Jordan, 1999). To foster self-regulation, students must be actively involved in monitoring and regulating their performance in the context of strategies and resources they choose, and how these influence progress against goals (Nicol and MacFarlane-Dick, 2006). The more self-regulating learners become, the more effective they are at generating and using internal feedback (self-assessment) to measure progress against personal goals, and the more effective they are at interpreting external feedback in relation to their goals (Butler and Winne, 1995). Students must understand and assume ownership of goals to measure progress effectively and achieve them.

The instructor's role

The instructor's role is to provide formative feedback that centres on learner self-regulation. Feedback concerns how the student's present state of learning relates to their goals, which must have some overlap with goals originally set by the instructor. Table 8.1 offers specific advice on effective feedback.

Models for self-regulated learning

There are several models or infrastructures through which educators can integrate SRL practices into curricula. Zimmerman's groundbreaking work on

---

Table 8.1 Seven principles of good feedback practice that facilitate self-regulation (Nicol and MacFarlane-Dick, 2006)

1	Helps clarify what good performance is	• Learner must have clear understanding of criteria for good performance • Exemplars of performance make the standard explicit
2	Facilitates development of self-assessment and reflection	• Self-assessment tasks are effective and structured opportunities for self-monitoring and judging progress against goals • Tasks might include self-assessment of performance with integrated tutor feedback; assessing strengths and weaknesses in own work before handing in to instructor; reflecting on achievements and selecting work to compile a portfolio
3	Delivers high-quality information to students about their learning	• Focuses on strengths and weaknesses and offers corrective advice • Directs students to higher-order learning goals • Helps students trouble-shoot their own performance and self-correct • Helps students take action against discrepancy between their intentions and resulting outcomes
4	Encourages teacher and peer dialogue around learning	• Dialogue provides students with opportunities to engage instructor in discussion about feedback; helps students develop an understanding of expectations, correct misunderstandings, and get immediate response to difficulties • Peer dialogue enhances sense of self-control over learning (peer language more accessible; peer discussion exposes students to different viewpoints, peer assessment helps develop detachment of judgement that can be transferred to self-assessment)
5	Encourages positive motivational beliefs and self-esteem	• Feedback that draws attention away from the task and toward self-esteem can have a negative effect on attitude, attribution, and performance • Motivation and self-esteem are more likely to be enhanced with many low-stakes assessment tasks and feedback geared to progress and achievement • Tasks might include allocating time for learners to redo assignments; automated testing with feedback; drafts and resubmissions

Table 8.1 Seven principles of good feedback practice that facilitate self-regulation (Nicol and MacFarlane-Dick, 2006)—cont'd

6	Provides opportunities to close the gaps between current and desired performance	• Provides opportunities to repeat the same 'task–performance–feedback' cycle to ensure that feedback has influenced performance • Helps learners recognise the next steps in learning and how to take them, during assignment production and related to next assignment • Tasks might include two-stage assignments where feedback on stage one improves stage two; incorporating specific 'action points' into feedback
7	Provides information to instructors that can help shape instruction	• To produce good feedback, instructors need good data on how students are progressing; review of and reflection on this data help them to support self-regulation in their students • Information about student progress becomes available when learning outcomes are translated into performances or products • Tasks might include using variants of the one-minute paper; having students identify where they are having difficulty as they hand in assignments; asking students to identify a 'question worth asking' they would like to explore

self-regulated learning developed a three-step model comprising forethought (task analysis and self-motivation); performance/control (self-control and self-observation); and self-reflection (self-judgement and self-reaction) (Zimmerman, 2000). While many educators agree that all learners self-regulate to some degree (Winne, 1997), Zimmerman believed that what separates effective SRL from ineffective SRL is the quality and quantity of SRL processes. The model on which the seven principles above were developed (Nicol and MacFarlane-Dick, 2006) comprises a series of steps that begin with the instructor assigning a task. Subsequent steps include the learner drawing on prior knowledge and motivation to construct an interpretation of the task and its requirements, formulating personal learning goals, and using strategies and tactics that produce internally and externally observable outcomes. Internal feedback (self-monitoring; self-assessment) permeates almost all of the steps; external feedback is compared with the learner's interpretation of the task, which is modified as needed to adjust future strategies and tactics (Nicol and MacFarlane-Dick, 2006).

White and Gruppen (2007) proposed a model adapted from Zimmerman's work (2000) comprising four major phases: planning (institutional and personal learning goals, motivation, and self-efficacy); learning (expectations and methods, epistemology, learning styles, learning strategies); assessing (self-assessment, external feedback); and adjusting (reflection, adjustment). This model views SRL as dynamic and contextual, with both learners and instructors having roles and responsibilities – some separate and some overlapping. External feedback is built into all phases.

In an engineering schools study, students were encouraged to develop habits for self-regulated learning by practicing planning, time management, self-reflection, and self-motivation (Jowitt, 2008). They were provided with information about tools and techniques that included self-evaluation, organising and transforming, goal-setting and planning, information seeking, self-monitoring, environment structuring, self-consequences (e.g. rewards for good performance), rehearsing and memorising, seeking social assistance (e.g. study groups), and reviewing records (e.g. grades). Although definitions of SRL and models for it might vary somewhat, there are many more similarities than differences. In general, medical educators agree that SRL is important for practicing physicians, include it in medical schools' goals for education, and commonly discuss it in literature on medical education.

Medical schools' role

If medical schools want their students to assume responsibility for learning, there are a few specific steps they can take. Intended learning outcomes of their curricula can include SRL skills and attitudes, which can be reinforced with opportunities for learning and practicing SRL, role modelling, and feedback pertaining to those outcomes. Learning SRL can be integrated across the educational programme rather than compressed into the clinical years. SRL can also be a structured activity which includes feedback. Increasing choices about and responsibility for learning will help students become more effective self-regulating learners (Hagen and Weinstein, 1991). When learners rely on others for their learning, they look for cues about what to learn and how to learn it; they focus on trying to figure out what teachers want from them and on what they will be assessed. This is poor preparation for independent, lifelong learning.

Self-assessment

A key element of self-regulated learning is self-assessment. Learners need detailed formative and summative feedback about their progress so they can gauge their self-assessments and make adjustments in order to reach learning or mastery goals. Although scores on quizzes and examinations are sufficient to tell learners whether they are memorising or comprehending information and concepts correctly, such scores tend to focus on lower-order cognitive skills that do not help learners achieve the higher-order skills of analysis, synthesis, and evaluation. We know that most learners do not possess inherent self-assessment skills (Baker, 1984)and that poorer performers tend to overestimate their performance while better performers tend to underestimate it (Eva and Regehr, 2005; Kruger and Dunning, 1999). Sullivan and colleagues (1999) acknowledged that 'In order for students to acquire lifelong learning skills, they must develop the ability to critically evaluate themselves'. Their study, similar to many medical school studies (e.g. Calhoun et al, 1984; Risucci et al, 1989), compared students' assessments of their performance with peer and tutor evaluations of their performance. Students were less able to identify their strengths and weaknesses than peers and faculty, leading the authors to conclude that, 'A possible explanation for these results is that students are not routinely taught self-evaluation skills in a traditional curriculum'. Self-regulated learning helps learners take responsibility for their own learning, change from a focus on external measures (e.g. faculty and grades) to a focus on learning, helps them monitor their own performance more effectively, and achieve at higher levels. Self-regulated learners can effectively use a broad array of measures – internal and external – to guide and enhance their own education in school, in residency, and in practice.

Learning principles and methods that support self-regulated learning and self-assessment

Principles

Learning objectives (or intended learning outcomes) should send a clear message to learners about the content (knowledge, skills, attitudes) faculty intend them to learn and how learning of it will be measured. Likewise, it is paramount that learners are clear on the pedagogic principles of the curriculum and the methods that will be used to deliver content. An inherent assumption of self-regulated learning is that both instructors and learners share accountability for learning – that is, both parties have explicit responsibilities. Two examples of educational principles that align with self-regulated learning and a joint (and in some ways also co-dependent) sense of responsibility are constructivism and adult learning (andragogy), topics that are also discussed in Chapter 2.

Constructivism

Constructivists believe that knowledge is developed within learners rather than transmitted by an instructor to a passive student. Learning occurs most effectively when the mind filters incoming information and connects that information to past experience and current need or relevance. Thus, learners find solutions by 'playing' with new information – revising, restructuring, and exploring new information as they place it in their own personal cognitive structures (Spigner-Littles and Chalon, 1999). Understanding and embracing constructivism in theory and principle is one thing; integrating it into the design of a curriculum, however, is another matter (Tenenbaum et al, 2001). Box 8.2 lists some elements of a constructivist approach.

Furthermore, instructors in a constructivist environment must have appropriate training and resources so they are prepared to create motivating conditions for students, take responsibility for creating problem situations for students to work through, foster acquisition and retrieval of prior knowledge, and create a social environment that emphasises the attitude of learning to learn (Phye, 1997). Instructors in constructivist settings need to learn how to guide and not tell, and to create and foster an environment in which

Box 8.2

Elements that indicate integration of constructivism

- Subject matter can be viewed through the context of students' personal experiences
- Subject matter is real, authentic (case studies, examples)
- Ample interaction between teacher and student is encouraged
- There is interaction and collaboration among students
- Students identify their own learning goals
- Educational methods are learner-centred
- Subject matter is evidence-based

students can make their own meaning rather than receive 'pre-packaged' meaning from teachers, not focus on one right answer but look for diversity in thought processes, modify previous notions of right and wrong, and loosen rigid standards and criteria (Airsian and Walsh, 1997). In such environments, students learn to think for themselves (instead of waiting for the teacher to tell them what to think), proceed with more autonomy and less direction from the teacher, express their own ideas in their own words, and revisit and revise knowledge constructions (Airsian and Walsh, 1997). The reward for integrating constructivism into a course or curriculum is that students learn to think more critically and creatively – they are able to analyse, predict, present theories, and engage in meaningful dialogue (Brooks, 1990). Constructivism lends itself extraordinarily well to SRL. SRL calls for students to assume increased responsibility for their own learning by creating personal goals that are challenging but achievable, looking inwardly for motivation to learn, experimenting with learning strategies to find which are most effective, comparing external feedback with self-assessment, and finally reflecting on performance and continuously and dynamically adjusting goals and plans (White and Gruppen, 2007).

Adult learning principles

The work of Malcolm Knowles focused on how adult learners differ from standard school-aged learners (Knowles, 1973). He was interested in how the development of individuals influenced their learning. He wrote about how earlier traditions of teaching and learning practiced by great teachers in ancient history – Confucius, Jesus, Socrates, Plato, and Aristotle, who

primarily taught adults with methods such as dialogue and learning by doing – were lost with the fall of Rome. It became common for children to be educated from the seventh century onwards and pedagogy (from the same stem as paediatrics) was based on obedience and efficiency. Other educators and researchers have provided evidence that, as individuals mature, the need to be self-directing, use personal experiences as a context for learning, and organise learning around life problems increases steadily and rapidly (Bower and Hollister, 1967; Bruner, 1961; White, 1959). Ultimately, Knowles (1984) identified the following characteristics of adult learners, who

- Are more self-directed: adults want to be actively involved in learning processes and can use personal goals to guide their learning,
- Need to connect personal experiences with new knowledge: adults learn most effectively when new knowledge can be connected with prior life experiences,
- Are goal-oriented: adults have a much clearer idea of what they want to achieve in a class, which guides their learning,
- Must see the relevance of or a reason to learn: adults must see the relevance of what they are learning to what they do, or want to do,
- Are practical: it is much less likely that adults will want to learn just for learning's sake – they will more likely want to learn something that is useful to them for their job,
- Need respect: adults bring a wealth of knowledge and experiences to learning environments; learning will be most effective when this is recognised and they are treated as equals.

As with constructivism, instructors must align their teaching practices with adult learning principles to achieve desired outcomes. Guidance from research includes the following (Zemke and Zemke, 1984):

- The learning environment should be physically and psychologically comfortable; avoid long periods of sitting and/or being lectured to,
- Self-esteem and ego are important attributes that support adult learning; create opportunities for them to risk a new behaviour safely in front of or with peers,
- It is critical to articulate and clarify expectations prior to getting into content,
- Tap into the experiences of adult learners; they will learn effectively from dialogue with respected peers,

- Concentrate on open-ended questions that foster critical thought and self-discovery, and draw out relevant learner knowledge and experience,
- Create opportunities that actively engage learners in learning processes so they can integrate new knowledge with existing knowledge,
- Adult learning environments need a different type of control from the instructor, which needs to be facilitative and ego-free,
- Facilitate diverse – minority and majority – opinions and solutions; make connections between various opinions and ideas (i.e. there are multiple solutions to problems, not just one right answer),
- Create opportunities for learners to apply new knowledge,
- Be flexible in choosing methods to meet learning objectives/outcomes.

Educational methods

Connecting principles with educational methods is key to building a bridge of understanding and shared accountability between teachers and learners. Just as it is important for educators to explain principles that underlie their expectations and educational approaches, learners need to understand and embrace the principles as well, so they are prepared to meet their teachers' expectations. As self-directed learners in training', students should be expected to set their own goals, use experts and resources to help them achieve their goals, be willing to take responsibility for their own learning and productivity, be able to manage their own time and projects, and assess themselves and their peers (Grow, 1991).

Teachers can conceptualise, construct, and model specific learning activities that encourage ongoing cognitive growth and acquisition of complex reasoning skills. Approaches that foster development and provide opportunities for development of self-regulating habits tend to be those with progressively increased emphasis on learners' participation and responsibility for their own and their peers' learning. Active learning methods such as collaboration and opportunities for learners to discuss and analyse ill-structured problems and controversial issues help foster advanced cognitive skills (Baxter Magolda, 1999; King and Kitchener, 1994). Other methods include small group discussion, cooperative projects, simulations, case studies, and role-playing (Meyers and Jones, 1993). Use of active learning methods requires more attention from the instructor than more passive methods. For instance, small groups must be carefully composed and their discussions carefully crafted based on explicit principles and intended outcomes.

In choosing methods that align with principles and reinforce expectations, instructors can keep the following seven guidelines, developed by Chickering and Gamson (1987), in mind:

1. *Encourage contact between students and faculty*: Knowing at least a few faculty members well enhances students' intellectual commitment,

2. *Develop reciprocity and cooperation among students*: Good learning is collaborative and social, not competitive and isolated,

3. *Encourage active learning*: Students do not learn effectively by listening to teachers, memorising packaged assignments, and spitting out answers,

4. *Give prompt feedback*: Knowing what you know and do not know (or what you can do and cannot do) focuses learning; with feedback, students can reflect on what they have learnt and what they still need to learn (self-assessment),

5. *Emphasise time on task*: Time plus effort equals learning; allocating realistic amounts of time will lead to more effective learning,

6. *Communicate high expectations*: Expect more and you will get more; high expectations are important for everyone – students and instructors,

7. *Respect diverse talents and ways of learning*: Individuals bring different talents and styles of learning to the learning environment; they need opportunities to show their talents in ways that work for them, and they can be pushed to learn in new ways that do not come as easily.

Finally, instructors should write clear and precise learning objectives that convey achievement expectations to students, but that also guide decisions about learning and assessment methods. Bloom's taxonomies for cognition (1956) and affect/attitude (Krathwohl et al, 1973) and Simpson's for psychomotor skills (Simpson, 1972) are excellent resources for writing learning objectives.

Faculty development: see also Chapter 19

Many instructors, especially in professional education, are not formally trained as educators (Wilkerson and Irby, 1998). Their professional degrees certify them to practice, as a result of which they can provide a critical element of professional education by role modelling. Comprehensive professional education, however, also requires specific educational competencies that include designing learning modules, choosing and executing appropriate and innovative teaching/learning and assessment methods, scaffolding/sequencing presentation of new knowledge and skills, and evaluating the effectiveness of those educational elements.

Guiding, not leading

Important links between active/collaborative learning methods (e.g. small group discussions, cooperative projects, case studies, role-playing) and self-regulation have been investigated (Bell and Kozlowski, 2008; DeRouin et al, 2004; Ivancic and Hesketh, 2000). There is agreement among researchers that SRL habits can (and should) be taught in formal educational settings (Pintrich, 1995) but, to be learnt effectively, they must be embedded or integrated into a curriculum (Cho, 2004). So, instructors have a critical role in learners' SRL development – see Box 8.3. In many active

Box 8.3

Teaching tips for facilitators in active learning environments (adapted from Tulane University, 2009)

- Prepare a plan for the small group discussion,
- Listen well and be patient,
- Be supportive of the group, individuals in the group, and the small group process,
- Make learning a shared responsibility; involve all participants, and monitor personal level of participation (do not lead – facilitate),
- Feel comfortable with silence. Learners need to think, and thinking takes time,
- Be prepared to re-focus the discussion,
- Take risks by expressing personal thoughts about a topic or case; honesty and authenticity will create a setting where all group members are comfortable expressing themselves,
- Do not be afraid to say, 'I don't know',
- Challenge, but do not threaten; ask thoughtful questions and involve learners but do not belittle or judge,
- Summarise progress or decisions reached when appropriate – during discussion or at the end of discussion.

learning environments, the instructor acts more as a facilitator than a lecturer, a role that is very different and in many ways more difficult. In discussions in which one of the goals is for students to tackle complex, ill-defined issues or problems (King and Kitchener, 1994), for instance, a facilitator needs to step away from the leading role and let students grapple with the problems or issues they are addressing.

The art of questioning

Effective questioning can promote effective learning (see Table 8.2). Planned carefully and posed thoughtfully, questions arouse curiosity, stimulate interest, clarify important concepts, role model and encourage thinking at more advanced cognitive levels, promote collaboration, confirm learners' grasp of the material, and help identify which learners are having difficulty. Good questions are the backbone of productive (and enjoyable) group discussion. The most productive questions open up a variety of responses and invite students to think about and respond to the material at a high level.

Bloom's taxonomy in the domain of cognition (Table 8.3) provides a very useful tool for writing learning objectives, which can also be useful in designing learning activities – including types of questions that facilitate learning. The taxonomy begins at a low level of expected outcome (knowledge – the recall of memorised information) and progresses through to a much more complex level (evaluation – assessing evidence and defending decisions). The level of the question should match the complexity of intended learning.

Classroom assessment: improving teaching and identifying students' needs

For more than a decade, leading educators and educational researchers have advised that a broader range of assessment tools is needed to connect assessment with learning. More open-ended performance tasks, the argument goes, help ensure that students are able to reason critically, solve complex problems, and apply knowledge in real-world contexts. That means expanding the assessment 'toolbox' to include observations, clinical interviews, reflective journals, projects, demonstrations, collections of student work, and student

Table 8.2 Tactics for effective questioning (after Davis, 1995)

What to do	How to do it
Ask one question at a time	Keep questions brief and clear
Avoid yes/no questions	Ask why or how questions – let students work towards answers
Pose questions that lack a single right answer	Ask 'Ill-structured' questions – they have a number of equally-plausible responses; students can generate their own hypotheses
Ask focused questions	Avoid overly broad questions that can easily lead students off-topic
Avoid leading questions	Leading questions can limit open, relevant discussion around the topic; also, do not answer your own question
After asking a question, wait silently for an answer	Be patient. Waiting is a signal that you want thoughtful participation. If a prolonged silence continues, ask learners what it means
Search for consensus on correct responses	When one student immediately gives a correct response, ask others what they think; get them involved in the discussion
Ask questions that require students to demonstrate their understanding	Instead of asking 'Do you understand how to take an appropriate family history?' (a yes/no question) ask, 'What are the key elements of an appropriate family history?' or 'What are the critical approaches to keep in mind when taking a family history?'
Structure questions to encourage student-to-student interaction	Relate what one student says with what another subsequently says; find links and make them clear for the students. Think-pair-share: pose a question or problem and ask students to discuss in pairs
Use questions to change direction of discussion	Clarify perspectives: 'In a few words, name the most important …' Move from specific to general: 'If you were to generalise …' Move from general to specific: 'Can you give some specific examples?' Acknowledge good points made previously: 'John, would you agree with Mary on this point?' Elicit or give closure: 'Beth, what two themes recurred in today's discussion?'

Table 8.3 Bloom's taxonomy with sample questions

Knowledge (simplest)	Recall; repeat *Sample*: List four major causes of pneumonia in immuno-compromised patients
Comprehension	Interpret; describe *Sample:* Explain the molecular basis of the polymerase chain reaction
Application	Use facts, rules, principles *Sample*: A 40-year-old patient has a persistent cough and a fever (39°C) for 3 days. A radiograph shows a right lower lobe lung infiltrate. Based on these findings, construct a differential diagnosis
Analysis	Subdivide to component parts; reveal underlying structure *Sample*: Compare and contrast the symptoms, pathophysiologic mechanisms, and complications between Crohn's disease and ulcerative colitis
Synthesis	Put together elements and hypothesise; predict *Sample*: A 53-year-old patient with hypertension, peripheral oedema, and shortness of breath is diagnosed with cardiomyopathy. His ejection fraction is 22%. What would be your diagnostic and therapeutic plan?
Evaluation (most complex)	Assess; justify *Sample*: Defend why you would order a test for subtype influenza A in a 24-year-old pregnant woman and not a 57-year-old healthy man

self-assessments. It also means that teachers 'must engage in a systematic analysis of the available evidence' (Shepard, 2000). A specific class of assessment methods, called Classroom Assessment Techniques (CATs), has been designed to involve teachers and students in continuous monitoring of student performance against course objectives (Haugen, 2005). CATs help students become more effective self-assessors and help faculty monitor links between effective (or ineffective) teaching and learning and make adjustments and improvements as part of a dynamic cycle. Without such monitoring, there can be significant gaps between what is taught and what is learnt. Instructors often assume that students are learning what they are teaching, only to be faced with disappointing evidence to the contrary when they grade tests, when it is too late to fix problems (Angelo and Cross, 1993). Also, as a result of practice with classroom assessment, faculty members become better teachers and improve their ability to help students become more effective self-assessing, self-regulating learners.

Learning management systems: lifelong tools for self-regulating learners

A growing number of educators are convinced that a learner-centred approach yields deeper and more cognitively advanced learning, which in turn makes knowledge more accessible throughout formal education and professional life (Shepard, 2000; Spencer and Jordan, 1999). This approach requires students to be actively involved in their own learning – taking increasing responsibility over time. However, managing learner-centred education can be complex for the learner and the institution. In the last few decades, as curricula have transitioned from teacher-centred learning to more and more student-centred learning, there has been a growing recognition that robust management tools can support and enhance learning. Many such tools have been developed and are in widespread use but continuous advances in computer technology – and continuously more facile learners – mean that there is still important work in progress.

Learning tools and guides

A number of systems have been developed over the years to provide students with tools they can use to guide their learning. Below are just a few examples:

Study guides

Study guides support learning by specifying learning outcomes, helping students develop their own personal goals and study plans, identifying appropriate learning resources and how they should be used, and providing students with self-assessment opportunities (Skelly and Quentin-Baxter, 1997). They are particularly useful in the context of discovery learning.

Scaffolded, integrated tool environments

These environments are designed to help novice learners engage in new, complex processes such as investigation of scientific phenomena (Quintana et al, 2004). Using a learner-centred design, developers have created tools that support novices by breaking down complex processes into individual steps.

'Proposal wizard'

Currently, this tool is specific to one programme (pharmacy graduate education) but it is applicable across disciplines and educational levels. It helps students through the logical stepwise process of building a (written) research project. They complete one step (online), receive feedback from an experienced faculty member, and then revise that step before moving on to the next one.

Course management systems

Online course management systems (e.g. Moodle, Blackboard, TRIO) have changed the face of education. Both 'home grown' and commercial systems provide educational programmes with enormous flexibility for learning to take place outside the physical environment of classrooms (i.e. distance learning). Instructors can post announcements, syllabi, instructions, resources (e.g. book chapters, journal articles), assignments, and questions. Students can access these postings, submit assignments, engage in 'chats' (with faculty and classmates), take exams, and collaborate on assignments/projects. Course management systems, like tools and guides, can support learner-centred approaches to education; however, they are actually teacher-centred systems in that they help instructors manage the many elements of their courses. While students can access learning tools and instruments, they generally cannot customise the site to manage their own learning over time.

Portfolios

Portfolios are not new in the educational world, particularly in disciplines such as art, architecture, and interior design. Since they have gone online, 'ePortfolio' systems have gained ground in medical education as effective tools, especially for helping students assume responsibility for learning, reflection, self-assessment, and formative/summative assessment. Although some are created for personal use only, most that are used in formal educational contexts are open to scrutiny beyond individual learners. They are used as longer-term repositories that reflect longitudinal development, reflection, and achievement of outcomes. Learners may be asked to select the work most representative of their development and achievements – this self-assessment is then linked with formative or summative feedback from faculty – see Box 8.4 (Challis, 2000).

Despite the growing popularity of portfolios among educators, concerns linger about the effectiveness of them in virtual learning environments beyond formal educational structures (i.e. are they effective tools for lifelong learning?) (Larsen and Lofgreen, 2007). Medical students have expressed concern about the additional time-related burden of using portfolios, particularly in the clinical years and when portfolios are used as journals for longitudinal reflective writing (Elango et al, 2005). It is critical that learners understand the purpose of a portfolio and how to construct one that meets their goals and expectations (van Tartwijk et al, 2008). Articulating clear expectations and providing specific instructions might preclude some current concerns about portfolios.

Box 8.4

Advantages of portfolios (Challis, 2000)

Portfolios:
- Encourage reflective learning and identification of learning needs.
- Are based on learner's own experience, connects theory with practice.
- Allow learners to use a range of learning styles.
- Foster assessment within an established framework of competencies and learning objectives.
- Provide evidence of learning from a range of contexts.
- Enable self-assessment, and both formative and summative feedback.
- Provide a model for lifelong learning and continuous professional development.

Comprehensive learning management system

An effective learner-centred learning management system (LMS) could help learners customise, manage, share, and regulate their learning, both in the shorter term (for instance, within a course, or within a degree programme) and the longer term (for instance, from the beginning of medical school, through postgraduate training, and into clinical practice). Such a system could be built on a logical model for self-regulated learning (SRL) (White and Gruppen, 2007). An appropriately robust LMS will ultimately provide individuals with a customisable, user-friendly, online system for

- Identifying and monitoring educational/ programmatic and personal goals and learning objectives,
- Identifying and engaging in appropriate learning strategies and activities,
- Collaborating on projects and presentations,
- Sharing resources,
- Organising, managing, and tracking resources that comprise learning or future professional endeavours inside and outside of formal educational structures,
- Completing and documenting self- and external assessments, and
- Modifying and designing future learning plans.

Ultimate LMS functionality would include creating, modifying, tagging, rating, sharing, and storing resources; chatting and collaborating with selected groups of others; journaling; and giving and receiving feedback to/from peers and faculty. Students would have a private space within the system, but would also be able to permit access at multiple levels (individual faculty and/or students, pairs or small groups of faculty and/or students, friends, potential residency directors or employers, etc.). The LMS is envisioned as a dynamic system of elements and activities associated with self-regulated learning that can be used by individuals at micro, macro, and mega levels, depending on status, activities, curriculum, and personal/professional interests (Forment et al, 2009).

Implications for practice

There have historically been boundaries between and among outcomes that learners should achieve in medical school, in residency, and in professional practice.

With changes in health care delivery, in what we know about effective education, in the vast and dynamic body of relevant information for medical practice, and in tools and technology that support education, these boundaries are fading. Advanced skills and habits that support effective learning can be acquired within the formal structures of education, when there are significant opportunities for modelling, practice, and feedback. Habits for self-regulated learning – so key to effective lifelong learning and high-quality health care – can be integrated into formal curricula, with specific outcomes articulated and appropriate tools, mechanisms, and methodologies available to support learner achievement. This chapter has presented some of the underlying theory and evidence related to self-regulated learning, along with suggestions for instruments, mentoring, feedback, principles, methodologies, and

faculty development that support mastery of effective SRL. Expectations of SRL already exist in residency programmes in the form of required self-assessment and individual learning plans; their effectiveness is extremely limited – as is effectiveness of physician self-assessment – because there has been no formal and longitudinal cycle of practice–feedback– adjustment within the educational programmes, and no faculty development to support the cycle. Almost every medical school publishes a formal statement of goals that include some mention of self-assessment and lifelong learning, yet curricula have yet to indicate how and where they can be learnt. This chapter is intended to provide some level of guidance as to how to think about formal integration and assessment of self-regulated learning into curricula across the continuum of medical education.

References

Airsian PW, Walsh ME: Constructivist cautions, *Phi Delta Kappan* 78:444–449, 1997.

Anderson G, Boud D, Sampson J: *Learning contracts: a practical guide*, London, 1996, Kogan Page.

Angelo T, Cross PK: *Classroom assessment techniques: a handbook for college teachers*, San Francisco, CA, 1993, Jossey-Bass.

Baker L: Children's effective use of multiple standards for evaluating their comprehension, *J Educ Psychol* 76:588–597, 1984.

Bandara I, Calvert G: General practitioners: uncelebrated adult learners – a qualitative study, *Educ Prim Care* 13:370–378, 2002.

Baxter Magolda MB: *Creating contexts for learning and self-authorship: constructive-developmental pedagogy*, Nashville, TN, 1999, Vanderbilt University Press.

Bell BS, Kozlowski SWJ: Active learning: effects of core training design elements on self-regulatory processes, learning and adaptability, *J Appl Psychol* 93(2):296–316, 2008.

Bloom BS: *Taxonomy of educational objectives, Handbook 1: the cognitive domain*, New York, NY, 1956, David McKay, Co Inc.

Bloom BS, Krathwohl DR: *Taxonomy of educational objectives: the classification of educational goals, by a committee of college and university*

examiners. Handbook 1: cognitive domain, New York, 1956, Longmans.

Boud D, Walker D: Promoting reflective learning in professional courses: the challenge of context, *Supporting lifelong learning*, vol 1, Perspectives on learning, Oxon, UK, 2001, Routledge.

Bower EM, Hollister WG, editors: *Behavioral science frontiers in education*, New York, 1967, Wiley.

Brooks JG: Teachers and students: constructivists forging new connections, *Educ Leadersh* 47:68–71, 1990.

Bruner JS: The act of discovery, *Harv Educ Rev* 31:21–32, 1961.

Butler DL, Winne PH: Feedback and self-regulated learning: a theoretical synthesis, *Rev Educ Res* 65(3): 245–281, 1995.

Calhoun JG, Woolliscroft JO, Hockman EM: Evaluating medical student clinical skill performance: relationships among self, peer, and expert ratings, *Proc Annu Conf Res Med Educ* 23:205–210, 1984.

Challis M: Portfolio-based learning: continuing medical education for general practitioners – a mid-point evaluation, *Med Educ* 31:22–26, 1997.

Challis M: AMEE medical education guide No. 19: personal learning plans, *Med Teach* 22:225–236, 2000.

Chickering AW, Gamson ZF: Seven principles for good practice in undergraduate education, *Wingspread J* 7(2), 1987.

Cho M-H: *The effects of design strategies for promoting students' self-regulated learning skills on student's self-regulation and achievement in online environments*. Presented at the Association for Educational Communications and Technology, Chicago, Illinois, 2004.

Davis D, Thomson M: A systematic review of the effect of continuing medical education strategies, *JAMA* 274:700–705, 1995.

Davis DA, Mazmanian PE, Fordis M, et al: Accuracy of physician self-assessment compared with observed measures of competence, *JAMA* 296 (9):1094–1103, 2006.

DeRouin RE, Fritzsche BA, Salas E: Optimizing e-learning: research-based guidelines for learner-controlled training, *Human Resource Management* 43:147–162, 2004.

Dewey J: *How we think: a restatement of the relation of reflective thinking in the educative process*, Boston, MA, 1933, University Press.

Elango S, Jutti RC, Lee LK: Portfolio as a learning tool: students' perspective, *Ann Acad Med Singap* 34:511–514, 2005.

Eva K, Cunningham J: How can I know what I don't know? Personalities, *Adv Health Sci Educ* 9:211–224, 2004.

Eva K, Regehr G: Self assessment in the health professions: a reformulation and research agenda, *Acad Med* 80 (10):S46–S54, 2005.

Fitzgerald JT, White CB, Gruppen LD: A longitudinal study of self-assessment accuracy, *Med Educ* 37(7):645–649, 2003.

Forment MA, Guerrero MJC, Gonzalez MAC, Peñalvo FJC, Severance C: In *Lecture Notes in Computer Science*, Volume 5736. Berlin, 2009, Springer, pp. 286–295.

Ghaye T, Lillyman S: *Learning journals and critical incidents: reflective practice for health care professionals*, Salisbury, UK, 1997, Mark Allen Publishing Limited.

Grant J: Learning needs assessment: assessing the need, *BMJ* 324:156–159, 2002.

Grow G: Teaching learners to be self-directed, *Adult Educ Q* 41:125–149, 1991.

Hagen AS, Weinstein CE: Achievement goals, self-regulated learning, and the role of the classroom context. In Pintrich PR, editor: *Understanding self-regulated learning*, San Francisco, CA, 1991, Jossey-Bass.

Haugen S, Becker D: Classroom assessment and accounting student performance, *International Journal of Innovation and Learning* 2(1):36–46, 2005.

Ivancic K, Hesketh B: Learning from errors in a driving simulation: Effects on driving skill and self-confidence, *Ergonomics* 43:1966–1984, 2000.

Jowitt WA: 2008, Promoting and monitoring self-regulated learning techniques in engineering schools, *Proceedings of the 2008 AaeE Conference*.

King P, Kitchener KS: *Developing reflective judgment: understanding and promoting intellectual growth and critical thinking in adolescents and adults*, San Francisco, 1994, Jossey-Bass.

Knowles M: *Self-directed learning: a guide for learners and teachers*, New York, NY, 1975, Association Press.

Knowles M: *Using learning contracts*, San Francisco, CA, 1986, Jossey-Bass.

Knowles MS: *The adult learner: a neglected species*, Houston, TX, 1973, Gulf Publishing.

Knowles MS: *Andragogy in action. Applying modern principles of adult education*, San Francisco, 1984, Jossey-Bass.

Krathwohl DR, Bloom BS, Masia BB: *Taxonomy of educational objectives, the classification of educational goals. Handbook II: affective domain*, New York, 1973, David McKay Co., Inc.

Kruger J, Dunning D: Unskilled and unaware of it: how difficulties in recognizing one's own incompetence lead to inflated self-assessments, *J Pers Soc Psychol* 77(6):1121–1134, 1999.

Larsen LJ, Lofgreen LB: *PLE and e-portfolio as learning tools in the educational system*, 2007, In Proceedings of the World Conference on E-Learning in Corporate, Government, Health Care and Higher Education pp. 2069–2076.

Lowenthal W: Continuing education for professionals: voluntary or mandatory? *J High Educ* 52(5):519–538, 1981.

McGrath D, Higgins A: Implementing and evaluating reflective practice group sessions, *Nurse Educ Pract* 6:175–181, 2005.

Marton F, Hounsell D, Entwistle N, Editors: *The experience of learning*, Edinburgh, Scotland, 1984, Scottish Academic Press.

Mathers NJ, Challis MC, Howe AC, et al: Portfolios in continuing medical education – effective and efficient? *Med Educ* 33:521–530, 1999.

Meyers C, Jones TB: *Promoting active learning: strategies for the college classroom*, San Francisco, CA, 1993, Jossey-Bass.

Nicol DJ, MacFarlane-Dick D: Formative assessment and self-regulated learning: a model and seven principles of good feedback practice, *Stud High Educ* 31(2):199–218, 2006.

Phye GD: *Handbooks of academic learning: construction of knowledge*, San Diego, 1997, Academic Press.

Pintrich PR: *Understanding self-regulated learning. New directions for teaching and learning, No. 63*, San Francisco, CA, 1995, Jossey-Bass.

Platzer H, Snelling J, Blake D: Promoting reflective practitioners in nursing: a review of theoretical models and research into the use of diaries and journals to facilitate reflection, *Teach High Educ* 2:103–121, 1997.

Quintana C, Reiser B, Davis EA, et al: A scaffolding design framework for software to support science inquiry, *Journal of the Learning Sciences* 13 (3):337–386, 2004.

Risucci DA, Tortolani AJ, Ward RJ: Ratings of surgical residents by self, supervisors, and peers, *Surg Gynecol Obstet* 169:519–526, 1989.

Schunk DH, Zimmerman BJ: *Self-regulation of learning and performance: issues and educational applications*, Mahwah, NJ, 1994, Lawrence Erlbaum.

Simpson EJ: *The classification of educational objectives in the psychomotor domain*, Washington, DC, 1972, Gryphon House.

Skelly G, Quentin-Baxter M: *Implementation and management of on-line curriculum study guides: the challenges of organizational change*, 1997, In Proceedings of CTICM Computers in Medicine Conference, Bristol, CTICM pp. 656–673.

Spencer JA, Jordan RK: Learner centered approaches in medical education, *BMJ* 318:1280–1283, 1999.

Spigner-Littles DA, Chalon E: Constructivism: a paradigm for older learners, *Educ Gerontol* 25:203–210, 1999.

Sullivan ME, Hitchcock M, Dunnington GL: Peer and self assessment during problem-based tutorials, *Am J Surg* 177:266–269, 1999.

van Tartwijk, van Rijswijk M, Tuithof H, Drieesen EW: Using an analogy in the introduction of a portfolio, *Teaching and Teacher Education* 24(4): 927–938, 2008.

Tenenbaum G, Naidu S, Jegede O, et al: Constructivist pedagogy in conventional on-campus and distance learning practice: an exploratory investigation, *Learn Instr* 11 (2001):87–111, 2001.

Wald HS, Davis SW, Reis SP, et al: Reflecting on reflections: enhancement of medical education curriculum with structured field notes and guided feedback, *Acad Med* 84(7):830–837, 2009.

Westberg J, Jason H: Fostering learners' reflection and self-assessment, *Fam Med* 26:278–282, 1994.

White CB: Smoothing out transitions: how pedagogy influences medical students' achievement of self-regulated learning goals, *Adv Health Sci Educ* 12(3):279–297, 2007.

White CB, Gruppen LD: Association for the Study of Medical Education: *Self-regulated learning in medical education*.

White RH: Motivation reconsidered: the concept of competence, *Psychol Rev* 66:297–333, 1959.

Wilkerson L, Irby D: Strategies for improving teaching practices: a comprehensive approach to faculty development, *Acad Med* 73 (4):387–396, 1998.

Winne P: Experimenting to bootstrap self-regulated learning, *J Educ Psychol* 88:397–410, 1997.

Zemke R, Zemke S: Thirty things we know for sure about adult learning, *Innov Abstr* 6(8):57–60, 1984.

Zimmerman BJ: Attaining self-regulated learning: a social cognitive perspective. In Boekaerts M, Pintrich PR, Zeidner Moshe, editors: *Handbook of self-regulation*, San Diego, CA, 2000, Academic Press.

Zimmerman BJ, Schunk DH: *Self-regulated learning and academic achievement: theoretical perspectives*, Mahwah, NJ, 2001, Lawrence Erlbaum.

Teaching and learning in small groups

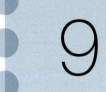

Reg Dennick   John Spencer

© 2011, Elsevier Ltd.
DOI: 10.1016/B978-0-7020-3522-7.00009-7

ABC
Glossary

Active listening A communication skill characterised by the deliberate act of maintaining eye contact and using appropriate body language when listening to an individual. In addition, a listener may reflect back what the speaker has said to indicate that their message has been completely received.

Andragogy; see also adult learning See main Glossary, p 337.

Assessment; formative See main Glossary, p 337.

Attention conflict Distraction from performing a task optimally by an individual in a group caused by giving attention to other group members.

Brainstorming A small group teaching activity in which individuals are encouraged to call out ideas in an informal and uninhibited way. Learners should be free to say what they like without interruption during the initial phase of the process. The technique is frequently used to generate a large variety of ideas, concepts, and information, which can then be processed and analysed in a more structured way. It is termed 'thought showering' in the United States.

Cognitive dissonance See main Glossary, p 337.

Constructive alignment A curriculum principle that emphasises the importance of mapping learning outcomes to teaching opportunities and learning experiences, which are then matched to assessment requirements and processes.

Constructivism See main Glossary, p 338.

Deep learning; see also approaches to learning See main Glossary, p 338.

e-facilitation; see virtual group The process by which a facilitator engages with a virtual group of learners 'on-line'.

Elaboration The cognitive process whereby learners expand their knowledge networks by making connections between elements of their knowledge and new information, frequently facilitated by active learning, application, and problem solving.

Evaluation apprehension A stressful feeling engendered in an individual within a group caused by being observed, assessed, or evaluated by other group members.

Experiential Learning Theory See main Glossary, p 338.

Facilitation The process whereby an individual helps or enhances the learning of others by organising appropriate learning resources or experiences and giving encouragement and feedback. Frequently associated with small group learning. Requires good interpersonal and communication skills and an ability to empathise with learners. More advanced facilitation skills are required to facilitate problem-based learning groups.

Feedback See main Glossary, p 338.

Forming A stage in small group dynamics during which members of the group come together for the first time.

ABC
Glossary (continued)

Free riding A strategy adopted by an individual in a group in which they reduce their contribution to the group product because they perceive other group members to be more competent.

Ground rules A set of working principles developed and/or approved by a small group of learners (e.g. a problem-based learning group) that guides their working activities and provides a framework to which all group members can adhere when conflict or other group problems arise.

Ice-breaking An activity designed to allow members of a newly formed group to introduce themselves to one another in an informal and often light-hearted way in order to reduce initial anxiety and develop group cohesion.

Learning outcomes See main Glossary, p 339.

Learning set A small group of students who meet on a regular basis to share knowledge acquired via self-directed learning and/or to engage in a group activity with a specific aim. Learning sets may also engage via virtual learning environments.

Maslow's hierarchy of needs See main Glossary, p 339.

Metacognition See main Glossary, p 339.

Norming A stage in group dynamics when group members have agreed on roles and are deciding how the group will engage with the task, activity or discussion.

Problem-based learning (PBL) See main Glossary, p 339.

Performing A stage in small group dynamics during which a group is actively engaged with an activity, task or discussion.

Process losses Potential losses of intellectual capacity due to inhibitory factors that might be operating in a small group. For example, some individuals might be inhibited from participating due to the presence of a more dominant group member, activities may be uncoordinated, or participants may lack appropriate motivation.

Professionalism See main Glossary, p 340.

Self-actualisation See main Glossary, p 340.

Seminar A teaching and learning session, usually midway in size between a small group and a lecture, during which there may be a presentation (often by a student) followed by a discussion. Seminars are often focused on advanced topics and include an element of interactivity allowing learners to engage in deep learning and the critical evaluation of evidence.

Social cognitive theory; see also self-efficacy See main Glossary, p 340.

Social inhibition Reduction in an individual's output in a small group due to the presence of others.

Social loafing The reduced contribution to a group task by an individual, who perceives that their input cannot be identified and consequently their involvement cannot be

ABC

Glossary (continued)

evaluated. This motivational loss becomes more prevalent as group size increases.

Storming A stage of small group dynamics when members of a group attempt to identify their roles and how they will work together.

Student-centred See main Glossary, p 341.

Surface learning; see also deep learning See main Glossary, p 341.

Syndicate group Small group of learners (e.g. 3–5) put together from a larger group for the purpose of carrying out a specific task or engaging in a particular discussion or activity.

Teacher-centred See main Glossary, p 341.

Time management The ability to use one's time effectively by prioritising and balancing the variety of activities one engages in during the working day.

Transferable skills See main Glossary, p 341.

Tutorial A small group session with a relatively small number of learners or even just one, usually focused on a particular topic, during which learners engage with questions and problems or discuss specific issues. Tutorials are designed to encourage deep learning by application, problem solving, and critical evaluation.

Virtual group; see e-facilitation A group of learners connected by means of computers and information technology engaging in group-orientated tasks and activities 'on-line'.

Zone of proximal development (ZPD) See main Glossary, p 341.

Outline

In the past two to three decades, there has been increasing disquiet about the didactic nature of much large group teaching and its tendency to encourage passive learning. Meantime, teaching and learning in small groups has gained prominence and become a major element of students' experience in classrooms and lecture theatres, workplace settings, independent study groups or learning sets, and, increasingly, on-line – so-called virtual groups. Yet, compared to large groups (see Chapter 10), small group teaching can be very costly in terms of human and physical resources and may be used inappropriately or ineffectually. Small group sessions need to be carefully planned to match tasks and methods with intended outcomes. Resource material needs to be developed, problems anticipated, and strategies for

dealing with them thought through. Consideration has to be given to evaluation of the session and assessment of learning. Of course, most of this applies to any learning situation but the point here is that small group teaching and learning (SGTL) is neither an easy option nor a panacea.

In this chapter, we discuss the definition of a small group, the benefits of teaching and learning in groups, and some theoretical perspectives both on the learning process and group functioning. The process of facilitation is explored in some depth, including theories of facilitation and the attributes of effective facilitators, and we consider the skills they need to deploy, particularly communication skills. The types of groups commonly encountered in medical education are then discussed, along with some of the problems that may arise, and the developmental stages groups pass through. A number of group techniques that can be used both to facilitate active involvement and to troubleshoot problems are outlined. Finally, 'virtual groups' are considered before we explore issues related to assessment and evaluation, and highlight some of the practical implications.

What is a 'small group'?

First, what is a *group*? A precise definition is not possible, but there is general agreement that a group can be said to exist, as more than just a collection of people, when the following features are manifest: a shared perception of being a group; shared aims; a degree of interdependence; a sense of cohesion; social organisation (e.g. norms, ground rules, and power relationships); and interactivity (Jaques and Salmon, 2007).

What about the *small* group? Andy Warhol famously quipped: 'One's company, two's a crowd, and three's a party'. He might have added that '*four or more is a small group*'! (http://posters.seindal.dk/p1813776_Threes_a_Party.html#similar – accessed October 2009)

Size *does* matter, although not as much as some might think (see later). The number of participants inevitably influences the quality and quantity of members' verbal contributions as well as their non-verbal communication. By general consensus, the optimum size for a small group meeting face-to-face is between five and eight participants. When there are more than 10 members, the interpersonal dynamics change and the quality and quantity of spontaneous interaction falls off. With a 'virtual' (on-line)

Table 9.1 Characteristics of small groups (adapted from Dennick and Exley, 1998)

Type of small group	Examples	Typical student numbers
Tutor-led small group teaching	Clinical sessions (bedside or in clinics)	2–4
	Tutorial	4–12
	Seminar	10–25
	Problem-based learning	8–12
Student-led small group teaching	Self-directed clinical sessions	2–4
	Tutorless tutorials	4–8
	Learning sets	4–8
	Self-help groups	4–8
Small group teaching in large groups	Syndicate work	10–200
	Group practicals	10–200
	Workshops	10–200
Virtual small groups	Virtual tutorials	4–15
	Email and social networking discussions	> 4

group, the equivalent number is up to 15 for a single facilitator (or 'e-moderator'). However, both face-to-face and 'virtual' groups can function productively and satisfactorily even if their size lies outside those limits; the tutor or facilitator just has to work harder! The classification in Table 9.1 links the type of small group teaching, the approach adopted, and the typical group size. See glossary for a definition of the terms used in it.

The educational benefits of small group teaching and learning

A fundamental aim of SGTL is to enable learners to talk and engage in a variety of collaborative activities, which enable them to go below the surface of a subject and question its fundamental concepts. Marton and Säljö (1976a,b) and Entwistle et al (1992) identified different strategies that may be adopted when learners are confronted by different learning environments. There is a tendency to adopt a 'surface' approach when involved in passive, didactic learning (like a traditional lecture) but a 'deep' approach when small group action prompts questioning, discussion, and interaction with subject matter. The result is 'deep learning', whereby facts, concepts, and principles are elaborated and restructured into a robust cognitive framework. Learners in a small group, at least in principle, can address all the domains of learning identified by Bloom and modified (in the knowledge domain) by Anderson and Krathwohl (2001) (*see* Table 9.3). Importantly, learners' assumptions and prejudices can be challenged and reflection promoted, leading to the development of appropriate personal and professional attitudes. Coles (1999) emphasised the importance of 'context' and 'elaboration' in learning, which group learning can certainly provide. Relevant problems can form the focus of learning, particularly in problem-based learning (PBL), and the talking and questioning that follow provide an ideal environment for learners to elaborate their learning and apply it to relevant contextualised tasks.

But deeply engaging with intellectual *content* is only one part of the purpose of group learning. Another equally important aim is the *process* of verbal interaction itself and the development of interpersonal and communication skills. Thus, SGTL has both content and process aims. Depending on the context and intended outcomes, process is as important as content (Box 9.1).

The content dealt with in group learning can range widely from discussing a topic in order to clarify understanding, through participating in PBL triggered

Box 9.1

Elements of small group teaching and learning

- Content
  - ○ Problem
  - ○ Context
  - ○ Knowledge
  - ○ Skills
  - ○ Attitudes
- Process
  - ○ Dialogue
  - ○ Questioning
  - ○ Collaboration
  - ○ Activity
  - ○ Interpersonal skills

by a scenario, to learning a practical skill with group feedback. Process outcomes, which are more generic than content ones, are chiefly related to interpersonal communication: presenting an argument, listening, responding, questioning, challenging, and being challenged. On the clinical side, reasoning (the ability to hypothesise, theorise, and deduce) is a skill that can be nurtured in small groups. The ability to handle scientific evidence cuts across content and process, as some understanding is required before analysis, synthesis, and critical evaluation can take place. Other important professional skills that can be acquired in group sessions are the ability to collaborate and work with others, function as part of a team, take personal responsibility, and develop leadership potential. Finally, questioning, challenging, and defending ideas in small groups promote reflection and contribute to both personal and professional growth. It should be emphasised that the sheer pleasure and enjoyment of learning in a human group is an end in itself! There is considerable anecdotal evidence that most students enjoy working in collaborative groups, and that this provides significant motivation for learning.

Groups provide an ideal environment for monitoring and supporting the learning of individuals. People cannot easily hide in a group and they can be given constructive feedback, whether they are struggling or thriving. The intimate nature of a group allows closer relationships to develop between learners and facilitators, who may find themselves in the role of counsellor or advisor.

The theoretical basis of small group teaching and learning

Educational theories

A variety of theories provide a rationale for learning in small groups (see also Chapter 2). A constructivist approach emphasises building on learners' existing knowledge in active learning environments, when old concepts can be challenged and new ones applied and elaborated (Dennick, 2008). Both Piaget's later work on socio-cognitive conflict (Richardson, 1998), and Vygotsky's writings stressed the part that social interaction plays in cognitive development. Vygotsky's 'zone of proximal development' – the gap between an individual's developmental level and their potential level – can be closed by

collaborating with more capable peers in groups (Wertsch, 1985). Experiential learning theory (Kolb, 1984) emphasises that reflection on experience leads to cognitive elaboration and subsequent action planning, which can be fostered by small group interaction. Social cognitive theory (Bandura, 1977) stresses the role of social interaction in learning, the hallmark of SGTL. The framework of Lave and Wenger (1991) describes how learners are inducted into 'communities of practice', again stressing the primacy of social learning. Communities of practice are environments in which learners engage in reflective practice as described by Schön (1983), a process encouraged and fostered by learning in groups.

The more intimate relationships between teachers and learners that develop in groups can be understood in terms of the humanistic theories of Rogers (1983) and Maslow (1968). These theories embed individuals in sets of social relationships that need to be optimised for effective personal development and learning to occur. Maslow's work highlighted the fundamental importance of creating supportive psychological and social environments. He suggested that each individual is motivated to fulfil basic needs (e.g. physiological) before moving on to address other, more complex needs (e.g. psychological); these levels are often portrayed as a 'hierarchy of needs' (Maslow, 1943). See Figure 9.1 (and later).

A significant amount of learning comes about through observing and reflecting on the thoughts and actions of others, and group learning is the ideal context for so-called vicarious learning. The discussion that follows observation promotes deep learning and in the context of professional or vocational education this also includes the acquisition of domain-specific language and concepts (McKendree, 2003). Dialogue thus enhances experience through what has been called a 'conversational apprenticeship' (McKendree et al, 1998).

A broader viewpoint on groups has recently been provided by a large interdisciplinary study, which has categorised a number of theoretical perspectives listed in Table 9.2. Each theoretical perspective is briefly described, the inputs, processes, and outputs of group activities are listed, and some of the main theoretical ideas and concepts that the perspective deals with are also listed (Pool and Hollingshead, 2005). Some of the concepts overlap with ideas in social psychology described later, but some are independent theoretical constructs in their own right.

Most recently, the language of complexity theory has been invoked to explain some of the processes

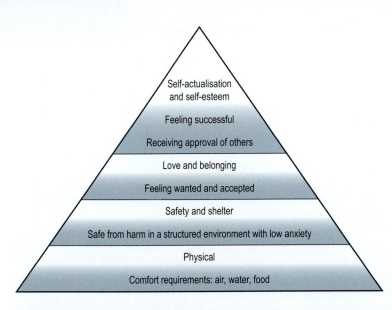

Figure 9.1 • Maslow's hierarchy of needs.

Table 9.2 Theoretical perspectives on groups (from Pool and Hollingshead, 2005)

Perspective	Input variables	Processes	Outputs	Theories and concepts
Functional: Focuses on the functions of inputs and processes in groups. Assumes groups are goal-oriented and that group performance can be identified and evaluated	Nature of task Internal structure of group Group cohesiveness Environment	Interactions Information processing Conflict management	Group effectiveness Productivity Quality Satisfaction with group outcome	Functional theory of group decision-making 'Groupthink' Collective information processing Goal setting
Psychodynamic: Psychoanalytic and humanistic approaches focus on the influence of emotional and unconscious processes on the rational and conscious processes of interpersonal interaction	History of the group and its members Unresolved problems Biological instincts	Facilitator–member dynamics Dependence and independence Group fantasies	Individual growth and development Group insight and understanding	Freudian psychoanalysis Humanistic psychology Psychodrama Field theory
Social identity: Explains group processes by reference to participants' social groups and the identity they build on this basis. Deals with the dynamics of in-groups and out-groups	Structure of society Social processes Socio-economic class and social identity	Shared identity Inter- and intra-group social comparisons Development and maintenance of group norms	Conformity Loyalty Collective action and protest	Social identity theory Self-categorisation theory Group culture In-groups/out-groups Social loafing
Conflict–power–status: Focuses on the dynamics of power and status in group interactions. Assumes that inequalities of power and resources generate conflict	Individual status outside group Resources Power and status within the group Interdependence of group members	Conflicts Conflict management Negotiation Consensus building	Redistribution of resources Achievement of members' interests Group performance Changes in status	Political science Social psychology Social exchange theory Power-dependence theory Game theory

Table 9.2 Theoretical perspectives on groups (from Pool and Hollingshead, 2005)—cont'd

Perspective	Input variables	Processes	Outputs	Theories and concepts
Symbolic–interpretive: An approach to understanding the social construction of groups and the use of symbols within groups to create meaning for their members, including how group processes are the products of symbolic activity	Conditions or stimuli for symbolic interpretations	Fantasy chaining Structuration Dialectics Sense-making Metaphor Narratives Rites and rituals	Common vision Group identity Group boundaries Group cohesion	Symbolic convergence theory Dialectical group theory Group decision-making Groups as communities
Feminist: Group dynamics and outcomes are a product of differences in male and female power, privilege, and motivations in social situations	Gender composition of group Individual gender perspectives Societal gender perspectives	Oppression and domination Unequal participation Male autocratic leadership Male control-oriented communication	A focus on interpersonal relationships within groups A focus on the division of power relations in groups and society	Oppression and domination Gender construction Individual difference theories Structural inequality theories
Social network: Groups are interlinked structures in larger social networks. Groups are seen as patterns of relationships (ties) among members (nodes)	Member characteristics Pre-existing networks Network structure and properties	Affiliation Exchange Diffusion Information flow	Task effectiveness and efficiency Cohesiveness Attitude and belief convergence	Graph theory and sociograms Emergence Social cliques Self-interest and social exchange Network 'ties' Homophily
Temporal: Groups are systems that change with time and group processes unfold in time as experiences accumulate	Group members' constructions of time Amount of time available	Change Development Sequencing and prioritisation of tasks in time Time management	Group development Improved performance over time Project completion	Sequential, cyclical, and punctuated equilibrium Structuration theory Action theory Complex systems
Evolutionary: Small groups are located between genes and culture. Natural selection has shaped the evolution of human cognitive and social behaviour and hence group behaviour	Individual-inherited tendencies for group behaviour	Co-operation Altruism Nurturing and teaching	Survival Reproduction	Evolutionary theory Sociobiology Group selection Reciprocal altruism Prosocial behaviour

and outcomes of small group learning. Mennin explored this in relation to PBL (Mennin, 2007), quoting Arrow et al: "Groups, are open complex systems that interact with smaller systems (group members) embedded within them and the larger systems (organisations, classes, and society) within which they are embedded. Groups have fuzzy boundaries that both distinguish them from and connect them to their members and embedding contexts" (Arrow et al, 2000). It can be argued that *all* groups (not just PBL groups) demonstrate features of a complex adaptive system; i.e. comprise a set of interdependent units – group members and facilitator – and are non-linear, adaptive, and self-organising.

The social psychology of groups

In addition to educational theories, there are some important social psychology theories that can be used to understand the nature of groups and their dynamics. First, there are theories about social influences in small groups, which deal with issues such as compliance, conformity, and obedience. Second, there are theories that explore concepts such as in-group/out-group behaviour, aggression, and prejudice (Avermaet, 2001). Third, and more important from a small group teaching perspective, there are theories that deal with group performance (Wilke and Wit, 2001). These are discussed in more detail since they illuminate group dynamics and practical facilitation issues. Social psychologists observe that group performance is optimal when members collaborate and use their collective resources effectively. However, as a result of so-called 'process losses', such as poor co-ordination of group activities or reduction in the motivation of group members, optimal performance is not always achieved. Process losses can be caused by someone's mere presence influencing another's performance, a phenomenon termed 'social inhibition'. This inhibition can itself be caused by 'evaluation apprehension' when an individual is concerned that their contribution will be criticised by other group members. Social inhibition can also be caused by 'attention conflict' when, for example, an individual's attention to a task is distracted by the presence or behaviour of other group members. It is self-evident on the other hand that individuals are often *positively* motivated by others' presence. Those inhibitory and activating factors affect different group members in different ways, depending on the nature of the group task; for example, whether

it is a simple one with a clear goal or a complex, open-ended one. Other factors in group working identified by social psychologists are 'social loafing', when an individual reduces their effort (a motivational loss) so that their contribution cannot be identified, and 'free-riding', when individuals who consider their contribution to be dispensable leave the work to other group members. Recognising those phenomena and being able to deal with their consequences are among the most important skills required of a group facilitator.

Conditions for successful SGTL: features of effective small groups

The educational benefits of SGTL can only be realized if the correct conditions are met. The skills of a facilitator, dealt with in a later section, are very important. Here, we describe the organisational, environmental, psychological, and interpersonal conditions for small group interaction to result in deep learning (Box 9.2). Failure to optimise the conditions results in group dysfunction and failure to achieve the full potential of the method.

Box 9.2

Conditions for successful teaching and learning in small groups
Preparation

Know your group

Develop appropriate aims and outcomes

Identify or create resources

Psychological conditions

Be aware of learners' needs

Anticipate problems

Physical conditions

Consider group size

Think about room layout and organisation

Interpersonal conditions

Warm up and break the ice

Create ground rules

Articulate the aims and outcomes (including transferable skills outcomes)

Clarify tasks

Preparation is everything

The old adage that *'by failing to prepare you are pre-paring to fail'*, attributed to Benjamin Franklin (http://www.quotedb.com/quotes/988 – accessed October 2009), is nowhere more relevant than in small group teaching. We now outline some condi-tions for effective SGTL.

Know your group

Facilitators should find out about the background of the group they will be tutoring, particularly the stage of the programme they are at. Letting people know you know (and care) who they are right from the beginning will greatly facilitate subsequent interper-sonal relationships.

Develop appropriate aims and outcomes

In a constructively aligned curriculum (Biggs and Tang, 2009), all learning experiences (lectures, seminars, practical sessions, self-directed learning, and small group teaching sessions) fit together into an integrated whole and are embedded in a matrix of learning out-comes. The facilitator should have a broad idea of what learning outcomes are appropriate for an individual ses-sion before it starts. They may be more or less well defined or they may develop as the session progresses, as in PBL when a set of intended learning outcomes is formulated through group debate (see later).

Identify or create resources

While many small group sessions can function without additional resources, some will require use of materials such as worksheets, handouts, video clips, envelopes, cards, pens, overhead transparencies, drawing pins, and flip charts. Reference books and, increasingly, the internet can be used to ensure that factual material under discussion is up to date and accurate. If the ses-sion is being used to introduce and rehearse practical skills, then appropriate equipment must be available.

Getting the psychological conditions right

SGTL is most likely to meet its goals if participants are physically, psychologically, spatially, and tempo-rally organised, bearing in mind Maslow's hierarchy of needs (see Figure 9.1, and later).

Physical conditions

Group size

The size of a group will influence any individual's ability to make a contribution. Conversation between two individuals will be limited to a modest exchange whilst eight people will contribute a greater variety of alternative viewpoints. But if the membership grows bigger still, individual contributions will be reduced and some people may find themselves inhib-ited. As stated earlier, evidence and experience sug-gest that the number that optimises interaction and the variety of knowledge, experience, and viewpoints available ranges from five to eight people. However, as McCrorie noted: 'group size is probably less important than what the group actually does' (McCrorie, 2006). Small group techniques can be incorporated into any teaching environment so long as large groups are broken up into smaller units to encourage interaction and active participation (see later).

Group arrangements

The physical arrangement of participants also influ-ences how they interact. The best arrangement is a circular or semicircular configuration of seats, which ensures that all participants can maintain eye contact with one another and the facilitator. Obviously this creates a potential challenge in respect of virtual groups (see later).

The position of the facilitator

A facilitator who physically joins the group is more likely to create an environment that encourages dis-cussion and interpersonal interaction. So, it is gener-ally best for the facilitator to join the circle. On the other hand, if one of the aims of the group session is to foster learners' autonomy (or if the facilitator finds the temptation to intervene too great), it may be bet-ter to sit outside the circle and function as observer and commentator.

Choice of room

The influence of venue on group functioning should not be underestimated. For example, a room may have particular associations in members' minds and may not be seen as entirely 'neutral' territory. Room size is also important. If there is a choice, smaller rooms are more suitable for small groups, but it is sometimes necessary for several groups to work simultaneously in a large room or even in a raked lecture theatre. The advantage of a circular grouping becomes apparent in such situations since group members in an inward-facing configuration can concentrate on their task without too much outside interference.

Interpersonal conditions

Group learning thrives on discourse, debate, discussion, and argument but learners need to feel comfortable engaging in those activities and will be inhibited from participating if the conditions are not right. First impressions are important and many potential problems (see later) can be avoided by the facilitator starting a session in an appropriate way. There are a range of activities that need to be carried out early in a session to create the right conditions and context for deep learning.

Introductions and ice-breakers

When people get together for the first time, there is often a period of embarrassment, insecurity, and even anxiety during which they attempt, consciously or subconsciously, to work out the 'pecking order' and dynamics. This process may be slight when members already know one another but will be a significant feature of newly formed groups' first moments together (especially mixed groups). Effective facilitators use appropriate introductory techniques to reduce anxiety and optimise self-confidence, helping ensure good interpersonal relations later on. The process of encouraging group introductions and facilitating an ice-breaking activity should reduce initial anxiety levels and make group members feel more comfortable. However, it is important that the facilitator is clear about the purpose of an ice-breaker, and articulates that to members. Ice-breakers have the potential to contribute more to a group process than simply to warm it up. They can be used, for example, to develop organisational or decision-making skills, or team working. They can thus be used strategically; in the words of one author "*. . . . they could be used irrespective of their icebreaking properties if they meet the needs of the course or session*" (Jones, 1991).

Ground rules

All groups have ground rules, the problem being that they are usually implicit and 'hidden' yet may

influence, for example, relationships within the group, not necessarily in a helpful way. Before moving into the main part of a group session, therefore, it is worthwhile establishing some *explicit* ground rules. This is particularly important with a new group, especially one that a facilitator will be working with over a period of time, or if sensitive subjects are to be discussed. Ground rules provide an attitudinal, behavioural, and procedural framework for all subsequent work. The facilitator can recommend a pre-existing set of ground rules, though getting members to generate their own will result in greater likelihood of adherence to them through 'ownership'. For this, they will probably value guidance and a facilitator's knowledge of rules that other groups have used successfully will be very useful (see Box 9.3).

Aims and outcomes

Students arrive at 'deep learning' by analysing assumptions they have about their knowledge and critically evaluating the meanings they are trying to construct. Thus, most of the aims and outcomes of SGTL are at higher levels of the cognitive and attitudinal domains. They should not, however, just be plucked out of the air. They should gradually be introduced as the context of the session is introduced and revealed. It is sometimes appropriate, however, for students to generate their own learning

Box 9.3

Suggested ground rules for groups

- All members should contribute ideas and opinions to the discussion as far as possible
- Respect other people's point of view
- Do not interrupt anyone when they are speaking
- Do not dominate the discussion; give others a chance to speak
- Criticise people's arguments, not their personality
- Listen to what other people are saying
- There are no 'stupid' questions
- Keep group discussions confidential outside the group
- Keep to the aims and outcomes of the session
- Try to remain focused on the specified tasks
- Members should feel responsibility towards achieving group aims
- Perform required preparation tasks outside the group
- Group members accept the ground rules

outcomes. That is a fundamental feature of PBL but may also occur in more traditional group settings. It is useful to discuss with learners if there are any specific outcomes they might like to achieve over and above those intended. Important outcomes may emerge during sessions and facilitators should be responsive enough to incorporate them.

Clarifying tasks

Tasks and activities direct the focus of a group and so the facilitator needs to give clear and unambiguous instructions. Group members need to know precisely what they are supposed to do, how long to take, what to do when they have finished, and what to do if they need help. Depending on the tasks and the number of groups involved, verbal explanations may be all that is required but using a flip chart or handout can be useful.

Facilitation

Facilitation has been defined as 'ensuring the right structures and processes exist for helping the group to meet its agreed objectives, and in helping the group members to identify and overcome problems in communicating with one another and in managing emotions' (Elwyn et al, 2001). In this section, we examine the facilitator's role, including attitudes towards learners and towards groups, aspects of communication such as questioning and giving feedback, and time management and organisation.

Attitudes towards individual learners

An effective facilitator will have an attitude that encourages participants to talk, debate, and question. A facilitator needs to be 'learner-centred', acknowledging learners' needs and their existing knowledge and skills, and building on them in an active, collaborative, and democratic way. They must recognise the autonomy of individuals and the responsibility they have towards their own personal growth and development. For some teachers, giving up their didactic 'transmitter of knowledge' role and adopting a more learner-centred approach is challenging. For others, it is a liberating acknowledgement of something they have always known: that people learn best when they are in control and, with appropriate support, take responsibility for their own learning. In the words

of Carl Rogers, *"As I began to trust students .... I changed from being a teacher... to being a facilitator of learning"* (Rogers, 1983). There is a spectrum of potential interventions from total control at one end to a completely 'hands-off' approach at the other. A facilitator must be flexible enough to move back and forth along this spectrum in response to the evolving aims and dynamics of particular groups.

The nature of learners

A fundamental issue concerns the status of human knowledge, a topic that is also covered in Chapter 2. Are we born with some innate knowledge and a 'human nature' encoded in the hardwiring of our brains? Or are we born with a mind that is a blank slate or 'tabula rasa' on which experience writes (Pinker 2002)? Are we the products of 'nature' or 'nurture'? The answers we give to those questions influence how we structure educational environments and how facilitators interact with learners. If we think learners are 'blank slates' we will assume we can mould and manipulate them as we please. If, on the other hand, we accept that human beings have a 'nature', then we will be more receptive to some of the developments in cognitive psychology and neuroscience that support constructivist teaching methods (Goswami, 2004).

Self-actualisation

As previously explained, Maslow (1968) argued that an important motivating factor in human behaviour is "the need to become as much as one can possibly become;" to self-actualise. Each person has a hierarchy of needs (Fig 9.1) that must be satisfied, ranging from basic physiological requirements to love, esteem, and finally, self-actualisation itself. Box 9.4 lists the tasks that face the facilitator in helping create the conditions for the needs to be met and, ultimately, self-actualisation to occur.

Carl Rogers, who also supported the concept of self-actualisation, developed his person-centred psychotherapeutic ideas to deal with the optimum type of human relationships that would lead to educational effectiveness (Rogers, 1983). His key principle was that individuals have a self-actualising tendency focused on achieving their own potential, and their individuality needs to be respected. Facilitators must demonstrate a positive and trusting attitude, personal genuineness, and empathy. Facilitation is about

Box 9.4

Maslow's hierarchy of needs and task for the facilitator

Needs	Tasks
Self-actualisation needs	Encourage personal growth through helping learners develop insight and self-awareness, openness to change, and problem-solving skills.
Self-esteem needs	Praise good work and new ideas but give constructive and specific feedback. Be optimistic and supportive.
Social needs	Adopt a caring attitude towards participants. Encourage groups to interact and bond by means of appropriate warm-up activities and collaborative tasks.
Safety needs	Treat participants with respect and honesty. Ensure that participants remain within a psychological 'comfort zone' with minimum anxiety, respecting personal privacy and confidentiality. Create ground rules.
Physiological needs	Make sure that rooms are big enough, well ventilated, and neither too hot nor too cold. Ensure that seats are comfortable. Participants need regular breaks for food, drink, and the toilet.

building relationships, the implication of which is that facilitators should engender a climate of trust, allow students to participate in decisions about their learning, and encourage curiosity and a desire to learn. In addition, facilitators should help students build confidence and develop self-esteem. All those attributes are ones that facilitators need if they are to run small groups successfully.

Student-centred learning

The ideas of Maslow and Rogers are also related to the concept of learner-centredness. The idea of child-centred education can be traced back to eighteenth- and nineteenth-century scholars, particularly Jean-Jacques Rousseau. It was also advocated by the American philosopher John Dewey (Dewey, 1916), who asserted that educational processes must start with and build upon the interests of learners; they must involve both thinking *and* activity; the teacher should be a guide and co-worker (i.e.

facilitator) rather than someone who prescribes rigid learning tasks (teacher-centredness); and the goal of education should be the personal growth of individuals. Those ideas resonate strongly with the concepts of client-centredness in psychotherapy and patient-centredness in clinical practice (Stewart et al, 2003). Acknowledging the importance of the learner's own cognitive framework as a platform for building further knowledge and understanding is a fundamental assumption of constructivist theories of learning (Dennick, 2008).

Adult learning

Medical education is aimed at adult learners, a type of teaching and learning for which Knowles (1990) coined the term 'andragogy'. Adults have needs and motivations that are different from those of younger learners and they approach learning situations with more mature expectations. From the point of view of group learning, adults have more life experiences to draw on in discussions. Facilitators therefore need to be aware that they are dealing with independent adults with rich personal backgrounds rather than dependent children with relatively little experience. The concept of the 'adult learner' has, however, been contested (Norman, 1999), as also discussed in Chapter 2. Andragogy is predicated on adult learners' ability to identify their own learning needs and monitor their progress in meeting those needs. There is, however, little empirical support they can do so reliably. Indeed, some people are notoriously inaccurate at identifying their learning needs and assessing their own performance (Eva and Regehr, 2008). Also, differences between the way adults and children learn may be less than previously thought, and so the concept that 'adult' learners are distinct from child learners is debatable.

Attitudes towards groups

Having dealt with individual attributes that are relevant to group facilitation, we now explore the attitudes facilitators might have towards the group. Lewin (1951) is one of the more important authors to have addressed this problem and his categorisation of facilitators as 'democratic', 'autocratic', or 'laissez-faire' is a useful starting point. Autocratic facilitators are authoritarian and control all the objectives and activities of groups and intervene constantly. *Laissez-faire* facilitators allow groups to decide what their objectives should be and what activities they will carry out, intervening minimally. Between those two extremes, democratic facilitators collaborate with groups on objectives and activities and only intervene to keep them orientated. Lewin found that groups operated best when conducted in a democratic manner. Facilitators, however, may adopt any of these roles in different situations and even during the same session.

John Heron has made an important contribution to understanding the structure and dynamics of group learning with his 'six dimensions' of facilitation (Heron, 1989). According to him, facilitators need to be aware of six independent influences on group processes that weave constantly through each session:

- Planning: What are the group's aims and how will they be achieved?
- Meaning: How are group members making sense of their experiences?
- Confronting: How does the facilitator deal with resistance and raise the group's consciousness?
- Feeling: How should feelings in the group be managed?
- Structuring: How can the group's learning experiences be structured?
- Valuing: How can individual autonomy be acknowledged and supported?

A fundamental question is whether the facilitator, the group, or a combination of the two decide on each of these dimensions. This leads to three modes of facilitation for each dimension, a classification reminiscent of Lewin:

- Hierarchical: complete facilitator control
- Co-operative: shared power with the group
- Autonomous: the group decides

Heron suggests that the most effective attitudinal stance for a facilitator is to value autonomy, co-operation, and hierarchy in that order as this acknowledges the personal autonomy of group members to self-actualise in collaboration with others, the facilitator taking responsibility to achieve group goals.

Communication in facilitation

The skills of initiating, structuring, and monitoring a group session have been described. However, in addition, effective communication skills are absolutely essential. The ability to listen, respond, question, and explain, and to be flexible constitutes a set of key communication skills that all facilitators should possess. These are similar to core skills for effective communication in a range of other contexts, not least doctor–patient interactions (Kurtz et al, 2005).

Active (or attentive) listening

Non-verbal communication is a key element of 'active' or 'attentive' listening. Maintaining eye contact and using appropriate facilitatory gestures, for example, nodding and making encouraging noises ("Uh-huh", "Go on", and so on) are essential micro-skills. Hand gestures may be used, consciously or unconsciously, to guide discussion (e.g. bringing in or shutting out a participant). Being attentive requires a focused awareness of oneself and one's surroundings, a kind of 'situational awareness'. It requires alertness to the presence of cues, both verbal and non-verbal, which indicate levels of engagement or discomfort of members. When there is an incongruity between verbal and non-verbal messages, the non-verbals have it! (Silverman et al, 2005). Responding appropriately to such cues is important and demands sensitivity and judgement. Paraphrasing and summarising (the discussion) are also useful tools that help both the learner and the facilitator.

Questioning

Learning is driven by questions, not answers. When learners are questioned, they have to think; whether they respond is another matter. Questioning serves a wide variety of functions: arousing interest and motivating learners; activating prior knowledge; diagnosing strengths and weaknesses; checking progress and understanding; assessing achievement; manipulating group dynamics by encouraging participation and discussion; encouraging deep-level thinking and active learning; modelling professional thinking and providing new insights; and reviewing and summarising (Sachdeva, 1996). Questions and questioning techniques can be categorised in a number of ways (Box 9.5).

Open and closed questions

Closed or 'convergent' questions are usually limited to a single answer and are thus directed at the lowest levels of cognitive activity, namely recall. They are useful in establishing facts and activating prior learning at the beginning of a session. Because they are generally straightforward and usually easy to answer, they are also useful in warming up learners

Box 9.5

Classification of question types

- Open and closed questions
- Questions aimed at different levels of the learning hierarchy
  - Creation
  - Evaluation
  - Analysis
  - Application
  - Understand
  - Remember
- Probing questions
  - Prompting
  - Justification
  - Clarification
  - Extension
  - Redirection
- Pivotal and emerging questions

before moving to more complex questioning. Open or 'divergent' questions, on the other hand, are of a higher cognitive order. They may have several possible responses or no fixed response. They may require learners to defend or justify a particular course of action or moral position, apply their knowledge in novel situations, or make judgements requiring the critical evaluation of evidence. They demand more elaborate and thoughtful answers and cannot usually be answered by simple recall. They elicit deep-level thinking and can focus, for example, on

application and problem-solving, analysis of complex concepts, creative speculation, and decision-making.

Questions aimed at different levels of the learning hierarchy

Bloom's revised taxonomy (after Anderson and Krathwohl, 2001), previously referred to, can be used to formulate different levels of questions in the cognitive domain of learning, see Table 9.3.

Probing questions

There will always be situations when facilitators need to ask questions to encourage learners to clarify or elaborate their initial responses. Those probing questions, and questioning sequences allow facilitators to ensure that deep-level thinking is taking place or to diagnose misunderstandings and take appropriate action. Such questions can be classified into the following types: prompting; justifying; clarifying; extending; and re-directing. A prompting question is used when a learner does not respond to a question or gives an incorrect or incomplete answer. The question might contain suggestions, clues, or a 'prompt' that will trigger the necessary response. Justification questions can be used when a learner has provided a correct answer without explaining why they chose it. If a learner has articulated an answer poorly or given an incomplete one, clarification can be sought. The student can be asked to re-phrase or elaborate their answer until the facilitator is satisfied they have answered the question satisfactorily. Extension questions ask learners to extend their thinking to new

Table 9.3 Questions aimed at different levels of the learning hierarchy

Cognitive level	Type and focus of questions	Examples of key verbs and specimen questions
Creation	Questions aimed at the creation of new ideas, concepts, or plans. Problem solving	Create; speculate; design; plan
Evaluation	Questions involving making judgements on the basis of standards, criteria, rules, or the critical evaluation of evidence	Judge; defend; evaluate the evidence for; justify
Analysis	Questions aimed at analysing assumptions, reasons, evidence. Problem solving	What are the assumptions? What is the evidence? How does this fit together?
Application	Questions aimed at applying or using knowledge in new situations or problems	How would you? What would you do in this situation?
Understand	Questions aimed at reformulating or explaining existing knowledge	Compare; contrast; explain; differentiate between
Remember	Questions aimed at recalling factual information	What is that called? Define; describe; give me an example of; list some of the causes of

situations. Their answers may give clues to the depth of their understanding. Finally, re-direction questions ask different students the same open-ended questions to generate a variety of responses and increase participation.

The questioning process

As well as having a good working knowledge of question types, facilitators need to be aware of the ways questioning can affect learners' behaviour. For example, simple closed questions activate prior learning at the beginning of a session and encourage participation, whereas open-ended and more complex questions might be used later in the session. So-called 'pivotal questions', incorporated prospectively into a questioning sequence, are usually planned ahead. Emerging questions, on the other hand, are not planned and reflect a facilitator's ability to adapt according to the particular demands of the situation. The facilitator's approach to asking and responding to questions may have powerful effects on group dynamics. They should generate an atmosphere of trust and co-operation, which will make members feel comfortable about asking and responding to questions and confident that they will not be ridiculed when they expose their lack of knowledge. The way in which questions are asked can have a significant impact. For example, people should be given plenty of 'think time' to respond before the facilitator either re-phrases the question or uses a prompting question. It is useful to tell students in advance that they are going to have plenty of time to think about their answers. There is evidence (Carin and Sund, 1971) that leaving a long silence after asking a question makes students more likely to respond and result in longer and more elaborate answers.

Responding to answers

How a facilitator responds to an answer is not only extremely important to the individual answering the question but also sends messages to the rest of the group about how they will be treated if *they* answer a question. A correct answer should be acknowledged and positive, supportive feedback given. If an answer is incorrect or incomplete, probing techniques discussed previously should be used. On no account should a facilitator use negative, sarcastic, or personally demeaning language. One can speculate (correctly, as it happens) that Albert Einstein suffered as a result of such an approach when he wrote "*Humiliation and mental oppression by ignorant and selfish teachers wreak havoc in the youthful*

mind that can never be undone and often exert a baleful influence in later life" (Einstein, 1934).

Socratic questioning

So-called 'Socratic questioning' is a form of questioning that brings together all the skills and types of question referred to earlier. It aims, through systematic dialogue, probing, and challenging understanding, to promote critical thinking. A facilitator poses a question, then responds to the answer with further questions. The dialogue evolves in an organic fashion but is not a free-for-all. Participants are helped to go beneath the surface of the topic and delve into the complexities of one or more fundamental ideas (https://www.criticalthinking.org/TGS_files/Socra ticQuestioning2006.pdf – accessed November 2009).

Giving feedback

Feedback, described as 'the lifeblood of learning', aims to close the gap between current and desired performance. It is as much about the future – feeding *forward* – as it is about the past. It is important because, as previously mentioned, self-assessment can be inaccurate with, on the whole, poor performers tending to overestimate their abilities, and good performers tending to underestimate (Regehr and Eva, 2006). Feedback is one of the areas of teaching, learning, and assessment that has a significant evidence base and general principles can be drawn from the literature to inform the process, whether the feedback is to a group or an individual. In terms of influences on learning, *specific* information about 'the task' – how to do it more effectively – focused on goals or intended outcomes appears to be more effective than rewards, marks and grades, punishment, or praise. Indeed, praise that is non-specific and targeted at the *person*, however well-intentioned and 'nice', may have an adverse effect. Furthermore, although people need and generally crave feedback, they may not be very good at receiving it, and it invariably invokes an emotional reaction. A host of defensive reactions have been described, including ignoring feedback, or arguing against it – 'shooting the messenger'.

Generally, then, constructive feedback should be: based on observation, not inference; descriptive and non-judgemental; specific and concrete; as succinct as possible; and linked, where possible, to goals or intentions. It should also be timely; feedback given at the wrong time and in the wrong way is worse than no feedback at all. Various models have been described for one-to-one feedback, such as the so-called Pendleton's rules and agenda-led, outcomes-based feedback (Kurtz et al, 2005), which can be adapted for group situations. An important principle is to ask the recipient what *they* feel is working well, then get them to consider things they might do differently. Elwyn et al (2001) suggested a set order for giving feedback to a group, giving priority to individual(s) first, followed by the group, and last the facilitator. Feedback is a key component of assessment and evaluation in groups – see later.

Time management, monitoring, and control

Facilitators have a responsibility to manage and direct the work of a group effectively and efficiently despite the often open-ended and potentially unstructured nature of their work. They should make clear during the introduction or setting of ground rules that the session has aims and outcomes, a focus on particular activities, a specific structure, and that it has to finish at a particular time. Facilitators perform a balancing act between being autocratic and hierarchical, and allowing autonomy and a *'laissez-faire'* attitude; they are essentially benign dictators in charge of the group's freedom! Good time management and organisation also induce confidence in the participants which translates into effective and efficient group dynamics. The facilitator needs to ensure that the group remains focused on the task(s), whilst keeping a watchful eye on group dynamics. It is important to monitor the group's achievement and progress and it may be useful to record it, either to strategically use the information or simply for 'the record'. For example, after a 'brainstorming' activity, the ideas generated may need to be recorded for subsequent analysis and prioritisation; during a discussion, opinions and questions might be listed to clarify issues, or guide further study. Finally, conclusions and action points of the group need to be recorded.

Closure

An important feature of all teaching sessions is closure, during which achieved outcomes can be summarised, conclusions emphasised, reflection promoted, and learners' sense of accomplishment nurtured. An effective facilitator will have the time management skills to ensure that there is time for closure. A useful technique is to ask members of the group to summarise the key points learnt, which can use 'pyramid' techniques (see later) or a facilitated discussion in which all group members participate.

Types of group

There are many types of small groups, each with its own particular dynamics and each requiring different approaches from the facilitator. We now look at several common types encountered in medical education, and consider how the conditions necessary to create effective group function can be applied.

'One-off' groups

This type of group, in which students do not necessarily know either one another or the facilitator and will not meet again, is familiar in clinical settings. The facilitator's key task is to 'warm up' participants and encourage them to talk to one another. There should be special emphasis on anxiety-reducing measures: friendly introductions, ice-breaking activities, non-threatening questioning to activate prior learning, and clear, unambiguous instructions and goals. Because the group will not convene again, it is worth saving time by recommending a set of ground rules rather than getting the group to generate them *de novo*. Such a group is likely to be very task-oriented, focused, for example, on a specific topic, but even so, will ignore group process and dynamics at their peril.

Regular groups

A common example is a PBL group meeting weekly during a whole semester. Members get to know one another and the facilitator, resulting in better group interactivity and collaboration. Introductions, ice-breaking, and ground rules can be tackled in the first meeting and minimised in subsequent sessions, leaving more time to work on subject matter. The regularity of meetings makes it possible to rotate roles and duties, such as chairing, recording, and summarising progress, demonstrating practical procedures or giving presentations, thus helping participants develop a range of useful skills. Seeing group members over an extended period allows an observant facilitator to monitor the development of interpersonal skills, depth of thinking, strengths and weaknesses in particular situations, and maturing of attitudes in individual learners. Sensitive, confidential feedback from the facilitator can enhance all those developments.

Potential disadvantages of regular small group meetings are that group members may develop antipathy towards one another, which might inhibit collaboration or cause outright conflict. However, a good facilitator who watches out for the development of such problems can hopefully prevent them arising or, if they do, can minimise their effects on group dynamics.

Mixed groups

The individual members of a mixed group differ from one another, for example, in terms of their knowledge, experience, or professional group. For example, a multi-professional group of health professionals might include medical students, doctors of varying levels of seniority, nurses, physiotherapists, and social workers. Working together in multi-professional or multi-cultural groups helps learners, in theory, accommodate one anothers' beliefs and cultural views, and challenges prejudice. Although there is significant potential for conflict, the tensions within such a group can also be fertile ground for creative learning. The most important issue for a facilitator is to acknowledge differences openly from the start and to stress the benefits that can result from diversity. Problems can then be viewed from the holistic perspective of multi-professional teams, which is much more analogous to professional practice (Becher, 1989); see also Chapter 4. Encouraging students to explore their different knowledge bases, values, and perspectives together can lead to much useful learning.

Peer-led groups

Learners have long gathered together spontaneously without a tutor or facilitator to study or revise, and self-help groups and learning sets (see Table 9.1) have become commonplace in postgraduate and professional settings. Now, student-led group working is gaining prominence as a formal component of undergraduate medical curricula (Ross and Cumming, 2009) not only in recognition of its inherent virtues but also as a pragmatic response to increasing student numbers, and because professional regulating bodies require graduates gain experience in areas such as leadership and teaching skills (General Medical Council, 2009). Many benefits are claimed for

so-called peer-assisted learning (PAL): it is self-evidently learner-centred; it can foster collegiality and collaboration; it can nurture the development of generic skills such as facilitation; and there are potential pedagogic gains – not least the value of learning through teaching, but also positive effects on motivation. More able students benefit from helping their less able peers, which leads to deeper and more lasting understanding (Biggs and Tang, 2009; Boud et al, 2001). There is, as well, convincing theoretical support for PAL from cognitive, affective, and organisational perspectives (see Ross and Cumming, 2009). Disadvantages include the learning being patchy or superficial, the potential for dysfunction and conflict within groups, and 'value for money' to the institution, given the amount of organisation and faculty support that some PAL schemes seem to require. There are many variations on the theme; for example, group members may all be at the same stage or senior students may act as facilitators, instructors, or mentors. It is important to recognise that not all students are suited to the role of tutor, so they have to be carefully selected, then trained and supported.

Problem-based learning groups

PBL, or perhaps less ambiguously 'problem-*first* learning' (Maudsley, 1999), is an instructional method in which a problem is the primary stimulus for learning (as opposed to the more traditional approach of theory first, problems later). The problem is, typically, a carefully crafted written scenario describing a problem such as clinical case which can only be fully understood by further enquiry. In small groups, with or without a tutor, learners explore the problem, identify gaps in their understanding, decide what they need to do to fill the gap – then fill it. This inquiry is carried out over a week or two, often supplemented by 'resource sessions' of one sort or another. A number of theories provide 'compelling support' for PBL (Albanese, 2007), including information processing theory, co-operative learning, self-determination, and control theory. The role of the PBL tutor has been described as a 'custodian of the group process and guide for discovery' (Maudsley, 1999). PBL has been the subject of a vast amount of research, often with conflicting findings. Notably, the debate about whether a facilitator should be a 'content' or 'process' expert is still unresolved, although intuition might suggest that a content expert with exemplary process skills would be the ideal. The research has been confounded by variable definitions of what constitutes 'content expertise'. However, Albanese has argued that the more important question is not whether content expertise is important, but what is the minimum expertise needed for effective tutoring (Albanese, 2007). He quotes a recent review article on the topic whose title, he contends, sums up the 'state of the art:' *Problem-based learning: the confusion continues* (Miflin, 2004).

One consistent finding in research, however, is that both learners and faculty enjoy PBL. There is a need for an on-going faculty development to sustain PBL programmes and prevent didactic, teacher-centred learning from dominating tutor interventions.

Challenging or dysfunctional groups

Conditions for effective group learning need to be maintained throughout a session. This involves monitoring the progress of the group as described earlier, and also monitoring the activity and contributions of individuals whose behaviour may affect group functioning, for better or worse. In all cases, 'prevention is better than cure'. The best way for a facilitator to deal with the challenge of a dysfunctional group is not to let it become dysfunctional in the first place.

Dysfunctional organisation

Groups become dysfunctional when facilitators do not pay attention to preparation, organisation, and monitoring, leaving group members anxious and reluctant to participate. Activities should be appropriate to the group's experience or maturity and the facilitator should check that activities are not too complex to be completed within the time available and not so simple that they leave time to spare.

Dealing with group conflict

Conflict is an essential, even desirable, feature of a group process since it exposes opinions and engages participants in debate. Participants challenging the assumptions of others may lead to conflict and even hostility. 'Cognitive dissonance', a state in which someone is confronted by a perception, idea, or fact that does not fit into their cognitive framework (Festinger, 1957), can be a powerful stimulus to learning. Acknowledging that disagreement may arise but that it is legitimate will help set the scene. Emphasising the importance of adhering to ground rules, not using *ad personam* arguments, and criticising peoples' arguments rather than them as individuals reduces the risk of hostilities. Another helpful ground rule is to get members to 'own' their comments ("*I* think . . . ." rather than "*Doctors* think . . . ." unless, of course, the assertion is evidence-based!). Sensitively monitoring debates helps facilitators prevent hostility but should conflict arise, it is important to establish the cause(s) at an early stage and encourage 'ownership' of the problem. Getting the group to write about issues on a flip chart or self-adhesive notes may help. It is also important for the facilitator to be alert to some of the 'games groups play', such as scapegoating (i.e. 'sacrificing' a group member by focusing on their behaviour and diverting attention away from group dynamics) or 'flight' (where the group goes into a state of denial of conflict, for example, by adopting distracting behaviours, changing the subject, trivialising issues through use of humour, etc.). Ideally, a skilled facilitator will use conflict creatively and help the group learn something from it.

Dealing with dominant group members

One of the commonest questions asked by group facilitators is 'How can I deal with the situation where one person dominates the discussion and prevents others from participating fully?' Reminding the group of ground rules about participation can help, supplemented by a gentle statement such as: '*John, you've made quite a lot of interesting points, can we hear from someone else?*' Breaking the group into smaller units or pairs to allow individuals to talk to one another should also prevent domination by one individual and give others an opportunity to discuss. If dominant behaviour still continues and threatens to disrupt the group, then stronger measures are called for. The use of peer pressure and group consensus are often more effective than requests from the facilitator. When such a situation has arisen, it is important to discuss it with the person outside the group. Ultimately, a facilitator has the responsibility of ensuring 'the greatest good for the greatest number' and might have to ask a challenging participant to leave the group.

Dealing with passive group members

Another common problem is a very quiet group, whose members seem reluctant to participate. The most important thing to do here is warm up the group and use ice-breakers that will help members feel comfortable with one another. That will be less effective when the problem is a boring, trivial, or overwhelmingly complex material, is either too advanced or too basic for the group, or if the facilitator has slipped into 'lecture' mode. Nonetheless it is important not to assume that a quiet group member is only superficially or passively engaged with the group's tasks. There may be a cultural explanation, such as the learner in question coming from a background in which deference to tutors and a seemingly passive approach to learning are the norm.

Dealing with a non-participating individual

Since one of the goals of SGTL is to develop interpersonal communication, complete non-participation is not an option, and this should be made clear to participants while framing ground rules. A non-participating individual might, of course, simply be very shy, unhappy, anxious, or ill. As with a passive group, cultural factors may also be relevant. It is the facilitator's role to make an individual diagnosis whilst maintaining group collaboration.

Dealing with cynical group members

Some participants, particularly those who strongly prefer passive or solitary learning or who enjoy didactic teaching and are simply focused on acquiring facts, will find group learning challenging. They may not understand that they will develop important interpersonal skills as a result of interacting within a group or that they will achieve deeper learning from engaging in discourse. One approach is to promote 'metacognition' through encouraging individuals to explore their underlying beliefs about learning, and how they learn. Rewarding cynical participants with positive feedback on their contributions can also help to bring down barriers.

Developmental stages of a group

Groups are 'developing and thriving organisms' (Jaques and Salmon, 2007). Tuckman described a four-stage developmental process – forming, storming, norming, performing – arguing that it is inevitable and necessary for a group to go through those stages in order to function effectively (Tuckman, 1965). While 'forming', group members are orienting themselves and checking out what is expected in terms of behaviour, tasks, and roles. Figuratively speaking, the main question at this stage is *'Why am I here?'* and group dependency is high (see Table 9.4). The 'storming' stage is characterised by conflict and polarisation as members attempt to change the group to meet their own needs. Conflicts such as role assignment, role strain, and role ambiguity may arise. The question here is *'Why should we do things this way?'* Although diversity within a group is more likely to generate tension and be more challenging for a facilitator, such groups are often more flexible, creative, and adaptable in the long term (Jaques and Salmon, 2007) and less prone to 'group think' if the tension can be harnessed. In the 'norming' stage, tensions are reconciled through negotiation, and perhaps, compromise. Group cohesion begins to develop, and

Table 9.4 The relative influence on members' behaviour of individual, group, and task needs, and dependency on the facilitator, during Tuckman's development stages (after Jaques and Salmon, 2007)

Stage	Individual needs	Group needs	Task needs	Dependency on facilitator
Forming	+++	+	+	+++
Storming	+++	++	+	++
Norming	++	++	++	+++
Performing	+	+	+++	++
Adjourning (ending)	++	+	+	++

energy and attention are increasingly focused on the group's aims and tasks, and group norms emerge and ground rules are established, the main question now being '*How shall we do things?*' Finally, in a group that is 'performing', members have settled into functional roles, and the group's energy is channelled into the task. That is not to say the group will go on to achieve its tasks effortlessly. In fact there needs to be a 'constant cycle of observation, reflection and intervention' (Elwyn et al, 2001) to avoid dysfunction. Tuckman later added a fifth stage, 'adjournment', recognising that groups that have existed over a period of time may go through a phase akin to mourning as the group winds down, tasks are completed, roles terminated, and dependency reduced. Other developmental models have been described; for example, a seven-stage model whose authors claim it is particularly pertinent to situations where the group leader has particular responsibility for effective functioning of the group (Jaques and Salmon, 2007).

It is important for facilitators and group members to understand that a group will experience these stages, sometimes with 'regression' to previous stages (e.g. if there are personality clashes or if the group has difficulty understanding the tasks). If the stages are negotiated successfully, the group will function more efficiently and harmoniously. Table 9.4 illustrates relationships between the needs of individuals, the group, and the task, and dependency on the facilitator in each of Tuckman's stages.

Group techniques

David Jaques described one of the key principles of effective facilitation as 'More structure, less intervention' (Jaques, 2003), and this can be achieved by building in exercises that demand participation and by breaking a group into smaller units to promote active participation. Although this chapter is not intended as a 'How to Do It guide', it is pertinent to describe briefly some of the techniques that can be used in this way.

Brainstorming

The purpose of brainstorming is to promote creative thinking, although it is also useful as an ice-breaker and for activating prior knowledge. Important principles are that: the problem or question should be clearly articulated; "anything goes" (within reason!);

and "quantity breeds quality", based on the notion that it is necessary to work through conventional ideas in order to reach original ones. It is important, however, that the generation of ideas is separated from their evaluation since the latter may stifle the creativity that is the hallmark of the technique. Despite its popularity, the technique has been criticised by social psychologists on a number of counts, including a contention that its creative potential is illusory and that other group methods such as nominal group technique (see later) are more productive (Elwyn et al, 2001).

Buzz groups

A buzz group is one of several structured methods of breaking down group into smaller units. Working in pairs or 3s, usually for just a few minutes, group members undertake a task ("Discuss the reasons why . . .") or tackle a problem. The task needs to be clear and achievable within the time allocated to it. Once the buzz has died down, the facilitator solicits feedback from the subgroups; for example, key points from the discussion using a technique such as a round robin ("One key point from each pair . . ."). The ideas generated can then be summarised, analysed or synthesised unless the method is used simply to 'unstick' a group or activate prior knowledge, when there is no need to use the generated material.

Snowball (or pyramids)

This technique builds on the buzz group principle, allowing ideas and concepts to be developed in a structured fashion through a progressive doubling of subgroup size, for example, from 2 to 4, then to 8, and so on. It is important, however, that each step-up demands a new level of challenge and is not merely a repeat of the previous task – boredom and hostility will ensue quickly if not!

Nominal group

A technique more commonly used in research and development that aims to identify and rank problems related to a predefined topic, a nominal group allows consensus to be reached fairly quickly, is pragmatic, and is efficient. The group is 'nominal' in that the interactions are highly structured, but it has been shown to generate a better range of ideas than brainstorming. It gives everyone a voice and overcomes problems of hierarchy (the technique was originally devised, appropriately enough, in the context of community development – Delbecq et al, 1986). Silent generation of ideas is followed by a 'round robin' (one idea per person), when all ideas are listed. Those ideas are then discussed, clarified, reworded, grouped, or broken down into simpler categories, before a series of ranking exercises, which prioritise the ideas. Obviously, a facilitator using this technique necessarily adopts a dominant and directive role.

Line-up

Line-ups are useful for swiftly surveying opinion or soliciting attitudes about a topic, when there is likely to be a range of views. Participants take up a position representing their views along a hypothetical line representing the possible range. Their reasons for choosing the position are justified and further discussed. Line-ups are useful for 'unsticking' a group (or waking one up!), with the clear benefit that it requires physical activity and considerable interaction as people negotiate their positions.

Role play

Role play is a powerful method for exploring different scenarios and experimenting with different approaches, particularly in the area of interpersonal communication, attitudes, and feelings (van Ments, 1999). It provides an opportunity for rehearsing new skills and can generate new insights, promote empathy, contextualise understanding, and integrate thinking and feeling. It can be thought of as 'a safe introduction to reality' – it is not the real thing, but almost (even though the scenario is a simulation and demands some suspension of disbelief, the thoughts and feelings evoked are perfectly genuine). Its use requires care, however, because it can distress individuals if misused and may damage group dynamics or trust. Facilitators need to be clear, therefore, why they are using role play, and what they intend to achieve. Roles need to be carefully prepared and clearly described. There should be adequate time for preparation and briefing, for enactment, for reflection and discussion, and finally for debriefing (the latter particularly when the role play has tackled an emotionally challenging issue). Many areas of learning can be explored using role play, focused on a role, a situation, and/or a task (Elwyn et al, 2000).

Fishbowl

The fishbowl is a technique commonly used with role play. Participants sit at the front or in the middle of a group, which observes the action. Whilst a role play is enacted, those 'outside' the bowl observe and then give constructive feedback on specific things they agreed to observe. There are many variations on the fishbowl theme, depending on the intended purpose of the session (see Jaques and Salmon, 2007).

Such techniques provide effective means for promoting interaction and participation. However, they should not be used simply for their own sake – it is important to think strategically about why and when a technique might be used, as well as how. The reader is referred to the Further reading at the end of this chapter for more extensive guidance on using these and other techniques.

Virtual groups

The globalisation of learning and advances in technology have increased the use of on-line learning, and thus of virtual groups, both synchronous (i.e. interacting in real time) and asynchronous. The main differences between face-to-face and virtual groups include: the obvious dependence on technology; the context, notably physical location; the timing and immediacy of interactions; and opportunities to record and archive discussions, and to monitor contributions. There are also obvious communicative differences resulting from lack of face-to-face contact, notably absence of non-verbal signals (despite the advent of videoconferencing using webcams). On-line discussion, however, may be of particular value for less assertive learners; also, it allows more time for participants, including the e-moderator, to consider their words, reflect on and review the discussion, and to formulate responses.

Despite the aforementioned points, it can be argued that there more similarities than differences between virtual and face-to-face groups, in terms both of factors that promote effective function and factors that detract from it. Most of the structured group techniques described earlier (and more extensively in other texts – see Jaques and Salmon, 2007) can be adapted for use on-line. Group dysfunction will, however, occur if members are not sufficiently involved in the discussion, or if tasks are not clear. Participants in virtual groups need 'to learn how to collaborate all over again', with communication lying 'somewhere between the formality of the written word and informality of the spoken' (Jaques and Salmon, 2007). Put another way, 'Working together on-line involves a hybrid of familiar forms of communication' (Elwyn et al, 2001). Planning is as crucial as in other contexts, and particular questions e-moderators should ask themselves include: How will members interact? How much input will be required from the e-moderator? Do I need to break group size down and, if so, what techniques will I use? and, Who will lead discussions, summarise them, and chase-up contributions?

Key requirements for effective function of virtual groups

Key requirements include thoughtful design of tasks, flexible facilitation, and technical support. As with face-to-face groups, the early stages are crucial, and time invested by the e-moderator in articulating objectives and clarifying tasks will be time well spent. Participants also need time to become acquainted with the technology and clear guidelines about modes of collaboration. Ground rules are as important as in other contexts, as are ice-breakers that encourage social interaction and personalisation of participants through, for example, short autobiographies.

In the absence of the social and contextual clues that influence face-to-face communication and group dynamics, the tasks faced by an e-moderator are somewhat different. They include: 'weaving', that is, synthesising and integrating various threads, and keeping the discussion moving; summarising; sorting and archiving material. Problems often arise because of delayed or muddled discussions, or poor time management (Jaques and Salmon, 2007).

Encouraging active participation is a continual challenge but can be achieved using so-called 'e-tivities'. A framework for crafting such activities has been proposed (Jaques and Salmon, 2007). An e-tivity should be as simple as possible; it requires an illustrative title and a stimulus or challenge, also known as 'the spark'. An invitation to respond is followed by the interactive element including responding to the postings of other group members, and provision of clear timelines. Finally, there should be a summary, possibly some feedback from the facilitator, a critique, and crucially, reflection.

The received wisdom is that a virtual group will function reasonably effectively, efficiently, and spontaneously with up to 15 members. Above that number, a facilitator will probably have to use similar techniques to those used in face-to-face groups to break down the group into smaller units for some or all tasks. For example, buzz groups can be created (using email or bulletin boards) that can then lead to snowballing, with the large group eventually reconvened to share and synthesise ideas.

A 5-stage developmental process has been described for virtual groups (Jaques and Salmon, 2007). Each stage requires mastery of specific competencies by participants, and demands different skills of the facilitator. The stages are as follows:

1. Access and motivation
2. On-line socialisation
3. Information exchange
4. Knowledge construction
5. Development

As with face-to-face groups, careful attention must be given by the e-moderator to question style and sequence. On-line interaction may lend itself particularly well to a Socratic approach, with evidence that critical thinking is promoted and sustained (Ya-Ting et al, 2005). The 'conversational apprenticeship' referred to earlier may also lend itself well to both asynchronous and synchronous discussions on bulletin boards and videoconferencing, respectively (McKendree et al, 1998).

Assessment and evaluation in groups

Assessment (of students) and evaluation (of the group) are interlinked; after all, the performance of individuals is the main influence on whether or not a group achieves its potential and intended outcomes.

Assessment

There are strong arguments in favour of delegating assessment to learners, with potential benefits for all parties, although learners will probably have to learn new skills to be able to do so effectively (Jaques and Salmon, 2007). Assessment in groups poses considerable challenges, although it is inevitably more transparent and somewhat more straightforward than the assessment of individuals. The reader is referred to Chapter 14 for a discussion of basic principles and concepts of assessment but, as with assessment in any situation, the choice of method will depend on the intended purpose. It will depend, for example, on whether the assessment is formative or summative and whether is to be used to grade members' contributions to diagnose strengths and weaknesses, or to predict future performance.

Assessment at the group level can focus on either the product (e.g. completion of tasks) or the process. Methods include participant self-report; and observation, either by the tutor or an external observer. A common focus for assessment of individuals is their contribution to the group's outputs, for example, completion of a project. There are a number of methods: allocation of a shared group grade (the best approach is probably to decide the criteria for allocation at the start of the project); a project-based examination; and oral or written reports (Jaques and Salmon, 2007). Assessment of an individual's contribution to group *process* is more problematic but, depending on the context, equally important. Criteria on which such assessments are based might include attendance, quantity or quality of learners' contributions, and how much support they gave to the process and others. Methods include tutor observation, process review, and reflective logs. Multi-source feedback is another useful approach (see Chapter 13).

Evaluation

Evaluation can serve many purposes (Elwyn et al, 2001). It can help members understand and reflect on the group process (e.g. in order to move towards a more advanced stage of development following a period of 'storming'), foster a culture of collaboration, provide feedback to facilitators, and be used in quality assurance. Evaluation may also be viewed as an integral part of the learning process, both for the tutor and the group members. Other considerations include who the evaluation is for and who should conduct it, whether or not it is formative or summative, and timing (e.g. as a continuous process, at the end of the session, or after a delay). The intended purpose (s) will guide what aspects are evaluated and which methods are used but, as with assessment, it can be targeted at many levels: the task, the group process, use of resources, organisation, intended outcomes. Methods include: observation (e.g. asking a colleague to observe the session and provide feedback about what worked well and what not so well); videotaping

the session for later analysis; using a structured group technique such as a buzz group to solicit feedback from the learners; a checklist, or questionnaire with rating scales and/or space for comments (e.g. how useful and interesting the session was, list 3 things learners got out of the session, and any (constructive) criticisms or suggestions for improving it); and descriptions, critical incidents, thoughts, and opinions about how the session went, for example, in a reflective log or portfolio. Review of group process should ideally be conducted at regular intervals. The method need not be complicated or take up too much time but will be useful at all stages of a group's 'life' (e.g. during the 'forming' stage, process review will provide feedback to the facilitator about effectiveness of their interventions, and to members about how the group is shaping up). Methods include asking learners what is working well and what not so well, for example, using a flip chart or post-it labels, or a more detailed checklist. The tutor leaving the room for a few minutes may catalyse a more honest review. A sociogram is a useful tool for evaluating contributions and providing insight into the process. It is essentially a map detailing who is talking and interacting with whom and how often, and may provide both qualitative and quantitative perspectives (Elwyn et al, 2001).

Evaluation, although intended to be positive, may be experienced as a negative process. It may be perceived as externally imposed, there may be a perception of evaluation 'overload', it may fail to identify problems or help a group move forward, and it may be divisive. Such problems and reactions may be prevented or forestalled by being clear from the start about the purpose, methods, and intended outcomes of evaluation.

Both assessment and evaluation in on-line groups may be carried out effectively and efficiently, and depending on a number of factors, may enable a more honest and thoughtful appraisal than with face-to-face groups.

Implications for practice

To organise a small group of students and give them a relevant and interesting task that makes them discuss, challenge, and elaborate their knowledge and attitudes is surely one of the most stimulating and exciting areas of teaching and learning. To engage with a group of learners who are controlling their own path through a learning activity expands one's role as a teacher from a provider of information to a facilitator of learning. This requires an approach to learners and learning involving flexibility and trust, plus a range of communication skills, particularly attentive listening, a repertoire of questioning techniques, and the ability to give constructive feedback. It also demands that certain conditions (organisational, physical, psychological, and interpersonal) are established at the start, and an effective facilitator will plan ahead and anticipate problems and challenges.

SGTL is also about *activity* and facilitators need to develop a repertoire of activities and exercises that encourage learners to interact, usually involving breaking the group into smaller units, whilst retaining a 'light touch' ("More structure, less intervention"!). Group size itself is ultimately less important than what the group gets up to, although the ideal might between 5 and 10 members (slightly larger for virtual groups). However, the most important activity that group members need to engage in is *talking*, and the ability of a facilitator to warm up or break the ice and set off a group talking with each other has to be a primary skill. Although SGTL may sometimes feel unstructured and may contain opportunistic and unplanned elements, facilitators must ensure that deep learning takes place in a time-managed environment by skilfully guiding and manipulating the group. The facilitator must not only attend to the requirements of the task but also to the needs of the group, both the individuals within it and the group as an organic whole. In this respect, the process is often as important as the intended outcomes and tasks; thus facilitators need to understand how groups develop and function, and the factors that may cause dysfunction. Thus, developing a range of strategies for dealing with challenges is important. Most of the principles and guidance described earlier apply to learning in virtual groups, albeit with a different emphasis, and some new skills are demanded of both the group members and the e-moderator.

Box 9.6 describes the features of an ideal small group.

We finish, appropriately, with the views of learners. A recent study of Canadian medical students' perceptions of small group teaching (Steinert, 2004) offers a pragmatic perspective on those factors associated with effective group function. They identified the following: being able to ask questions and think things through; having their understanding

Box 9.6

An ideal small group

An ideal group knows exactly what it is supposed to be doing and works collaboratively towards deep learning goals that have been agreed between its members. It has been warmed up by a facilitator, who has made sure its members have introduced themselves, decided on ground rules, are aware of the context and the goals of the session, and feel comfortable with and understand the activities they are to undertake. Group members engage in deep-level discussions or carry out challenging tasks and activities that push them to the edge of their knowledge and experience. The facilitator keeps them on track by asking judicious questions and managing time expertly. Closure is achieved at the end of the session when all outcomes have been met and summarised verbally. And pigs are to be seen flying past the window! This situation, whilst ideal, is the one to be aimed for by good group facilitators.

checked out; working as a team and learning from one another; being able to apply content to 'real-life' situations; and learning to solve problems. In addition, they thought that a good tutor promoted thinking and problem-solving, was not threatening, encouraged interaction, did not lecture, highlighted clinical relevance, and 'wanted to be there'. Effective tutors were obviously interested in teaching and created an atmosphere conducive to learning. They also acted as guides in helping students see links between current material and 'the big picture', and facilitated reflection. Students' messages to tutors included those shown in Box 9.7.

Box 9.7

Students' advice to tutors about running an effective group (from Steinert, 2004)

Be excited to be there
We are there to learn, not to be drilled
Remember we are only students
We all come from different backgrounds
Tell us when you do not know
Please do not lecture in the small group
Relax!

References

Albanese M: *Problem-based learning. Understanding medical education*, Edinburgh, 2007, Association for the Study of Medical Education.

Anderson LW, Krathwohl DR: *A taxonomy for learning, teaching, and assessing*, Boston, 2001, Longman.

Arrow H, McGrath JE, Berdahl JL: *Small groups as complex systems: formation, coordination, development, and adaptation*, Thousand Oaks, CA, 2000, Sage Publications, Inc quoted in Mennin S: Small-group problem-based learning as a complex adaptive system, *Teach Teach Educ* 23:303–313.

Avermaet EV: Social influence in small groups. In Hewstone M, Stroebe W, editors: *Introduction to social psychology*, Oxford, 2001, Blackwell.

Bandura A: *Social learning theory*, New Jersey, 1977, Prentice Hall.

Becher T: *Academic tribes and territories, intellectual enquiry and the cultures of disciplines*, Buckingham, 1989, Society of Research into Higher Education and Open University Press.

Biggs J, Tang C: *Teaching for quality learning at university*, Buckingham, 2009, Society for Research into Higher Education and Open University Press.

Boud D, Cohen R, Sampson J: *Peer learning in higher education: learning from and with each other*, London, 2001, Kogan Page.

Carin AA, Sund RB: *Developing questioning techniques: a self-concept approach*, Columbus, OH, 1971, Charles E. Merrill.

Coles C: Is problem-based learning the only way? In Boud D, Feletti G, editors: *The challenge of problem-based learning*, 2nd ed., London, 1999, Kogan Page.

Delbecq AL, van de Ven AH, Gustafson DH: *Group techniques for program planning. A guide to nominal group and delphi processes*, Middleton, WI, 1986, Green Briar Press.

Dennick RG: Theories of learning: constructive experience. In Matheson D, editor: *An introduction to the study of education*, ed 3, London, 2008, Routledge.

Dennick RG, Exley K: Teaching and learning in groups and teams, *Biochem Educ* 26:11–115, 1998.

Dewey J: *Democracy and education*, New York, 1916, Macmillan.

Einstein A: Almanak van het Leidsche Studentencorps. (Leiden: Deosburg-Verlag, 1934). In Calaprice A, editor: *The expanded quotable Einstein*, Princeton, 2000, Princeton University Press, p 69.

Elwyn G, Greenhalgh T, Macfarlane F: *Groups. A guide to small group work in healthcare, management, education and research*, Oxford, 2001, Radcliffe Medical Press Limited.

Entwistle N, Thompson S, Tait H: *Guidelines for promoting learning in higher education*, Edinburgh, 1992, Centre for Research on Learning and Instruction, University of Edinburgh.

Eva KW, Regehr G: "I'll never play professional football" and other fallacies of self-assessment, *J Contin Educ Health Prof* 28(1):14–19, 2008.

Festinger L: *A theory of cognitive dissonance*, Stanford, 1957, Stanford University Press.

General Medical Council: *Tomorrow's doctors 2009*. London, 2009, GMC.

Goswami U: Neuroscience and education, *Br J Educ Psychol* 74:1–14, 2004.

Heron J: *The facilitators' handbook*, London, 1989, Kogan Page.

Jaques D: Teaching small groups. ABC of learning and teaching in medicine, *BMJ* 326:492–494, 2003.

Jaques D, Salmon G: *Learning in groups. A handbook for face-to-face and online environments*, ed 4, Oxford, 2007, Routledge (ISBN 978-0-415-36526-0).

Jones K: *Icebreakers: a sourcebook of games, exercises and simulations*, London, 1991, Kogan Page.

Knowles M: *The adult learner: a neglected species*, Houston, 1990, Gulf Publishing.

Kolb DA: *Experiential learning*, New Jersey, 1984, Prentice Hall.

Kurtz S, Silverman J, Draper J: *Teaching and learning communication skills in medicine*, ed 2, Oxford, 2005, Radcliffe Medical Press.

Lave J, Wenger E: *Situated learning: legitimate peripheral participation*, Cambridge, 1991, Cambridge University Press.

Lewin K: *Field theory in social science*, New York, 1951, Harper & Row.

McCrorie P: *Teaching and leading small groups*, Edinburgh, 2006, Association for the Study of Medical Education.

McKendree J: Focus: better learning through discussion, 2003. LTSN-01 Newsletter No 1. Available at: http://www.medev.ac.uk/external_files/pdfs/01_newsletter/LTSN011.pdf. Accessed November 2009.

McKendree J, Stenning K, Mayes T, et al: Why observing a dialogue may benefit learning: the vicarious learner, *J Comput Assist Learn* 14(2):110–119, 1998.

Marton F, Säljö R: On qualitative differences in learning – I. Outcome and process, *Br J Educ Psychol* 46:4–11, 1976a.

Marton F, Säljö R: On qualitative differences in learning – II. Outcome as a function of the learner's conception of the task, *Br J Educ Psychol* 46:115–127, 1976b.

Maslow AH: A theory of human motivation, *Psychol Rev* 50(4):370–396, 1943.

Maslow AH: *Toward a psychology of being*, New York, 1968, Van Nostrand Reinhold.

Maudsley G: Roles and responsibilities of the problem based learning tutor in the undergraduate medical curriculum, *BMJ* 318:657–661, 1999.

Mennin S: Small-group problem-based learning as a complex adaptive system, *Teach Teach Educ* 23:303–313, 2007.

Miflin B: Problem based learning. The confusion continues, *Med Educ* 38:921–926, 2004.

Norman G: The adult learner: a mythical species, *Acad Med* 74:886–889, 1999.

Pinker S: *The blank slate*, London, 2002, Allen Lane.

Pool MS, Hollingshead AB: *Theories of Small Groups: interdisciplinary perspectives*, Thousand Oaks, CA, 2005, Sage Publications.

Regehr G, Eva K: Self-assessment, self-direction, and the self-regulating professional, *Clin Orthop Relat Res* 449:34–38, 2006.

Richardson K: *Models of cognitive development*, Hove, 1998, Psychology Press.

Rogers C: *Freedom to learn for the 80s*, New York, 1983, Merrill.

Ross MT, Cumming AD: Peer-assisted learning. In Dent JA, Harden RM, editors, ed 3: *A practical guide for medical teachers* (Ch 18), Edinburgh, 2009, Churchill Livingstone.

Sachdeva AK: Use of effective questioning to enhance the cognitive abilities of students, *J Cancer Educ* 11:1, 1996.

Schön D: *The reflective practitioner: how professionals think in practice*, New York, 1983, Basic Books.

Silverman J, Kurtz S, Draper J: *Skills for communicating with patients*, ed 2, Oxford, 2005, Radcliffe Medical Press.

Steinert Y: Student perceptions of effective small group teaching, *Med Educ* 38:286–293, 2004.

Stewart M, Belle Brown J, Weston WW, et al: *Patient-centred medicine. Transforming the clinical method*, ed 2, Oxford, 2003, Radcliffe Medical Press.

Tuckman BW: Developmental sequence in small groups, *Psychol Bull* 63:384–399, 1965.

van Ments M: *The effective use of role play*, ed 2, London, 1999, Kogan Page.

Wertsch JV: *Vygotsky and the social formation of mind*, Cambridge, MA, 1985, Harvard University Press.

Wilke H, Wit A: Group performance. In Hewstone M, Stroebe W, editors: *Introduction to social psychology*, Oxford, 2001, Blackwell.

Ya-Ting CY, Newby TJ, Bill RL: Using Socratic questioning to promote critical thinking skills through asynchronous discussion forums in distance learning environments, *Am J Distance Educ* 19(3):163–181, 2005.

Further reading

There is a website associated with the book at: www.learningingroups.com

Kindred M, Kindred M: *Once upon a group*, Southall, 1998, 4M Publications (ISBN 0 9530494 2 6).

Exley K, Dennick R: *Small group teaching: tutorials, seminars and beyond*, London, 2004, RoutledgeFalmer (ISBN 0-415-30717-1).

Hare AP, Blumberg H, Davies MF, et al: *Small group research: a handbook*, ed 2, Norwood New Jersey, 1994, Able Publications (ISBN 0 893916927).

Teaching and learning in large groups: lecturing in the twenty-first century

10

Tim Dornan   Rachel H. Ellaway

CHAPTER CONTENTS

ABC

Glossary

Advance organiser A statement explaining in advance what subject matter will follow and/or how it will be structured.

Buzz group Small group activity convened *ad hoc* within a plenary session for active learning through interaction between a small group of learners.

Cognitive scaffolding See main Glossary, p 338.

Collaborative technologies Tools and systems through which users can collaborate on shared tasks, typically based on shared content creation or manipulation and shared communication.

Delivery A metaphor applied to lecturing, which suggests that the lecture or its content is an object to be passed on to participants.

Epistemic curiosity Intellectual arousal that can be provoked by discussion or debate, motivates the quest for knowledge, and is relieved when knowledge is acquired.

Information and communication technology (ICT) Any technology that allows its users to manipulate information and/or communicate with other users.

Large group event See plenary session.

Lecture See plenary session.

Lecturer A term used as shorthand for people who lead/facilitate a plenary session and who may do many things other than 'deliver a lecture'.

Minute paper See main Glossary, p 339.

Plenary session Includes 'lecture' and 'large group event;' a many (learners) to one or several (teachers) event, where the number of learners is great enough (12 or more) to prevent leadership being invested in a small group activity.

© 2011, Elsevier Ltd.
DOI: 10.1016/B978-0-7020-3522-7.00010-3

Most people tire of a lecture in ten minutes; clever people can do it in five. Sensible people never go to lectures at all.

Stephen Leacock (1922)

Outline

This chapter is an overview of recent literature aiming to define whether, why, and how the large group oral tradition continues to have a valued place in the medical curriculum. It reviews features of the large group genre that are specific to medicine and presents opposing opinions about the value of the genre. It summarises recent research evidence from the medical domain and tries to find what makes large group teaching most effective.

Having established that charisma and the ability to tell a good story can have a powerful impact on an audience, it suggests that excellent lecturers should continue to lecture despite the growing challenges to this medium. It considers the affordances of new educational technologies and how they can enrich the large group genre. It suggests how to evaluate large group events, and lists useful publications.

There are many assumptions embedded in the terms 'lecture' and 'large group'. This chapter follows Biggs and Tang's (2007) lead in using the neutral term 'plenary session' to mean a many (learners) to one (teacher) event, where the number of learners is great enough (12 or more) to prevent leadership being invested in a 'small group' activity of the type described in Chapter 9. The term 'lecturer' is used throughout this chapter to mean a facilitator of such a plenary session. Like any good facilitator, an effective lecturer will use techniques ranging from eloquent rhetoric to the appropriate use of silence and is very likely to engage learners into active learning (possibly in small [buzz] groups) for at least part of the allotted time. This chapter is applicable across the undergraduate–postgraduate-continuing education spectrum but has a conscious bias towards undergraduate education because that is where plenary sessions are more often used and abused.

Introduction

Large group teaching has as long a history as medical education itself. Until textbooks came into being, the only way of acquiring a breadth of medical knowledge was to study all the primary sources oneself or attend lectures (Small and Suter, 2002). The oral tradition has survived the advent of the textbook and, more recently, the self-directed learning movement, which spawned policy documents calling for a move away from a 'transmissive' style of medical education.

Now that Web technologies (General Medical Council, 1993) offer increasingly sophisticated alternatives to individuals assembling at a single location at a single time to hear a single person speak, a society concerned about greenhouse gas production might reasonably argue that the lecture should at last be consigned to history. But even if technology-mediated alternatives finally win the day, should we not identify what has made large group teaching, and in particular the lecture, such an enduring educational medium, and use that insight to help make best use of the new opportunities afforded us?

The large group genre

Learners in historical paintings are typically depicted clustering around a master, who is holding forth as he conducts a practical demonstration. Changes over time have changed the genre to the one we know today. Rather than gentleman scholars and curious lay people, audiences for plenary sessions are registered learners who are quite narrowly focused on a particular course of study. Despite medical school expansion and the use of audio–visual technology, contemporary learners in plenary sessions still sit in tiered ranks akin to those adopted in Padua and Leiden centuries ago. Freshly executed criminals are no longer available and, even if they were, would not be made welcome in lecture theatres by the custodians of health and safety, so practical demonstrations have generally given way to verbal and pictorial representations of subject matter. The historical 'theatre in the round' has given way to an auditorium centred on a lectern and screen. The hanging skeleton and clinical couch may still be there but the couch is used less as doctors become more scrupulous about exposing patients' peculiarities to several hundred pairs of eyes; audio–visual technology has demoted the skeleton to a passive onlooker.

The one constant feature of the large group genre is the central position of the lecturer, though today lecturers are more likely to be anonymous reproducers of didactic facts than scholars extending the boundaries of their discipline (as depicted in historical medical art). Medicine is a huge, knowledge-rich discipline, which leads staff and learners to regard lectures as a way of defining a curriculum within the curriculum. Even more important, lectures are often taken as an examination syllabus with attention focused not so much on intellectually stimulating aspects of the subject matter as on specifics that might later be tested. Plenary sessions do not need to be that way. Exemplary medical practitioners and non-clinical scholars can communicate excellently and use plenary sessions both to role model what learners aspire to be and to make their otherwise tacit knowledge and professional values explicit. In that way, plenary sessions can expose large numbers of learners to an iconic figure they might not otherwise encounter. Exemplary lecturers typically have both personal charisma and good humour, tell stories about their professional experiences, express compassion, and link relevant theory to practice in an intellectually stimulating way (McKeachie, 2006).

Perspectives on plenary sessions

Laurillard (2002) represented effective university teaching as an 'iterative dialogue between teacher and learner focused on the topic goal' and asked why the lecture ('a very unreliable way of transmitting the lecturer's knowledge to the learner's notes') had not been scrapped. In her words,

'The lecturer, meeting a class for the first time, must guide this collection of individuals through territory they are unfamiliar with towards a common meeting point, but without knowing where they are starting from, how much baggage they're carrying, and what kind of vehicle they are using. This is insanity. It is truly a miracle and a tribute to human ingenuity that any student ever learned something worthwhile in such a system'.

Laurillard's preoccupation was with the need for higher education to cater justly and effectively for geographically dispersed learners from particularly heterogeneous backgrounds. If current admission policies and medical school cultures persist, however, medicine may continue to be an exception to her rule. The uniform and high entry criteria for medicine discussed in Chapter 16 allow lecturers to make reasonably safe assumptions about the capabilities and prior knowledge of their learners, conditions Laurillard regarded as prerequisite to successful lecturing.

Custers and Boshuizen's (2002) detailed exposition of the psychology of learning took a more positive view. Whilst acknowledging that

'Many educational and curricular innovations of the past 50 years owe their origins and popularity to widespread dissatisfaction with the conventional techniques of expository verbal instruction, in particular classroom lecturing'

the authors drew attention to the lack of experimental evidence that the lecture 'is an inefficient or ineffective means to present facts or meaningful generalisations'. To the contrary, they quoted evidence that:

'A lecture can be effective and efficient, particularly if given by an expert in the domain because it enables learners to embed new knowledge in a meaningful context'.

The stance of 'lecture bashing', they concluded, is driven by social and political rather than educational factors. If we accept their arguments, we should make a well-established genre work to best effect rather than demonise it.

Biggs and Tang (2007), although not writing specifically about medical education, overviewed what is known about lectures. Long periods of unbroken monologue by the lecturer make no greater demand on learners than to jot notes. The snag is that sustained and unchanging low-level activity lowers concentration, whilst the complexity of medicine's subject matter requires high-level and persistent engagement. Good concentration can typically be sustained for only a quarter of an hour, though it can be restored by brief rest periods or changes in the nature of the activity, such as discussing the subject matter with another learner. Moreover, retention can be enhanced greatly by reviewing the content towards the end or very soon after the lecture. Again, this means getting learners to engage actively with subject matter rather than leaving the learners to absorb it passively. Simple and well known as these pedagogic techniques are, how well embedded are they in practice?

Research in the medical education domain

To access the evidence base behind plenary sessions, we searched four major general medical and five medical education journals for relevant articles published in the years 2007–2008. Many publications were uninformative because they used an unspecified plenary format as the control condition for some novel educational intervention. Twelve articles could be characterised as empirical research. Six examined how to enhance traditional lectures by including active learning techniques or adopting non-standard presentation formats; three showed benefit (Bye et al, 2007; Forgie, 2007; Koklanaris et al, 2008) and three did not (Birgegaard et al, 2008; Duggan et al, 2007; Selby et al, 2007). Three articles claimed benefit for various applications of ICT, including video-linking to a remote subject expert (Kelly et al, 2008), making available podcasts of plenary sessions (Pilarski et al, 2008), and adding aural material to visual material in a Web-delivered lecture (Ridgway et al, 2007). Two articles clarified learners' reasons for attending plenary sessions and the effect of electronic media on that choice; learners still wanted plenary sessions (Billings-Gagliardi and Mazor, 2007; Mattick et al, 2007). One article found no measurable difference in students' learning between Web-delivered instruction and attendance at a plenary session (Davis et al, 2008). Based on this review, the current research effort is adding rather limited new knowledge about whether, why, and how the large group oral tradition can continue to have a valued place in the medical curriculum. The next step is to examine whether the knowledge we already have is being applied to best effect.

Techniques

Procedurally, a description of how to conduct a plenary session should consider what the lecturer should do before, during, and after the event – preparation, delivery, and evaluation.

Preparation: choosing subject matter and a format

The main preparatory task is to choose appropriate content. The subject matter that is best suited to a plenary session is at the cognitive levels of analysis, synthesis, and evaluation rather than recall. Put differently, a lecturer's task is to give good explanations rather than recount facts. If an explanation is good enough, acquisition and retention of facts will take care of themselves because the intellectual

scaffolding provided will help learners retain information they encounter outside as well as during the plenary session. Intellectually stimulating explanations may also motivate learners to study in their own time. Explanations need not be complex – indeed, they should be as simple as possible whilst retaining the essential ideas to be communicated. The challenge of distilling complexity down to clear and simple explanations makes lecturing an intellectually rewarding activity. Objectives need not be restricted to knowledge; plenary sessions can have a strong impact on learners' attitudes such as their level of motivation and value systems. Skills objectives, however, can rarely be achieved in a plenary setting beyond laying knowledge and attitudinal foundations for them. A skilled lecturer will choose subject matter that provides variety and interest and match it with an equally varied set of methods and styles. The topics of explanation and cognitive scaffolding are so important that they are revisited under 'Content', (page 162).

The following reflective questions can help in planning a plenary session:

- If learners take just two or three points away from this event, what would I like them to be?
- What other learning outcomes are relevant and achievable?
- How does the subject matter of this event fit with the course as a whole and how can I explain that to learners?
- Of the possible subject matter, what must I include and what would I like to include for variety and interest?
- What format(s) would be most appropriate?
- How can I promote active learning during the event?
- What audio–visual aids do I need?
- Who else do I need to speak to/alert/engage in my planning?

It can be useful to pose those questions to learners and fellow staff at the planning stages either through informal conversation or through, for example, an open email inviting suggestions. Box 10.1 gives a more complete list of preparatory steps for a plenary session.

On the day: the importance of personality and craft

Custers and Boshuizen (2002) qualified Flexner's aphorism that 'a lecturer is a textbook plus a personality'

Box 10.1

Preparing for a plenary session

The brief
- Obtain a clear brief such as the course learning objectives to be covered
- Find out what else is covered in the course and how this event fits into the whole
- Find out from fellow staff and learners what they would like covered
- Ask other lecturers in the course for their lecture plans and/or slides

Objectives
- Think of the one thing you would like learners to take away, if they were to take away nothing else
- Identify attitudinal and behavioural as well as knowledge objectives
- Include skills objectives only if they are truly amenable to plenary instruction
- Pitch knowledge objectives at the level of understanding rather than factual recall

Subject matter
- Prioritise what is to be covered
- Be selective and realistic

Methods
- Choose a structure and format(s)
- Choose methods that match the objectives
- Consciously plan for variety
- Think how to engage learners actively, for example, by spending a few minutes discussing the subject matter with the person next to them or forming a buzz group

Timing
- Schedule about 10 minutes' less content than is timetabled to allow for a late start and prevent over-runs
- Allow 1 minute per slide
- Allow time to pause at points during your presentation

Audio–visual aids
- Aim for simplicity and clarity
- Carefully test the use of any advanced aid such as video or a live participant
- Prepare handouts and/or make slides available to reduce the pressure on learners to take notes

Rehearsal
- If you are inexperienced or the event is a particularly important one, rehearse it, preferably with people who can give critical feedback

Evaluation
- Plan to obtain data on the effectiveness of the event

---

with the wry comment that 'in practice, the personality is often missing'. It could be argued there is not much a lecturer can do about their personality. Perhaps not, but they can put across whatever personality they have to best effect. That means, quite literally, coming across to learners as a person through the use of humour, through understanding learners' perspectives and difficulties with the subject matter, and through the choice of language. Personality also comes across in a lecturer's ability to project attitudes onto an audience. It has been asked 'Which of us can be inspirational day on day?' (Custers and Boshuizen, 2002) People who struggle to be inspirational should be steered away from lecturing and those who can inspire should be excused the occasional bad day. The best lecturers transmit their enthusiasm, interest in the subject matter, and compassion and pathos. It is not unheard of for subject matter that would otherwise be regarded as boring or irrelevant to be given meaning by an inspirational lecturer. When feedback shows that a lecturer is making inspirational material boring or irrelevant, a curriculum leader should select either a different lecturer or a format more suitable than the plenary one to deliver the subject matter in question.

Closely allied to personality is the rhetorical craft of lecturing. In Laurillard's words (Laurillard, 2002):

'The point of a lecturer's presence must be to use their oral presentation skills to enable learners to see the subject from their perspective, to see why they are enthusiastic about it.'

To reconcile that argument with the previous one that a lecturer's personality comes across in their ability to understand learners' perspectives, the rhetorical skill of an effective plenary session is to show a perspective on subject matter that makes their way of knowing accessible and interesting to learners. Effective lecturers are faithful to their topic and give the critical perspectives of people at the cutting edge; they show the active working of scholarly minds (Biggs and Tang, 2007). When a lecturer has a researcher's knowledge of a subject matter, they can augment the presentation with personal perspectives on knowledge, including the process of constructing and validating it (Biggs and Tang, 2007), though there is a danger that their enthusiasm for the topic will exceed their ability to see it from an audience's perspective. Practitioners, likewise,

Box 10.2

Leading a plenary session as 'craft'

Put across your personality
- Use humour judiciously
- Demonstrate understanding of learners' perspectives and difficulties with subject matter
- Choose language that forges a personal connection between yourself and your audience

Project attitudes
- Do not be afraid of showing emotion
- Project enthusiasm and interest in the subject matter

Use rhetorical skills
- Show why you are enthusiastic about the subject matter; help others share your enthusiasm but do not get carried away by it
- Use rhetoric to open up interesting and informative perspectives

  ○ The critical perspective of the scholar
  ○ A practitioner's perspective, bridging theory and practice
- Be a good raconteur

Make your plenary session aesthetically pleasing
- Show what is elegant and pleasing about your topic and how it makes sense of the world by giving it appropriate:
  ○ Relevance
  ○ Structure
  ○ Story line
  ○ Audio–visual aids
  ○ Narrative style
  ○ Means of learner engagement

---

may need to restrain their enthusiasm for the minutiae of the topic and simply help their audience bridge the gap between 'dry' theory and a world of practice they aspire to enter. Judicious use of illustrative case examples and anecdotes has a clear role to play.

Laurillard also emphasised the aesthetic dimension of lecturing; the lecturer should help the learner see what is elegant or pleasing, and how it makes sense of the world. The good lecturer is not just a humane expert but a good story teller. They use a narrative model of delivery and informal language to bring subject matter to life (Box 10.2). Narrative has great power as a medium of communication. The well-delivered plenary session should be, quite literally, both an unfolding story and a thing of beauty.

Delivery

Procedural rules

Assuming that a presentation has more complex rules than 'I speak and you listen', those rules need to be shared with the audience, perhaps coupled with an outline of how the allotted time will be used. When will there be opportunities for questions? Are members of the audience encouraged to stop the flow of the presentation? If they are not able to hear or do not understand something, how will they signal it? Are there breaks in the presentation for learners to 'buzz' with the people sitting next to them or in ad hoc groups? How will the audience know that time is up? What report-back will be expected?

Presentation style

The presentation should be a clear and logical exposition of subject matter, making explicit links between theory and practice. Enough words are used to make it very clear and not to depend overmuch on the audience's ability to fill gaps in the discourse but the presentation is concise and free of verbiage. It is articulated clearly and in an audible voice, using amplification if it is available. Feedback and exaggeration of consonants by speaking too close to a microphone are very distracting but, if those are avoided, the extra audibility afforded by using, for example, a radio microphone can do a lot to gain and sustain an audience's attention. Because it is essential to speak at a consistent distance from it and in a consistent direction, a lectern microphone can be tricky to use, particularly if the speaker has to turn round and point to slides.

The presentation should not be delivered at such a speed that the audience cannot follow it and should not be so slow as to be boring. The pace varies according to the complexity of the subject matter; it slows to give due emphasis to very important points, while moving quite quickly over prosaic details. The speaker makes a conscious effort to vary the manner and style of the presentation. Likewise, expression is added to a presentation by moving away from the

Box 10.3

Delivering a plenary presentation effectively

Procedural rules
- Explain in advance:
  - How time will be used
  - When questions will be invited
  - How to signal difficulty hearing or understanding
  - How any active learning will be managed during the event

Presentation
- An exposition of subject matter that is:
  - Clear
  - Logical
  - Comprehensive enough to avoid misunderstanding or doubt
  - Concise
  - Well paced
  - Varied in tone, pace, emphasis, movement, and body language
  - Punctuated with effective use of silence

Amplification
- Appropriate use of the available room amplification, preferably using a radio-microphone

Make and keep eye contact with the audience

---

lectern – perhaps moving over to the opposite side of the podium to encourage questions or answers from learners farthest away. Used sparingly, body language and movement add considerably to a speaker's self-expression. Used excessively, they make the presenter a figure of fun. Judicious variation in style is used to avoid monotony. Also, judicious use of silence punctuates the spoken discourse. Finally, eye contact is a useful tool. It is hard to project personality into thin air so it is helpful to fix different members of the audience with your gaze at different moments of the presentation (always provided you are far enough away not to intimidate them) so you direct your rhetoric towards a single, real person and pay attention to getting your message across to them (Box 10.3).

Structure and process

Objectives

Having established clear aims and objectives in advance, it is good practice to communicate them at the beginning and relate subject matter to them on a number of occasions during the presentation.

Assuming that slides are being used, the first one (s) after the title slide show the aims and objectives. The same slide can be revisited during the presentation to make the link between subject matter and objectives explicit.

'Navigation'

A well-prepared plenary presentation should have the sort of explicit and clear navigation you would expect of a good Web site. After the slide of objectives comes a slide setting out the layout of what is to come. The same slide can be used to punctuate the presentation and show the audience where they are in it, perhaps with all the headings except the one for the next section greyed out. Colour or icons on the slides can be used to make the learners' cognitive navigation even more explicit, though that ploy could also make the presentation unnecessarily fussy. A presenter can help their audience navigate through the nitty-gritty of the presentation by using 'advance organisers' and summary statements, such as 'what I will explain in the next section is . . .;' or 'what I hope I have made clear is that . . .'.

Managing attention

Continuous periods of exposition of subject matter should not exceed the 15 minutes of the typical learner's attention span. One technique is to punctuate a presentation every 10–15 minutes with a short period of active learning. For instance, learners can be posed a question to discuss in groups of two or three so as to review what they have learnt in the preceding phase and think about it critically. At the end of the presentation, they can be asked to tell the person sitting next to them what they think the key points of the presentation were. The aim of such interludes is to clear and refresh short-term memory, renew motivation, and actively construct learning rather than transmit it passively. Periods of active learning can usefully be followed by question and answer sessions, the effectiveness of which can be increased by leaving a 2–3 second pause between asking a question and soliciting an answer. A gap between receiving an answer and responding to it is also of value. Setting aside time for note-taking and incorporating it into the pauses and learning activities described above can be beneficial though it is important to make the intention to do so clear at the start of the event. Learners' ability to concentrate on what is being said is greatly increased by a handout of the slides to be shown or an assurance that the slides will be made available for download afterwards. Handouts should provide enough space to write notes during the presentation.

Finishing

There is an oft-cited aphorism that effective communication entails 'saying what you are going to say, saying it, then saying what you have said'. Having helped learners construct their understanding of the subject matter, it is important to summarise the same subject matter, emphasising key 'take-home' messages in one or two final slides. Once the presentation has finished, it can be deflating to invite a lecture theatre full of learners to ask questions, particularly if all the allocated time has gone and lunch beckons. An alternative is to build in time for them to 'buzz' about the lecture. An effective way of getting less articulate members of a group involved in a plenary debrief is to invite them to shout out, one at a time, even single words they were just discussing with their neighbour. The presenter can simply repeat them, add a word or two, comment, or pose questions related to what learners said. A more formal way of setting up a question and answer session would be to invite 'buzz groups' to formulate questions then answer them in a plenary discussion (Box 10.4).

Content

An analogy between the construction of a building and the construction of knowledge may serve to explore how content works best in a plenary session. The walls of a building are made up of many bricks, which equate to factual knowledge. To erect the building, a structural framework of pillars and beams is needed, which equates to the conceptual framework of the subject matter. Supplying just the factual bricks of a topic results in a formless heap that is overwhelming; moreover, facts are available in any textbook, so the learner has to reconcile this new formless heap with other more or less formed ones given or read before or after. So, a plenary session that concentrates primarily on presenting facts does no more than any readily available textbook and likely overwhelms the learner with formless detail that has to be reconciled with other learning. It is human nature for lecturers to be preoccupied with putting across the factual 'canon' of their topic. Having done so, they feel that they have given their subject matter due attention and discharged their responsibility to learners. They can then interpret shortcomings in learners' subsequent knowledge as a lack of attention or diligence. But that is not good lecturing.

The conceptual structure of a topic is what a lecturer should concentrate on. Provided with a robust

---

Box 10.4

Structuring a plenary session

Opening
- Introduce yourself and your topic
- State the objectives

Navigation
- Explain the layout of the presentation
- Introduce each section, relating it to the structure of the whole
- Revisit the objectives showing how subject matter relates to them
- Preview and summarise the subject matter with advance organisers and summary statements

Managing attention and cognitive load
- Do not present continuously for any longer than 15 minutes
- Punctuate with learning activities alone, with the person sitting next to the learner, or in 'buzz groups' of more than two learners such as:
  - ○ Free conversation
  - ○ Active review of the subject matter

- ○ Framing questions
- ○ Stretching legs and taking a comfort break
- Allow pauses between:
  - ○ Posing a question to the plenary group and inviting an answer
  - ○ Receiving an answer and responding to it

Handouts and note-taking
- Give learners a handout of the slides, which they can annotate
- Build time for note-taking into pauses in the presentation so learners can concentrate on the narrative

Concluding
- Summarise the presentation, with due emphasis on key points
- Allow time for reflection and questions

Encourage questions by allowing learners first to review the content with one or two other learners and identify what they are clear about and what they do not understand structure, learners will assemble the bricks of knowledge with little difficulty. In fact, prior learning will likely have equipped them with large prefabricated sections, waiting for a suitable structure to adhere to. A feature of experts is their possession of highly compiled knowledge structures, which allow them to apply complex subject matter to their practice effectively and without cognitive overload. The term 'cognitive scaffolding' describes teachers' use of such structures to reduce their learners' cognitive load when acquiring subject matter. An effective teacher can provide quite a simple conceptual structure that makes a whole morass of subject matter more easily assembled into a building with little effort on the part of the learner. So, the question to would-be lecturers is this: 'Are there simple conceptual frameworks that can open up your field of expertise to needy learners and make otherwise overwhelming detail assemble itself into robust conceptual structures?' If so, perhaps those can be the two or three things learners should take away from this session'. Knowledge that is orientated towards performance is much more useful than knowledge that is not.

Cognitive insights into large group learning

The construction metaphor might imply that there is a single building whose construct is passed (albeit at the level of explanation rather than fact) from teacher to learner. In fact, cognitive psychology emphasises not just the active construction but also the individual nature of knowledge. The lecturer passes on a framework for learners' understanding. The goal, then, is to help learners establish, elaborate, link and, ultimately, apply their own conceptual structures.

The preceding text has described how the lecturer can use advance organisers, cognitive scaffolding, summaries of subject matter, social interaction, questioning, and projection of positive attitudes to help learners build knowledge and tell stories. Lecturers can also include precise elaborations and analogies in their teaching. They can ask learners to consider reflectively, rework, and integrate new material into their existing cognitive structures by making notes and reformulating presented material into their own words. They can ask learners to verbalise their learning by explaining it to a neighbour in the lecture theatre. They can generate 'epistemic curiosity' by provoking discussion and debate. They can encourage learners to reflect on their learning and

refine the descriptions and explanations offered by the lecturer. They can make a question from the floor the business of a whole class, not just a dialogue between a single learner and the lecturer. They can use positive responses to learners' questions to increase motivation, confidence, and reward. They can use learners' questions to gain insight into how learners are thinking about a topic and they can use their own enthusiasm and real-world examples to give a topic vicarious relevance that enhance learners' interest in it.

A drawback of plenary sessions is that learners' learning may remain contextually bound to the lecture theatre in which it was learnt. That problem may be addressed by linking theory to experience; for example, by appealing to learners' own prior experience or by using analogy. A thoughtful lecturer asks their learners to draw on their prior experience and share it in a small group or plenary discussion. They may also ask learners to anticipate contexts in which the learning may be applied in the future (Box 10.5).

Supporting materials

Slides are a valuable adjunct to a spoken discourse. They scaffold the presentation and the subject matter it addresses, keep the lecturer on track, and make it possible to use pictures and diagrams to supplement explanations. The combination of visual and spoken material can be a virtuous one if they are mutually reinforcing. Moreover, computer-generation of slides allows learners to have copies of them either as a download or as a paper handout to maximise attention during the event and allow for personal notes combined with pre-prepared material. Video and other complex media may be effective but there is one just distracting or inappropriate audio–visual failure for every slick and effective presentation using such media. It is generally best to be parsimonious in the use of audio–visual aids and concentrate on learning rather than entertainment. Box 10.6 gives some general guidance about preparing slides and Chapter 16 discusses learning resources of all kinds in more detail.

Evaluation

There are two main categories of evaluation information that can be obtained about plenary sessions: information about process and information about

Box 10.5

The content of a plenary session

Subject matter
- Concentrate on explanations; the simpler and more general the better
- Use facts to illustrate principles but leave the 'bulk acquisition' of facts to individual study
- Orientate learning towards practical application

Processes
- Help learners establish, elaborate, and apply their own conceptual structures
- Help learners build knowledge by including in your discourse:
  - Advance organisers
  - Cognitive scaffolding
  - Summaries of subject matter
  - Precise elaborations and analogies
  - Projection of your own positive attitudes
- Intersperse the discourse with periods of active learning to promote:
  - Curiosity
  - Reflective reworking and integration of new material into learners' existing cognitive structures
  - Greater understanding on your part of learners' level of understanding and difficulty
- Make learning active by encouraging:
  - Social interaction between learners
  - Formulation of explanations and questions
  - Note-taking
  - Discussion and debate
- Promote retention and transfer by linking:
  - Prior experience to the current discourse
  - The current discourse to anticipated future experiences and actions

Box 10.6

Slides

Visual effect
- Aim for a good contrast between the text and background colour
- Format the material carefully for a good aesthetic effect
- Use as much of the frame as possible and use a large font
- Ensure the material can be read easily from the back of the lecture hall
- Avoid excessive use of colour and garish colour schemes
- Be consistent and keep to a single visual style throughout

Animations and cartoons
- Just because the facility to animate is provided in your software, you do not have to use it
- Simple, uncluttered slides where the whole content appears simultaneously are ideal
- Occasional cartoons may be helpful but they tend to be overused and are a poor substitute for well-presented factual material

Content
- A well-chosen picture can say 1000 words; a poorly chosen or irrelevant one just distracts and irritates
- About six lines of text are as much as can easily be taken in from one slide
- Well-chosen and -prepared graphs or line drawings can communicate complex information clearly and, used sparingly, emphasise simple, important messages

General
- Vary the way you present information within a consistent overall format – for example, some bullet lists, some diagrams, and some graphs, but with a consistent colour scheme and fonts
- Allow no more than one data slide (i.e. excluding title slides) per minute of the presentation

what has been learnt. Information may be gathered in the form of numbers, words, or both. Evaluation forms are nicknamed 'happy sheets' because of a tendency to enquire about satisfaction, often with process aspects of an event rather than its educational effectiveness. Numerical ratings are attractive because they allow summative comparison between different components of an event or between different events; however, they can be hard to interpret because of the lack of any benchmark against which to compare them and because inadequate response rates introduce unquantifiable biases. Textual responses may not support summative judgements as conclusively as numerical ones but are of greater formative value. When learners are asked to support their numerical responses with explanatory textual statements, event organisers can make both summative and formative judgements.

It can be argued that the most important information to gather is what participants have learnt from a plenary session. The technique known as a 'minute paper' is singled out for description here because it can so easily and effectively be adopted. At the start of the event, every participant is given a sheet of paper with questions (such as those listed in Box 10.7) printed on it, allowing plenty of space for written comment. Although it is optimistically

Box 10.7

Typical wording of a 'minute paper'

Questions, of which these four are just an example, are evenly spaced on a single side of A4 to help respondents reflect on what they have learnt and have yet to learn, and how they will apply their learning. The final one obtains formative feedback on the event. All participants' papers are handed in at the end, and (if resources permit) cumulated into a qualitative evaluation of the event and emailed to participants to remind them of what they have learnt and show them what others have learnt.

- Something I have learnt today ...
- Something that is unclear or I would like to know more about ...
- Something I will do as a result of today ...
- Feedback to the lecturer (strengths and/or suggestions for change) ...

named a 'minute paper', typically 5 minutes are scheduled at the end of the event for participants to write something under each heading. In addition to crystallising what they have actually taken away from the event, the minute paper identifies areas for further learning, and encourages learners to make a commitment to pursuing those goals. Finally, it obtains a qualitative evaluation of strengths and weaknesses of the event for formative purposes. From a cognitive perspective, completing the minute paper is not just an act of evaluation but an act of learning because the learner has to verbalise what has been learnt, what is yet to be learnt, and how this event links to future actions and intentions. If time permits, the lecturer can ask members of the audience to share what they have written so that other participants can have the benefit of learning from others' learning as well as from their own. If learners hand in their papers as they leave, the lecturer can cumulate what has been written on them into a summary evaluation with an extremely high response rate that can be compared with the objectives of the event and used to refine the same presentation on future occasions. The cumulated data from all the minute papers can be returned to learners as a synthesis of the event they took part in to refresh and keep alive their learning and allow them to compare it with what others have learnt.

Training as a lecturer

Chapter 19 discusses faculty development. Suffice it to say here that there is substantial evidence that teaching skills can be learnt and teachers value learning them (Steinert et al, 2006). Not everyone can be funny or inspiring but many can become clearer, more confident lecturers. The art of leading

a plenary session can be effectively taught in a workshop, short course, or longitudinal programme. It is consolidated through experience and can be enhanced by feedback from co-teachers, peer observers, and/or students (Steinert et al, 2006).

The future of 'the lecture'

Chapter 16 defines 'affordances' as 'the things a resource can do or might do', and divides learning resources into four categories. Type A includes information and knowledge resources, which have quite recently made a variety of media richer and more readily available to medical educators; however, Chapter 16 also reminds us that such resources are relatively passive and/or low in interactivity. Moreover, it states that 'the use of a learning resource can never be causal'. Simply making learning resources available to learners will not guarantee any kind of result, a caution of which Custers and Boshuizen's (2002) lecturer without a personality is apparently unaware. Type B includes environments that contain or provide context and can assuredly be both active and interactive. Type C includes the hardware and software 'tools that act on the world' and make Type A resources available for instance in lecture theatres. Type D resources support simulation and include 'wetware', another name for us members of the human race! In line with Chapter 7, which argues for the importance of learning environments, we suggest that the most interesting affordances of technology lie in the way we put Type C resources to Type B purposes: that is, create context for learning. As for the subject matter, a theme that runs throughout this book is that human Type D 'wetware', in all its complexity, is an unrivalled learning resource.

If information and communication technology (ICT) can make Type D resources available in lecture theatres, do we need lecturers at all? Assuredly yes, we submit, if we accept that personality, craft, and interactivity promote learning. And does the lecturer need to be there in person? An excellent lecturer who is present in the flesh may have more impact than an excellent one who is only virtually present, though a streamed excellent lecturer will likely have more impact than a weak or dispassionate one who is present in person. Key concepts here are 'economies of presence' and the power of ritual, performance, and direct physical participation in effecting and affecting learning.

There are a number aspects of plenary sessions that are changing as a result of technological support and remediation:

- *Augmented Presentation Space:* technology extends or changes the nature of the physical space in which a plenary session takes place. Podium computers and data projectors can help make the visual presentation more dynamic and amplified public address systems and radio microphones allow of larger audiences. Technology may also enhance control from the podium through the use of visualisers, dual projection, and other multimedia techniques. Networked video connections allow remote events to be streamed into the lecture hall, allowing 'real-time' access to a remote expert to add their experience and expertise to the learning environment. For example an operating theatre or other environment where aseptic precautions, patient sensitivities, or other considerations prevail can be connected to a lecture theatre. The surgeon who is performing a remote procedure can add interactivity to the event by answering or asking questions. Where expertise is scarce and learners are geographically dispersed, this is a potentially cost-effective augmentation of a learning environment.
- *Augmented Interaction Space:* this involves adding dimensions of interactivity to an otherwise passive learning environment. For example 'audience response systems' (more commonly called 'clickers') make it possible to check participants' knowledge and opinions before, during, and/or after a presentation, allowing individuals to 'normalise' their responses against a peer group as well as generating a sense of curiosity and increased attention. Judicious use of clickers can add humour and variety, collectively make

choices, or identify learning needs in order to redirect the plenary session to address them. Augmented interactivity can also be afforded by learners using collaborative tools such as wikis or shared online whiteboards. Microsoft's OneNote is particularly well suited to such collaboration as it allows multiple subscribing users to create and shape meaning and shared knowledge, using a range of integrated tools. There are two interesting challenges arising from this kind of learner collaboration during plenary sessions:

- To what extent is learner attention distracted from the presentation by such collaboration? Many lecturers are nonplussed by learners using computers during lectures; are they paying attention, emailing, using Facebook, or playing games? Managing these multimodal 'sidebar' conversations for more overt educational purposes may at least allay these kinds of concerns.
- Should the lecturer have access to the collaboration during the lecture or afterwards? If they do, then they can observe and diagnose problems as they arise. However, learners typically combine social interactions with work and may wish to keep these away from scrutiny for reasons of privacy or unwillingness to share less than favourable comments about, for instance, the lecturer.

- *Augmented Location and Distribution:* this involves the use of technologies to break down barriers of geography and location to involve multiple sites and distributed groups of learners in what previously required collocation. There are a number of ways this might happen:

- Breakout rooms may help to accommodate greater numbers of learners than in the space in the primary lecture theatre – a particular problem as student cohorts continue to grow. In this case a direct video link of the podium and/or the slides can provide the next best thing to 'being there'.
- Videoconferencing involves room-to-room, venue-to-venue connections and can allow a lecture to be given simultaneously to multiple groups of learners in different locations. There is still some social assembly at each linked venue but the sense of presence can be significantly attenuated in remote locations unless lecturers adapt their style of presentation to the medium and pay particular

attention to the learners not collocated with them.

– Web conferencing involves the connection of individual computers to each other or a central point. This allows learners and lecturer to hold different kinds of events without being constrained by physical space, though they are exchanged for the constraints of the software and hardware they are using.

• *Augmented Time:* asynchronous access to lectures means that at least the presentation part of the plenary session can be recorded and made available to learners whenever they choose to view or review it. Many institutions now provide many of their lectures in that way. This raises a number of challenges, particularly for those students for whom this is the only engagement they have with the lecture.

The use of such learning resources in plenary sessions, as well as other settings, is more fully explored in Chapter 16. Economies of scale, reduction in travel, and mitigation of environmental impact come at the cost of technical support, without which the most promising education technologies will fail. Support is necessary but not sufficient because use of new technology for plenary education is a learnable skill, over and above the skill of lecturing without it. Organisations and individuals who want to benefit from the affordances of new technology need to consider implications for faculty development, the subject of Chapter 19.

Beyond the use of technology are the ways that professions, societies, and cultures change over time. Michael Wesch and 200 of his students at Kansas State University produced "a short video summarising some of the most important characteristics of students today – how they learn, what they need to learn, their goals, hopes, dreams, what their lives will be like, and what kinds of changes they will experience in their lifetime" (Wesch, 2009).

Implications for practice

There are many metaphors in and of educational practice. This chapter has argued that the commonly used transmission metaphor – expressed in the language of 'delivering', 'giving', and 'presenting' – tacitly focuses a plenary session on knowledge transfer to the exclusion of performance and experience, features of the participation metaphor (Chapter 2). It has suggested ways plenary session can be improved and enhanced by more critical engagement with the multidimensional nature of the medium. It has tried to show the potential richness and diversity of this technique. Key messages are:

• Interaction with peers, teachers, and patients, one-to-one and in groups, provides an all-important social milieu for learning medicine.

• Learning is an active, constructive process.

• Teaching and learning must take account of the contexts in which they are conducted and will eventually be applied.

One reason the large group genre is so enduring and seductive to programme leaders is that it can be impersonal, passive, and decontextualised. Yet, current opinion and evidence reviewed in this chapter show that human chemistry at a personal level, active, constructive learning, and contextualisation are as important here as in other learning activities. It has shown how those qualities can be incorporated into the genre. Large group teaching is not a 'quick fix' and neither are the new technologies, though they can add value to large group learning. On the other hand, Laurillard's dismissal of lectures as an outmoded pedagogic medium is also questionable given the nature of the learners and subject matter of medical education (Laurillard, 2002). We predict and rather hope large group learning will endure though there is plenty that lecturers must do to raise our game – and many questions for education researchers to pursue in support of excellent large group medical education.

References

Biggs JA, Tang C: *Teaching for quality learning at University*, ed 3, Maidenhead, 2007, Open University Press.

Billings-Gagliardi S, Mazor KM: Student decisions about lecture attendance: do electronic course materials matter? *Acad Med* 82(10):S73–S76, 2007.

Birgegaard G, Persson E, Hoppe A: Randomized comparison of student-activating and traditional lecture: no learning difference, *Med Teach* 30:819, 2008.

Bye A, Connolly AM, Netherton C, et al: A triangulated approach to the assessment of teaching in childhood

epilepsy, *Med Teach* 29:255–725, 2007.

Custers EJFM, Boshuizen HPA: The psychology of learning. In Norman GR, van der Vleuten C, Newble DI, editors: *International handbook of research in medical education*, Dordrecht, 2002, Kluwer, pp 163–203.

Davis J, Crabb S, Rogers E, et al: Computer-based teaching is as good as face to face lecture-based teaching of evidence based medicine: a randomized controlled trial, *Med Teach* 30:302–307, 2008.

Duggan PM, Palmer E, Devitt P: Electronic voting to encourage interactive lectures: a randomised trial, *BMC Med Educ* 7:25, 2007.

Forgie S: The enteric jazz band lecture: enhancing active learning, *Med Educ* 41:509, 2007.

General Medical Council: *Duties of a doctor*, London, 1993, General Medical Council.

Kelly N, Gaul K, Huynh H, et al: Quality trumps face-to-face presence when delivering lectures in a distributed multi-site medical education programme, *Med Educ* 42:225, 2008.

Koklanaris N, MacKenzie AP, Fino ME, et al: Debate preparation/ participation: an active, effective tool, *Teach Learn Med* 20:235–238, 2008.

Laurillard D: *Rethinking university teaching. A framework for the effective use of learning technologies*, ed 2, Abingdon, 2002, Routledge Falmer.

McKeachie WJ: *Teaching tips: strategies, research and theory for college and university teachers*, Boston, MA, 2006, Houghton Mifflin.

Mattick K, Crocker G, Bligh J: Medical student attendance at non-compulsory lectures, *Adv Health Sci Educ Theory Pract* 12:201–210, 2007.

Pilarski PP, Alan Johnstone D, Pettepher CC, et al: From music to macromolecules: using rich media/podcast lecture recordings to enhance the preclinical educational experience, *Med Teach* 30:630–632, 2008.

Ridgway PF, Sheikh A, Sweeney KJ, et al: Surgical e-learning: validation of multimedia web-based lectures, *Med Educ* 41:168–172, 2007.

Selby G, Walker V, Diwakar V: A comparison of teaching methods: interactive lecture versus game playing, *Med Teach* 29:972–974, 2007.

Small PA, Suter E: Transitions in basic medical science teaching. In Norman GR, van der Vleuten C, Newble D, editors: *International handbook of research in medical education*, Dordrecht, 2002, Kluwer, pp 337–363.

Steinert Y, Mann K, Centeno A, et al: A systematic review of faculty development initiatives designed to improve teaching effectiveness in medical education: BEME Guide No 8, *Med Teach* 28:497–526, 2006.

Wesch M: *A vision of students today*, 2009. Available at: http://www.youtube.com/watch?v=dGCJ46vyR9o Accessed September 22.

Further reading

Angelo TA, Cross KP: *Classroom assessment techniques: a handbook for college teachers*, ed 2, San Francisco, 1993, Jossey-Bass.

Learning and teaching clinical procedures

Roger Kneebone   Debra Nestel

CHAPTER CONTENTS

ABC

Glossary

Contextualising learning See main Glossary, p 338.
Hybrid simulation The seamless linking of simulators (e.g. bench top urinary catheter model or virtual reality endoscopy simulator) with simulated patients.
SP (simulated patient) See main Glossary, p 341.
Technical skills Psychomotor and dexterity skills and requisite knowledge required for performing procedures.

Outline

This chapter focuses on educational issues around learning, teaching, and assessing clinical procedures. We limit our scope to procedures carried out on conscious patients and exclude surgical operations. We start with a brief historical overview, reviewing key drivers which are changing the landscape of clinical care and health care education. We identify changes to procedural skills training, highlighting the move from

DOI: 10.1016/B978-0-7020-3522-7.00011-5

apprenticeship models to competency-based curricula, and shifts from doctor-focused and task-focused care to patient-centred and team-based approaches. We allude to themes in contemporary medical curricula, framing the emergence of skills centres as a central factor in the teaching and assessment of procedural skills. We summarise procedural skills assessments including the simulation-based objective structured clinical examination (OSCE), objective structured assessment of technical skills (OSATSs), and the direct observation of procedural skills (DOPS) in workplace-based assessments. The next section outlines selected theories relevant to skills-based teaching. Here, our aim is to raise awareness of the extensive literature which bears upon our topic, without providing a comprehensive critique. Much of the chapter deals with simulation, whose role in procedural skills training is key but whose uncritical acceptance has led to problems. A critique of current approaches identifies key limitations. From this, we put forward our own 'learner-centred, patient-focused' approach to procedural skills training, using hybrid simulation. We use the integrated procedural performance instrument (IPPI) as an example of how to consider strengths and limitations of innovative approaches. We conclude by proposing a 'layered learning' approach. This combines scenario design, hybrid simulation, and contextualised training within a learner-centred framework that includes patients as they would exist in real clinical practice.

Introduction

Medical education has witnessed many upheavals during its long history and recent years have been characterised by continual flux (Calman, 2007; Ludmerer, 1999). There has been a series of profound changes during the twentieth century, punctuated by influential reports (Flexner, 1910; General Medical Council, 1947, 1957, 2003; Medical Education Committee of the British Medical Association, 1948). From the perspective of procedural skills, the change from apprenticeship to competency-based programmes has been especially influential.

The historical apprenticeship approach to learning and teaching clinical procedures

In the apprenticeship model, medical students went on a prolonged 'journey', stretching from undergraduate training to their postgraduate years. This extended time frame was crucial because it allowed them to absorb a particular way of practising medicine that was heavily based on their master's style. This approach flourished in an era that has now passed, where patients routinely spent days or weeks in hospital for routine procedures and where a culture of learning 'on' patients was widely accepted. In the United Kingdom, this took place within consultant-led 'firms' which were stable and relatively independent, and where medical students were treated as inexperienced but legitimate members of a community of practice (Lave and Wenger, 1991; Wenger, 1998). Procedural skills (such as taking blood, intravenous cannulation, and inserting urinary catheters) formed part of a learner's routine duties; they were learnt under the tutelage of junior doctors and integrated within clinical care. Again, the culture of the time meant that patients were generally acquiescent in a system where being 'practised on' was the norm.

Apprenticeship under pressure

The contemporary climate is radically different. The number of medical students has greatly increased, placing further pressure on dwindling opportunities for clinical experience. At the same time, the ethical climate has changed profoundly, and it is no longer acceptable for unskilled novices to practice on patients. Progressively more limited working hours have fragmented the traditional 'firm' structure, forcing a change towards shift systems. And the dizzying pace of technological development has meant that patients no longer spend many days in hospital but are processed through specialist units as rapidly as possible. As a result, the slow process by which learners gradually acquired a range of procedural skills is a thing of the past. There is growing concern that a mismatch between book knowledge and procedural skills experience leads graduating doctors to lack confidence in what they can do. Many clinicians in the current climate are graduating with minimal real-world clinical experience (Boots et al, 2009; Cave et al, 2007; Wu et al, 2008) and this mismatch is even more challenging for them. Contemporary developments around revalidation and relicensing of registered practitioners make this debate relevant to professionals at all stages of their career.

Competency-based education

The notion of competencies has exerted a powerful influence on educational thinking. The move towards competency-based programmes is, in part, a response to the changing influences described in the previous paragraph. Such programmes set out specified learning outcomes, stating explicitly what learners are expected to know and be able to do at graduation, and providing learners at the start of their medical education with a clear sense of where they are going (General Medical Council, 2003). In theory at least, making it clear what competencies are expected should help new doctors meet the demands of their roles in a complex health service. The notion of competency-based education has particular relevance for clinical procedures, which are 'observable' and therefore 'measurable'. However, defining competencies is more difficult than might at first appear. One particular challenge is accounting for the variability of clinical practice. Although a new doctor might be expected to perform a procedural skill competently (e.g. suturing), outcomes are often written in broad terms and assumed to be generic. Suturing varies in complexity and is affected by many factors (the depth and site of the wound; availability of suitable equipment and facilities; and characteristics of the individual patient). 'Generic' skills do not necessarily transfer through different contexts. Across higher education, a key driver of competency-based education is the production of 'workforce ready' graduates. A further limitation of this approach is its focus on achieving minimum standards of safe practice. Although baseline competence is a *sine qua non*, there is a strong case for pursuing excellence rather than minimal competence (Tooke, 2008). Finally, in competency-based education, there is a risk that a long list of individual competencies may overshadow the 'whole' professional practitioner (de Cossart and Fish, 2005). In clinical practice, the whole is much greater than the sum of its parts. A reductionist approach can result in educators becoming overfocused on fine-grained components, causing learners and teachers to lose sight of the bigger picture.

Fragmentation of curricula

At the same time, there is increasing emphasis on professionalism, patient safety, and a range of other attributes which medical students are expected to develop. These learning outcomes are codified in the United Kingdom by the General Medical Council, and all medical schools have to adopt them (Box 11.1). We will return to this tension between fragmented skills and whole-patient care in a later section. One consequence of the competency movement has been the splitting off of procedural skills into a separate educational stream. Medical curricula are now often built around themes, one of which is 'clinical skills'. Learners are expected to develop a repertoire which is aligned with the GMC's specifications. The learning and teaching of procedural skills has acquired an identity of its own. Although this has helped focus attention on clinical skills training, it becomes removed from the broader context in which the skills are performed in clinical practice. Factors shaping procedural skills training are summarised in Box 11.2.

Teaching of procedures

Simulation is steadily gaining ground as a means of learning procedural skills in a safe setting. In the United Kingdom, skills centres, which provide a range of bench top models, are now a part of every university and most hospitals. Although most are fairly unsophisticated, a spectrum of simulators is available, with highly complex mannequins and virtual reality systems becoming more widespread. High cost puts more complex ones beyond the reach of undergraduate training. See the following references for an overview of simulators in procedural skills (Bradley, 2006; Kneebone and Bello, 2005; Maran and Glavin, 2003; Vozenilek et al, 2004; Windsor, 2009). The aim is that all learners should receive an initial introduction to the techniques of clinical procedures away from actual patients, in a setting where they can master the basics and make mistakes without causing harm. Many current simulators are fairly crude representations of body parts, such as models for practising venepuncture or urinary catheterisation. The focus is on the equipment and techniques of each procedure, and the patient is 'absent'. Such decontexualised learning runs the risk of oversimplification, implying that there is always one 'correct' way to perform any procedure. Simulation of this kind is becoming widely accepted as an alternative to learning at the bedside, developing its own identity as an educational approach. This has obvious benefits, such as allowing novices to learn and practice the basics of a practical procedure in a protected setting where undivided attention can be given to the learner and where patient care is not in jeopardy. But there is a danger that simulation may be seen as an alternative rather than an adjunct to clinical practice.

Box 11.1

Clinical and practical skills the UK General Medical Council expects of new doctors

Clinical and practical skills

- Take and record a patient's history, including their family history
- Perform a full physical examination and a mental-state examination
- Interpret the findings from the history, the physical examination, and the mental-state examination
- Make clinical decisions based on the evidence they have gathered
- Assess a patient's problems and form plans to investigate and manage these, involving patients in the planning process
- Work out drug dosage and record the outcome accurately
- Write safe prescriptions for different types of drugs
- Carry out the following procedures involving veins:
  - i   Venepuncture
  - ii Inserting a cannula into peripheral veins
  - iii Giving intravenous injections
- Give intramuscular and subcutaneous injections
- Carry out arterial blood sampling
- Perform suturing
- Demonstrate competence in cardiopulmonary resuscitation and advanced life-support skills
- Carry out basic respiratory function tests
- Administer oxygen therapy
- Use a nebuliser correctly
- Insert a nasogastric tube
- Perform bladder catheterisation

Communication skills

Graduates must be able to communicate clearly, sensitively, and effectively with patients and their relatives, and colleagues from a variety of health and social care professions. Clear communication will help them carry out their various roles, including clinician, team member, team leader, and teacher.

Graduates must know that some individuals use different methods of communication, for example, Deafblind Manual and British Sign Language.

Graduates must be able to do the following:

- Communicate effectively with individuals regardless of their social, cultural, or ethnic backgrounds, or their disabilities
- Communicate with individuals who cannot speak English, including working with interpreters

Students must have opportunities to practise communication in different ways, including spoken, written, and electronic methods. There should also be guidance about how to cope in difficult circumstances. Some examples are listed as follows:

- Breaking bad news
- Dealing with difficult and violent patients
- Communicating with people with mental illness, including cases where patients have special difficulties in sharing how they feel and think with doctors
- Communicating with and treating patients with severe mental or physical disabilities
- Helping vulnerable patients

http://www.gmc-uk.org/education/undergraduate/undergraduate_policy/tomorrows_doctors.asp#Clinical%20and%20practical%20skills

Assessment of procedures

In former times, there was little or no assessment of procedural skills within undergraduate education. There was a widespread assumption that new graduates would have acquired the skills they needed for clinical practice by the time they finished their course. As evidence to the contrary began to emerge, simulation began to be used increasingly for assessment of procedural skills, providing a proxy for clinical observation. One of its attractions was the ease with which components of a procedural skill could be isolated and examined. Several approaches are in use:

Objective structured clinical examination

OSCEs have been widely used for over three decades for formative and summative assessment. There are several excellent descriptions of the process and reports of validity and reliability (Harden, 1990; Harden and Gleeson, 1979; Hodges, 2003; Regehr et al, 1999; Reznick et al, 1998; Townsend et al, 2001). Although there are variations in OSCEs, learners usually work through a series of stations, in each of which they perform a task. This may form part of a procedure, examination, communication, or other clinical activity. The task may involve a real patient or a simulated patient (SP), simulator kit, medical equipment, patient records, or other relevant items.

Box 11.2

Factors shaping learning and teaching in procedural skills

- Competency-based education
- Larger cohorts of medical students
- Increased range of settings for learning
- Skills centres or skills labs
- Team-based training
- New practitioner roles
- Expanded role for nursing and allied health professionals
- Patient empowerment
- Ethical imperatives to train in simulation
- Patient safety movement
- Working Time Directives
- Increased range of procedural skills simulators
- Advances in simulator technology
- Accessible audiovisual recording
- Improved understanding of educational theory
- Requirements of professional organisations (e.g. General Medical Council)

The format is formal, with whistles and bells signalling when learners start and finish stations. An assessor (examiner) is present at each station, recording judgements on paper forms. SPs may also be requested to make judgements (Cleland et al, 2009; Homer and Pell, 2009; Whelan et al, 2005). Feedback to learners often depends on the purpose of the OSCE, high stakes assessments usually offering limited feedback while formative assessments provide a richer learning experience (Nestel et al, in press). The number and length of stations varies widely, with published examples from 4 to 30 stations, each lasting between 5 and 20 minutes. Although the literature contains many descriptions of OSCEs, there are few references to an underpinning theoretical framework. Tasks are often reduced to component parts, using these as representations of the whole. On Miller's pyramid for assessing clinical competence (Miller, 1990), the OSCE addresses the 'shows how' of isolated tasks. Although this may be an important component of mastering technique, we argue that it is also important for learners to practise and be assessed on any skill in the context in which it will be used.

Objective structured assessment of technical skill

This influential approach, developed by Reznick's Toronto group, addresses the technical aspects of

surgical procedures (Faulkner et al, 1996; MacRae et al, 2000; Martin et al, 1997; Regehr et al, 1998; Reznick and MacRae, 2006; Szalay et al, 1998). A series of procedural stations (using bench top models or human cadavers) allows learners to be directly observed as they carry out operative procedures. A combination of checklists and global rating scales is used to make judgements about the skills observed. The use of global assessments by experts has proved to be especially valuable. Expert judgements allow for variation in individual technique (a major criticism of the reductionist OSCE approach). OSATS has been extensively validated and is widely used for assessing 'technical' surgical skill.

Direct observation of procedural skills

There has been a major shift within postgraduate education towards assessment in the workplace (Norcini, 2003; Norcini and Burch, 2007). For procedural skills, this has been through DOPS, where doctors are observed and assessed as they conduct procedures on selected patients (Box 11.4). The Foundation Programme for junior doctors in the United Kingdom is usually undertaken in the first 2 years after medical school (The Foundation Programme, 2010a). Foundation doctors are expected to undertake a series of work-based assessments covering a spectrum of knowledge, attitudes, and skills relevant to practising as a junior doctor. The assessments include case-based discussions, observations of junior doctors performing clinical examinations and procedural skills, and multi-source feedback. For procedural skills, a nominated assessor observes the junior doctor performing a selected procedure on a patient (Box 11.3). In real time, the assessor uses a six-point rating scale on a generic rating form – DOPS (The Foundation Programme, 2010b). The form consists of 11 items (Box 11.4). Foundation doctors arrange their own assessments, selecting which procedure they will be assessed on from the Foundation Programme curriculum and choosing a suitable patient and assessor. This work-based assessment represents a significant shift in procedural skills education for junior doctors, ensuring that actual practice is observed. That is, the highest point ('does') on Miller's pyramid. The DOPS form provides a framework relevant to many procedures, encouraging systematic thinking about skills and encouraging dialogue between learner and assessor with the intention of supporting learning. A key aim is to encourage junior doctors to take

Box 11.3

The procedural skills doctors in the UK Foundation Programme are expected to undertake in workplace-based assessments

- Venepuncture
- Cannulation
- Blood cultures (peripheral)
- Blood cultures (central)
- Intravenous infusion
- ECG
- Arterial blood sampling (radial/femoral stab)
- SC injection
- ID injection
- IM injection
- IV injection
- Urethral catheterisation
- Airway care
- NG tube insertion

Box 11.4

Criteria for assessment on the direct observation of procedural skills form

1. Demonstrates understanding of indications, relevant anatomy, technique of procedure
2. Obtains informed consent
3. Demonstrates appropriate preparation pre-procedure
4. Appropriate analgesia or safe sedation
5. Technical ability
6. Aseptic technique
7. Seeks help where appropriate
8. Post-procedure management
9. Communication skills
10. Consideration of patient/professionalism
11. Overall ability to perform procedure

responsibility for managing their learning in the clinical environment.

There are, of course, limitations. Although doctors are encouraged to sample widely from possible procedures, assessors, and patients, it is likely that a narrow sample is often chosen. It seems natural, for example, that doctors being assessed should choose to demonstrate a straightforward procedure on a co-operative patient. Doctors' responses to challenging situations and behaviours are therefore rarely

captured. Yet it is those very challenges that become crucial in clinical care. There are anecdotal reports of inaccurate recording of forms, unwillingness of assessors to report underperformance, and difficulties using the observation as a learning opportunity. The latter relates to limited time, knowledge of the purpose of the assessment, and teaching skill. However, the Foundation Programme provides a formal curriculum structure in what had often been an unstructured and service-oriented experience for junior doctors, providing first steps towards supportive monitoring of doctors' continuing professional development in a diverse health service.

Theory

In order to make rational choices about how best to learn, teach, and assess procedural skills, it is necessary to have an awareness of relevant learning theory. Such theories have emerged from many disciplines, including education, psychology, sociology, philosophy, and anthropology. Chapter 2 is wholly devoted to learning theory but we identify here theories which we believe are especially relevant to a discussion of procedural skills. We do not attempt to be comprehensive or to provide a formal critique of these positions. Learning theories are often classified as behaviourist, cognitivist, or constructivist. Like most classifications, there is overlap. *Behaviourism* is mainly concerned with learning manifested as changes in behaviour. The environment is seen as critical for shaping learning, and issues of contiguism (proximity of learning to application) and reinforcement (awards or punishments) are central to promoting learning. Unlike behaviourism, where factors external to the individual are seen as of primary importance, *cognitivism* outlines an individual's capacity to influence learning through memory (information processing), prior knowledge, and experience. *Constructivism* also focuses on individuals but not on 'memory'. It emphasises the ways in which individuals create new knowledge for themselves by engaging with others through talk, activities, and problem-solving. It emphasises, also, the social environment within which learning occurs.

Expertise

It is clear that expertise does not just 'happen'. Indeed, it has become a mantra that its acquisition in any field requires sustained deliberate practice over many years. Ericsson's pivotal work (Ericsson, 2004, 2005) has done much to highlight the crucial role of practice in the development of elite performance across a range of domains and disciplines. It is clear, for instance, that all international performers have engaged in a minimum of 10,000 hours of deliberate practice – not just doing, but doing with the express intention of improving. Traditional models of expertise, especially around procedural tasks, are based on a sequential process with defined stages (Dreyfus and Dreyfus, 1986; Fitts and Posner, 1967). Although the details vary according to which model is used, the learner progresses from a cognitive stage (learning what is to be done), through an associative stage (learning how to do it), and finally to an automatisation stage (where it falls from conscious awareness). Although this provides helpful insights into the acquisition of surgical skill, it leaves unanswered questions. The final stage of expertise demands particular attention. Cognitivists describe automaticity as the effortless completion of tasks, where the learner no longer has to think about steps in completing the task or procedure. This reduces demands on their cognitive capacity and enables them to deal with other stimuli. The concept is often illustrated with driving skills. As a newcomer to driving, it can be completely overwhelming simply to steer the car at low speed, let alone accelerate, brake, and indicate. Reversing and parking may seem far too complex. With practice, however, these component skills come together, allowing the driver to process the broad range of stimuli with which they are confronted. In clinical practice, learners commonly block out what are seemingly obvious cues as they focus on completing steps in a clinical procedure they are learning. If the procedure is taught 'out of context', then the learner does not have an opportunity to rehearse the skill as it might be performed in real practice, surrounded by the range of factors that can impinge on the clinician's performance.

An alternative framing is the distinction between routine and adaptive expertise. Routine experts become good at performing the same task over and over again. Adaptive experts, on the other hand, remain alive to the complexities of their setting and continually challenge themselves to come up with creative solutions to new circumstances. Although routine expertise is essential, especially for repetitive tasks, we must not lose sight of the need for adaptive expertise. It is in the real world that adaptive expertise is required, where the unexpected is the norm. According to Bereiter and Scardamalia, adaptive experts reinvest their freed-up attentional resources into progressive problem-solving, setting out to find situations which go beyond what they already know (Bereiter and Scardamalia, 1993, 2003; Scardamalia and Bereiter, 2003). As they become more comfortable with tasks which initially required all their attention, they are able to extend their learning in different directions. Returning to the motoring parallel, the novice's attention is at first wholly absorbed by trying to co-ordinate key controls and functions. As those become more familiar, they can concentrate more on managing the traffic and learning to read the road. However, once this in turn becomes second nature (automatised), most people use their freed-up attentional resources to do things unrelated to driving – listening to the radio, for example, or talking to other people in the car. But those who wish to become professional drivers channel these attentional resources into extending their range of driving skills rather than dissipating them in other activities. They seek out ways to corner at speed without losing control, to recover from a skid, and so on. In terms of clinical expertise, any educational framework should allow learners to continually develop and hone their skills at the *edges* of their existing competence, aiming to achieve excellence.

Experiential learning

There are two ways of thinking about 'experiential learning'. One relates to deliberately providing learners with an experience (learning activity) which enables them to gain knowledge and skills. The second relates to learning which occurs simply as the result of 'living'. Of course both are important, but it is the former which teachers can influence directly. Kolb and Fry (1975) describe a learning cycle which individuals may enter at any point. Key waypoints include 'concrete experience' (learner does something that produces an outcome), 'observation and reflection' (learner makes sense of what they have done, especially the particular circumstances that led to the outcome), 'forming abstract concepts' (learner extracts key elements of the action and the outcome to predict what might happen next time), and 'testing in new situations' (learner tests their prediction). This cycle is continuous and allows an individual to build a progressive repertoire of knowledge and skills. It follows that the more experiences learners have the more likely they are to learn.

However, we know that experience is only one of the variables that influence learning. The cycle has obvious application to teaching and learning procedural skills, especially training that provides opportunities for 'concrete experiences' in simulated settings.

Reflection

Schön's concepts of reflection-in-action (immediate 'thinking on your feet') and reflection-on-action (later analysis of actions in the light of outcome, prior experience, and new knowledge) describe the responses of practitioners to unexpected events (Schön, 1983, 1987a,b). Schön argued that practitioners seek to place new and unexpected experiences within a personal framework by identifying similar past experiences and then give consideration to possible outcomes by selecting new actions. Reflection-on-action is obviously a process that could be facilitated by peers and teachers, as it takes place after the event, but reflection-in-action requires an immediate response, especially in emergency clinical situations. Although Schön's approach is criticised by theorists, reflection-on-action is widely embodied in training programmes (e.g. portfolios, critical incident reports, etc.). Much literature focuses on what teachers know and how they might impart their knowledge to learners. But of course there is more to learning than the acquisition of propositional knowledge or psychomotor skills.

Boud et al extends Schön's concept of reflection-on-action, highlighting that it is important for teachers to work with learners' experiences. Boud argues that it is especially important to explore adult learners' experiences in order to help locate new knowledge and skills within their breadth of experience (Boud et al, 1996). Boud describes a 'critical reflective' approach which is 'context conscious'. 'Critical reflection' promotes and values both learning content and process. This approach includes both cognitive and affective elements of learning. In order to locate new knowledge and skills in a learner's experience, the process of learning must be active. The teacher designs the learning experience to make use of what the learner brings and takes from the interaction. The teacher also acknowledges the role of the environment in which learning takes place (the 'learning milieu'). Vicarious and experiential learning merge imperceptibly, and 'observing' and 'doing' both offer potential value in supporting learning. Another feature of Boud's approach is that

it is highly structured, addressing three elements: returning to the experience, attending to feelings, and then re-evaluating the experience. In re-evaluation, he further describes:

- Association (relating new information to that which is already known)
- Integration (seeking relationships between old and new information)
- Validation (determining the authenticity for the learner of the ideas and feelings which have resulted)
- Appropriation (making knowledge their own, Boud et al, 1996).

Vygotsky and the zone of proximal development

A useful framework for simulation-based learning is provided by Vygotsky (1978; Wertsch and Sohmer, 1995). Working with young children in the early twentieth century, he identified the critical role of social interaction in learning. Although formulated decades before simulation became established, Vygotsky's notion of the zone of proximal development (ZPD) is useful in conceptualising how learners gain and absorb skills. The ZPD highlights the importance of learning supported by peers and what he termed 'more knowledgeable others'. Vygotsky defines it as:

> the distance between the actual development level as determined by independent problem solving and the level of potential development as determined through problem solving under adult guidance or in collaboration with more capable peers.
>
> (Vygotsky, 1978)

The ZPD is therefore an intermediate zone between what learners can do on their own and what they cannot do at all. Here, the role of a teacher is crucial because it enables learners to gain and internalise knowledge and skills for themselves. The zone of current development is where the learner currently 'resides' and where tuition can move learning forward. From there, the learner can move with assistance from a 'more knowledgeable other' to their ZPD. From a contemporary standpoint, the ZPD can be thought of as a 'learning space', populated not only by teachers but also by educational resources such as simulation and e-learning (Boud et al, 1996; Schön, 1983, 1987a).

Several theorists have extended Vygotsky's work, developing the importance of instructional conversation between the learner and teacher. Bruner described the concept of 'scaffolding', where it is as important for teachers to know when to step back from supporting learners as it is to provide that support (Bruner, 1986, 1990, 1991; Wood, 1998). Tharp and Gallimore point out that learning is not static but prone to decay, and that when skills are lost, the learner must loop recursively back through earlier phases (Tharp and Gallimore, 1988, 1991).

Communities of practice

The ZPD focuses on learning by individuals but clinicians do not learn or function in isolation. Lave and Wenger's work on communities of practice and learning highlights how newcomers gradually become part of a professional group, and how learning and clinical practice both take place through gradual absorption into a shared activity with common goals.

> Learning viewed as situated activity has as its central defining characteristic a process that we call *legitimate peripheral participation*. By this we mean to draw attention to the point that learners inevitably participate in communities of practitioners and that the mastery of knowledge and skill requires newcomers to move toward full participation in the sociocultural practices of a community. 'Legitimate peripheral participation' provides a way to speak about the relations between newcomers and old-timers, and about activities, identities, artefacts, and communities of knowledge and practice. It concerns the process by which newcomers become part of a community of practice. A person's intentions to learn are engaged and the meaning of learning is configured through the process of becoming a full participant in a sociocultural practice. This social process includes, indeed it subsumes, the learning of knowledgeable skills.
>
> (Lave and Wenger, 1991)

Chapter 2 contains a more detailed discussion of Lave and Wenger's theoretical perspective but, for present purposes, their work makes it clear that procedural skills must be part of a wider picture of teamworking and shared approaches to learning and to practice.

Activity theory

Several authors provide stimulating and often challenging perspectives on medical education, drawing on literature around activity theory and actor network theory (Bleakley, 2006a,b; Bligh and Bleakley, 2006; Engestrom, 2001; Engestrom et al, 1999; Lingard, 2007). Activity theory provides a framework for considering ways in which people act. Derived from the work of Vygotsky and other influential scholars in the former Soviet Union, the framework provides a way of looking at the production and shaping of knowledge by individuals within social systems. It is easy to see applications within clinical settings, especially highly specialised and contained ones (e.g. operating theatres). Again, the topic is covered more fully in Chapter 2 but its significance to this chapter is the importance of viewing individuals in the context of the dynamic social environment in which they reside and that individuals' thoughts are influenced by those around them as they shape their environment too.

Threshold concepts

Elsewhere, it has been argued that personal development as a clinician involves transitions (Kneebone, 2005). Such transitions include developing from a medical student to a doctor and from a registrar to a consultant. Meyer and Land's work on threshold concepts is illuminating here (Meyer and Land, 2003, 2005). According to their approach, threshold concepts provide new ways of looking at a subject. Such concepts tend to be challenging and require learners to reconfigure their views of the world. This process can be uncomfortable and lead to a sense of alienation and anxiety. This is especially evident in health care education, where part of the development process as a clinician involves coming to terms with thresholds. Dealing with uncertainty, with ambiguity, and with lack of confidence is part of every clinician's experience, but such feelings are seldom expressed. According to Meyer and Land, many teachers become ensnared by 'enchantment', providing an oversimplified version of a complex reality in the hope of helping learners. In fact this can be counter-productive, leading to long-term difficulties in mastering complex domains and interfering with deep understanding. We return to the concept of transition later.

Patient-centred learning and simulated patients

The role of real patients

A significant proportion of undergraduate medical education takes place within clinical care provided by the health service of the country in which it takes place. Taking the United Kingdom as an example, the National Health Service (NHS) placed medical education alongside health care provision at its inception, seeing education as one of its fundamental components and expecting patients to participate and be 'taught and learned on' (General Medical Council, 1947, 1957). The role of patients in learning and teaching procedural skills has traditionally been passive (Howe and Anderson, 2003; Spencer et al, 2000; Wykurz, 1999). Learners have been guided by clinicians, with the patient's contribution limited to simply being present. The same language is less likely to be used to describe the role of patients in medical education today. Although the UK GMC and other regulatory bodies encourage active roles for patients in undergraduate education, each patient's choice is now paramount. This has triggered a radical shift in the relationship between patients and clinicians, with major implications for education. Practices that were once commonplace (e.g. vaginal examination of anaesthetised female patients without their consent) are no longer acceptable (Coldicott et al, 2003; Nestel and Kneebone, 2003). This is especially the case with invasive procedures, where there is real risk of causing harm. With the advent of patient-centred care and acknowledgement of patients' own expertise, medical educators have to find ways to represent patient perspectives in curricula. As societal values change, educators must respond by developing methods acceptable to the public. High-profile cases of medical malpractice and doctors' unprofessional behaviours have focused a spotlight on the medical profession. Medical education has also come under scrutiny from within and outside the profession. Most medical curricula now have lay or patient representation which include considering the acceptability of programme content and educational methods, and of raising the profile of patient perspectives. The ethics of patient involvement in medical education are fully explored in Chapter 1.

The role of simulated patients

For many years, SPs have worked as 'substitutes' or 'proxies' for real patients, an approach which offers many benefits. SPs are trained to portray patients and to provide feedback to learners. They have the potential to raise the profile of patient perspectives, especially as they relate to communication and other professional behaviours (Bokken et al, 2009; Cleland et al, 2009; Nestel and Kneebone, 2009).

Additional benefits of trained SPs include having scenarios that pose predetermined levels of challenge reflecting curriculum goals, the opportunity to tailor learning to individual learner needs, and the provision of standardised scenarios to assess learners in a range of clinical skills (Adamo, 2003; Barrows, 1968; Boulet et al, 2009; Hoppe, 1995; Ker et al, 2005; Nestel et al, 2006). The use of SPs offers major benefits in 'grounding' procedural skills training in holistic practice.

Simulation

We have argued earlier that simulation allows learners to gain procedural skills within a changing clinical landscape where traditional methods of learning on patients are no longer acceptable. We also alluded to some of the difficulties and dangers which may follow an uncritical acceptance of simulation. We have highlighted some theoretical positions that we believe can help develop a more integrated approach to simulation; one which helps to bridge the gap between formulaic, impoverished model-based training and the richness and unpredictability of clinical practice. We now move on to a critique of current simulation-based training.

Benefits of simulation

A key advantage of simulation is that it allows procedural skills to be practised and assessed outside the clinical arena, away from the complexities of actual care. This reductionist approach ensures safety. Yet there is increasing acceptance that clinical practice must be holistic and patient-centred, integrating clinical knowledge and skills with professionalism, communication, and patient safety. At the heart of this tension is confusion about what is meant by clinical and procedural skills. From one viewpoint, clinical skills encompass history taking, physical examination, and the skills of performing diagnostic and therapeutic procedures. From another, clinical skills are perceived as procedural skills which are learnt and assessed in a skills lab setting. To us, procedures are simply another form of clinical encounter. At the centre of this encounter lies a technical intervention which requires specific kinds of knowledge and dexterity. But that intervention must take place within a wider arc of care, which starts by ensuring that the patient understands and consents to the procedure and which ends with agreeing a plan for future action. Fragmentation of this process into isolated components can lead to over-focusing on the technical elements of the procedure.

Current approaches to assessment tend to exacerbate this imbalance. Learners who ask 'Shall I show you how I do it for the OSCE, or how I do it on the ward?' are highlighting an artificial distinction which has grown up between skills centres and clinical practice. The link between skills taught in centres and actual clinical practice is not readily grasped by learners. The limitations of widely available simulators (crude body parts) entrench this view further, suggesting that all venepunctures are the same. So, the attractions of simulation (bench top models) lead to a distorted perception of what clinical skills are about, and 'skills' become synonymous with labs in skills centres rather than patients.

Reconciling expert and novice perspectives

Somewhere in all this, the link between skills labs and real clinical practice becomes lost. This is probably because experts (for whom the skills labs trigger a wealth of clinical experience) make assumptions about novices (who have not yet gained that clinical experience, and who therefore engage with skills lab models at a completely different level). Kneebone has used the *ha-ha* as a metaphor for the difference in perspective between experts and novices (Kneebone, 2009). The ha-ha is a device used in eighteenth-century English landscape gardening. A deep ditch surrounds a country house and its garden, separating them from the surrounding parkland with its deer and cattle. Viewed from the house, this ditch is invisible, providing a powerful illusion that the house is in the midst of untamed nature. Seen from the park, however, the ditch is very evident, presenting an unscalable barrier. According to this metaphor, experts are in the house, looking out at novices in the park and wondering why they do not simply walk across and join in. From the novices' perspective, however, they are separated from the experts by a gulf which they cannot yet cross.

In the case of procedural skills, experts (who design the training that the novices undertake) have often lost sight of where the key challenges lie during the earlier stages of learning. Because of their extensive experience with a wide variety of patients, experts no longer find *any* example of cannulation

especially challenging. For the novice, on the other hand, there is a huge difference between an 'easy' and a 'difficult' cannulation. This difference in perspective lies behind some of the problems we see with conventional skills-based training. It is therefore important to return to first principles when designing educational programmes aimed at novices, ensuring that notions of simplicity and relevance reflect learners' perspectives as well as those of their teachers and mentors. Observation, peer feedback, and clinical expert supervision are all characteristic of contemporary approaches to the development of procedural skills.

Today, a significant proportion of medical education is delivered in the service arena, where there is a focus on the delivery of safe and cost-effective care to patients. There has been a shift from the traditional distinction between pre-clinical and clinical phases of medical curricula to curriculum designs in which early clinical placements are commonplace. The breadth of health services in which medical students are educated has also expanded. These changes influence the potential timing and settings for procedural skills education. Clinical skills are seen as crucial and are taught early in the curriculum. For obvious reasons, novices cannot practice on patients and so they are exposed to skills labs early on. Learners come to associate clinical skills, skills labs, and OSCEs.

Managing danger and experiencing risk

This issue of managing danger is central here. At one level, it is clearly essential to protect patients from unnecessary risk of harm, especially when undergoing invasive procedures. Yet, from the learner's point of view, recognising and managing danger is an essential element of becoming an effective clinician. If that sense of danger is stripped out of simulation-based training, how are learners to recognise premonitory signs of trouble and gain insight into their own capacities and responses? It seems to us that effective simulation should be able to recreate in the learner those real-world experiences of uncertainty and fear which are an inseparable component of clinical care. Only by doing so can learners recognise such responses in themselves, and develop the skills and maturity to deal with them effectively.

Too great an emphasis on simulation as a proxy for the real world holds more subtle dangers too. Although it may appear self-evident that initial learning in a safe environment is desirable, clinical practice is inherently risky. Managing such risk is crucial to becoming a mature and flexible practitioner, and dealing with uncertainty, ambiguity, anxiety, and even fear, is part of this process. A risk-averse culture that shies away from any potential danger could have a counter-productive effect, resulting in doctors who are ill-equipped for the realities of practice.

Simulation of clinical procedures therefore offers an alternative to clinical reality which is safe but does not reflect the complexities of authentic practice. Most educators are compelled to work within the limitations of existing models, whose crudeness dramatically reduces the correspondence with clinical reality. This reductionist approach is driven partly by a need to simplify a complex picture and to measure what is most easily measured. Yet a balance needs to be struck between swamping a novice with unmanageable levels of complexity before they have grasped the basics, and creating a sense of infantilism which prevents the learner from developing expertise to cope with a complex and sometimes dangerous reality. Workplace-based assessment, on the other hand, provides selective glimpses into authentic clinical practice but cannot sample the wide range of potential clinical challenges which a clinician should be expected to manage. Partly this is because there are such large numbers of medical students. Partly it is because most observed procedures are carried out on relatively straightforward patients, and so do not address the difficulties and challenges which require true expertise.

Procedural skills training, especially at a novice level, usually takes place within institutions which have to cater for large numbers of learners. Institutions and learners have different agendas. Immediately there appears a tension between the needs of the individual learner to experience individuality and clinical complexity, and the needs of the institution to create conditions of reproducibility and consistency. One major criticism of model-based simulation is that it does not recreate the variability of clinical experience, assuming for example that all instances of venepuncture are similar. In a sense, this is a conflict between validity and reliability. Ideally, every individual's learning experience would be based on unique encounters with real patients but set in a context which optimises learning. From an institutional standpoint, however, there is increasing pressure to provide a controlled and reproducible exposure for all learners within a given cohort, allowing teaching to be planned and resourced and

providing the conditions for formative and summative assessment in an equitable setting which meets the requirements of the curriculum. So, if there are limitations to skills centre practice, how might these be overcome? In the next section, we describe an approach we have developed, which addresses some of those issues.

Learning and teaching procedural skills

In the first section of this chapter, we outlined historical approaches to learning and teaching procedural skills, introduced key conceptual frameworks, and described the now well-established role of clinical skills centres for practising specific techniques on bench top models. We pointed out the combination of pressures and constraints acting upon clinical education. In this section, we make the case for integrating technical skills with other crucial aspects of clinical care and explore possible solutions, which use simulation in innovative ways.

Traditional model-based teaching of procedural skills places the technical aspects of each procedure at the heart of learning. The rationale for this approach lies in the need to build a foundation of technical mastery. And of course such mastery is essential. The question that follows logically is whether technical mastery alone is sufficient. Practice using isolated bench top models offers obvious benefits, especially to novices. At the earliest stages of learning, it is obviously essential to grasp the basics of technique, the instruments and equipment that are being used, and the fundamentals of each procedure. By practising the technical components of a procedure away from the pressures of clinical care, learners (so the argument runs) can give their undivided attention to the task in hand, without fear of causing damage. In one sense, all simulation relies upon simplification. Simulation demands the abstraction of key elements of real life and their representation in a format that allows learning to take place.

But simplification is a double-edged sword. In real life, attention is never undivided, and technical skills cannot be isolated from their clinical context. Too much emphasis on the technical can mask the fact that practising procedures is only relevant because procedures are carried out on patients. A defining characteristic of clinical practice is its complexity. Although much educational energy is directed towards learning 'generic' skills of history taking, physical examination, and diagnosis, each clinical encounter is unique and must be managed on its merits. The technical elements of procedures carried out on conscious patients are only one part (although a crucially important part) of a wider clinical encounter which includes communication, professionalism, and much else besides. Addressing this complexity is a key challenge. This applies as much to invasive procedures as to any other area. Inserting an intravenous cannula, for example, might be seen as a straightforward procedure requiring relatively low levels of expertise. That is true of inserting a cannula in a co-operative patient with 'easy' veins but certainly not true when it comes to inserting a cannula in an elderly, demented, and unco-operative patient with low blood pressure. Being able to do the first does not imply an ability to do the second. To conceive of the procedure simply as 'cannulation' is to oversimplify a complex picture.

Patient-focused simulation

Invasive procedures occupy a special position in clinical education, as they can cause harm. The dangers of inexpert attempts to take blood, insert a urinary catheter, or perform a lumbar puncture are obvious. Sooner or later, of course, every learner must perform their first procedure on a real patient but there is a strong argument for getting as far along the learning curve as possible before this happens. In that sense, the advantages of simulation are obvious. From the patient's perspective, it is not acceptable to be used as a guinea pig for a purely technical exercise. This raises the question of how preliminary integration can be achieved. We propose a conceptual model which shifts the emphasis from a technical skill *per se* to a clinical encounter which involves a procedure. The technical element, although no less important, becomes modulated by the clinician–patient relationship. For this purpose, we require a proxy for clinical practice which satisfactorily represents all the key elements of the encounter.

As a focus for discussion, we use our own work on patient-focused (hybrid) simulation (Higham et al, 2007; Kneebone et al, 2002, 2003, 2005, 2006a). For several years, we have been exploring the potential of combining SPs with bench top models to create realistic quasi-clinical encounters which combine the benefits of simulation (safety, the opportunity for repeated practice, a framework for feedback and assessment) with the complexities of clinical practice. In our initial work, we aligned existing bench top models with SPs to create the illusion of performing a procedure on a real person (Figures 11.1 and 11.2). The model acted as a proxy for that part of the patient on which the procedure was performed, while the SP acted as a proxy for the whole person. Rather to our surprise, we discovered that integrating the two proxies could create high levels of perceived realism despite the apparent crudeness

Figure 11.1 • Preparing the simulated patient.

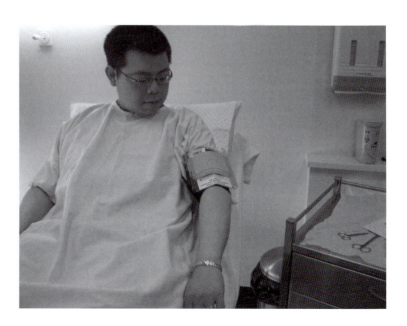

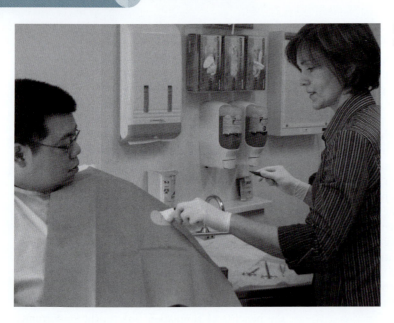

Figure 11.2 • Preparing the area for simulated treatment.

of the technical model. This high level of tolerance to apparently unrealistic elements raises important issues about priorities within simulation design. The crucial factor appears to be the presence of a real person within a procedurally focused encounter. In ways we are still exploring, this seems to break down the 'skills lab mentality', foregrounding the clinical nature of the encounter, and moving it away from being seen as a technical exercise.

As highlighted earlier, there is an extensive literature on SPs. Much has also been written about the wide variety of models and computer simulators which are now available. Much less has been written about the intersection zone between SPs and bench top models. We see hybrid simulation as a means to reconcile some of the imbalances of clinical care (where the patient's needs are paramount and the learner becomes subsidiary) and skills centre activity (where the learner's needs are central but the patient 'disappears'). Our model provides a balance between those two drivers, ensuring that additional elements (such as other clinical team members) can be provided.

Integrated procedural performance instrument

After exploring the concept of patient-focused simulation (PFS) in various settings and with a range of procedures, we developed the IPPI. This consists of eight 10-minute scenarios built around the clinical procedures expected of new medical graduates and set out in *Tomorrow's Doctors* (General Medical Council, 2003; Box 11.1). These included intravenous cannulation, urinary catheterisation, injections, suturing, and venepuncture. We have reported the IPPI concept elsewhere (Kneebone et al, 2006b, 2008; Leblanc et al, 2009; Moulton et al, 2009; Nestel et al, 2008a) and now use our experience with this technique as a focus for discussion. Each procedure was performed within a clinical encounter which specified the clinical scenario, the patient's role, and what the participant (junior doctor) was required to do. Each patient's role was played by SPs (professional actors) and was designed to reflect situations which new graduates might be expected to deal with. Alongside the technical procedure were specific challenges relating to communication, patient safety, and professionalism. These included patients who were distressed, hostile, visually or aurally impaired, unable to speak English, or accompanied by anxious relatives. The procedures themselves were performed on models attached to or aligned with SPs, using the hybrid approach described earlier. Each participant rotated through all eight scenarios. Encounters were recorded using a small video camera. There was no observer physically present in the scenario room. Each encounter was rated by expert clinicians, by the SP (acting as a proxy for the patient), and by the participant themselves. A combination of global ratings, checklists, and free text comments was used. Because the primary purpose was formative, participants were able to access their assessments via the web and review each of their videotaped performances.

We set out to create a panel of tasks which, taken together, would sample a range of clinical skills required at a given level of experience. We wished to create scenarios which moved away from the OSCE, with its tacit assumption that there is a formulaic set of steps which, if memorised and displayed, will satisfy the examiners. Instead, we tried to offer clinical situations where there was no single right answer, but rather a need to make choices and follow up their consequences. From the perspective of educational design, this posed a problem. From a practical point of view, it is clearly unacceptable to provide a set of free-range scenarios with no guidance on how to conduct them. On the other hand, too rigid a framework would constrain the very sense of authenticity and real-world uncertainty we were trying to achieve. We therefore designed scenarios to provide a consistent format (10-minute scenario) and a standardised opening gambit, but considerable latitude for how the encounter might evolve. Rather as the pieces on a chessboard start each game in the same positions but rapidly develop a unique disposition, simulations of this kind begin from a standard opening but can then develop in many possible directions depending on the relationship between the patient and clinician.

This unpredictability raises obvious potential difficulties. What might happen, for example, if a clinician lacked the skills and insight to defuse a hostile situation caused by an abusive patient? It is certainly better to address such issues within a simulation than a real encounter, but situations must not go out of control or result in physical violence. By using professional actors, we were able to set limits in advance, ensuring that the scenario would be terminated if a certain point was reached. The actors' detachment and professionalism provided a backstop which allowed us to trade realism against safety. We aimed for each scenario to be a managed microcosm of clinical reality, where participants could display a range of skills and behaviours while experiencing a range of feelings. In particular, we wished to create conditions for displaying adaptive expertise. Although individual scenarios might be challenging or upsetting, our aim was to provide these within a supportive overall matrix where participants' educational needs were our priority. The primary focus of the IPPI is procedural skills but we believe that this integrated

approach allowed us to sample a wide range of relevant behaviours.

To gain further insights, we explored learners' responses to both a formative OSCE and the IPPI immediately prior to a high stakes OSCE (Nestel et al, 2009). Learners valued both assessments, identifying that they met different needs. The OSCE prepared learners for their forthcoming exam, while the IPPI prepared them more for clinical practice, since it was perceived as 'holistic' and included 'patients'. Learners reported that the IPPI provided an opportunity to 'think on their feet' while dealing with a patient's problems. Almost all learners thought this was good preparation for their future as a doctor, providing them with an opportunity to work beyond their limits and explore boundaries of their competence which they were unable to do 'safely' in real practice. Learners did not believe that their course had prepared them for the IPPI style of assessment, and reported that the IPPI scenarios forced them to think and be creative. The IPPI seemed to be providing a means of moving between 'routine' and 'adaptive' expertise.

Since it is acknowledged that assessment drives learning, medical educators need to design assessments that reflect the needs of safe and effective clinical practice. Our experience with this study confirms the widely held view that learners adjust their learning to task-focused assessments. Contextualised and patient-focused assessments are more likely to align learning with real clinical practice, in line with the values underpinning *Good Medical Practice* (GMC, 2006) and the NHS.

A continuum of learning

We have previously put forward a conceptual model of simulation as complementing clinical practice rather than taking place in isolation from it (Kneebone et al, 2004). Instead of an impermeable barrier between the clinical and simulated settings, we see a porous membrane, which allows simulation to reflect and support specific aspects of clinical practice (Figures 11.3 and 11.4). Current developments are placing such an approach within reach. We now suggest a continuum model for procedural skills (Figure 11.5). On the left are isolated bench top models, allowing novices to become oriented to a new procedure and learn its basics. On the right lie complex simulations designed to challenge learners by recreating real-world situations with no right

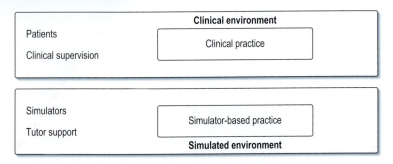

Figure 11.3 • An impermeable barrier between the clinical and simulated settings.

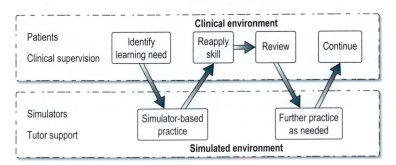

Figure 11.4 • A porous barrier between the clinical and simulated settings.

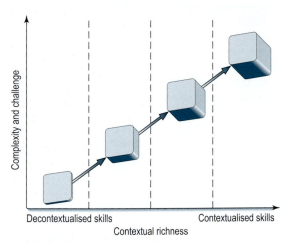

Figure 11.5 • Patient-focused simulations can be designed to reflect complexity and challenge against contextual richness.

or wrong answers. Between those poles lie a range of intermediate stages. Towards the left are formulaic, prescriptive settings whose primary focus is technical skill, while towards the right lie non-linear encounters which reflect the realities of clinical work. All are provided within a supportive, learner-centred setting which allows for feedback and debriefing and is sensitive to each participant's individual requirements and level of development. Such a continuum would allow the needs of learners to be

systematically mapped against their level of clinical experience. In the initial stages of training, or when learning a new procedure, learners would spend time towards the left. As their skills and confidence increased, they would spend more time within a quasi-clinical context towards the right.

Transitions

We have alluded earlier to the work of Meyer and Land on threshold concepts, highlighting how they may relate to issues of transition between states (between the medical student and doctor, for example, or registrar and consultant). We described their notion of 'enchantment', where oversimplified pictures of complex realities may be presented by a teacher with the misguided intention of aiding learning. There is a danger that such a strategy may backfire, providing an incomplete and partial view that interferes with full understanding. In our view, oversimplification of clinical procedures by over-focusing on models for technical tasks can lead to a similar enchantment, providing learners with a false sense of security which is abruptly overthrown when they are confronted by real patients. For this reason, simulation should set out to recreate all the necessary components of complex clinical encounters, rather than stripping them down to simple components. Simulation, if imaginatively designed and rigorously applied, can support learners in crossing the many thresholds which straddle the path to maturation as a competent and caring clinician. Such a model would take into account the transitions described earlier.

Layered learning

We end by proposing a conceptual model for simulation-based learning of procedural skills. The touchstone of clinical learning must be the real world of patient care. Simulation can only be useful if it is an adjunct to clinical experience. Without clinical care as its aim, simulation loses all meaning. Such care is, of course, driven by the needs of individual patients; the learning which takes place around such care must necessarily be subordinate to the care itself. The clinical needs of the patient must always take priority over the educational needs of the learner. This of course affects the balance between what may be desirable educationally and what is acceptable clinically. It may therefore be useful to consider what compromises can and should be made in order to achieve the best of both these worlds. This onion-like model consists of concentric layers which mediate between clinical and educational agendas (Figure 11.6). The model's core is the learner's interaction with a patient while performing an invasive procedure. The simulation sets out to recreate as accurately as possible the characteristics of a real clinical encounter. Conceptually, therefore, a real patient stands at the focal point. In reality, of course, compromises have to be made to maximise the educational benefits and minimise the risk of harm (to the patient and learner). These compromises take several forms and can be seen as a series of protective layers surrounding the 'idea' of the real patient.

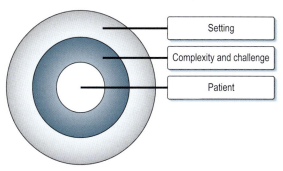

Figure 11.6 • The 'onion model' of layered learning.

Layer 1: the patient

First is the need to represent patients themselves. Presenting a real person (in the form of an SP) provides a high level of face validity and overcomes many of the problems around engagement and willing suspension of disbelief which beset the use of mannequins. A drawback is that the SP is not really a patient and may not respond authentically in a given scenario. This can be overcome to a large extent through rigorous role development and SP training. Although SP roles are often based on individual or 'combinations' of patients, they are usually crafted by clinicians and educators (Morris, 2006; Nestel and Kneebone, 2009). This is often a result of the pressure to produce new roles for teaching and assessment purposes. These composite roles may therefore be quite different from the authentic experiences of individuals. We know that those who deliver health care experience it differently from those who receive it. Therefore, we must take care that SP roles reflect authentic rather than clinician-interpreted experiences. Real patients can contribute directly to the development of SP roles and scenarios (Black et al, 2006; Nestel et al, 2008b). In our experience, involving real patients in scenario design has been salutary for SPs, clinicians, and educators involved in the process of role development and SP training. The line between authenticity and drama is a fine one, requiring careful management (Nestel and Kneebone, 2009).

Alongside the patient must be a convincing representation of the interventional procedure. In essence, an appropriate model is attached to or aligned with the SP. In order to minimise the task of suspending disbelief, the conjunction should be as realistic as possible. Careful design ensures that no harm can result to the SP, even from clumsy or inexpert intervention. As described earlier, technology in this area is developing rapidly and new approaches to link physical models with SPs are starting to emerge (see later). This combination of SP and model provides a working proxy for a real patient. In this sense, the actual patient is protected by a representation of that patient. At least two aspects of patient safety must be ensured. One is safety from physical harm, ensured as described earlier. The other is safety from any mental distress which might be caused by the conditions of education (as opposed to clinical care). Such distress might include: tiredness (from repeated encounters with many learners); anxiety (if inexperienced learners mistakenly suggest the presence of cancer or other serious disease); unwillingness to offend (if invited to give feedback); learner reaction to feedback; and pressure to comply with being 'taught on' (especially within the power gradient around clinical care).

Layer 2: complexity and challenge

The second layer refers to the level of challenge and complexity which is presented. As has been alluded to earlier, even an apparently simple procedure can become challenging if the patient or their circumstances are perceived as difficult. Such challenges might include patient behaviour (aggression, hostility, anxiety, confusion, or intoxication), environmental problems (missing, malfunctioning, or unfamiliar equipment), team working issues (dysfunctional relationships with colleagues), or personal issues (tiredness and lack of confidence in own skill). Simulation offers the opportunity to address those elements and ensure that they are aligned appropriately. This high degree of control allows simulations to be calibrated according to the level of challenge required by individual learners and to be used sequentially to build up an evolving picture of skills.

Layer 3: the setting

The final layer relates to the educational setting within which an encounter takes place. Such settings should support a learner-centred approach which provides opportunities for experience, feedback, and developing a systematic approach to the acquisition of skills. From the institution's point of view, learners must be able to practice as required, and their learning must be scheduled within the practical constraints of the curriculum.

Using SPs as a mirror for clinical encounters can satisfy many of these desiderata. SPs are able to 'sit on their own shoulder' while playing a role, monitoring the learner's response as well as providing detailed and systematic feedback tailored to the needs and capacities of individual learners. Locating simulations within purpose-designed facilities allows video recording to be used. This has a powerful effect in consolidating learning and allowing learners to view their own performance as others have seen it. This provides additional resources for documenting the acquisition of expertise and building up longitudinal portfolios. Such issues lie beyond the scope of this chapter, but are likely to become increasingly

prominent. This deliberate design allows safeguards to be embedded, ensuring that scenarios can be monitored and stopped if they are generating unduly high levels of anxiety or provoking potentially destructive behaviours.

Future directions

In our view, a major limiting factor in the development of effective simulation has been the limited availability of satisfactory models for procedural practice. Interesting possibilities are now emerging. Imaginative use of prosthetics techniques from the film and television industries seems likely to create new solutions to the limitations of current simulators. It seems likely that hybrid simulation will be developed widely in the future, offering increasing levels of realism and engagement. We are now, for example, working towards much higher levels of perceived realism through the use of sophisticated materials which can be seamlessly joined to SPs. This concept of seamlessness between realistic models and SPs eliminates much of the artificiality of crude simulators, creating a 'believable patient' where both the person and the procedure are sufficiently convincing to engage clinicians. This minimises obstacles to suspending disbelief and makes it much easier to engage with the scenario as a clinical encounter. Crucially, this approach allows bespoke simulations to be developed in response to educational need, rather than being constrained by which models are available for use.

Implications for practice

In this chapter, we have outlined key issues affecting how procedural skills are learnt, taught, and assessed. Providing learner-centred education within an increasingly embattled health care system creates new complexities and challenges for which solutions must be found. We have put forward a conceptual model and described practical ways of encouraging excellence while protecting patients from harm. Procedural skills must take their place within a wider curriculum, supported by all the elements of educational design which underpin health care education. We end on a note of caution. However seductive the attractions of simulation, our touchstone must remain clinical practice. Simulation cannot be an end in itself but must serve an educational need.

At the heart of every simulation lies a patient, either explicitly or implicitly. Simulation can only ever be an adjunct to clinical experience, never a substitute. The challenge is to ensure that simulation remains rooted in clinical experience and does not develop into a self-referential universe which loses touch with reality (Bligh and Bleakley, 2006). Technology has much to offer in expanding what simulation can offer. But it must remain a tool in the service of education.

References

Adamo G: Simulated and standardized patients in OSCEs achievements and challenges 1992–2003, *Med Teach* 25:262–270, 2003.

Barrows HS: Simulated patients in medical teaching, *Can Med Assoc J* 98:674–676, 1968.

Bereiter C, Scardamalia M: *Surpassing ourselves: an inquiry into the nature and implications of expertise*, Chicago, IL, 1993, Open Court.

Bereiter C, Scardamalia M: Learning to work creatively with knowledge. In E. De Corte et al, editors: Unravelling basic components and dimensions of powerful learning environments, 2003, EARLI Advances in Learning and Instruction Series.

Black S, Nestel D, Horrocks E, et al: Evaluation of a framework for case development and simulated patient training for complex procedures, *Simul Healthc* 1:66–71, 2006.

Bleakley A: Broadening conceptions of learning in medical education: the message from teamworking, *Med Educ* 40:150–157, 2006a.

Bleakley AA: A common body of care: the ethics and politics of teamwork in the operating theater are inseparable, *J Med Philos* 31:305–322, 2006b.

Bligh J, Bleakley A: Distributing menus to hungry learners: can learning by simulation become simulation of learning? *Med Teach* 28:606–613, 2006.

Bokken L, Linssen T, Scherpbier A, et al: Feedback by simulated patients in undergraduate medical education: a systematic review of the literature, *Med Edu* 43:202–210, 2009.

Boots R, Gegerton W, McKeering H, et al: They just don't get enough! Variable intern experience in bedside procedural skills, *Internal Med J* 39:222–227, 2009.

Boud D, Keogh R, Walker D: Promoting reflection in learning. In Edwards R, Hanson A, Raggat P, editors: *Boundaries in adult learning*, New York, 1996, Routledge.

Boulet J, Smee S, Dillon G, et al: The use of standardized patient assessments for certificate and licensure decisions, *Simul Healthc* 4:35–42, 2009.

Bradley PP: The history of simulation in medical education and possible future directions, *Med Educ* 40:254–262, 2006.

Bruner JS: *Actual minds. Possible worlds*, Cambridge, MA, 1986, Harvard University Press.

Bruner JS: *Acts of meaning*, Cambridge, MA, 1990, Harvard University Press.

Bruner JS: The narrative construction of reality, *Crit Inq* 18:1–21, 1991.

Calman K: *Medical education, past, present and future*, Edinburgh, 2007, Churchill Livingstone Elsevier.

Cave J, Goldacre M, Lambert T, et al: Newly qualified doctors' views about whether their medical school had trained them well: questionnaire surveys, *BMC Med Educ* 7:38, 2007.

Cleland J, Abe K, Rethans J: The use of simulated patients in medical education. AMEE Guide No 42 Medical Teacher 31(6):477–486, 2009.

Coldicott Y, Pope C, Roberts C, et al: The ethics of intimate examinations – teaching tomorrow's doctors. [Commentary]: Respecting the patient's integrity is the key. [Commentary]: Teaching pelvic examination – putting the patient first, *BMJ* 326:97–101, 2003.

De Cossart L, Fish D: *Cultivating a thinking surgeon*, Shrewsbury, 2005, tfm Publishing.

Dreyfus H, Dreyfus S: *Mind over machine: the power of human intuition and expertise in the era of the computer*, Oxford, 1986, Basil Blackwell.

Engestrom Y: *Expansive learning at work: toward an activity-theoretical reconceptualisation*, London, 2001, Institute of Education.

Engestrom Y, Miettinen R, Punamaki R, editors: *Perspectives on activity theory*, Cambridge, 1999, Cambridge University Press.

Ericsson K: Deliberate practice and the acquisition and maintenance of expert performance in medicine and related domains, *Acad Med* 79: S70–S81, 2004.

Ericsson K: Recent advances in expertise research: a commentary on the contributions to the special issue, *Appl Cognit Psychol* 19:233–241, 2005.

Faulkner H, Regehr G, Martin J, et al: Validation of an objective structured assessment of technical skill for surgical residents, *Acad Med* 71: 1363–1365, 1996.

Fitts P, Posner M: *Human performance*, Belmont, CA, 1967, Brooks/Cole Publishing Co.

Flexner A: *Medical education in the United States and Canada: a report to the Carnegie Foundation for the Advancement of Teaching*, New York, 1910, Carnegie Foundation for the Advancement of Teaching.

General Medical Council: *Recommendations as to the medical curriculum*, London, 1947, HMSO.

General Medical Council: *Recommendations as to the medical curriculum*, London, 1957, GMC.

General Medical Council: *Tomorrow's doctors*, London, 2003, General Medical Council.

GMC: *Good medical practice*, 2006.

Harden RM: Twelve tips for organizing an objective structured clinical examination (OSCE), *Med Teach* 12:259–264, 1990.

Harden RM, Gleeson FA: Assessment of clinical competence using an objective structured clinical examination (OSCE), *Med Educ* 13:41–54, 1979.

Higham J, Nestel D, Lupton M, et al: Teaching and learning gynaecology examination with hybrid simulation, *Clin Teach* 4:238–243, 2007.

Hodges B: Validity and the OSCE, *Med Teach* 25:250–254, 2003.

Homer M, Pell G: The impact of the inclusion of simulated patient ratings on the reliability of OSCE assessments under the borderline regression method, *Med Teach* 31:420–425, 2009.

Hoppe RB: Standardized (simulated) patients and the medical interview. In Lipkin M, Putnam S, Lazare A, editors: *The medical interview*, New York, 1995, Springer-Verlag.

Howe A, Anderson J: Involving patients in medical education, *Br Med J* 327:326–328, 2003.

Ker JS, Dowie A, Dowell J, et al: Twelve tips for developing and maintaining a simulated patient bank, *Med Teach* 27:4–9, 2005.

Kneebone RL: Clinical simulation for learning procedural skills: a theory-based approach, *Acad Med* 80: 549–553, 2005.

Kneebone R: Perspective: simulation and transformational change: the paradox of expertise, *Acad Med* 84:954–957, 2009.

Kneebone R, Bello F: Technology in surgical education. In Taylor I, Johnson C, editors: *Recent advances in surgery*, vol. 28, London, 2005, Royal Society of Medicine Press.

Kneebone R, Kidd J, Nestel D, et al: An innovative model for teaching and learning clinical procedures, *Med Educ* 36:628–634, 2002.

Kneebone RL, Nestel D, Moorthy K, et al: Learning the skills of flexible sigmoidoscopy – the wider perspective, *Med Educ* 37(Suppl. 1):50–58, 2003.

Kneebone RL, Scott W, Darzi A, et al: Simulation and clinical practice: strengthening the relationship, *Med Educ* 38:1095–1102, 2004.

Kneebone RL, Kidd J, Nestel D, et al: Blurring the boundaries: scenario-based simulation in a clinical setting, *Med Educ* 39:580–587, 2005.

Kneebone R, Nestel D, Wetzel C, et al: The human face of simulation: patient-focused simulation training, *Acad Med* 81:919–924, 2006a.

Kneebone R, Nestel D, Yadollahi F, et al: Assessing procedural skills in context: exploring the feasibility of an Integrated Procedural Performance Instrument (IPPI), *Med Educ* 40:1105–1114, 2006b.

Kneebone R, Nestel D, Bello F, et al: An Integrated Procedural Performance Instrument (IPPI) for learning and assessing procedural skills, *Clin Teach* 5:45–48, 2008.

Kolb D, Fry R: Toward an applied theory of experiential learning. In Cooper C, editor: *Theories of group process*, London, 1975, Wiley.

Lave J, Wenger E: *Situated learning. Legitimate peripheral participation*, Cambridge, 1991, Cambridge University Press.

Leblanc R, Tabak D, Kneebone R, et al: Psychometric properties of an integrated assessment of technical and communication skills, *Am J Surg* 197:96–101, 2009.

Lingard L: The rhetorical 'turn' in medical education: what have we learned and where are we going? *Adv Health Sci Educ Theory Pract* 12:121–133, 2007.

Ludmerer K: *Time to heal*, Oxford, 1999, Oxford University Press.

MacRae H, Regehr G, Leadbetter W, et al: A comprehensive examination for senior surgical residents, *Am J Surg* 179:190–193, 2000.

Maran N, Glavin R: Low- to high-fidelity simulation – a continuum of medical education? *Med Educ* 37:22–28, 2003.

Martin JA, Regehr G, Reznick R, et al: Objective structured assessment of technical skill (OSATS) for surgical residents, *Br J Surg* 84:273–278, 1997.

Medical Education Committee of the British Medical Association: *The training of a doctor: a report of the Medical Education Committee of the British Medical Association*, London, 1948, HMSO.

Meyer J, Land R: *Threshold concepts and troublesome knowledge: linkages to ways of thinking and practising within the disciplines, Enhancing Teaching and Learning Environments in Undergraduate Courses*, Edinburgh, 2003, School of Education, University of Edinburgh.

Meyer J, Land R: Threshold concepts and troublesome knowledge 2: epistemological considerations and a conceptual framework for teaching and learning, *High Educ* 49:373–388, 2005.

Miller G: The assessment of clinical skills/competence/performance, *Acad Med* 65(9):S63–67, 1990.

Morris P: The patient's voice in doctor's learning. In Thistlethwaite J, Morris P, editors: *The patient doctor consultation in primary care: theory and practice*, London, 2006, Royal College of General Practitioners.

Moulton C, Tabak D, Kneebone R, et al: Teaching communication skills using the integrated procedural performance instrument (IPPI): a randomised controlled trial, *Am J Surg* 197:113–118, 2009.

Nestel D, Kneebone R: Please don't touch me there: the ethics of intimate examinations: integrated approach to teaching and learning clinical skills, *BMJ* 326:1327, 2003.

Nestel D, Kneebone R: Authentic patient perspectives in simulations for procedural and surgical skills, *Acad Med*, 85(5):889–893, 2010.

Nestel D, Kneebone R, Black S: Simulated patients and the development of procedural and operative skills, *Med Teach* 28 (4):390–391, 2006.

Nestel D, Bello F, Kneebone R, et al: Remote assessment and learner-centred feedback using the Imperial College Feedback and Assessment System (ICFAS), *Clin Teach* 5:88–92, 2008a.

Nestel D, Cecchini M, Calandrini M, et al: Real patient involvement in role development evaluating patient focused resources for clinical procedural skills, *Med Teach* 30:534–536, 2008b.

Nestel D, Kneebone R, Carmel N, et al: Formative assessment of procedural skills: students' responses to the Objective Structured Clinical Examination and the Integrated Performance Procedural Instrument, *Assess Eval High Educ*, 34:1–13, 2009.

Norcini J: ABC of learning and teaching in medicine: work based assessment, *BMJ* 326:753–755, 2003.

Norcini J, Burch V: Workplace-based assessment as an educational tool: AMEE Guide No. 31, *Med Teach* 29:855–871, 2007.

Regehr G, MacRae H, Reznick RK, et al: Comparing the psychometric properties of checklists and global rating scales for assessing performance on an OSCE-format examination, *Acad Med* 73:993–997, 1998.

Regehr G, Freeman R, Hodges B, et al: Assessing the generalizability of

OSCE measures across content domains, *Acad Med* 74:1320–1322, 1999.

Reznick R, MacRae H: Teaching surgical skills – changes in the wind, *N Engl J Med* 355:2664–2669, 2006.

Reznick RK, Regehr G, Yee G, et al: Process-rating forms versus task-specific checklists in an OSCE for medical licensure. Medical Council of Canada, *Acad Med* 73:s97–s99, 1998.

Scardamalia M, Bereiter C: Knowledge building. In J. Guthrie, editor: Encyclopedia of education, New York, 2003, Macmillan Reference.

Schön D: *The reflective practitioner: how professionals think in action*, London, 1983, Temple Smith.

Schön D: *Educating the reflective practitioner*, San Francisco, CA, 1987a, Jossey-Bass.

Schön DA: *Educating the reflective practitioner: toward a new design for teaching and learning in the professions*, San Francisco, CA, 1987b, Jossey-Bass.

Spencer J, Blackmore D, Heard S, et al: Patient-oriented learning: a review of the role of the patient in the education of medical students, *Med Educ* 34:851–857, 2000.

Tharp R, Gallimore R: *Rousing minds to life*, Cambridge, 1988, Cambridge University Press.

Tharp R, Gallimore P: A theory of teaching as assisted performance. In Light P, Sheldon P, Woodhead M, editors: *Learning to think*, London, 1991, Routledge.

The Foundation Programme 2010a: http://www.foundationprogramme. nhs.uk/pages/foundation-doctors (accessed May 24, 2010).

The Foundation Programme: 2010b. http://www.foundationprogramme. nhs.uk/pages/home/key-documents #foundation-programme-curriculum (accessed May 24, 2010).

Tooke J: *Aspiring to excellence*. Independent Inquiry into Modernising Medical Careers, Aspiring to Excellence: Final Report of the Independent Inquiry into Modernising Medical Careers, London, 2008.

Townsend AH, McIlvenny S, Miller CJ, et al: The use of an objective structured clinical examination (OSCE) for formative and summative assessment in a general practice clinical attachment and its relationship to final medical school examination performance, *Med Educ* 35:841–846, 2001.

Vozenilek J, Huff J, Reznek M, et al: See one, do one, teach one: advanced technology in medical education, *Acad Emerg Med* 11:1149–1154, 2004.

Vygotsky L: *Mind and society: the development of higher mental processes*, Cambridge, MA, 1978, Harvard University Press.

Wenger E: *Communities of practice. Learning, meaning, and identity*, Cambridge, 1998, Cambridge University Press.

Wertsch J, Sohmer R: Vygotsky on learning and development, *Hum Dev* 38:332–337, 1995.

Whelan G, Boulet J, McKinley D, et al: Scoring standardized patient examinations: lessons learned from the development and administration of the ECFMG Clinical Skills Assessment (CSA®), *Med Teach* 27 (3):200–206, 2005.

Windsor J: Role of simulation in surgical education and training, *ANZ J Surg* 79:127–132, 2009.

Wood D: *How children think and learn*, Oxford, 1998, Blackwell.

Wu E, Elnicki D, Alper E, et al: Procedural and interpretive skills of medical students: experiences and attitudes of fourth year students, *Acad Med* 83:s63–s67, 2008.

Wykurz G: Patients in medical education: from passive participants to active partners, *Med Educ* 33:634–636, 1999.

Further readings

Dieckmann P, editor: *Using simulations for education, training and research*, Lengerich, 2009, PABST.

Kneebone RL: Practice, rehearsal, and performance: an approach for simulation-based surgical and procedure training, *JAMA* 302 (12):1336–1338, 2009.

Learning and teaching in workplaces

12

Pim W. Teunissen   Tim J. Wilkinson

CHAPTER CONTENTS

ABC

Glossary

Codified knowledge See main Glossary, p 339.

Context See main Glossary, p 340.

Community of practice (CoP) See main Glossary, p 340.

Cultural knowledge Knowledge about social relationships, norms, and values that impacts on interactions within a group of people.

Curriculum in action See main Glossary, p 340.

Curriculum, intended See main Glossary, p 340.

Experienced curriculum See main Glossary, p 340.

Implicit learning See main Glossary, p 341.

Informal education/learning See main Glossary, p 341.

Intersubjectivity When members of a team understand each others' preferences and idiosyncrasies, they can work together without the need for constant interpersonal negotiation.

Learning See main Glossary, p 341.

Medical (education) workplace See main Glossary, p 341.

Personal knowledge What individuals bring to situations that enables them to think, interact, and perform.

Self-efficacy See main Glossary, p 342.

Tacit knowledge See main Glossary, p 343.

Outline

Whether we like it or not, the main purpose of workplaces is getting a job done rather than learning. Yet, workplaces are rich learning environments and

DOI: 10.1016/B978-0-7020-3522-7.00012-7

getting jobs done entails a lot of learning, a tension that creates both opportunities and challenges. Workplace learning and teaching is pivotal throughout the medical continuum, from medical student clerkship placements to trained practitioners' continuing professional development. Sometimes learning is serendipitous and messy; at other times it is planned and systematic. Learning *on* the job is increasingly being complemented by learning *at* the job, which includes formal teaching sessions, meetings with supervisors, personal reading, and personal reflection that have always been part of medical workplaces. This chapter considers what we really mean by learning *on* the job and what can be done to enhance it. It is complementary to Chapter 7, which discusses learning environments. Because workplace learning is so pivotal, learning *at* the job is spread over many other chapters: Chapters 9, 10, and 11 consider small and large group and skills learning. Chapters 8, 13, and 18 consider individual tuition at the job, including the identification of learning needs, reflective learning and appraisal, and guiding career progression. Chapter 19 considers how to develop learners and teachers for their respective roles in clinical education. This chapter first considers, from an educational viewpoint, what a workplace is. It then separates out, from both practical and theoretical standpoints, the components and processes of workplace learning. Finally, it puts them back together into a complete system and considers how the workings of that system can be enhanced.

Features of learning in medical workplaces

Learning in context

A medical education workplace has been defined as 'any place where patients, learners, and practitioners come together for the conjoint purpose of providing medical care and learning' (Dornan et al, 2009). This broad definition helps make explicit that when we use the term learner we are not just referring to medical students – in continuous professional development, for example, the practitioner is the learner. What is common to all learning, however, is that workplaces where learning occurs are similar to the complex environments in which learners must apply the skills, knowledge, and attitudes that they develop. For trainees, it is similar to the context in which they will work later. For practitioners, it is identical to the context where they must apply their learning. Therefore, workplaces present learners with both learning opportunities and possible learning outcomes. This is an important feature of workplace learning. There is good evidence showing that we are better able to recall and apply knowledge and skills in places that are similar to those where they were learnt; learning is also most effective when it meets immediate needs and is directly applicable (Rogoff, 1990; Slotnick, 1999). However, the advantages of immediacy and context can be offset by workplaces providing limited time to prepare, brief, reflect, and debrief – features that are important to make the most of learning experiences. Another disadvantage is that busy workplaces can disjoin practice from theory. The dominance of 'this is how we do it around here' over 'let's make our practice evidence based and theoretically underpinned' has brought workplace and apprenticeship learning into some disrepute, though recent advances in our understanding of how learning occurs in workplaces and how it can be enhanced have started something of a renaissance in apprenticeship models (Rogoff, 1995; Sheehan et al, 2005; Teunissen et al, 2007).

Triadic relationship

The primary focus of health care workplaces is on patient care, whereas the primary focus of traditional classroom contexts is on the learner and teacher. Learning in health care workplaces therefore changes these two-way relationships to three-way teacher–learner–patient relationships (Dornan et al, 2007). Attention to patients' needs is of foremost importance, a value that is shared between teacher and learner but which imposes on the teacher the dual obligation of attending to the patient's needs and to the learner's needs. This triadic relationship is self-evident when a patient is physically present but the immediacy of a patient's needs very easily dominates even when just a teacher and learner are in the same room. Patients' unpredictable needs can turn the best-prepared teaching session to chaos but can, equally, present powerful learning opportunities at the most unexpected moments. While this triadic relationship can cause tensions, it can also be used to advantage by all parties. For example, many valuable learning opportunities arise when a teacher and learner are both puzzled over a patient's problem. Arriving at a solution to this problem can help the learning of both the teacher and learner and help the health of the patient. While classroom learning is often planned and explicit, workplace learning is more opportunistic and covert. Understanding how this triadic learning relationship occurs can help all parties recognise opportunities and make the most of them when they arise.

Processes and outcomes are hard to control

Another characteristic of workplace learning and teaching is that the education actually being offered (the curriculum in action) does not fully coincide with the curriculum on paper, or intended curriculum, of a formal education programme. And the curriculum that is experienced – what trainees actually learn – is different again and will even differ between two individuals who share the same experiences (Lempp and Seale, 2004; Remmen, 1999). Furthermore, access to role models is a feature of workplaces that has a powerful influence on what people actually learn, particularly their acquisition of 'tacit' knowledge (knowledge that is learnt and applied almost unconsciously) and covert knowledge (Eraut et al, 2000; Polanyi, 1974). Daily interaction with other co-workers also contributes important knowledge despite both parties remaining unaware that learning and teaching are going on (Lave and Wenger, 1991). So, workplaces have very powerful effects on learning, much of which is positive, but only some of which is overt. Workplaces support a type of learning that simply cannot take place in other contexts and much of what is learnt will be remembered and applied. However, there are factors that may inhibit learning of good habits and/or promote good learning of bad habits. While some of it seems to happen effortlessly under our noses, aspects of workplace education can be improved by making it more explicit.

Table 12.1 outlines some advantages and disadvantages of workplace learning. The next section analyses in finer detail some theories of workplace learning followed by the constituent parts of workplace learning and the ways in which they interact.

Theoretical perspectives on workplace learning

Just as doctors need to understand the pathophysiology of diseases to care for patients, an understanding of the concepts of participation and cognition helps understand workplace learning. There are many theoretical perspectives (Cheetham and Chivers, 2005), ranging from cognitivist views of how experts transfer their knowledge and skills to learners, to socio-cultural perspectives on how learning arises from interactions among members of workplace 'communities of practice' (CoP) (Bleakley, 2006; Slotnick, 2001; Swanwick, 2005; Wenger, 1998). Theoretical underpinnings of medical education are considered more fully in Chapter 2 but three of them – concepts around informal learning, social cognitive theory, and communities of practice theory – provide useful perspectives on workplace learning and deserve a brief overview at this point. Subsequently, workplace learning is broken down into three constituent parts: 'tasks', 'contexts', and 'learners'. Those three interrelated parts are common to different theoretical perspectives on workplace learning and teaching.

Concepts around informal learning

Much learning at work, even in an educational context, occurs outside the formally organised and delivered curriculum. Informal learning has been described by Eraut as taking place 'in the spaces surrounding activities and events with a more formal educational purpose' (Eraut, 2004). From an educational viewpoint, informal learning appears to be unstructured, unintended, and opportunistic. Informal learning is closely linked to implicit or tacit learning. Reber describes implicit learning as 'the acquisition of knowledge, independent of conscious attempts to learn and in the absence of explicit knowledge about what was learned' (Reber, 1993). According to Eraut, it is hard to understand learning at work because of several factors. First, informal learning is largely invisible because much of it is taken for granted and not recognised as learning. Second, the resulting knowledge is either tacit or regarded as part of a person's general capability rather than something that has been learnt. Lastly, discourse about learning is predominantly about propositional, codified knowledge, and people have difficulty describing the more complex aspects of their work and the nature of their expertise. So, although informal learning and the use of tacit knowledge are probably the largest part of the learning process in workplaces, the characteristics of informal learning make its identification difficult. To study and understand learning in workplaces, Eraut asks three questions about this type of learning: What is learnt?

Table 12.1 Advantages and disadvantages of workplace learning

Features of workplace learning	Advantages	Disadvantages
Learning occurs in context	Learning is more easily applied and recalled	Workplace demands may limit available time
Learning has immediate relevance	Learning can be applied directly	Time spent preparing and reflecting can be limited
Learning can be unpredictable	Learning can occur at any time	Hard to prepare
Learning content can be unstructured	Learning can be directly related to needs	Hard to be systematic so gaps may be left or there may be duplication
Learning is from experience	Learning is powerful	Not all experiences are good experiences; some learning is from mistakes
Learning from patients	Results and feedback can be immediate and direct	Learning may impinge on patient safety issues
Learning is determined by case mix	The case mix forms a *de facto* curriculum that covers common problems	Important but uncommon problems may be omitted
Learning depends on relationships with work colleagues	Learning can be individualised and motivating when relationships are positive	Learning can be inhibited or threatening when relationships are negative
Learning from role models	Helps professional identity and role development	Not all role models are good role models
Learning from colleagues	Applicability is immediate; experience of others offers additional perspectives	Practice can dominate over theory; underpinning theory and evidence base may be lost; bad habits are perpetuated
Learning may be covert and outcomes tacit	Consciousness is reserved for more strenuous tasks; helps to develop fluidity in performance	Some influences may be unfavourable; tacit knowledge is hard to teach to others; learners are not aware of learning processes and outcomes

How is it learnt? And what are the factors that influence learning? (Eraut, 2004).

What is learnt?

Eraut distinguishes three types of knowledge outcomes. Codified knowledge is the kind of academic knowledge that can be found in nearly all workplaces in the form of textbooks, organisation-specific or specialty-specific protocols, records, correspondence, manuals, etc. Secondly, cultural knowledge plays a key role in workplace activities, which is knowledge about social relationships, norms, and values that impact on interactions within a group of people. According to Eraut, much uncodified cultural knowledge is 'acquired informally through participation in social activities; and so much is often taken for granted that people are unaware of its influence on their

behavior'. As a counterpart to these two types of socially shared knowledge, Eraut identifies 'personal knowledge' as 'what individuals bring to situations that enable them to think, interact and perform'. This includes personalised versions of codified knowledge, but also knowledge of self, people, situations, attitudes, and emotions. In his terms, skills require a combination of personal and cultural knowledge. Competence is then defined as meeting other people's (often implicit) expectations, making it a much more problematic concept in terms of defining competence as an educational outcome and in its assessment.

How is it learnt?

Given the fact that so many learning outcomes go unnoticed, studying how people learn in workplaces is challenging. Eraut's approach to this problem is to describe four types of activity through which learning occurs: participation in group activities, working alongside others, tackling challenging tasks, and working with clients. In all of these activities the quality of relationships is essential. Billett also takes participation in workplace activities to be central to understanding workplaces as learning environments (Billett, 2004a). Moreover, he stresses the importance of how and what activities and interactions workplaces afford learners. Additionally, he acknowledges the active role learners play in choosing how they participate and in what activities they participate. Billett stresses that an individual's participation is 'not *ad hoc*, unstructured or informal' (Billett, 2004b). He introduces the concept of the 'workplace curriculum' to indicate that learners' participation is highly structured, albeit usually not on educational grounds. The organisation of tasks is usually directed towards the goals of particular workplaces, for instance the efficient provision of health care. Billett argues that 'workplaces will invite workers to engage and learn, insofar as that participation serves its goals and/or the interests of those within it, that is the continuity and/or development of the workplace or affiliates or individuals within it' (Billett, 2006). The opportunities for engagement afforded to learners and the way in which they choose to participate will influence the quality of a workplace as a learning environment. In taking this view, Billett explicitly introduces power and control as important regulators of opportunities. Fuller and Unwin (2003) have pursued a line of research in which they have looked at the opportunities and challenges learners experience in a workplace. Based on several case studies in vocational training programmes in the United Kingdom, they identified differences in participatory practices that could be located on a continuum from a 'restrictive' to an 'expansive' working environment (Fuller and Unwin, 2003). 'Expansive' workplaces offer a broad range of possible learning activities, provide gradual transition from peripheral participation to more full participation, provide support and guidance to learners, and recognise learners' status within a community among others. 'Restrictive' workplaces lack these characteristics. Such restriction can arise from a number of influences, such as the attitudes of co-workers, the 'queue' of other learners that may take precedence, the value the workplace puts on the personal development of others, or physical constraints that limit informal interactions among co-workers. They argue that an 'expansive' approach leads to 'a stronger and richer learning environment' (Fuller and Unwin, 2003).

What factors influence workplace learning?

Eraut's third question concerns factors that influence learning in workplaces. There are many factors that impact on learning in one way or the other. Most of them influence how learners decide on which activities to participate in and factors that influence how learners interpret their experiences. Such factors can be grouped into three broad categories: factors associated with the activity itself, factors related to an individual learner's characteristics, and contextual factors. These three categories are discussed in detail later in this chapter. At this point we limit ourselves to an illustration of how factors that impact on learning are interrelated. Eraut highlighted the importance of confidence that arises from meeting the challenges in one's work (Eraut, 2004). Confidence in this situation seems integrally related to Bandura's concept of self-efficacy (Bandura, 1994); it is a context-specific perception and relates to the ability to execute a specific task or to fulfil a particular role. Confidence relates strongly to the perceived quality of relationships in the workplace; tackling challenging tasks will be easier when learners feel appropriately supported in doing so. Support and confidence lead to social inclusion in teams and engenders commitment. To develop confidence in tackling new tasks, feedback and appreciation of the value of the work are also critical. Again, workplace learning reveals a complex interrelatedness among concepts such as confidence, commitment, context, challenge, and value of work, and feedback and support in performing tasks.

Social cognitive theory

Another theoretical perspective relevant to understanding workplace teaching and learning is social cognitive theory. This perspective sheds light on how interactions between people and their environments lead to behaviour and behavioural change. Therefore, it places greater emphasis on cognitive aspects of learning than socio-cultural perspectives do. The main proponent of social cognitive theory has been the psychologist Albert Bandura. Drawing on research on learning and self-efficacy, social cognitive theory has gradually developed over the past 50 years. Central to social cognitive theory is personal agency. People are the producers and products of the social systems in which they operate (Bandura, 2001). They try to 'make good judgments about their capabilities, anticipate the probable effects of different events and courses of action, size up sociostructural opportunities and constraints, and regulate their behaviour accordingly' (Bandura, 2001). Bandura identified intentionality, forethought, self-reactiveness, and self-reflectiveness as core features of personal agency (Bandura, 2001). Intentions are cognitive representations of future courses of action to be performed. Individuals can motivate themselves and choose between courses of action because they anticipate certain consequences of their own behaviour. The surgeon who plans to add a new surgical technique to the range of procedures he is qualified in can intentionally look for courses and opportunities to develop the necessary new skills. Forethought is another hallmark of personal agency. For example, when attending to a woman in labour who previously suffered from postpartum haemorrhage, a resident in obstetrics will actively lead the third stage of labour (when the placenta is delivered) because he or she will have confidence in being able to influence the outcome. Intentions and forethought are influenced by an individual's beliefs, values, goals, and personal knowledge structures. According to Bandura, the relative stability of one's intentions explains why individuals can display considerable self-directness and do not necessarily change a course of action even if it leads to unrewarding outcomes (Bandura, 2001). Some learners will continue to be proactive in seeking learning opportunities if they believe that these experiences will help them obtain their goals, even in a situation where their initiative is not reciprocated.

Self-regulatory behaviour

In guiding learners to develop appropriate action possibilities, the concepts of self-reactiveness and self-reflectiveness are personal qualities that have received considerable attention in medical education. They stem from the realisation that the outcome of events, especially if other people are involved, is only partly the result of one individual's agentic actions. Therefore, when engaged in tasks, individuals 'cannot simply sit back and wait for the appropriate performances to appear' (Bandura, 2001). To make sure that you perform appropriately, you need to regulate your thoughts and actions in the ongoing flow of events. Based on personal standards of appropriate behaviour, individuals use self-monitoring and self-guidance to react and respond to events (Bandura, 2001). Such self-regulatory aspects of behaviour are receiving increased attention within

medical education as an alternative way of conceptualising self-assessment (Eva and Regehr, 2007). The concept of self-assessment is discussed in Chapter 8. Gradually, through practice, proficient modes of action are developed that are suited to similar situations and the execution of these actions becomes automated. Self-reflectiveness will then help learners continue to learn from the outcomes of events by judging 'the correctness of their predictive and operative thinking against the outcomes of their actions, the effects that other people's actions produce, what others believe, deductions from established knowledge and what necessarily follows from it' (Bandura, 2001). From a teacher or supervisor perspective, this means that a trainee's lifelong learning may be enhanced by taking time to understand the learner's motivations and aspirations.

Self-efficacy

A central premise underlying Bandura's work is that the factors involved in the motivation and guidance of behaviour are all 'rooted in the core belief that one has the power to produce effects by one's actions' (Bandura, 2001). This belief, if related to a specific task, is called perceived self-efficacy (Bandura, 1997). Perceived self-efficacy judgements influence the tasks trainees choose to participate in, how they self-regulate, and how they self-evaluate their performance (Bandura, 2005). It thereby influences trainees' experiences and shapes their future participation in the clinical workplace. Four distinct sources contribute to self-efficacy beliefs. First, mastery experience is the most influential source of self-efficacy beliefs (Pajares, 1997). Outcomes interpreted as successful raise self-efficacy, those interpreted as failures lower it (Bandura, 1997; Pajares, 1997). If you have done ten venepunctures successfully, you will believe that you can do the eleventh one successfully too. If you learnt something from a particular interaction or activity, you will be more confident in making future attempts. The second source is vicarious experience of the outcomes produced by the actions of others. Role models and peers are particularly relevant to judgements about the self (Bandura, 2005). If your peers are all able to do venepunctures, you are more likely to believe that you can do them as well. However, when your peers all fail to perform a procedure only senior staff members can perform, your self-efficacy beliefs will probably drop. A third source of self-efficacy, whose effects are not as strong as mastery or vicarious experiences, is verbal persuasion by others. It is usually easier to weaken self-efficacy beliefs through negative appraisals than to strengthen such beliefs through positive encouragement (Bandura, 1997). We are more motivated when told what we did right, not just what we did wrong, and we are more likely to be successful if a supervisor has confidence in us. Fourth, physiological states such as anxiety, stress, and arousal can influence self-efficacy beliefs.

Communities of practice theory

As a third theoretical perspective on workplace learning and teaching, we discuss Lave and Wenger's work on CoP and legitimate peripheral participation. It is a prime example of the sociocultural theorising that is finding its way into medical education (Lave and Wenger, 1991; Swanwick, 2005; Wenger, 1998). In essence, Lave and Wenger conceptualised learning as 'an integral and inseparable aspect of social practice' (Lave and Wenger, 1991). It is valuable for understanding learning and teaching in the workplace because it offers a lens through which the development of relative newcomers (e.g. medical students and interns) within an existing group of practitioners (e.g. medical wards or departments) can be analysed. Central to this socio-cultural view on learning is the concept of 'participation'. According to Lave and Wenger, participation is the key to understanding how learners develop within a community. Questions such as what opportunities do learners get or create to participate, with whom do they participate and on what tasks, and what do they take out of their participation are crucial in this view on learning. Lave and Wenger's work specifically focused on the relation between novices and experts in CoP. A CoP is a 'set of relations among persons, activity, and world, over time' that is the result of collective learning in the 'pursuit of a shared enterprise' (Lave and Wenger, 1991; Wenger, 1998). Because newcomers participate alongside more experienced community members, this stimulates an exchange of knowledge and a negotiation of meaning between members, resulting in the ongoing reproduction of a CoP. After studying a number of apprenticeship situations, from tailors in West Africa to the US. Navy quartermasters, Lave and Wenger proposed legitimate peripheral participation as a descriptor of how practices are made accessible to newcomers (Lave and Wenger, 1991). Initially, newcomers are introduced into a CoP by allowing them to observe, for example,

in an operating theatre or outpatient clinic. This is followed by allowing them to participate in low-risk tasks (such as a physical examination) or by letting them perform tasks under close supervision. What counts as a low-risk or simple task will depend on the expertise of the newcomer and supervisor. This type of introduction into a CoP can be described as peripheral participation. It has to be accompanied by enough legitimacy to really engage newcomers. The newcomer has to feel that he or she is allowed to be there. If, for whatever reason, a CoP does not open up, then 'inevitable stumblings and violations' become a 'cause for dismissal, neglect, or exclusion' rather than opportunities to learn (Wenger, 1998). Through their participation in a CoP, newcomers will develop along personal trajectories towards the kind of full participation that is characteristic of experts. Research on learning in the operating theatre and on trainees' participation in internships suggests that situated learning theories, and the specific focus of legitimate peripheral participation on the development of newcomers, can be valuable for understanding medical workplace learning (Deketelaere et al, 2006; Lyon, 2004; Sheehan et al, 2005).

We have discussed three theoretical perspectives particularly relevant to workplace learning. However, as stated before, there are many educational perspectives that can be applied to workplace learning and teaching in medical education. Moreover, theories from the social sciences, ranging from social psychology to transition psychology and medical sociology, may also help us to understand aspects of learning and teaching in the workplace as well. We now provide a framework to break down workplace learning into three constituent parts: 'tasks', 'contexts', and 'learners'. These three interrelated parts are common, in varying compositions, to different perspectives on workplace learning and can help identify differences between them. The next section analyses the constituent parts of workplace learning and the ways they interact in finer detail.

Constituent parts of workplace learning

Tasks

Workplace learning can be analysed by understanding three components and their interactions. The first of these parts is 'tasks'. Medical students, residents, specialists, general practitioners, and other health care workers have different but complementary responsibilities whilst sharing the common purposes of providing a high standard of care, being cost-effective, and educating themselves and others. The participation of learners in a medical workplace is mainly dictated by the demands of patient care. Understanding the importance of what tasks people participate in and how the sequencing of tasks affects different individuals and groups is crucial to workplace learning. It then becomes possible to look at the way in which teams share tasks and different individuals within them interpret tasks, as this will eventually influence their learning (Eraut, 2004; Teunissen et al, 2009). Consider, for example, the endoscopic removal of a gallbladder. The surgeon-in-training is concerned about the anatomy of the abdomen and the steps needed to remove the gallbladder. The operating nurse focuses on the same steps but with a different aim than the surgeon. The anaesthetist has different concerns again. As each of them repeats different tasks with different colleagues and different patients over time, they follow paths that are both different from and linked with that of others. A practical implication of this is that a teacher may expect a certain task to lead to a particular set of learning outcomes, but it should not be assumed that everyone will learn, or would even wish to learn the same things from the same activities.

Contexts

The second component of workplace learning is context. The circumstances in which a task is undertaken are divided here into a physical and a social context.

Physical context

The term physical context refers to the physical setting in which a task occurs as well as the artefacts used to perform the task. Outpatient clinics, operating theatres, wards, and general practitioners' surgeries are just some settings whose differences influence learning in important ways. Research on expertise has shown that people incorporate contextual information in the concepts and mental models they develop (Hatala et al, 1999). This kind of information can help them recognise the symptoms and signs of certain diseases. The differential diagnosis for a patient in Western Europe with a high fever will be different if he or she has been to a region where malaria and dengue are endemic. Physical context

can hinder learning as well. Irrelevant contextual information can lead to wrong judgements (Teunissen et al, 2009) and differences in physical context can act as barriers to the transfer of learning between contexts (Hamstra et al, 2006). For example, it is most likely that what are learnt in an operating theatre are psychomotor skills and decision making, whereas what are learnt in an outpatient clinic are most likely to be diagnostic and management skills. General practice will most likely provide opportunities to learn about interventions that have longer-term outcomes or that affect people other than the patient. While any of these types of learning can occur in any context, it is important to recognise that some contexts are more likely to provide some types of learning opportunities than others.

Physical context can also influence the dynamics of learning environments. Consider, for example, the arrangement of chairs during morning rounds. Do doctors and medical students sit around the same table or are the doctors on the front row and medical students at the back? Another example is the availability of suitable medical equipment. A monitor on which students can see what the specialist is seeing makes a crucial difference to what they can learn from the laryngoscopic examination of the vocal cords and glottis. Such differences in the physical context give strong messages about the roles and value learners have in a group: whether they are to participate in discussions or just to watch and listen (Tan, 2009). So, physical context shapes learning (Lave and Wenger, 1991).

Social context

Just as physical factors shape learning, so do the people involved in a task and the social meaning system of which they are part. Doctors, nurses, secretaries, and cleaners, each with their own responsibilities and expertise, share the common goal of providing high-quality patient care. As stated earlier, such a group is called a 'community of practice' (Wenger, 1998). As gatekeepers of a practice, these co-workers determine the tasks learners can learn from. Everyone involved in a task is a potential learner and anyone can be a gatekeeper. The ways in which co-workers interact can facilitate or inhibit the learning of all parties. Whilst a medical student is the person who is present explicitly as a learner, a clinical supervisor or others who are present may learn vicariously from the same encounter. Significant learning opportunities are lost when senior staff monopolise interesting tasks and relegate juniors to menial ones. Simple, inclusive actions can have profound impacts on the learning opportunities tasks offer: for example, 'You see this patient first and I'll see her with you later' versus 'Come watch me see this patient'; or even 'I've seen this patient, can you please arrange the following tests (but I'm not telling you why they need to be done)'. Moreover, giving learners an opportunity to engage with different tasks and different members of a community of practice will stimulate their engagement and motivation. Furthermore, a 'queue of learners' can also influence opportunities – a senior doctor may give higher priority to the learning needs of the senior trainee than to a medical student or nurse.

A second feature of the social context is the way people working with (or around) each other recognise each other's role and input, develop customs and traditions, and share a common meaning system. Workers function better when they understand how others like to function and vice versa. For instance, newcomers learn how their seniors use jargon and abbreviations. By reciprocating the same jargon and abbreviations a trainee may strengthen the relationship with the senior colleague but alienate and worsen their relationship with more junior colleagues. This can also apply to role modelling – if a trainee imitates the behaviours of a senior colleague, the opportunities to learn from that colleague may be strengthened. If the behaviours being imitated, however, are negative or harmful, this strengthening of opportunities may be at the cost of good patient care. From those examples, it is easy to see how the social context can perpetuate desirable, or undesirable, behaviours through feedback loops; such influences may often not be made explicit. Likewise, a supervisor needs to be aware that seeing junior staff imitate their behaviour is not necessarily an endorsement that the behaviours are appropriate. Such positive or negative role modelling is a powerful influence on learning. We are well attuned to picking up subtle cues from others around us – hearing or reading how something should be achieved can easily be overpowered by seeing someone in authority, or who is perceived as expert, do something else. This may lead to tensions, but also powerful learning opportunities, that can often be capitalised on by good debriefing – either formally with a mentor or, not uncommonly, with co-workers in informal settings.

Thirdly, co-workers can directly affect the learning outcomes of tasks (Teunissen et al, 2007). In a setting where a clinical teacher tries to educate a resident or medical student, he or she does this by highlighting specific aspects of a task at hand, giving instructions, and feeding back on a learner's performance (Irby, 1994). In doing so, the teacher shapes which aspects of the task and the learner's behaviour are subjected to reflection and lead to permanent changes in the way the learner will think or act (Hattie and Timperley, 2007).

Learners

The third and final component of workplace learning is the actual learner. Within a community of practice, every member of the community is a potential learner. Conceptually, individual learners are part of the social system of a workplace, but they deserve to be discussed as individuals with unique characteristics and ways of doing things that shape their contribution to patient care and their role in a community of practice. Understanding some of the ways individuals differ is necessary if we are to understand workplace learning. Furthermore, the outcomes of learning and the decisions they inform apply to individuals, as much as they apply to the social systems in which they operate.

The outcomes of workplace learning depend not just on the experiences and prior knowledge learners bring, but importantly on how they use their experiences and knowledge to interpret tasks. Main influences on the interpretation of tasks are a learner's:

- frame of reference
- role as active participant, not just an interpreter of events
- emotions and physical states

Frame of reference

There is a wide range of learners in workplace settings: from medical students to trained professionals engaging in continuous professional development. In what way do those individuals differ? The literature on clinical reasoning provides part of the answer. Clinical reasoning focuses on 'the processes doctors use to arrive at an initial diagnosis based on history and physical examination' (Norman, 2005). Clinical reasoning is usually researched by conducting experiments that incorporate individuals with different amounts of experience. As Mylopoulos and Woods state, 'the underlying assumption is that experts and novices differ in terms of the cognitive mechanisms that organise their knowledge and affect their decisions' (Mylopoulos and Woods, 2009). The notion that each learner brings a unique set of capabilities to a situation that allows him or her to think, interact, and perform is called personal knowledge by Eraut (1994). To optimise workplace learning, understanding a person's past experiences and current frames of reference help set attainable educational goals (Sandars, 2005).

Social psychology research conducted in the medical domain has shown that individuals' personal knowledge is used selectively to interpret tasks. Depending on the situation, certain categories of personal knowledge or certain concepts are more salient than others and can potentially influence interpretations, learning, and subsequent behaviours. Teunissen et al (2009) investigated this by using a research technique from social psychology called 'priming'. A priming effect occurs when a mental concept activated in one situation is preferentially applied in another, unrelated, situation, because its accessibility has been enhanced through that activation. Teunissen et al asked obstetric gynaecologic residents to participate in a number of ostensibly unrelated tasks. One of the experiments concerned residents' patient management decisions. A total of 50 residents with different levels of experience were randomised to two groups and asked to participate in word tasks. This consisted of several items, each presenting a set of words. Participants were instructed to underline the words that would make a correct sentence. In one experimental condition, these 'priming' sentences conveyed action (e.g. 'we deal with it'), and in the other they conveyed holding off (e.g. 'it won't be removed'). Subsequently, all residents were presented a paper case of a 37-year-old woman with menorrhagia (heavy menstrual bleeding) and asked to decide between a strategy of watchful waiting or hysterectomy. Being primed to act or hold off yielded significantly different responses in the decisions of year one and year two residents. The decisions of year three and year four residents showed a similar but less marked tendency. In neither experiment was an effect of priming found on residents in the final years of specialist training. Teunissen et al concluded from their experiments that, without residents being aware, context (such as an immediate prior experience unrelated to the case now at hand) influenced residents' constructions of a work-related situation by activating mental concepts, which in turn affected how residents experienced situations. The strength of the effect in their specific example varied with residents' levels of experience, indicating the importance of a person's prior experience. The results show how aspects of an individual's frame of reference can, even unconsciously, influence interpretations, learning, and behaviour. It again highlights the interplay between tasks, individuals' frame of reference, and the physical and social context in which the task takes place.

Learners as active participants

Individuals are not just interpreters of tasks; they are also active participants who contribute to the way tasks evolve (Sheehan et al, 2005). Learners come to workplaces with certain goals and intentions in mind, which may or may not be in line with formal learning goals laid down in a curriculum. Understanding the behaviour of learners and seeing how their behaviour creates or inhibits learning opportunities and leads to learning outcomes allows teachers to guide their development by discussing and attuning goals and organising tasks in such a way that learners actually meet those goals. The work of Bandura on social cognitive theory provides a helpful perspective in understanding learners' personal agency where notions of intentionality and forethought explain learners' motivations to pursue hard-to-reach learning goals. For instance, medical students have to complete a range of clinical rotations in areas they will never practise in. They nevertheless know that, to reach their goal (i.e. graduate as a medical doctor), they will have to pass all rotations. Motivating students is a challenge that requires at least some knowledge of the goals and intentions individuals bring with them to a workplace. It means that clinical teachers need to know what tasks their practice offers and how those tasks can serve individuals with different learning goals. Understanding that a learner's behaviour is partly the result of intentions and anticipated outcomes can also serve as a basis for reflection.

Emotions and physical states

Emotions pervade our lives and are therefore always part of learners' interpretations (Illeris, 2002). They can stem from a good (or bad) working relationship within a health care team or from the emotions inherently coupled to life events such as birth, sickness, and death. According to Illeris, besides being a social and cognitive process, 'all learning is simultaneously an emotional process [...], that is, a process involving psychological energy, transmitted by feelings, emotions, attitudes, and motivations which mobilise and, at the same time, are conditions that may be influenced and developed through learning' (Illeris,

2002). A supervisor who always makes a learner feel nervous or rushed will not encourage learning as well as one who creates an environment where questions are encouraged and positively reinforced. Moreover, there is strong evidence from laboratory studies that sleep deprivation impairs mood, cognitive, and motor performance (Pilcher and Huffcutt, 1996). The impact that learners' physical states might have on their performance and learning is also demonstrated in research on self-efficacy. All these notions illustrate the importance of creating safe learning climates in order to encourage learning (Boor et al, 2008).

Going back to the range of learners within workplace settings, it is clear that the learning outcomes for a medical student in an outpatient clinic are very different from the medical specialist whom he or she is shadowing. The medical student has a different frame of reference with regard to clinical conditions compared to the specialist. Moreover, when working up a patient, students may be more concerned with how their performance will be assessed, guiding their (proactive) behaviours accordingly, whereas the specialist is concerned with treating the patient. And the fact that students are assessed by the specialist creates a power difference leading to emotions that can influence behaviour and learning.

Tying the three factors together; optimising learning in the workplace

We have discussed tasks, the physical and social contexts in which tasks are performed, and characteristics of the learner to explain the dynamic interplay that gives rise to workplace learning outcomes. Those factors are distinct but also highly interdependent. As a consequence, efforts to promote workplace learning can be directed to a variety of starting points, any of which may act to encourage active participation of the learner.

Intersubjectivity

Participation has beneficial consequences for individuals in that it facilitates effective learning, positive working relationships, and effective work performance. A key outcome of individuals working and communicating together effectively is the development of intersubjectivity. This means all members of a health care team understand each other's preferences and idiosyncrasies so that they can work together without the need for constant interpersonal negotiations, which can be reserved for dealing with novel tasks or problems. Intersubjectivity doesn't just happen and the behaviours that promote it are learnable. A person joining a team for the first time will not automatically know the preferences of other team members and misinterpretation of these preferences can alienate that person from the learning environment. This alienation can occur for experienced practitioners joining a new team but is even more probable for novice practitioners – not only does the novice have more to learn in general but also he or she must learn the skills required to detect the preferences of other team members. Add to this high levels of anxiety and it can be seen that there can be a potent mix of factors to inhibit good learning (Sheehan et al, 2005). One of the defining characteristics, or markers, of ineffective workplace learning is lack of participation. This is where a learner seems passive, unwilling to learn or just does what he or she is told (Wilkinson and Harris, 2002). One could be tempted to conclude that the problem lies solely with the learner but the previous sections have highlighted the importance of the context and task. Some contexts invite more participation than others. Research into this area has highlighted the crucial importance of the supervisor–learner relationship in enabling the acceptance of a learner and allowing the learner to participate fully in a team. This is an example of the impact of social context on individual learners; the clinical supervisor or a mentor can help a learner navigate his or her way through the initiation stages of joining a functioning team.

Promoting participation

Health care teams are naturally motivated to have as their highest priority the provision of high-quality care to their patients. Sometimes this can be at the expense of paying attention to relationships within the team. Intersubjectivity can arise in teams that have been working together for some time – but even for such teams, tensions can remain whereby some members work around others, avoid each other or undermine each other's decisions. Intersubjectivity requires those tensions and differences to be made explicit. A new team member will experience them to an even greater degree and any lack of resolution can impact adversely on learning, particularly if that new team member is a novice. One solution to this is to pay attention not only to patient care but also to team tasks; sports teams do not just focus on the task (playing the game), but also on team functioning (practice). Similarly, in clinical settings, learning does not just arise from the task, but also from the team's effective functioning.

Learners in health settings are active peripheral participants needing to integrate into a social learning environment. This integration requires actions on the part of both the learner and supervisor because neither alone can effect the transition. A reticent or unconfident learner, however, may not attract enough attention from a busy supervisor. Likewise, a supervisor who is busy or who seems aloof may make a learner feel that he or she is not allowed to seek attention. In such cases, bringing the learner into the social learning environment is more challenging and requires actions on the part of both learner and supervisor. Often this occurs in an iterative fashion – if either the learner or supervisor makes a move to show interest, the other party is more likely to reciprocate. For example, if the learner shows interest and asks pertinent questions, the supervisor will start to engage with the learner. Once the learner sees this engagement, he or she will

be more likely to make more enquiries. Alternatively, it could be the supervisor who makes the first move and, provided the learner reciprocates, the supervisor will be more likely to engage further. These tentative initial steps can then build on each other in a self-reinforcing cycle. Before long, conversations begin and dialogues ensue. It is through conversing, and 'thinking aloud', that learners come to understand the supervisor's idiosyncrasies and improve their clinical reasoning. It is the dialogue, the language, and the behaviours that give the experience meaning for the learner. Discussion and joint problem-solving, debate over decisions, and consideration of options are all important activities that promote participation and learning. The place of conversations around patient care, such as over morning coffee, and between all members of a team should not be underestimated as a medium for their engagement in the reciprocal process of workplace participation.

Sheehan, Wilkinson, and Billett used individual interviews and a focus group to gather data about interns' experiences in clinical rotations within a New Zealand hospital setting. Based on their data, they drafted a model (Figure 12.1) for participation

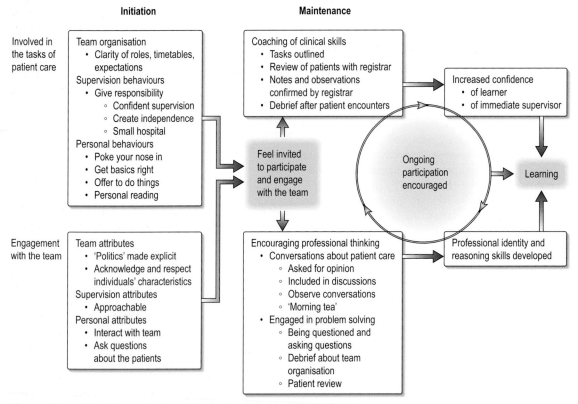

Figure 12.1 • Model for optimal participation in clinical settings.

in clinical settings that identifies two critical components: the tasks of patient care and engagement with the clinical team. Those two components are further divided into two aspects: initiation and maintenance. A reinforcing cycle of activities that promote and encourage effective participation and learning results from all four factors working well.

Initiation

As the Sheehan et al model also shows, one of the first steps to promote a positive learning environment is to get off to a good start by providing an effective initiation or orientation. A workplace is so familiar to supervisors that it is easy to forget it is new and foreign to most learners. Furthermore, each supervisor will have idiosyncrasies – these can be discovered by trial and error or, preferably, by discussions soon after a learner arrives into a new context. Sometimes orientation relates only to the physical environment, or to employment matters; however, to foster effective learning, it also needs to promote an early, effective supervisor–learner relationship. In practical terms, newly arrived trainees need to be provided with practical information on timetables, specific aspects of patient care related to the setting, clarification of the roles of the trainees, and a clear description of others' expectations of their performance on the attachment. The idiosyncrasies of other team members should be made explicit. In turn, trainees are expected to be enquiring but also to show initiative by reading around problems. Once this initiation phase has been satisfactorily completed, the maintenance phase can then occur, where ongoing review and feedback relating to patient care take place alongside activities to promote and encourage interactions within the team. Attention should be paid not only to the performance of trainees in relation to patient care but also to making time for interaction between team members, thus highlighting the significance of co-participation in workplace learning.

Team interactions

The importance of interactions between team members in promoting learning is well recognised. Richards, when discussing learning from physician colleagues, observed that self-directed, workplace learning involved more interactions with colleagues than did formal learning (Richards, 1986). Jennett

et al (1988) tested the effectiveness of a range of teaching methods in continuing medical education and found that those involved in small group discussions with peers learnt significantly better. Modelling by a respected peer has a positive effect (Stross et al, 1983). Studies in occupational therapy show that debriefing with peers in fieldwork practice helps learners appraise themselves and discuss confusing issues (Mackenzie, 2002). Studies in nursing reveal that similar practices boost confidence to apply knowledge and skills (Davies, 1995). These studies all provide evidence that interactions with peers or more experienced counterparts combine with everyday practice to promote learning on the job.

A communication hierarchy, which can arise if there are too many people in a team, can be a barrier to engagement; for example, when a medical student's learning needs have to take lower priority than the learning needs of more senior staff. Despite this, a learner's passive observation still has a place. Observing the practice of others or listening to other team members puzzling over a problem can be a valuable learning experience, provided the learners still feel entitled to be present as Lave and Wenger's 'legitimate peripheral participants' (Lave and Wenger, 1991). This learning opportunity can be capitalised on further by discussing the role of the novice student in advance and agreeing a limited set of topics for debriefing afterwards. For students, this turns a passive meeting into an active learning opportunity (Irby and Wilkerson, 2008).

Effective feedback

Drawing upon apprenticeship learning, Collins and Newman devised a model of learning for reading, writing, and mathematics that they termed cognitive apprenticeship (Collins et al, 1989). According to their model, the expert (a teacher) modelled, coached, and scaffolded the learner before withdrawing support incrementally until the learner could achieve independent performance. This approach is clearly analogous to practices proven to be successful in medicine and gives a central role to effective feedback in guiding learners' development. Ende stresses that formative feedback is a tool to keep learners on course and involved and suggests that, without it, 'the sense of being adrift in a strange environment is amplified' (Ende, 1983). Irby emphasises that such feedback requires interactive thinking and improvisation by supervisors because they must simultaneously identify a patient's problems and their learners' levels of understanding. He notes that excellent teachers 'incorporate the whole team in discussion' (Irby, 1992). Able clinicians and teachers can also include the patient as part of this whole team.

Several reviews and meta-analyses show that providing learners with effective feedback is difficult. Up to 38% of studies of the effect of feedback show negative effects on performance (Kluger and DeNisi, 1996). Hattie and Timperley (2007) published a synthesis of 12 meta-analyses (consisting of 196 studies and 6972 effect sizes) on the effectiveness of feedback. Their synthesis shows that feedback can only build on previous experience. So if a task is new to a learner, instructions will be more important than letting them try and then giving feedback on what went right and wrong. When giving feedback, both learners and teachers should bear in mind that the verbal and non-verbal information contained within feedback can be targeted at different levels with different results. In general, effective feedback is directed at tasks or parts of tasks and not at the person performing the task. For example, giving feedback to a resident who has just finished doing rounds should focus on concrete examples of what the resident did. Such feedback can often be preceded by asking the resident to explain to the supervisor the considerations that were weighed up before deciding on a plan of action. Understanding the reasoning behind decisions helps with the coaching of clinical reasoning. When there seems to be a recurrent problem with running late on rounds, the teacher can also focus on what it takes to strike a balance between paying attention to individual patients and being fair to the whole group of patients. Such comments give the resident insight in what went well and what can be improved. On the other hand, either positive or negative general comments such as 'You're good in doing rounds' or 'You're too slow, you should speed up your rounds' is ineffective as feedback (Hattie and Timperley, 2007). Such comments do not provide any clues as to what to keep doing or what actions should be changed. So, effective feedback provides timely, concrete suggestions on what to keep doing and on what to change. It helps learners to see where they are going, how they are getting on, and where they want to aim for next.

Formative feedback paired with reflection is even more powerful as this allows the assimilation and reordering of concepts and a consideration of meaning. The exploration of the meaning and implications of experiences and action in the hands of the skilled facilitator keeps discussions on higher levels, avoiding the repetition of mundane facts and more importantly growing team understanding and cohesion (Branch and Paranjape, 2002). The skills involved in these tasks should not be underestimated and have important implications for faculty development. A good doctor is not automatically a good teacher or provider of feedback. Likewise, reflection may not occur automatically for new practitioners. While reflection can be a self-directed, private activity, it is also a cognitive process that can be modelled and promoted by supervisors and mentors.

Conclusion

This chapter has discussed clinical workplaces as learning and teaching environments. Essentially, all workplaces present those working in them, from seasoned professionals to those who have just entered them, with an overwhelming range of learning opportunities. The nature of a particular workplace will influence learning objectives, processes, and outcomes; large parts of what workers learn will be overt and not marked as learning. Because of workplaces' unique abilities to offer learners opportunities to learn in a context very similar to the one in which they will ultimately function, medical training will always be partly situated in the clinical workplace. There are some specific features of clinical workplaces that set them apart from in-school medical education; learning in health care workplaces requires the negotiation of a three-way teacher–learner–patient relationship and, because the clinical workplace's main purpose is patient care, educational processes and outcomes are harder to control.

The features of learning and teaching in clinical workplaces make this a research area that can be analysed through many different theoretical lenses. This book offers numerous perspectives relevant to workplace learning and this chapter has discussed in more detail 'concepts around informal learning', 'social cognitive theory' including self-efficacy as a driver of learners' proactive behaviour in workplaces and ultimately their learning, and 'communities of practice theory', including legitimate peripheral participation as a descriptor of learners' participation. To put different theoretical angles into perspectives and allow readers to analyse any workplace, workplace learning has been broken down into three constituent parts: 'tasks', 'contexts', and 'learners'. Understanding the importance of what tasks people participate in is crucial to workplace learning. After doing so, it becomes possible to look at the way in which teams share tasks and different individuals within them interpret tasks. The social and physical context in which tasks are performed is an often overlooked but crucial component of understanding workplace learning and teaching. Finally, there are individual influences on the interpretation of tasks, such as a learner's frame of reference, his role as an active participant in a community, and his emotions and physical states.

Implications for practice

First and foremost, in letting learners participate in health care teams it is crucial that patients' needs are attended to. Understanding some of the workings of workplaces allows for an attempt to optimise workplaces as educational environments. This chapter discussed the importance of creating intersubjectivity, where learners are part of a team whose members understand each other's preferences and idiosyncrasies so that working together can occur without the need for constant interpersonal negotiations. If done properly, this will stimulate meaningful learning, some of which will be overt. Aspects of workplace learning and teaching may benefit from making more explicit what is being done and why. In doing so, understanding a person's past experiences and current frame of reference will help in optimising workplace learning. Overall, the opportunities for engagement afforded to learners and the way in which they choose to participate will influence the quality of a workplace as a learning environment. In the current landscape of medical education where teaching hospitals need to balance the training of a large number of future health professionals with providing cost-effective health care, more research on what opportunities lead to what kind of learning outcomes would be particularly valuable.

High-quality workplace education can be achieved through meaningful participation, which in turn requires learners to be initiated with care within a workplace and its community of practitioners. In practical terms, newly arrived trainees should be provided with practical information, clarification of their roles as trainees, and a clear description of what is expected of them. When the initiation phase is over, ongoing learning opportunities and engagement with different members of a community of practice will stimulate ongoing engagement, commitment, and motivation. These processes relate strongly to the confidence trainees need to develop in their capabilities; tackling challenging tasks will be easier when learners feel appropriately supported in doing so. Making space for informal dialogues, including learners within the team, and promoting effective (not simply positive) feedback, will stimulate team interaction and add to the learning potential of workplaces. Ultimately, workplace learning boils down to people showing a genuine interest in each other, their development as practitioners, and their patients.

References

Bandura A: Self-efficacy. In Ramachaudran VS, editor: *Encyclopedia of human behavior*, vol 4, New York, 1994, Academic Press, pp 71–81.

Bandura A: *Self-efficacy. The exercise of control*, New York, 1997, W.H. Freeman and Company.

Bandura A: Social cognitive theory: an agentic perspective, *Annu Rev Psychol* 52:1–26, 2001.

Bandura A: Guide for constructing self-efficacy scales. In Urdan T, Pajares F, editors: *Self-efficacy beliefs of adolescents*, Greenwich, CT, 2005, Information Age Publishing, pp 307–337.

Billett S: Learning in the workplace: reappraisals and reconceptions. In Hayward G, James S, editors: *Skills, knowledge and organisational performance*, Bristol, 2004a, Policy Press, pp 149–170.

Billett S: Workplace participatory practices: conceptualising workplaces as learning environments, *J Workplace Learn* 16(6):312–324, 2004b.

Billett S: Constituting the workplace curriculum, *J Curricul Stud* 38:31–48, 2006.

Bleakley A: Broadening conceptions of learning in medical education: the message from teamworking, *Med Educ* 40(2):150–157, 2006.

Boor K, Scheele F, van der Vleuten CP, et al: How undergraduate clinical learning climates differ: a multi-method case study, *Med Educ* 42 (10):1029–1036, 2008.

Branch WT, Jr., Paranjape A: Feedback and reflection: teaching methods for clinical settings, *Acad Med* 77 (12):1185–1188, 2002.

Cheetham G, Chivers G: *Professions, competence and informal learning*, Cheltenham, UK, 2005, Edward Elgar.

Collins A, Brown JS, Newman SE: Cognitive apprenticeship: teaching the crafts of reading, writing and mathematics. In Resnick LB, editor: *Knowledge, learning and instruction*, essays in honor of Robert Glaser, Hillsdale, NJ, 1989, Erlbaum & Associates, pp 453–494.

Davies E: Reflective practice: a focus for caring, *J Nurs Educ* 34(4):167–174, 1995.

Deketelaere A, Kelchtermans G, Struyf E, et al: Disentangling clinical learning experiences: an exploratory study on the dynamic tensions in internship, *Med Educ* 40(9):908–915, 2006.

Dornan TL, Boshuizen HP, King N, et al: Experience-based learning: a model linking the processes and outcomes of medical students' workplace learning, *Med Educ* 41 (1):84–91, 2007.

Dornan TL, Boshuizen HP, Gick R, et al: *A review of the evidence linking conditions, processes and outcomes of clinical workplace learning. BEME Collaboration*, 2009, Available at: http://www.bemecollaboration.org/beme/files/reviews%20in%20progress%20docs/Dornan%20Protocol.pdf. Accessed September 2009.

Ende J: Feedback in clinical medical education, *JAMA* 250(6):777–781, 1983.

Eraut M: *Developing professional knowledge and competence*, London, 1994, RoutledgeFalmer.

Eraut M: Informal learning in the workplace, *Stud Conti Educ* 26 (2):247–273, 2004.

Eraut M, Alderton J, Cole G, et al: The development of knowledge and skills at work. In Coffield F, editor: *Differing visions of a learning society*, vol I, Bristol, 2000, Policy Press, pp 231–262.

Eva KW, Regehr G: Knowing when to look it up: a new conception of self-assessment ability, *Acad Med* 82(10): S81–S84, 2007.

Fuller A, Unwin L: Learning as apprentices: creating and managing expansive learning environments, *J Educ Work* 16(4):407–426, 2003.

Hamstra SJ, Dubrowski A, Backstein D: Teaching technical skills to surgical residents: a survey of empirical research, *Clin Orthop Relat Res* 449:108–115, 2006.

Hatala RA, Norman GR, Brooks LR: Influence of a single example on subsequent electrocardiogram interpretation, *Teach Learn Med* 11 (2):110–117, 1999.

Hattie J, Timperley H: The power of feedback, *Rev Educ Res* 77 (1):81–112, 2007.

Illeris K: *The three dimensions of learning. Contemporary learning theory in the tension field between the cognitive, the emotional and the social*, Roskilde, Denmark, 2002, Roskilde University Press.

Irby DM: How attending physicians make instructional decisions when conducting teaching rounds, *Acad Med* 67(10):630–638, 1992.

Irby DM: What clinical teachers in medicine need to know, *Acad Med* 69 (5):333–342, 1994.

Irby DM, Wilkerson L: Teaching when time is limited, *BMJ* 336 (7640):384–387, 2008.

Jennett PA, Laxdal OE, Hayton RC, et al: The effects of continuing medical education on family doctor performance in office practice: a randomized control study, *Med Educ* 22(2):139–145, 1988.

Kluger AN, DeNisi A: The effects of feedback interventions on performance: historical review, a meta-analysis and a preliminary feedback intervention theory, *Psychol Bull* 119:254–284, 1996.

Lave J, Wenger E: *Situated learning: legitimate peripheral participation*, Cambridge, 1991, Cambridge University Press.

Lempp H, Seale C: The hidden curriculum in undergraduate medical education: qualitative study of medical students' perceptions of teaching, *BMJ* 329(7469):770–773, 2004.

Lyon PM: A model of teaching and learning in the operating theatre, *Med Educ* 38(12):1278–1287, 2004.

Mackenzie L: Briefing and debriefing of student fieldwork experiences: exploring concerns and reflecting on practice, *Aust Occup Ther J* 49 (2):82–92, 2002.

Mylopoulos M, Woods NN: Having our cake and eating it too: seeking the best of both worlds in expertise research, *Med Educ* 43(5):406–413, 2009.

Norman GR: Research in clinical reasoning: past history and current trends, *Med Educ* 39(4):418–427, 2005.

Pajares F: Current directions in self-efficacy research. In Maehr ML, Pintrich PR, editors: *Advances in motivation and achievement*, vol 10,

Greenwich, CT, 1997, JAI Press, pp 1–49.

Pilcher JJ, Huffcutt AI: Effects of sleep deprivation on performance: a meta-analysis, *Sleep* 19(4):318–326, 1996.

Polanyi M: *Personal knowledge: towards a post-critical philosophy*, Chicago, 1974, University Of Chicago Press.

Reber AS: *Implicit learning and tacit knowledge: an essay in the cognitive unconscious*, Oxford, 1993, Oxford University Press.

Remmen R: *An evaluation of clinical skills training at the medical school of the University of Antwerp*, Belgium, 1999, University of Antwerp.

Richards RK: Physicians' self-directed learning: a new perspective for continuing medical education III, *Phys Self-Dir Learn Proj Mobius* 6 (4):1–14, 1986.

Rogoff B: *Apprenticeship in thinking. Cognitive development in social context*, New York, 1990, Oxford University Press.

Rogoff B: Observing sociocultural activities on three planes: participatory appropriation, guided appropriation, and apprenticeship. In Wertsch JV, Del Rio P, Alvarez A, editors: *Sociocultural studies of mind*, Cambridge, 1995, Cambridge University Press, pp 139–164.

Sandars J: An activity theory perspective, *Work Based Learn Prim Care* 3 (3):191–201, 2005.

Sheehan D, Wilkinson TJ, Billett S: Interns' participation and learning in clinical environments in a New Zealand hospital, *Acad Med* 80 (3):302–308, 2005.

Slotnick HB: How doctors learn: physicians' self-directed learning episodes, *Acad Med* 74 (10):1106–1117, 1999.

Slotnick HB: How doctors learn: education and learning across the medical-school-to-practice trajectory, *Acad Med* 76 (10):1013–1026, 2001.

Stross JK, Hiss RG, Watts CM, et al: Continuing education in pulmonary disease for primary-care physicians, *Am Rev Respir Dis* 127(6):739–746, 1983.

Swanwick T: Informal learning in postgraduate medical education: from cognitivism to 'culturism', *Med Educ* 39(8):859–865, 2002.

Tan N: Learning in surgery: practice meets theory, *Clin Teacher* 6 (1):34–37, 2009.

Teunissen PW, Scheele F, Scherpbier AJJA, et al: How residents learn: qualitative evidence for the pivotal role of clinical activities, *Med Educ* 41(8):763–770, 2007.

Teunissen PW, Stapel DA, Scheele F, et al: The influence of context on residents' evaluations: effects of priming on clinical judgment and affect, *Adv Health Sci Educ Theory Pract* 14(1):23–41, 2009.

Wenger E: *Communities of practice: learning, meaning, and identity*, Cambridge, 1998, Cambridge University Press.

Wilkinson TJ, Harris P: The transition out of medical school – a qualitative study of descriptions of borderline trainee interns, *Med Educ* 36 (5):466–771, 2002.

Learning from practice: mentoring, feedback, and portfolios

13

Erik Driessen   Karlijn Overeem   Jan van Tartwijk

CHAPTER CONTENTS

ABC

Glossary

Coaching; see mentoring.

Competence An integrated body of knowledge, skills, and (professional) attitudes enabling proficient performance in certain real-life settings.

Mentoring (coaching or supervising) One-to-one learning activity with the goal of stimulating the learning and professional development of a learner.

Metacognition See main Glossary, p 341.

Multi-source feedback (also known as 360-degree feedback) A type of performance assessment that provides feedback on various tasks and behaviours from various reviewers. Ideally, it gathers information from people who are qualified and have credibility to judge clinical practice such as: (1) peers familiar with a similar domain of practice; (2) members of the health care team such as nurses, physicians assistants etc.; (3) patients as the recipients of health care.

Personal development plan A list of educational needs, development goals, and actions and processes, compiled by learners and used in systematic management and periodic reviews of learning.

Portfolio See main Glossary, p 341.

Reflection; reflective learning See main Glossary, p 342.

Supervising; see mentoring.

Outline

In this chapter, we focus on learning from practice in medical workplaces, for which self-directed assessment seeking and reflection are critical and a mentor

© 2011, Elsevier Inc.
DOI: 10.1016/B978-0-7020-3522-7.00013-9

is of great importance. First, we introduce two exemplar routines for learning from practice that mentors can use to stimulate self-directed assessment seeking and reflection. Next, we elaborate on strategies for providing feedback. Finally, we describe instruments that can be used for self-directed assessment seeking and reflection: multi-source feedback (MSF) and portfolios.

Introduction

Constructivist theories are dominant in the contemporary learning sciences and underlie many educational reforms. In constructivist theories, the view of *learning* is that people *construct* knowledge and understanding by interpreting information, processes, and experiences, building on what they already know (Bransford et al, 2000). This implies that what people consider "reality" is in fact their own construction of reality based on their personal knowledge. It is this personal reality that guides a person's actions and perceptions. Bransford and his colleagues emphasise that constructivism is a theory of knowing and *not* a theory of pedagogy (teaching). However, it does have major consequences for teaching. A logical extension of the view that new knowledge must be constructed from existing knowledge is that teachers need to pay attention to incomplete understandings, false beliefs, and naive renditions of concepts that learners may have about a given subject. Teachers then need to build on these ideas in ways that help each student achieve a more mature understanding. If students' initial ideas are ignored, the understandings they develop can be very different from those that the teacher intends (Bransford et al, 2000, p 10). This does not imply that teachers should never tell students anything directly (teaching by telling can be very effective in some situations) but Bransford and his colleagues emphasise the importance of helping people take control over their own learning. People must learn to recognise when they understand and when they need more information. They refer to people's abilities to predict their performances on various tasks and monitor their current level of mastery and understanding as *meta-cognition*. Teaching practices congruent with a meta-cognitive approach to learning include those that focus on self-assessment and reflection.

Self-assessment, which is considered in detail in Chapter 8, is widely propagated in the field of medical education as a tool for improvement. It is a self-regulatory proficiency that is powerful in selecting and interpreting information in ways that provide feedback (Hattie and Timperley, 2007). Generally, effective learners create internal feedback and cognitive routines while they are engaged in academic tasks. Less effective learners have minimal self-regulation strategies and they depend much more on external factors (such as the teacher or the task) for feedback. Learners with well-developed self-assessment skills can evaluate their levels of understanding, their effort and strategies used on tasks, their attributions and opinions of others about their performance, and their improvement in relation to their goals and expectation. Recent reviews, however, highlight that, for cognitive (information neglect and memory biases) and socio-biological reasons (doctors being adaptive to maintain an optimistic look on themselves), the adequacy of self-assessment as an individually conducted internal activity is limited (Davis, et al, 2006; Loftus, 2003). Eva and Regehr (2008) propose that learners make better use of external information about their performance by *self-directed assessment seeking*, which they describe as a process by which one takes personal responsibility for looking outward and explicitly seeking feedback and information from external sources of assessment data to direct performance improvements that can help validate one's self-assessment.

Reflection (see also Chapter 2) is a strategy which Eva and Regehr describe as "a conscious and deliberate reinvestment of mental energy aimed at exploring and elaborating one's understanding of the problem one has faced (or is facing) rather than aimed at simply trying to solve it" (Eva and Regehr, 2008, p 15). Hatton and Smith (1995) distinguish three types of reflection. The first type is concerned with the means to achieve certain ends. The second type is not only about means but also about goals, the assumptions upon which they are based, and the actual outcomes. The third type of reflection is referred to as *critical reflection*. Here, moral and ethical criteria are also taken into consideration. Judgements are made about whether professional activity is equitable, just, and respectful or not. Hatton and Smith emphasise that these three types of reflection should not be viewed as hierarchical. Different (educational) contexts and situations lend themselves more to one kind of reflection than to another. Other authors writing about reflection emphasise the impact of reflection on action. Among them Schön's work on reflection by professionals is undoubtedly the most influential (Schön, 1983). He distinguished between reflection-in-action and reflection-on-action. *Reflection-in-action* implies conscious thinking and modification during task performance. *Reflection-on-action* implies what we recently described as "letting future behaviour be guided by a systematic and critical analysis of past actions and their consequences" (Driessen et al, 2008, p 827). Most learners tend to find reflecting on their own learning difficult. For example, students arriving at university fresh from secondary education are not used to reflecting deliberately on their learning. Outside the domain of medical education, there is substantial evidence that it takes considerable effort for learners to learn to reflect on their actions or learning (Ertmer and Newby, 1996). Korthagen et al (2001) observed that some resistance was common when students were first introduced to reflective learning because their prior experiences were with education in which the *transfer* of knowledge was the goal. Thus, students' images and expectations of education tend not to be in keeping with learning from reflection.

Mentoring gives a push in the right direction by asking the right questions and thus focusing the learner's thinking processes. Mentors can also help learners with self-directed assessment seeking. Of course they can give feedback on performance themselves but they can also show learners where else to seek for information and how to present it. Finally, after self-directed assessment seeking and reflection, they can help learners identify and define learning goals. An effective mentor can have a positive influence on maximising the learner's performance and developing their talent (Jowett and Stead, 1994). A mentor needs to be good at providing constructive feedback, helping learners think about themselves by asking questions and confronting them with discrepancies, and creating a challenging but safe learning environment (Driessen et al, 2008).

In the next section, we introduce two examples of routines for learning from practice that mentors can use to stimulate self-directed assessment seeking and reflection.

Routines for learning from practice

Various routines for learning from practice have been proposed in previous publications (e.g. Kolb, 1984; Korthagen et al, 2001; NHS, 2001). All of them have

in common that they include experience and reflection, and most of them also include a phase of systematic evaluation. In this section we describe two of those routines: the National Health Service (NHS) appraisal routine and Korthagen's model for cyclic professional development. We use description of the latter to formulate suggestions for mentors aiming at stimulating their mentees' self-directed assessment seeking, reflection, and deliberate practice.

Appraisal

In 2001, the UK National Health Service (NHS, 2001) introduced an appraisal routine for consultants and general practitioners. This routine was defined as "a structured process of self-reflection". Appraisal sets out to enhance professional development and learning. It invites doctors (called "appraisees") to review their professional activities comprehensively and to identify areas of strength and need for development. The essence of appraisal is a confidential conversation, led by a trained appraiser (the term that is used for a mentor in appraisal procedures), supported by preparatory documentation such as a portfolio which is based on the General Medical Council's (GMC) components of good medical practice (General Medical Council, 2006). Since 2007, MSF tools (see later) have also been introduced to inform NHS consultant appraisal. The appraisal conversation should be followed by a period of reflection, after which the appraiser gives feedback. Then, an action plan is agreed, which the appraiser can use to steer development and learning (see Figure 13.1).

Early research findings have shown that the majority of appraisees feel encouraged and supported in their professional development by the appraisal process (Boylan et al, 2005). The most significant perceived benefit has been the opportunity to reflect on individual performance with a supportive colleague. There are, however, repeated concerns about time, confusion with revalidation, and worries about covering health and probity queries (Lewis et al, 2003). Reported changes in performance have included: being more reflective, updating medical bags, and improved record keeping. It is not yet clear whether appraisal truly meets expectations and leads to an improvement of patient care, not least because appropriate outcome measures are not yet available.

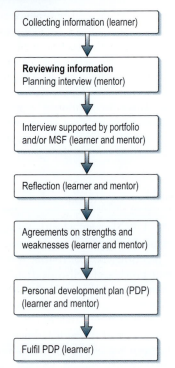

Figure 13.1 • Seven steps of appraisal (adapted from Conlon, 2003).

The ALACT model

Korthagen et al (2001) developed a model for cyclic professional development, aimed at stimulating reflection on experience. They refer to this model as the "ALACT model", named after the first letter of the five phases they distinguished, namely *Action, Looking back on action, Awareness of essential aspects, Creating alternative methods of action,* and *Trial* (Figure 13.2).

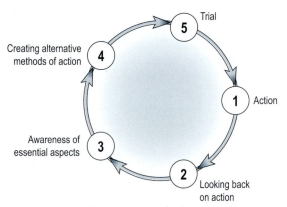

Figure 13.2 • The ALACT model (from Korthagen et al, 2001, with permission).

Action

The cycle starts with an action undertaken for a specific purpose (e.g. to develop a specific competence). Learners can be helped to improve their existing routines and, concurrently, acquire new ones by pre-selecting experiences from which they can learn, for example a mixture of patients who are more or less easy to diagnose.

Looking back on action: self-assessment seeking behaviour

The ALACT cycle then moves to the stage where learners look back on a previous action, usually when that action was not successful or something unexpected happened. This looking back on action is assumed to be accompanied by an evaluation of whether the goals were realised and the learner's part in this. In many cases this can be regarded as a form of self-assessment.

The role of mentors is to encourage learners to seek information about their performance from various sources. Information can come from external sources like assessments, practice guidelines, or formal feedback. Careful scrutiny of their own performance may be challenging for learners. Effective mentors have an important role in creating a safe environment by distinguishing between learners as individuals and their performance. If learners feel unsafe, they will be reluctant to acknowledge learning needs. Mentors need to help learners focus on descriptions of what happened and stimulate learners to be concrete. When learners give more general evaluations about a situation and their performance, mentors should ask questions such as, "What went well?", "What went wrong?", "How did you solve that?", and "What effect did it have?" Furthermore, it is important that the mentor stimulates learners to take a broader perspective than their own. To realise this, Korthagen et al propose questions for mentors such as:

• What did you want? What do you think the patient/your colleague/the nurse wanted?
• What did you think? What did the others think?
• What did you do? What did the others do?
• What emotions did you experience? What emotions did the other people involved experience?

Awareness of essential aspects: reflection

After conclusions have been drawn about the quality of performance and the characteristics of the situation, the next step in the ALACT model is to foster awareness of essential aspects. In this phase, learners try to develop a new and better *understanding* of what has happened: that is, they *reflect* on their performance. In this phase, a mentor is also essential to ensure that learners integrate external feedback into their self-concepts. The mentor can help the learner examine the data, see patterns, and identify cause–effect associations. Two strategies that are effective in making learners aware of essential aspects are confrontation and generalisation. A mentor can confront the learner with discrepancies between: self-assessment and external feedback; verbal and non-verbal expressions; how the learner sees himself and how the mentor sees the learner; and what the learner says he does and what he actually does. This confrontation can lead to an "Aha-moment", which is a catalyst for reflection. Communication strategies a mentor can use include statements such as:

- I read in your portfolio that you are happy with the result but, as we talk about it, your face tells a different story,
- You write here that this is what you want to achieve, but you are pleased with your results even though they do not match your goals,
- You do not actually do what you say you want to do.

Mentors can also help learners see general patterns. Because of their experience and a certain distance, it is easier for mentors to recognise patterns in the data. Learners are often too immersed in one situation to see similarities with other situations. Questions that help learners generalise across experiences are

- What similarities and differences do you recognise between what is happening now and what happened in other situations?
- When do those things happen?
- Do you recognise the feedback and do you see similarities with your self-assessment?
- Do you recognise a pattern?

The perspective of reflection can be on means, goals, or moral/ethical perspective (see earlier). The mentor can focus on the *means* a learner used to achieve a goal and try to understand why the strategy was successful or not. A mentor can ask questions like: "Which strategies did you consider?", "Why did you select this strategy?", "Which are the advantages and disadvantages of the strategy you used?", "Which part of your strategy was effective and which part was not effective?", "Why was it effective or not?", and

"Would this strategy have been more or less effective in a different situation?" The perspective can also be on whether the learner had selected a suitable *goal* for this particular situation, leading to questions such as: "What did you want to achieve?", "Were you successful?", "What do you consider successful?", "Why is this particular goal important?", and "Why did you pursue this goal?" Finally learners may consider what they want to achieve from a moral or ethical perspective. A mentor can stimulate moral or ethical reflection by asking questions like: "Do you think patients/patients' families/medical colleagues/nurses/administrators are satisfied with these outcomes?" "What are their primary interests?"

Creating or identifying alternative methods of actions

Reflection may trigger a search for alternative strategies or abandonment of original goals. It is important to explain (new) goals and alternative strategies. Reflection (awareness of essential aspects), stimulated by mentoring, is often not enough to induce behavioural change by itself. Barriers to change often comprise diverse personal, professional, and contextual factors. Goal setting, follow-up, and reminders are important strategies that can be used by mentors to motivate learners to improve their actual daily practice. The fact that people who are less oriented to goals and outcomes are less likely to take positive steps to change has been highlighted (Shute, 2008). Ericsson's research predicts that expertise will grow not just from the weight of experience but also from engaging in activities specifically designed or selected to improve performance (Ericsson, 2006).

The mentor has an important task here. Learners who work with a mentor set more specific goals and improve more than those who do not work with a mentor (Smither et al, 2003). A personal development plan (PDP), which records what was agreed between mentor and learner about what should be done differently and which goals should be achieved can be useful. This PDP can be on the agenda at the next meeting between mentor and learner, when what has already been achieved and what areas still need work can be discussed. A problem is that plans in PDPs are often too vague. It is therefore important that mentors stimulate learners to be concrete. To ensure future change in practice, mentors need to commit learners to: (1) identify the goals, (2) develop a SMART (Specific, Measurable,

Box 13.1

SMART criteria for learning plans

- Specific (straightforward, not ambiguous)
- Measurable (It is clear under which conditions the goals are achieved)
- Acceptable (The goals should be acceptable to all stakeholders)
- Realistic (The learner should be able to achieve the goals)
- Time-bound (It should be clear when the goal is to be achieved)

Acceptable, Realistic, and Time-bound) plan to achieve their goals (Box 13.1), (3) explore ways that can impede improvement, and (4) provide ways to overcome barriers.

Trial

The last step in the ALACT cycle is trialling, which starts a new cycle in the spiral of professional development. It is well known that, although adequate goals are set, feedback is not necessarily followed by change. Barriers such as lack of time and support, or even the perceptual belief of negative consequences of changed behaviour, can impede the implementation of change. If, as a mentor, you are convinced that goals are SMART, you should help learners to identify barriers that might stand in the way of improvement. Mentors and learners should also consider whether any additional resources are needed to overcome the barriers explored. Even when changes in practice are made, learners can relapse into old routines and improvements can decline because of lack of time, resources, and information. Reminders have been shown to be very effective in preventing relapse into old routines and decline of performance improvement. Reminders are meant to prevent busy, sometimes forgetful students or doctors from falling back into routines when their workloads are heavy. Mentors can organise such reminders, which do not need to be cumbersome; a 10-minute phone call asking how things are going at this moment can be effective.

Providing feedback

We have seen that feedback is essential for stimulating reflection. In this section, we highlight the goals of formative feedback and factors that are essential for it to exercise its full effects.

Goals of formative feedback

Before mentors can stimulate learners to reflect on and learn from their experiences, learners should have information about their performance with respect to those experiences. In other words, learners should receive feedback on their performance in particular situations. In general, formative feedback should address the accuracy of a learner's response to a problem or task and may touch on particular errors and misconceptions (Shute, 2008), the latter representing more specific or elaborated types of feedback. Formative feedback should also permit the comparison of actual performance with some established standard of performance. The main purpose of feedback is, therefore, to reduce the discrepancy between current and desired practices or understandings (Hattie and Timperley, 2007). In some cases, mentors will provide feedback before the phase of promoting reflection starts. In others, learners have already received the feedback from clinical supervisors or teachers.

Providing formative feedback

Several meta-analyses have found that feedback generally improves learning; however, there is wide variability in its effects and there are gaps in the literature, particular relating to how task characteristics, instructional contexts, and learner characteristics interact to mediate its effects. In other words, we simply do not know "what feedback works". Nevertheless, a recent review (Shute, 2008) has given some insights. In Table 13.1, we summarise some important conditions under which feedback is well known to improve learning and performance. In order for feedback to fulfil its purpose, three fundamental questions for the learner need to be addressed (Hattie and Timperley, 2007):

- Where am I going?
- How am I going?
- Where to next?

To address the first question, clearly defined goals should be available and learners should have clear understanding of desired practice or competence. Without goals, they are less likely to engage in properly directed action. The second question requires

Table 13.1 Formative feedback guidelines to enhance learning (things to do) (adapted from Shute, 2008)

Prescription	Description
Focus feedback on the task, not the learner	Feedback to the learner should address specific features of his or her work in relation to the task, with suggestions on how to improve
Provide elaborated feedback to enhance learning	Feedback should describe the what, how, and why of a given problem. This type of cognitive feedback is typically more effective than verification of results
Present elaborated feedback in manageable units	Provide elaborated feedback in small enough pieces that it is not overwhelming and discarded. Presenting too much information may not only result in superficial learning but also may invoke cognitive overload
Be specific and clear with the feedback message	If feedback is not specific or clear, it can impede learning and frustrate learners. If possible, try to link feedback clearly and specifically to goals and performance
Keep feedback as simple as possible (based on learner needs and instructional constraints)	Simple feedback is generally based on one cue. Keep feedback as simple and focused as possible. Generate only enough information to help students and not more
Reduce uncertainty between performance and goals	Formative feedback should clarify goals and seek to reduce or remove uncertainty in relation to how well learners are performing on a task and what needs to be accomplished to attain the goal(s)
Give unbiased, objective feedback	Feedback from a trustworthy source will be taken more seriously than other feedback, which may be disregarded
Promote a "learning" goal orientation via feedback	Formative feedback can be used to alter goal orientation – from a focus on performance to a focus on learning. This can be facilitated by crafting feedback, emphasising that effort yields increased learning and performance, and mistakes are an important part of the learning process

concrete information from an assessment of performance. It is essential that clearly defined indicators of whether a task has been completed are available. The final question informs the learner what actions need to be taken to close the gap between actual and desired performance. Therefore, an action plan is necessary, giving specific information about how to proceed.

How effectively feedback addresses the three questions for learners is dependent on what aspects of performance are addressed. There are four foci for feedback:

- About the task
- About the process of the task
- About self-regulation
- About the self as a person.

Feedback on a *task*, often called corrective feedback or knowledge of results, is the easiest type to give and consequently the most frequently given. It should concentrate on performance of a task rather than the knowledge required to perform it. Feedback that focuses on the *process* underlying a task encourages a deeper appreciation of performance. Such feedback is relevant to the detection and correction of error and helps learners develop a facility for self-feedback. Feedback that focuses on *self-regulation* addresses the interplay between commitment, control, and confidence. It addresses the way students monitor, direct, and regulate actions toward learning goals and implies a measure of autonomy, self-control, self-discipline, and self-direction. Learners' attributions of success and failure can have more impact than *actual* success or failure. In other words, feedback that does not explain the cause of poor performance or relate poor performance to identifiable circumstances is likely to engender personal uncertainties and decrease performance. It is essential that a supervisor directs feedback to observed performance, while being aware of the impact it has on the learner's self-efficacy, such that attention is directed back to the task, leading learners to invest more effort in it. Feelings of self-efficacy are important mediators in feedback situations. From their major review, Kluger and DeNisi (1996) concluded that feedback is effective to the extent to which it directs information to enhanced self-efficacy and to more effective self-regulation. Finally, feedback that focuses on the *person* of the learner usually does not have any educational value. It concentrates on the personal attributes of the learner and does not contain any task-related information, strategies to improve commitment to the task, or a better understanding of self or the task itself. This focus of feedback is usually not very effective. Rather, its impact can have an adverse effect on learners, particularly when negative feedback is at a personal level.

Emotional reactions to feedback

Published research shows that people are poor at self-assessment (Davis et al, 2006). Self-directed assessment seeking, which can for instance take the form of MSF (see later), may be more accurate. Studies have shown, however, that external feedback from peers and others that is inconsistent with self-perceptions may be discounted and not used to inform one's self-assessment. Learners who overrate themselves report more negative reactions to feedback and view it as inaccurate (Brett and Atwater, 2001). Negative (emotional) reactions to negative feedback, which may reflect transitory mood states, influence how learners use feedback. Mentors have an important role to play in this process. Emotion is one of the themes inherent within the processes of reconciling, assimilating, accepting, and using external feedback. It is important for mentors to acknowledge emotional reactions during the process of giving feedback (Sargeant et al, 2008).

Multi-source feedback

MSF, also known as 360-degree feedback, is a type of assessment that includes feedback on performance from various reviewers. It was originally developed for managers in the business sector in response to an increasing demand for managerial and professional performance in complex environments. MSF has

the potential to provide feedback on a broad range of competencies (particularly generic ones) from people who can observe performance directly. Generic competencies in the medical domain include: communication with patients; collaboration and communication with clinical colleagues; aspects of professionalism; and management. A strength of MSF, compared to a single assessment by one assessor, is that several assessments are aggregated, increasing the reliability of the rating. Moreover, observations are (at least ideally) based on a greater period of time than a single encounter, thus improving the validity of the assessment. When used effectively, MSF can generate structured feedback, which can facilitate the different steps of the reflective process. MSF is especially effective at informing learners about their performance (Step 2 of Korthagen's ALACT cycle) and making them aware of their strengths and weaknesses (Step 3).

MSF is being used on an increasingly large scale in medicine for both summative as well as formative purposes in undergraduate, postgraduate, and continuing education settings. Residency programmes in the United States and all Foundation Programmes in the United Kingdom use multi-source evaluations to assess their residents and fellows (ACGME, 2009; NHS, 2009). In the Netherlands and the United States, MSF is used to assess undergraduate students during their clerkships. In Canada, a programme has been developed to assess the performance of physicians routinely, with the primary purpose of improving the quality of medical practice. This programme also provides a way of identifying doctors for whom detailed assessment of practice performance or medical competence is needed (Hall et al, 1999).

Research on the impact of MSF on future clinical practice is still in its infancy and relies predominantly on doctors' self-reports of changes. A randomised controlled trial compared subsequent MSF ratings between one group of residents who received an MSF report and a control group who did not. The trial showed that nurse ratings increased for the MSF group compared to the group who did not receive MSF reports. The difference in change between ratings was statistically significant for communicating effectively with the patient and family (35%), timeliness of completing tasks (30%), and demonstrating responsibility and accountability (26%). Other researchers have shown that between 61% and 72% of doctors report a change in behaviour as a consequence of receiving MSF. For one-third of doctors, however, MSF does not seem to add any value.

Procedure

MSF systems vary in terms of: purposes, number of assessors, content of the questionnaires, frequency of evaluation; and mechanism for feeding back to learners. Ideally, MSF is used to gather information from qualified people, who have the credibility to judge clinical practice, such as (1) peers familiar with a similar domain of practice; (2) members of the health care team; and (3) patients as the recipients of health care. In this section we will refer to persons who give feedback as "raters".

With most MSF tools, learners complete a self-assessment questionnaire using the same items as the peer questionnaire. This allows a mentor to contrast the learner's self-assessment with collated external assessments and signal inconsistencies. Earlier, we wrote that mentors should do this in step 3 of the ALACT cycle: identifying essential aspects

(Korthagen et al, 2001). This exercise can be especially helpful for learners who lack insight into difficulties they are having, and learners who lack confidence and rate themselves less well than their colleagues.

Next, questionnaires are developed for the different categories of rater: for instance, patients, colleagues, and supervisors. Items are included relating to domains best observed by the group in question. For example, patient questionnaires include more items addressing communication, while co-workers' questionnaires mainly include items about collaboration (examples of questions are given in Box 13.2). In the example in the Box, completion of one questionnaire takes on average 5 minutes. A learner who is going to be assessed using MSF is usually sent a pack containing the rater questionnaires. In some systems, learners receive a password for a web-based system where they can select their raters. Raters are expected to return the completed forms or respond via a web-based system within a couple of weeks.

All ratings are aggregated and compiled in a feedback report that includes mean scores for each reviewer group on all the items, and also tables

---

Box 13.2

Examples of questionnaire items of multi-source feedback (available on www.par-program.org)

Patient Questionnaire

Based on ALL OF YOUR VISITS to your doctor's office, how do you feel about your doctor's attitude and behaviour towards you? My doctor:
(1 = strongly disagree, 2 = disagree, 3 = neutral, 4 = agree, 5 = strongly agree)

Spends enough time with me	1	2	3	4	5	Unable to assess
Shows interest in my problems	1	2	3	4	5	Unable to assess
Treats me with respect	1	2	3	4	5	Unable to assess
Talks with me about treatment plans	1	2	3	4	5	Unable to assess

Co-worker Questionnaire

Compared to the doctors I know, this one:
(1 = among the worst, 2 = bottom half, 3 = average, 4 = top half, 5 = among the best)

Communicates effectively with patients	1	2	3	4	5	Unable to assess
Is courteous to co-workers	1	2	3	4	5	Unable to assess
Accepts responsibility for patient care	1	2	3	4	5	Unable to assess
Is available to patients	1	2	3	4	5	Unable to assess

Colleague Questionnaire

Compared to the doctors I know, this one:
(1 = among the worst, 2 = bottom half, 3 = average, 4 = top half, 5 = among the best)

Communicates effectively with patients	1	2	3	4	5	Unable to assess
Maintains the quality of medical records	1	2	3	4	5	Unable to assess
Critically assesses diagnostic information	1	2	3	4	5	Unable to assess
Handles transfer of care	1	2	3	4	5	Unable to assess

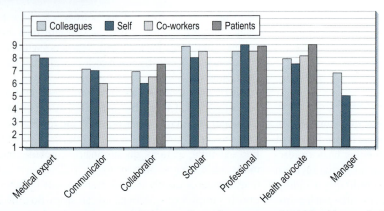

Figure 13.3 • Example of an MSF report (from Overeem et al, 2007, with permission).

and graphs to compare learners' scores with group scores. The total number of respondents is also documented in the report. In many systems, the feedback report contains free text comments as well (see Figure 13.3 for an example of an MSF report).

Web-based systems for the application of MSF are relatively new in medicine. A few countries have implemented them for use with clerks, registrars, and practising doctors. Studies in business have shown that using electronic MSF systems does not influence the consistency of the raters or the feedback scores themselves. It has been found that online feedback mechanisms promote anonymity, which increases learners' perceptions of trust in the authenticity of their feedback.

Quality of MSF

Validity and reliability

Content validity of MSF is established by mapping questionnaires to one of the frameworks that have been developed for medical students, doctors in training, and fully trained doctors (such as Good Medical Practice in the United Kingdom or CanMeds; Frank et al, 1996). By showing instruments' ability to discriminate between specialties and levels of experience, studies have also shown that MSF instruments have construct validity (Overeem et al, 2007).

The reliability of assessment instruments concerns their internal consistency and stability (inter-rater reliability, intra-rater reliability, or generalisability). Generally, instruments applied with MSF have reasonable internal consistency, with Cronbach's alpha varying from 0.83 to 0.98 (Overeem et al, 2007).

The generally accepted threshold of reliability for high-stakes judgement is a generalisability coefficient of 0.8. For formative purposes, a generalisability coefficient of 0.7 is appropriate. Achieving this level is influenced by the size of the group of respondents. For example, more patients than nurses or peers are required in order to achieve reliable results. Overall, reasonably reliable results can be achieved with the assessments of 8–12 peers or co-workers and 15–25 patients.

Rater credibility

Learners receiving MSF are more likely to use the feedback when they perceive their raters to be well informed about their practice. To ensure that credible raters are selected – raters who have been able to observe the learner's behavior for an extended period of time – learners should be involved in selecting them. Although it may seem counter-intuitive, there is evidence that this procedure does not distort ratings (Overeem et al, 2007).

One general assumption of MSF is that ratings reflect a rater's best and specific judgement about a learner and the dimension on which the learner is being assessed. This assumption needs further attention as researchers have pointed out that there is a tendency in peer ratings towards leniency to minimise bad feelings. Further, there is evidence that there is a "halo effect" exists in MSF (Mount and Scullen, 2001), whereby a rater perceives one factor to be of paramount importance and rates the learner based on this one factor. Rater training programmes have been developed to eliminate common rating errors such as halo effect and rater leniency. Research to date, however, is inconclusive about the effect of such programmes on rater accuracy (Mount and Scullen, 2001). Nevertheless, an important condition for valid and credible feedback is that raters understand what they are supposed to do and what happens with their feedback. Further, raters should be assured of the anonymity and confidentiality of the process so their ratings are credible. In addition, an anonymous feedback procedure is required whereby only mentors can gain access to raters' identities and everyone involved must have clear information about the confidentiality and safety of the procedures.

Specificity

Effective assessment feedback is specific in nature. A qualitative study with 15 family physicians in Canada showed that mailed MSF reports, which contained only numerical scores, were often inadequate to point towards useful improvements. Narrative comments in which respondents provide more specific explanations of their ratings and suggestions to improve performance are more informative and satisfactory to learners (Overeem et al, 2010). Research has also shown that recipients of feedback pay more attention to comments than quantitative ratings (Brett and Atwater, 2001). Raters should be encouraged to be constructive rather than destructive when making comments.

Mentoring MSF

Emotional reactions are the main impediment to using raters' judgements to support personal advancement. Recipients of negative MSF, first timers in particular, go through phases of shock, anger, and rejection of results before being able to accept it. A decline in subsequent multi-source evaluations has even been described (Brett and Atwater, 2001). Mentors can help MSF recipients through the stages of acceptance, as we have described earlier. Mentors must be especially sensitive to emotional reactions when: (1) feedback is largely negative, (2) incongruity exists between (inflated) self-ratings and ratings from others, (3) feedback concerns personal character traits instead of behaviour, and (4) feedback is judgemental. The utility of MSF for reflection and performance improvement depends enormously on the mentor facilitating the feedback. Mentors should take care not to focus on minutiae or isolated adverse comments in MSF reports. Rather, the discussion of feedback should identify areas of strength and weakness and, very importantly, help the learner identify where developmental work would be useful.

Steps 4 and 5 of the ALACT cycle create an ideal opportunity for goal setting, continuous feedback, and follow-up. Learners can inform people in their working environment about their improvement goals and seek feedback to foster their continuing efforts. Studies have shown that feedback recipients who perceive support from co-workers hold more positive attitudes towards the feedback system and are more involved in job development (Maurer et al, 2002). Table 13.2 overviews the factors that promote successful use of MSF.

Table 13.2 Factors promoting the success of MSF	
Factor	**Recommendation**
Implementation	An anonymous feedback procedure is required whereby only mentors can gain access to ratings. Ensure that everyone involved has clear information about procedures that guarantee confidentiality and safety. Make protected time and resources available
Content of MSF	Include narrative comments in the questionnaires. Provide learners with feedback reports that combine statistical data with narrative comments
Credibility and specificity of MSF	Provide clear information for raters about the criteria for credible and specific feedback. Let learners choose their raters so they include people who have observed performance
Mentoring	Provide mentoring by trained teachers, supervisors, or peers. Ensure that mentors are trained in how to encourage reflection and goal setting, and are sensitive to emotional reactions
Follow-up	Focus on the output of an MSF process. Formulating concrete goals for change and arranging follow-up interviews advances the use of MSF for practice improvement

Portfolios

Portfolios vary in their content and format but, basically, they report on work done, feedback received, progress made, and plans for improving competence. Portfolios may be digital or paper-based and content may be prescribed or left to the students' discretion. They can hold copies of materials, tests, photographs, observation reports, videotapes, handwritten notes, reports of evaluations, and so forth. Compared to assessment instruments like paper-and-pencil tests, OSCEs, and Mini-Clinical Examinations, portfolios offer an opportunity for assessors to see the wide range of a student's work and consider the limitations and opportunities of varying performance contexts when making judgements.

Portfolio as a multi-purpose instrument

Portfolios are promoted as an excellent instrument for authentic assessment as well as to stimulate reflective thinking. Working on a portfolio can activate reflection, because collecting work samples, evaluations, and other types of illustrative materials compels learners to look back on what they have done and analyse what they have and have not accomplished (ALACT Step 2: Looking back on action). Another way in which portfolios can stimulate reflective thinking is written reflections, the inclusion of which is usually mandatory. Examples are: reflective journals or diaries, reflective essays, mission statements, self-evaluations, and descriptions of steps taken to achieve improvement. In many cases, portfolios are assembled over a long period of time. That is why they can be used as an instrument to support planning and monitoring in professional development (ALACT Step 4: Creating alternative methods of action). One way to do so is to document learning objectives and the trail of related learning activities and accomplishments. Portfolios that are primarily geared to assessment will remain organised around artefacts and other kinds of materials, which provide "evidence" of competencies. Portfolios that are primarily used to monitor and plan students' development will give overviews centre stage. Portfolios whose primary objective is to foster learning by stimulating learners

to reflect on and discuss their development will be organised around learners' reflections.

Inevitably, these developments have widened the applicability of the label "portfolio" to a broad range of instruments. Some portfolios might as well be labelled "Personal Development Plan" or "Reflective Essay". Because of that tremendous variety, critical appraisal of the strengths and weaknesses of different systems is advisable before deciding which one to implement in a particular setting. The question to be answered is whether a certain portfolio is fit for its intended purpose. Just like shoes, portfolios come in different shapes and sizes (Spandel, 1997); and just as someone else's shoes are unlikely to fit comfortably, portfolios tailored to one particular institution may not fit into the educational configuration(s) of another institution. An ill-fitting portfolio will inevitably be discarded sooner or later. The triangle in Figure 13.4 helps clarify the nature of a portfolio to determine whether it is appropriate for its intended purpose. It does so by positioning the portfolio where it is most likely to achieve its intended principal objectives.

Obviously, a portfolio can achieve more than one goal. When it serves a combination of goals, its position in the triangle will shift towards the centre as its strengths are distributed more evenly across evidence, overviews, and reflections. In practice, the majority of portfolios are not situated at one of the corners of the triangle. A notable exception is PDPs.

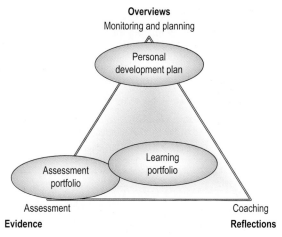

Figure 13.4 • Purposes and content of portfolios (van Tartwijk and Driessen, 2009).

The use of portfolios in medical education

Since their introduction in medical education in the early 1990s, portfolios have been increasingly used in all stages of the medical education continuum: in undergraduate medical education; postgraduate specialist training; and the continuing medical education (CME) of practising doctors. Portfolios in medicine have been subject of much educational research (Buckley et al, 2009; Driessen et al, 2007; Tochel et al, 2009), which confirms the theory-based notion that a portfolio has the potential to be a useful instrument to develop and assess competencies that are difficult to develop or assess with other instruments; especially reflective skills or performance in the workplace. However, the success of portfolios is conditional on fulfilment of certain prerequisites (Table 13.3).

Mentoring

The single most decisive factor is mentoring. If no provision is made for learner–mentor contacts in which portfolio content can be discussed and feedback given, all the time and effort expended on the portfolio will probably be wasted. First, as previously discussed, many learners are initially reluctant to engage in reflection because its purpose is not self-evident. A teacher, supervisor, or mentor is needed to convince learners that reflection is worthwhile. Second, reflection does not come naturally to most learners. As stated earlier, mentors have a supportive role to play in the various steps of the reflective process.

A systematic review showed that portfolio processes often fail to include adequate support and mentoring despite evidence of its positive impact (Driessen et al, 2007). There were also examples of portfolios being used without training or giving them time to perform their mentoring task properly. It was concluded that, although mentoring is possible without a portfolio, it is hardly possible to use a portfolio to promote reflection without mentoring (Driessen et al, 2007; van Tartwijk and Driessen, 2009).

A portfolio:

- Provides mentors with insight into learners' experiences and learning;
- Stimulates students to undertake the first reflection steps (i.e. self-assessment and analysis);
- Collates and integrates self-assessment with external assessments and other information sources, and gives mentors insight into possible discrepancies;
- Helps students set an agenda for personal development planning and meetings with mentors.

Table 13.3 Implementing portfolio learning

Factor	Recommendation
Goals	Clearly introduce the goals of working with a portfolio Combine goals (learning and assessment)
Introducing the portfolio	Provide clear guidelines about the procedure, the format, and the content Be cautious about problems with information technology
Mentoring/interaction	Provide mentoring by either teachers, trainers, supervisors, or peers
Assessment	Incorporate safeguards in the assessment procedure, such as intermittent feedback cycles, involvement of relevant resource persons (including the student), and a sequential judgement procedure Use assessment panels of 2–3 assessors depending on the stakes of the assessment Train assessors Use holistic scoring rubrics (global performance descriptors)
Portfolio format	Use a hands-on introduction with a briefing on the portfolio's purpose and procedures Keep the portfolio format flexible Avoid being overly prescriptive about the portfolio content Avoid too much paperwork
Position in the curriculum	Integrate the portfolio in other educational activities in the curriculum Be moderately ambitious for early undergraduate portfolio use

The format of portfolios

Another important point is that a portfolio must be "lean". Both learners and mentors have an aversion to large portfolios whether on paper or screen. There are too many instances of portfolios comprising a huge collection of materials, which indicates lack of clarity on the part of teachers as well as learners about the objectives. Because of such uncertainty, learners are sometimes advised to produce extensive portfolios, but there are good reasons to require selective and purposeful collection of materials. All parties involved stand to gain from portfolios that are tailored to their intended purposes so designers should create portfolios that are fit for the objectives to be achieved. When summative assessment is the sole objective of a portfolio, students can be asked to include only materials related to the competencies to be assessed and mark which parts of the portfolio have special relevance to which specific competencies (so-called captions). In that way, assessors do not have to peruse the full contents but can focus on what is relevant to the assessment.

When the portfolio's objective is to promote reflection, an open structure based on clear guidelines is preferable. When portfolio content is too rigidly prescribed, however, reflections tend to become superficial and students may even make up topics. A study in teacher training showed that trainees reflected more superficially on topics that were less important for their day-to-day practice (Mansvelder-Longayroux, 2006). It is therefore essential that learners have opportunities to adjust the content of portfolios to the experiences they have in day-to-day learning practice. On the other hand, it is important that students, for whom a portfolio is new, are offered support and clarity as to what is expected from them. This can be achieved by organising a portfolio along the lines of professional roles or a competency profile (e.g. the CanMeds roles: Frank et al, 1996), supported by guiding questions. Further guidance can be offered by a well-informed mentor, who introduces the portfolio and explains the objectives and how they can be attained.

Position in the curriculum

A rigidly predefined structure becomes even more counterproductive when learners do not have enough new experience on which to reflect. Since reflection starts by looking back on action, learners must encounter enough new events to provide objects of reflection. In the absence of new events, students reflect for the sake of reflecting and may resort to fantasy. In the early stages of medical school, the curriculum is mainly theoretical and students have few real practical experiences. Therefore, a portfolio used in the early undergraduate curriculum years should not be too ambitious.

Ever since the introduction of portfolios, a controversial issue has been whether or not it is acceptable to have a single portfolio serving both summative assessment and reflection. An argument against this dual function is that assessment jeopardises the quality of reflection and detracts from the portfolio's value in supporting effective mentoring. Learners may be reluctant to expose their less successful efforts or reflect on strategies for addressing weaknesses if they believe they are at risk of having "failures" turned against them in summative assessments. Unassessed portfolios, on the other hand, do not "reward" learners for the time and energy they have invested in them, which leads to them taking the portfolio and associated learning activities less seriously. We favour the middle ground and agree with the observation by Snyder and colleagues that: "The tension between assessment for support and assessment for high stakes decision making will never disappear. Still, that tension is constructively dealt with daily by teacher educators throughout the nation" (Snyder et al, 1998). Striking the right balance between support and judgement is the challenge facing mentors with whom students talk about their portfolios.

Assessment

Portfolios are seen by many as subjective and not suitable for high-stakes decisions. Early reports suggested we needed to temper our expectations for achieving strict psychometric criteria of validity and reliability because portfolios are individualistic and non-standardised. Low inter-rater reliabilities in portfolio assessment were a particular cause for concern. Educational developers responded by standardising assessment procedures to an excessive degree, with concomitant drawbacks. It was Snadden (1999), who asked for the first time whether we should continue trying to fit non-standardised portfolios to psychometric criteria. Webb et al (2003) came up with the idea of using criteria derived from qualitative research. Instead of a quantitative psycho-metric approach which looked at consistency across repeated assessment, a qualitative approach would add information to the judgement process until saturation was reached. Assessment procedures based on qualitative research criteria can incorporate safeguards, such as intermittent feedback cycles, involvement of relevant resource persons (including learners), and a sequential judgement procedure. It is also recommended that portfolio assessment procedures make use of: holistic scoring rubrics; small groups of trained assessors; and specific rater training expertise, including benchmarking and discussion between assessors.

Some final thoughts

The clinical workplace is an indispensable learning environment for the starting doctor. Doctors learn to put in practice all the knowledge and skills they acquired at medical school there and merge it into what one could refer to as competence. Research findings consistently show that teacher characteristics such as experience (Rivkin et al, 2005), scores on certification exams (Ferguson, 1991), and teacher training (Angrist and Lavy, 2001; Steinert et al, 2006) have a major impact on student learning. The strategies and tools available to teachers are also very important. In this chapter, we have introduced some of the tools and strategies the clinical teacher can use in the role of a mentor. Teaching tasks, however, have to compete with other tasks such as patient care and, sometimes, research. An investment of teaching time is an absolute requirement for successful use of the instruments we have presented.

Implications for practice

Self-assessment through "self-directed assessment seeking" and reflection, particularly "reflection-on-action", are important elements of learning from practice. Routines to facilitate learning from practice, such as the UK NHS appraisal process and the ALACT model for cyclical CPD, depend upon the input of a mentor who can support these processes since there is good evidence that, generally speaking, people are poor at self-assessment and many do not naturally reflect. A good mentor creates a safe environment in which to ask challenging questions of the learner, using techniques such as confrontation and generalisation. They support the learners' reflection, whether focused on means, goals, or ethical and moral perspectives. They provide constructive feedback, pointing the learner towards sources of information about their performance, facilitate goal-setting, possibly through creation of a SMART PDP, and help with follow-up including providing reminders about proposed actions.

Although research has not yet fully answered the question "What feedback works?", guidelines for providing formative feedback have been described. These help the learner address the key questions, "Where am I going?", "How am I going?", and "Where to next?", and may focus on the task, the process, self-regulation, or the person. Generally, feedback that focuses on the *person* does not have any useful value, and if critical or negative may be damaging. There is always an emotional component to peoples' reactions to feedback and mentors must recognise and work with this.

MSF has shown potential to provide people with useful information about a wide range of competencies, including strengths and weaknesses. Validity and reliability can be enhanced through procedures such as blueprinting and ensuring an appropriate number of respondents, and factors promoting success of MSF have been identified. The structured feedback provided can support reflection and action, and although research on its effect on future performance is still at an early stage, MSF seems to be acceptable to users. Mentors play an important role in helping people make the most of the process.

Portfolios are effective instruments both for promoting reflection (in support of professional development), and for assessment, although there are potentially conflicting issues that may jeopardise use of a single portfolio for both purposes. A wide variety of formats and approaches have been described and it is important to critically appraise strengths and weaknesses in the context of intended purpose before adopting a particular model. Notwithstanding the differences, the essential element in all portfolios is the documentation and collation of learning, usually in the form of written artefacts. The content of a portfolio must be kept to a minimum, and learners need support in how to use it. Again, the support of a mentor appears to be the most important factor in a portfolio's effectiveness.

References

ACGME: *Homepage of the Accreditation Council for Graduate Medical Education*. Available at: http://www.acgme.org/. Accessed October 16, 2009.

Angrist JD, Lavy V: Does teacher training affect pupil learning? Evidence from matched comparisons in Jerusalem public schools, *J Labor Econ* 19 (2):417–458, 2001.

Boylan O, Bradley T, McKnight A: GP perceptions of appraisal: professional development, performance management, or both? *Br J Gen Pract* 55:544–545, 2005.

Bransford J, Brown AL, Cocking RR: *How people learn: brain, mind, experience, and school*, Expanded ed, Washington DC, 2000, National Academy Press.

Brett JF, Atwater LE: 360 degree feedback: accuracy, reactions, and perceptions of usefulness, *J Appl Psychol* 86(5):930–942, 2001.

Buckley S, Coleman J, Davison I, et al: The educational effects of portfolios on undergraduate student learning: a Best Evidence Medical Education (BEME) systematic review: BEME Guide No. 11, *Med Teach* 31 (4):282–298, 2009.

Conlon M: Appraisal: the catalyst of personal development, *BMJ* 16 (327):389–391, 2003.

Davis DA, Mazmanian PE, Fordis M, et al: Accuracy of physician self-assessment compared with observed measures of competence: a systematic review, *JAMA* 296 (9):1094–1102, 2006.

Driessen EW, van Tartwijk J, Van der Vleuten CPM, et al: Portfolios in medical education: why do they meet with mixed success? A systematic review, *Med Educ* 41(12):1224–1233, 2007.

Driessen EW, van Tartwijk J, Dornan T: The self-critical doctor: helping students become more reflective, *BMJ* 336:827–830, 2008.

Ericsson KA: The influence of experience and deliberate practice on the development of expert performance. In Ericsson KA, Charness N, Feltovich PJ, et al, editors: *The Cambridge handbook of expertise and expert performance*, New York, 2006, Cambridge University Press, pp 683–704.

Ertmer PA, Newby TJ: The expert learner: strategic, self-regulated, and reflective, *Instr Sci* 24(1):1–24, 1996.

Eva KW, Regehr G: "I'll never play professional football" and other fallacies of self-assessment, *J Contin Educ Health Prof* 28(1):14–19, 2008.

Ferguson RF: Paying for public education: new evidence on how money matters, *Harvard J Legis* 28(2):465–498, 1991.

Frank J, Jabbour M, Tugwell P, et al: *Skills for the new millenium: report of the societal needs working group*, Ottawa, 1996, Royal College of Physicians and Surgeons of Canada.

General Medical Council: *Guidance on good medical practice*, 2006. http://www.gmc-uk.org/guidance/good_medical_practice/index.asp. Accessed September 23, 2009.

Hall W, Violato C, Lewkonia R, et al: Assessment of physician performance in Alberta: the physician achievement review, *CMAJ* 161:52–57, 1999.

Hattie J, Timperley H: The power of feedback, *Rev Educ Res* 77(1):81–112, 2007.

Hatton N, Smith D: Reflection in teacher education: towards definition and implementation, *Teach Teach Educ* 11(1):33–49, 1995.

Jowett V, Stead R: Mentoring students in higher education, *Educ Train* 36:20–26, 1994.

Kluger AN, DeNisi A: The effects of feedback interventions on performance: a historical review, a meta-analysis, and a preliminary feedback intervention theory, *Psychol Bull* 119(2):254–284, 1996.

Kolb DA: *Experiential learning: experience as the source of learning and development*, Prentice Hall, 1984, Englewood Cliffs, NJ.

Korthagen FAJ, Kessels J, Koster B, et al: *Linking theory and practice: the pedagogy of realistic teacher education*, Mahwah, NY, 2001, Lawrence Erlbaum Associates.

Lewis M, Elwyn G, Wood F: Appraisal of family doctors: an evaluation study, *Br J Gen Prac* 53:454–460, 2003.

Loftus EF: Our changeable memories: legal and practical implications, *Nat Rev: Neurosci* 4:231–234, 2003.

Mansvelder-Longayroux DD: *The learning portfolio as a tool for stimulating reflection by student teachers*, Leiden, 2006, Leiden University.

Maurer TJ, Mitchell D, Barbeite FG: Predictors of attitudes toward a 360-degree feedback system and involvement in post-feedback management development activity, *J Occup Organ Psychol* 75:87–107, 2002.

Mount MK, Scullen SE: Multisource feedback ratings. In London M, editor: *How people evaluate other in organisations*, Mahwah, NJ, 2001, Lawrence Erlbam Associates, Chapter 7.

NHS: *NHS appriasal toolkit*, 2001. Available from https://www.appraisals.nhs.uk/menu.html. Accessed October 15, 2009.

NHS: *Homepage of the Foundation Programme*. Available from www.foundationprogramme.nhs.uk. Accessed October 16, 2009.

Overeem K, Faber MJ, Arah OA, et al: Doctor performance assessment in daily practice: does it help doctors or not? A systematic review, *Med Educ* 41(11):1039–1049, 2007.

Overeem K, Lombarts MJMH, Arah OA, et al: Three methods of multisource feedback compared. A plea for narrative comments and co-workers' perspectives, *Med Teach*, 32 (2):141–147, 2010.

Rivkin SG, Hanushek EA, Kain JF: Teachers, schools, and academic achievement, *Econometrica* 73 (2):417–458, 2005.

Sargeant J, Mann K, van der Vleuten CPM, et al: Directed self-assessment: practice and feedback within a social context, *J Cont Educ Health Prof* 28(1):47–54, 2008.

Schön D: *The reflective practitioner: how professionals think in action*, New York, 1983, Basic Books.

Shute VJ: Focus on formative feedback, *Rev Educ Res* 78(1):153–189, 2008.

Smither JW, London M, Flautt R, et al: Can working with an executive coach improve multisource feedback ratings over time? A quasi-experimental field study, *Pers Psychol* 56:23–44, 2003.

Snadden D: Portfolios – attempting to measure the unmeasurable?

[Commentary], *Med Educ* 33 (7):478–479, 1999.

Snyder J, Lippincott A, Bower D: The inherent tensions in the multiple uses of portfolios in teacher education, *Teach Educ* Q 25(1):45–60, 1998.

Spandel V: Reflections on portfolios. In Phye GD, editor: *Handbook of academic learning: construction of knowledge,*

San Diego, 1997, Academic Press, pp 573–591.

Steinert Y, Mann K, Centeno A, et al: A systematic review of faculty development initiatives designed to improve teaching effectiveness in medical education: BEME Guide No. 8, *Med Teach* 28(6):497–526, 2006.

Tochel C, Haig A, Hesketh A, et al: The effectiveness of portfolios for post-graduate assessment and education:

BEME Guide No. 12, *Med Teach* 31(4):299–318, 2009.

van Tartwijk J, Driessen EW: Portfolios for assessment and learning: AMEE Guide No. 45, *Med Teach* 31 (9):790–801, 2009.

Webb C, Endacott R, Gray MA, et al: Evaluating portfolio assessment systems: what are the appropriate criteria? *Nurse Educ Today* 23:600–609, 2003.

Assessing learners

14

Valerie Wass   Julian Archer

CHAPTER CONTENTS

ABC

Glossary

Assessment See main Glossary, p 339.

Assessment; formative See main Glossary, p 337.

Competency See main Glossary, p 340.

Context specificity Commonly defined by the observation that an individual's performance on a particular problem or in a particular situation is only weakly predictive of the same individual's performance on a different problem or in a different situation.

Educational impact The effect of assessments on learning.

Evaluation See main Glossary, p 340.

Reliability See main Glossary, p 342.

Summative assessment See main Glossary, p 343.

Triangulate Comparing and integrating observations made using different assessment methodologies to form an overall judgement of competency.

Continued

© 2011, Elsevier Ltd.
DOI: 10.1016/B978-0-7020-3522-7.00014-0

Glossary (continued)

Utility of an assessment method A conceptual design model using multiplicative, differentially weighted functions of five variables (educational impact, validity, reliability, acceptability, and cost) to define the utility of an assessment method, or a programme of assessment, in a given situation.

Validity See main Glossary, p 343.

Outline

This chapter first explores theoretical frameworks and concepts underpinning our understanding of assessing learners in medicine. The rationale for the current philosophy, which moves clinical competency assessment away from examinations alone towards a more developmental formative approach to assessment, is explained. The principles needed to understand test design are then reviewed to provide a framework for the development of assessment programmes. The range of available assessment tools and the evidence base for their use is subsequently discussed. Basic psychometric principles essential to the evaluation and quality assurance of the assessment process are outlined. The chapter concludes with a look to the future.

A fundamental truth

Assessment drives learning. As educationalists, we may be uncomfortable with this statement. The curriculum learning outcomes and teaching delivery should be decided before the appropriate assessment methods are selected. Yet, we face a reality. What influences any student most is not the teaching but the assessment. The dominant impact of assessment has long been recognised. Derek Rowntree stated, 'If we wish to discover the truth about an educational system we must first look to its assessment procedures' (Rowntree, 1987). That does not negate the content of other chapters in this book. Assessment must mirror the philosophy and learning intent of the curriculum. The importance of harnessing assessment design to achieve appropriate learning cannot be too strongly emphasised. All assessments must have intrinsic educational impact on learners and teachers.

The challenge of assessing learners in medicine: important theoretical concepts

It is important to understand how to maximise the educational influence of assessment. Views on how to measure the competency of health professionals are changing in an attempt to do this. The increasing acknowledgement that assessment is integral to learning, and not a process that happens at the conclusion of learning, creates potentially conflicting issues for the health professions. We highlight four: (i) balancing competence with aspiration to excellence, (ii) recognition of the learner's rate of progression from novice to expert, (iii) the balance between formative and summative agendas, and (iv) difficulties in weighing reliability and validity within clinical assessment methodology.

Competence versus excellence

Competency-based curricula are increasingly being introduced in medical education, as outlined in Chapter 6, and there is an increased focus on technical qualifications. Some believe that this approach undermines medical professionalism and fails to provide the appropriate learning platform for continuing professional development. Instead, it fosters a 'tick box', 'can do' mentality. Trainees perceive that they have achieved competence when they pass an assessment and do not recognise that they need to improve their skills further through apprenticeship and practice. The aim to 'do better' may be lost. The United Kingdom Royal College of Physician's (RCPs) report (RCP, 2005) reviewing the challenges to the medical profession in the twenty-first century emphasised the need to aspire continually to excellence. It raised serious concerns that current assessment trends towards competency were failing us. Even more seriously, there is a risk of generating 'incompetency' if learners perceive prematurely that they have achieved 'competency'. They can fail to recognise that the judgement of competency pertains only to a point in time. The need to set goals for further development is lost (Hodges, 2006). That tension has to be acknowledged as you read through the content of this chapter.

To achieve a new developmental culture and move away from end point examinations and final competency assessments, we need to bring assessment more into the centre of the learning process (Shepard, 2000), as argued above. That would concur with Vygotsky's (1978) concept of a 'zone of proximal development'. Each learner is on a progressive, developmental pathway of expertise. At a particular moment in time, with a mentor's guidance, they need to understand not only what they are capable of performing independently but also how they can improve. Continually resetting their goals can foster an aspiration to do better. This requires a change in assessment culture for both students and tutors. In a competitive assessment world, high scores are of paramount importance; in a more developmental world, which encourages educational feedback, students will not necessarily score high. In the current culture, they can be uncomfortable with low scores. Tutors who are used to linking judgements with a numerical grade that can be defended will have to review their approach to assessment. Emerging evidence shows many tutors have difficulty giving constructive feedback rather than assigning a score or ticking off a competency. A fundamental change in practice is needed, which requires time and training resources.

There is increasing recognition, according to Lave and Wenger's theory (1991), that learning and the development of an identity of mastery occur simultaneously as students become increasingly adept at participating in a community of practice. If we are to understand why some students struggle to achieve competence and how to motivate others towards goals of excellence, then attention should be paid to the concept of legitimate peripheral participation. More theoretical understanding is needed of how students socialise into and communicate within a community of practice and how they develop competence as part of a social group. This almost certainly impacts on how they develop the institutional socially acceptable language, become accustomed to explaining their reasoning, and receive the feedback necessary to move across competency towards excellence. Herein may also lie an explanation of differences seen in performance across gender and ethnicity (Wass et al, 2003a).

Novice to expert

Clinical competence is a complex construct. We define competency as 'the ability to handle a complex professional task by integrating the relevant cognitive, psychomotor, and affective skills'. Inevitably, by the very nature of these three components, 'knowledge,

skills, and attitudes', multiple assessment methods must be used. The resulting observations can then be compared and integrated to create an overall picture of an individual's competence: a process termed 'triangulation'. This is not that easy, particularly if assessment is set in the context of continuous professional development, as discussed above.

Vygotsky's concept of a zone of proximal development highlights the importance of interactive assessments to explore where the student is placed in their progression from novice to expert. The pathway of learning diagnostic reasoning is, to a significant extent, dependent on expertise resultant on clinical experience. The move from a novice to an expert involves a complex cognitive process (Schmidt and Norman, 2007). The rather laborious data gathering process, on which hypothetico-deductive diagnostic reasoning is initially built, changes with time. A shift in the structuring of knowledge is intrinsic to the growth of expertise. For novices, a clinical case appears as a series of isolated symptoms and signs, which must be related to finite pathophysiological concepts. Similarly, a skill is learnt as a stepwise series of distinct procedural steps. Knowledge then becomes progressively assimilated into diagnostic labels, a process termed 'encapsulation'. As more clinical experience is gained, a further shift occurs as patterns of disease recognition, called 'illness scripts', develop. These are more narrative than factual, derive from everyday clinical practice, and almost completely 'bypass' the original building stones with which a novice works. They are cognitive entities containing relatively little basic knowledge and scaffolded from direct patient encounters, a product of growing clinical experience. Not surprisingly, 'illness scripts' can be very individual as clinical experience is so varied. If, for example, you have witnessed a significant thromboembolic episode in a young girl on the contraceptive pill, then pattern recognition when dealing with patients with headaches taking the pill will weigh towards more serious causes than for clinicians who have not. Similarly when learning skills, practice is essential to allow the initial rather pedantic stepwise checklist of tasks to become automatic and integrated.

A learner's position on the novice to expert pathway affects both their performance and the judgements of those assessing them. A medical student just starting clinical placements will be in the first stage of diagnostic reasoning, using a checklist of items to gather data, examine a patient, or demonstrate a skill. An experienced assessor will have developed a global, integrated approach and have difficulty reverting to explicit analysis of inexpert performance. As Eraut (2004) points out: 'expert performance is often tacit; identifying aspects of different disciplinary practices is in itself a significant task'. A useful model in understanding the novice to expert pathway, which provides a framework for assessing across the undergraduate postgraduate continuum, is that of Dreyfus and Dreyfus (1986). Table 14.1 outlines the stages and implications for testing as knowledge and skills move from basic knowledge, where there is little situational perception and situational judgement, through to the holistic, intuitive approach of experts. This 'mismatch' between reasoning processes of a novice and those of an expert explains some of the dilemmas faced when assessing learners in medicine.

Table 14.1 Novice to expert: stages of progression						
Level	Stage	Characteristics	How knowledge, etc., is treated	Recognition of relevance	How context is assessed	Decision-making
1	Novice	Rigid adherence to taught rules or plans Little situational perception No discretionary judgement	Without reference to context	None	Analytically	Rational
2	Advance beginner	Guidelines for action based on attributes to aspects (aspects are global) Characteristics of situations recognisable only after some prior experience Situational perception still limited All attributes and aspects are treated separately and given equal importance	In context			
3	Competent	Coping with crowdedness Now seems actions at least partially in terms of longer-term goals Conscious, deliberate planning Standardised and routinised procedures		Present		
4	Proficient	Sees situations holistically rather than in terms of aspects Sees what is most important in a situation Perceives deviations from the normal patterns Decision-making less laboured Uses maxims for guidance, whose meanings vary according to the situation			Holistically	
5	Expert	No longer relies on rules, guidelines, or maxims Intuitive grasp of situations based on deep tacit understanding Analytic approaches used only in novel situations or when problems occur Vision of what is possible				Intuitive

Adapted from Dreyfus (1981) and Dreyfus and Dreyfus (1984).

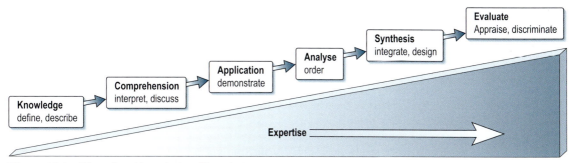

Figure 14.1 • Hierarchy of knowledge: Bloom's taxonomy.

Assessment methods must be tailored to accommodate shifts in reasoning which develop implicitly with experience. Although medical students and residents are among the most frequently tested groups in higher education, it is surprising how often the assessment methods still focus primarily on low-level skills. If we expect our future clinicians to be excellent, we must begin to test across the education continuum at increasingly higher skill levels or, indeed, use assessment to drive its development. It is important both to identify a trainee's position on the novice to expert pathway and encourage a higher level of reasoning.

Bloom's taxonomy of knowledge (Figure 14.1) provides a means of illustrating why this is important. Bloom (1965) defines increasing levels of complexity; initially defining basic facts, then applying these to clinical situations, before progressing towards analysis, and finally evaluating clinical events. It is relatively easy to test basic factual knowledge; it is not uncommon to find postgraduate examinations still assessing at this level. Yet, even at undergraduate level, novices need encouragement to 'interpret' basic facts in a clinical context and apply them to simple clinical scenarios. Assessment should be designed at increasingly higher levels of the taxonomy towards 'synthesis' and 'evaluation'. In the postgraduate arena, audit and critical appraisal become more appropriate assessment tools. Designing assessments to achieve this can be challenging. It is essential to ask the question repeatedly: 'Is this assessment appropriate to the cognitive level of the trainee as they progress towards clinical expertise?'

Summative versus formative

There are conflicting commitments within medical curricula. Throughout undergraduate and postgraduate 'training', there is a strong obligation on the part of institutions to ensure that their learners become 'safe'

to practise in health care. There is an absolute necessity to protect patients. Minimum levels of competency for progression in training are required. This summative approach is potentially threatening and, as we have discussed, may be counter-productive in supporting learners' progression from novice to expert. Some are concerned that 'licensing tests' can impact negatively on learning because they detract from the safe educational environments we strive to create. Examinations drive learning too narrowly towards the licensing test. Training towards minimum competency can conflict with the overriding commitment to education and lifelong learning. The latter requires a more 'formative' approach to assessment, with regular constructive feedback to trainees to ensure that they set personal goals for improvement.

The focus in the past has been very much on serial examinations and the summative assessment of learners. The need for a social constructivist approach to the assessment of clinicians is increasingly acknowledged (Rust et al, 2005). This view argues that knowledge evolves and is shaped through increasing participation within communities of practice (Lave and Wenger, 1991). Assessment needs to be constructively aligned with the environment in which trainees learn, that is, the apprenticeship foundation of medicine. We face a compelling need to change to a formative approach and foster continuous professional development in workplaces. There has been a strong initiative to replace summative examinations with more formative assessment programmes, which reflect the socio-cultural milieu of the curriculum (van der Vleuten and Schuwirth, 2005). The socio-cultural approach creates a further tension for tutors within the pressures of their working day. Tutors are being asked to collaborate formatively with trainees and give regular feedback on performance. At the same time, they may be asked to make summative judgements on the trainee's competence to practise. These roles entail very different power relations, which can be difficult to enact side by side, a dilemma that cannot be ignored.

There have been two significant consequences of this increasing move towards formative assessment. First, in an attempt to acknowledge assessment as developmental, confusion has evolved in the assessment discourse. Appraisal (see Chapter 13), essentially a confidential process focused on personal professional development, is increasingly seen as a potential vehicle for summative assessment. This is potentially damaging, threatening the educational potential of a feedback culture across the medical education continuum. The fundamental principle of supporting learning through feedback is in the systematic, supportive manner in which it is facilitated (Jamtvedt et al, 2003). Introducing a summative element threatens this. Learners can be confused by a language that uses appraisal outcomes, understood as confidential, to inform assessment processes such as revalidation. Whereas assessment can usefully inform appraisal, we believe appraisal cannot realistically inform assessment, by the very nature of its confidentiality. A second consequence is the use of 'formative' and 'summative' as dichotomous terms. Formative assessment risks are aimed only at the generation of educational feedback to support and develop learners, with little emphasis on psychometric principles. Psychometric preoccupation with reliability is viewed as the preserve of summative assessment – ensuring that pass/fail decisions are robust. As a result, feedback on performance is rarely given after summative assessment beyond a pass/fail decision. Continuing to view formative and summative assessment as separate processes is not progressive. Learners, whether they pass or fail, are entitled to expect detailed feedback on their performance. We argue that all assessments must be able to demonstrate reliable psychometric properties, whatever their purpose, so more attention must be paid to the development of psychometrically robust formative tools. If the main aim is to provide feedback, then the information given must be both valid and reliable. Research is urgently needed to address this cultural change as we move away from the formative–summative dichotomy.

Validity and reliability

The fourth challenge lies in addressing tensions that exist when ensuring that an assessment is both valid and reliable. There are trade-offs between reliability

and validity, which inevitably impact on developing more formative assessment programmes. It is important to explore theoretical understanding of these two concepts and how they relate to each other. Intrinsically, by the very nature of assessment, a test cannot be valid unless it is reliable. Yet, without validity, the purpose and value we place on the educational impact of assessment would have little meaning.

Validity

Validity is defined as 'the strength of conclusions and inferences which can be drawn from the outcomes of an assessment'; that is, 'Has the test effectively measured what it was intended to measure?' All assessments require evidence of validity. It is a conceptual term though, based on hypothesis. Its interpretation can be potentially confusing for two reasons. First, validity can only be evaluated retrospectively once performance data on a test have been collected. It cannot be measured at the planning stage, a common misconception. For example, an objective structured clinical examination (OSCE) station on the physical examination of a real patient's varicose veins may be designed and perceived as a valid test of a skill. If, on the day, the patient cancels and an adult with normal legs is substituted, the station has inadvertently lost its validity. Various pieces of information on a test can only be collated and analysed when the assessment has been completed. Whether the original intentions (as hypothesised) have been met or not must be decided after a test. Moreover, any conclusions are only applicable to that particular test in that specific cohort of learners.

Second, a series of facets were identified (Table 14.2) against which the validity of a test could traditionally be assessed. That rather pragmatist view of validity is now changing. According to a more contemporary conceptualisation, one unitary concept, 'construct validity', is offered (Downing, 2003b). The single term embraces all the multiple sources of evidence needed to evaluate and interpret the outcomes of an assessment. This approach was originally conceptualised by Messick (1989). It enables us to move away from the traditional individual descriptive 'facets' outlined in more detail below and focus more on sources of evidence available to validate assessment processes. This approach will be outlined in more detail later in the chapter.

Reliability

Reliability is, by comparison, a more 'concrete' parameter. It can be measured quantitatively, as

Table 14.2 Traditional facets of validity

Type of validity	Test facet being measured	Questions being asked
Face validity	Compatibility with the curriculum's educational philosophy	What is the test's face value? Does it match up with the educational intentions?
Content validity	The content of the curriculum	Does the test include a representative sample of the subject matter?
Construct validity	The ability to differentiate between groups with known difference in ability (beginners versus experts)	Does the test differentiate at the level of ability expected of candidates at that stage in training?
Predictive validity	The ability to predict an outcome in the future: for example, professional success after graduation	Does the test predict future performance and level of competency?
Consequential validity	The educational consequence of the test	Does the test produce the desired educational outcome?

described later in the chapter. It can be defined as the reproducibility of assessment data or scores, over time or occasions (Downing, 2004). Although usually distinguished from validity, reliability is a pre-condition for validity. If an assessment is not suffi-ciently reliable, then the evidence required to estab-lish validity becomes inaccurate. Reliability is usually (and correctly) said to be a necessary but not 'suffi-cient' condition for validity. Measurements or judge-ments may be reliable in the sense of being consistent over time or over judges but still be off-target (or invalid) if they have not actually measured what you set out to measure. Reliability and validity are, in a sense, intertwined and need to be balanced against each other, along with other parameters dis-cussed above (Figure 14.2).

The traditional, artificial separation of validity and reliability fuels the formative versus summative debate. Where educational supervision and feedback are of paramount importance, as in formative assess-ment, attention to the validity of judgements made by tutors and the constructive potential of their feed-back takes precedence. Yet, this must not be entirely to the exclusion of reliability. The emphasis on improvement must be based on robust as well as valid feedback. If a decision-making function is also placed on the process, then the defensibility required of the judgements places greater weight on reliability. Little is known to date on how assessments can be com-bined (if indeed they can) to balance validity with reliability. The importance of trying to achieve a greater understanding of this might well emerge as we move away from the defensibility of examinations

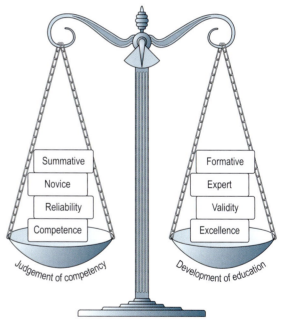

Figure 14.2 • Balancing development of education and judgement of competency.

to explore more developmental assessment pro-grammes in workplaces.

These theoretical concepts (Figure 14.2) should be kept in mind as the chapter proceeds to outline the fundamentals of assessment design. There is no gold standard for the assessment of any facet of clinical competence. At best, robust frameworks balance the formative approach needed to inform self-monitoring with the stringent judgements required to assure that trainees are competent for safe clinical practice. Increasingly, programmes must be designed to offer more flexibility, more formative feedback, and longitudinal assessment. Testing must adapt to levels of expertise and involve all stakeholders in setting standards and quality assurance.

The principles of designing assessments

This chapter opened by stating the fundamental, if uncomfortable, truth that assessment drives learning and must mirror the philosophy and learning intent of a curriculum. This truth is often lost as assessment methodology is driven by convenience, cost, or the latest fad. To avoid losing that truth, assessments must be carefully designed, following key principles.

Context specificity

Perhaps the most important evidence to emerge over the years is that all competencies are context bound and not generic, a principle that is fundamental to assessment design. It was once assumed that some skills, such as communication, were generic. If you communicated well on one occasion, you were 'a good communicator'. The ability to communicate was a personality trait. There is now ample evidence that this is not the case. Professionals do not perform consistently from task to task. Explaining a medical condition to a patient may be done well when one particular patient has one particular diagnosis. With varying diagnoses and different patients (e.g. explaining a more complex diagnosis to an angry patient), the individual's performance will vary. Performance on one case does not generalise to the 'universe' of cases and patients. The concept of a 'generically good communicator' does not exist.

Given our definition of competency, which emphasises *integration* of cognitive, psychomotor, and affective skills, this is not surprising. Communication skills and professional behaviours are contextually bound by the knowledge required for that particular situation. An individual's performance on a particular problem or situation only weakly predicts their performance on a different problem or situation. Although most of us believe that individuals have stable personality traits, research has clearly demonstrated that it is not true. The 'traits'

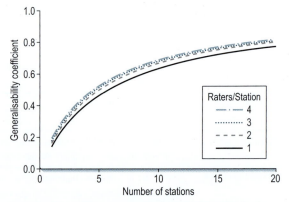

Figure 14.3 • The reliability of the OSCE. Statistics demonstrating how reliability (generalisability coefficient) improved as station number was increased and the number of raters on each station was increased (from Swanson et al, 1999, with thanks to David Swanson).

individuals exhibit are context-dependent. The situation (i.e. the context) should be considered a better predictor of behaviour than personality.

Two important lessons have been learnt. First, sampling of content must be wide. That was the main catalyst for developing OSCEs and for the demise of the long case. We now understand why sufficient testing time is essential in order to achieve adequate case specificity (reliability across cases), as shown in Figure 14.3, based on data published by Swanson et al (1995). A generalisability coefficient of 1.0 would indicate 100% test reproducibility (see below in section on measuring reliability). In reality, as Figure 14.3 demonstrates, that is rarely achieved because other variables such as examiner performance or poor standardisation of cases impact on tests. A coefficient of >0.8 is the pragmatic aim for most high-stakes tests of clinical competency. Based on that level, at least 14 OSCE cases are needed. Increasing the number of judges improves reliability to a significantly lesser extent (Figure 14.3). Second, more psychometric analyses of traditional methods, such as long cases and orals, have been published, which show that all methods are relevant provided the test is long enough to sample adequately. Sufficient testing across a range of contexts is essential (Figure 14.4). We have been released from the stringencies of examinations. Multiple assessment tools can, if planned appropriately using a sufficient range of contexts, be combined to assess individual performance more validly grounded in the reality of workplaces. (Wass et al, 2001c; van der Vleuten and Schuwirth, 2005).

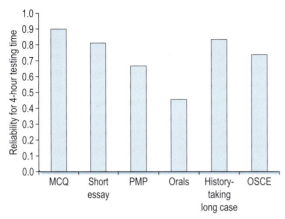

Figure 14.4 • Reliability of different assessment methods over 4-hour testing time (MCQ, Norcini et al, 1985; Short essay, Stalenhoef-Halling et al, 1990; PMP, Norcini et al, 1985; Orals, Swanson, 1987; Long case, Wass and Jolly, 2001; OSCE, Newble and Swanson, 1996).

Blueprinting

It follows that tests must be carefully planned against intended learning outcomes and curriculum content, a process known as 'blueprinting'. Assessments must validate all the objectives set by a curriculum because students inevitably focus on learning what is tested. Clinical competency is multifaceted. The learning outcomes required, sometimes defined as knowledge, skills, and attitudes, cannot realistically be assessed by a single test format. To assess clinical competence, a battery of different tests is needed. No single one can be valid, given the complexity of clinical competency itself. All tests must use a method that is appropriate to the learning outcome being tested. A multiple choice question (MCQ) may be a valid test of knowledge but not of communication skills, where an interactive test is required. Context specificity must be addressed and integrated into the framework to ensure an appropriate range of case scenarios are used. A blueprint is essential to overcome this complexity (Boursicot et al, 2007). It specifies not just what to assess but also how to assess it. For undergraduate curricula, where core content is more homogeneous, that is easier than for more broadly defined postgraduate curricula (Tombeson et al, 2000). To improve assessments, there is now a move for more detailed definition of their content. Conceptual frameworks to plan assessment programmes are essential and can be designed even for generalist collegiate tests. The assessment programme of the UK Royal College of General Practitioners (Rughani, 2007) provides an example.

Miller's model of competence assessment

Over the past 20 years, 'Miller's triangle' has provided an invaluable framework for planning clinical competency assessments (Miller, 1990). The model, shown in Figure 14.5, considers progression towards expertise as learners become more knowledgeable. They begin by assimilating knowledge ('knows'), then apply knowledge ('knows how'), before acquiring skills ('shows how'), and finally move to 'does': that is, performance in the workplace. Miller's model can be used to demonstrate the appropriateness of testing methods to competencies being measured. Mapping assessment tools against 'the triangle' has increasingly highlighted the lack of robust methods to assess performance (the apex of the triangle). As discussed above, the need to adjust test methodology to developing expertise has tended to be overlooked. There has been reconsideration of Miller's model. It implicitly assumes that competence, demonstrated under controlled conditions, predicts practice in the real world. Several studies have shown differences between doctors' performance in controlled high-stakes assessments and the reality of their actual practice (Rethans et al, 1991; Southgate et al, 2001). Knowledge is a prerequisite for competence (Ram et al, 1999b), but not sufficient alone to predict application in practice. Other influences related both to the individual (stress, health) and systems (conditions of practice) also have a significant impact on performance. Competence ('shows how') sheds light on performance but does not fully illuminate it, which Miller's model lacks the flexibility to reflect. Rethans et al (2002) suggested inverting the triangle to place greater weight on performance and modify it to highlight additional individual and system-related influences.

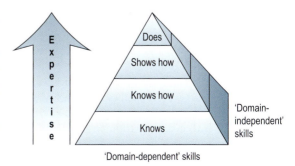

Figure 14.5 • Miller's triangle (modified).

They offered a useful reflection of the challenges faced when moving assessment from the relatively controlled environment of the medical school to the reality of postgraduate training in the workplace.

Our version of Miller's triangle is a three-dimensional pyramid (Figure 14.5), emphasising that blueprints must acknowledge 'domain-independent' skills – ones that are not specific to medicine but nevertheless essential facets of professional behaviour. We have added the third dimension because it is increasingly recognised that the two-dimensional (triangle) knowledge model favoured the use of unduly simply summative methodologies. It served as a good planning design but pulled us away from integration. Flexner's definition of an ideal test (Flexner, 1910) captures the essence of the problem. 'There is only one sort of licensing test that is significant, namely a test that ascertains the practical ability of the student confronting a concrete case to collect all relevant data and to suggest the positive procedure applicable to the conditions disclosed. A written examination may have some incidental value; it does not touch the heart of the matter.' Miller has offered a model of identifying how assessments can be combined at different levels of cognition to achieve Flexner's aim. Professional values must be integrated into the model in order to effectively capture performance.

The utility equation

No assessment tool is perfect. When designing assessment, it is important to acknowledge and weigh logistics. The practicalities of delivery cannot be ignored. The need to balance the concepts described above (Figure 14.2) to address the purpose of a test and reflect the philosophy of the training programme is essential. Choice is generally a compromise. The 'utility equation' (van der Vleuten, 1996) provides useful guidance for matching test method to the competency being assessed in the context of the curriculum:

$$\text{Utility} = \text{Reliability} \times \text{Validity} \times \text{Feasibility} \times \text{Acceptability} \times \text{Educational Impact}$$

The equation highlights the importance of balancing educational impact with reliability and validity when designing an assessment. Summative tests place more weight within the equation on reliability; formative tests lean more towards educational impact and validity. In addition, van der Vleuten has highlighted the inevitability of addressing the feasibility

of implementation. To achieve optimum reliability and validity, an individual needs theoretically to be assessed *ad infinitum*. That is never possible. Feasibility is intrinsic to assessment delivery. Reliability at this aspirational level is impractical. The time available, recruitment of assessors, administrative requirements, and financial restrictions all impact on test design. Similarly, test validity is undermined if collective acceptance of its theoretical framework is lost due to poor implementation. Constraints of practicality should be explicitly acknowledged. At the same time, assessment proposals must be acceptable to those involved: students, assessors, teachers, and institutions. Acceptability needs to be addressed when balancing assessment decisions.

No test can score uniformly high on all five parameters. Some trade-off is inevitable to ensure the purpose of an assessment is achieved. Utility counterbalances the selection of assessment methods, supporting delivery of a comprehensive, robust, and educationally transparent assessment package. We emphasise again the importance of educational impact. This should be at the heart of the endeavour. Too often, the educational benefits of assessments are lost. All assessors have a responsibility to make assessment a source of learning. Its place in the equation is fundamentally important.

Assessment formats through the continuum

The move away from examinations to more flexible assessment programmes, alongside the increasing aspiration to assess learners in workplaces, offers greater freedom to engage with available assessment tools, both traditional and new (van der Vleuten and Schuwirth, 2005; Wass et al, 2001c). There has been a historical tendency to adopt the latest trend and drop established methods, without reference to any evidence base. As psychometric information has emerged, it has become increasingly clear that the application of a test is more important than the method itself (Figure 14.4). Whatever the format, test length and its consequence, breadth of sampling, is critical (Figure 14.4). More emphasis can be placed on validity, provided context specificity, and hence reliability, are addressed. Now we accept that assessment must be contextual, a range of tools has become available. Expansion of methodological choice allows educational goals to be achieved at the relevant curriculum level of competency. Embedding different methods across the curriculum achieves that, provided they are sufficiently representative and carefully blueprinted. Logistic considerations, neatly summarised by the utility equation, can be balanced across programmes rather than confined to examinations. Methods can be tailored to trainees' progress along the novice-to-expert pathway, ensuring that assessments are delivered at the relevant point in time on the curriculum map and appropriate feedback is given. The choice of 'what' method and 'when' presents the challenge. Table 14.3 (modified from Epstein, 2007) summarises the properties of these different formats. Miller's model (Figure 14.5) shapes the following discussion of available methodologies.

The assessment of 'knows, and 'knows how'

From the start of undergraduate curricula, increasing emphasis is being placed on testing 'knows how' – that is, applying knowledge to problem solving – rather than 'knows' – that is, straight, factual knowledge recall (Figures 14.1 and 14.5). Problem solving is not a generic skill. It is closely linked to knowledge and is context-specific. A candidate's problem-solving ability is inconsistent across different tasks. As in all areas of clinical competence testing, inter-case reliability becomes an issue (van der Vleuten, 1996). This is more easily solved for written formats, where a large number of questions can be covered relatively quickly. As more complex approaches to assessment have evolved, pure knowledge tests have been criticised for their lack of validity. Yet, they remain a reliable and feasible way of assessing core knowledge. They retain a firm place in undergraduate and postgraduate training programmes and, arguably, in continuing professional development. Scores on pure knowledge tests can predict clinical performance. Studies by the American Board of Internal Medicine (ABIM) (Ramsey et al, 1989) showed a correlation between performance on the ABIM certification examination (a pure multiple-choice test) and performance in practice 10 years later, as assessed by peer ratings. More recently, Norcini et al (2002) linked data on all heart attack cases in Pennsylvania to certification by the ABIM. Physicians certified by this knowledge test had a 19% lower case fatality rate than those who were not. There was a 0.5% increase in mortality in their

practice for every year post graduation. That is consistent with knowledge decreasing as experience lengthens (Choudhry et al, 2005). Performance on pure knowledge tests appears to relate positively to health outcomes and negatively to experience.

Multi-choice knowledge tests

Tests of factual recall can take a variety of formats. Multiple choice methods remain the most widely used. They provide a large number of question items across multiple content areas and are relatively easily administered. These tests, if long enough, successfully address context specificity and have high reliability. As discussed, every effort must be made to ensure they challenge the learner at the 'knows how' level. To do that, a range of question formats have evolved: single best answer, extended matching, short and long menus of options, and short or long essays are examples (Schuwirth and van der Vleuten, 2003). Currently, the single best answer format is favoured. The correct response to a clinical scenario is selected from a series of options (usually 5). A notable limitation of multiple choice formats is that question items, at the applied knowledge level, are challenging and time consuming to write (Epstein, 2007). The delivery of tests can be modified to drive learning in the direction of the curriculum. The progress test, where all learners sit the same knowledge test simultaneously regardless of the point in the course they have reached, is an example of this (Muijtjens et al, 1998). Progress testing sets out to monitor growth of knowledge over time.

Written knowledge tests

It is hypothesised that validity improves when students are asked to explore subjects in more depth. Difficulties arise with complex scenarios, such as ethical ones, which are highly relevant to clinical practice but lack a clear 'single best' answer. Writing options that are sufficiently homogeneous and do not 'cue' candidates towards the correct answer is difficult (Schuwirth and van der Vleuten, 2004). When developing new formats, one of the key aims has been to reduce cueing. Traditional essays are notoriously unreliable (Frijns et al, 1990). Structuring essays can both preclude cueing and engage more complex cognitive processes. In terms of utility, though, the gain on validity and educational impact of essays is offset by a loss of reliability. Breadth of content is reduced and inter-rater agreement can be poor unless

Table 14.3 Examples of assessment methods in common usage

Method	Area of enquiry	Advantages	Disadvantages
Written			
Multiple choice questions (MCQs): single best or extended matching	Knowledge	Valid – large content, reliable yet feasible	Hard to construct, can result in cueing (question leads to answer), cue answer often and hard to make clinically applicable
Key feature	Clinical reasoning, knowledge application	Combines problem-solving questions with computer marking	No evidence that performance in test correlates with performance in the workplace
Short answers	Problem solving, clinical reasoning	Assessment of problem solving such as clinical investigations	Reliability reliant on assessor interpretation
Essays	Synthesis and analytical skills	Assesses higher-order cognitive processes	Assessor dependent again, often little case sampling so rarely very reliable
Direct observations			
Objective structured clinical examination (OSCE)	Clinical skills, some attitudes, and behaviours	Can be focussed on desired educational outcomes, multiple tasks and assessors support reliability	Can be perceived as artificial with 'quick fire' stations, checklist approach often used for marking can discriminate against the more expert candidate who uses shortcuts
Oral examinations (vivas)	Knowledge and some clinical reasoning	Often in-depth discussions, which explore some subject matter well	In-depth but little breadth, rarely reliable as few cases and difficult to standardise marking
Case-focused assessments (mini-CEX, DOPS, etc.)	Clinical and communication skills	With real or simulated patients. Tests real interactions in a structured format with opportunity for feedback	Competence rather than performance – so best performance not necessarily everyday
Standardised patients	Procedural skills, behaviours and if 'mystery shopper' – performance	Realistic, assesses many areas simultaneously	Expensive to train and reaccredit high-standard patients
Multi-source feedback (MSF)			
Colleague feedback	Clinical and psychosocial skills	Multiple sources of assessment data, captures true performance data	Concerns about leniency bias, therefore, credibility
Patient feedback	Psychosocial skills	Appears one of the most important sources of feedback in medicine	Doubts about validity of feedback – patients rarely identify poor performance
Portfolios	Reflective practice, collation of assessment data from any or all other formats	May facilitate profiling of an individual from multiple sources of data	May distract from individual source measurement characteristics, time consuming, not a reliable form of assessment in its own right

examiner training is provided using detailed marking schedules. The process is time consuming. This threatens feasibility and acceptability.

Key-feature questions, developed to assess decision-making skills and avoid cueing, offer one of the better solutions (Farmer and Page, 2005). These require short 'uncued' answers to clinical scenarios but restrict the candidate's response to a predetermined number of key statements. That makes it possible to cover more contexts. Script-concordance items present a case (e.g. *vaginal discharge*), add a piece of clinical information (*dysuria*), and ask the student to assess the degree to which the new information alters the probability of a diagnosis or clinical outcome (*Chlamydia-related pelvic inflammatory disease*) (Charlin and van der Vleuten, 2004; Epstein, 2007). There is evidence that such questions provide some insight into practical clinical judgement (Brailovsky et al, 2001). Similarly, computer simulations can replace written scenarios and raise the level of clinical testing by sequentially adding information into a scenario (Cantillon et al, 2004). In the past, these simulations have been complicated. Dynamic and complex situations have been created which require large resources rarely available to those delivering clinical curricula. The need for short simulations, which both cover context specificity and stimulate rather than cue responses, remains a challenge for those developing computer formats.

Orals

The 'knows how' of ethical situations and attitudinal issues, the domain-independent skills we emphasised in relation to Miller's model (Figure 14.5), remains difficult to assess. Traditionally, orals were used (Wass et al, 2003b), predicated on the belief that face-to-face encounters are needed to assess the more domain-independent aspects of professional behaviour. Two recent reviews highlight the difficulties orals present (Davies and Karunathilake, 2005; Memon et al, 2009). Criticism centres on (i) the use of discourse, which can selectively disadvantage certain candidates (Roberts et al, 2000), (ii) the logistics of extending the process sufficiently to address context specificity (Wass et al, 2003b), and (iii) the 'halo' effect. The latter is important to assessment in general. Assessors, after making their first judgement, tend not to change their minds. If a candidate

performs poorly on the first question, then assessors carry this impression ('halo') forwards. Subsequent questions also tend to be judged unfavourably (Swanson, 1987). One of the most striking examples of assessment being poorly informed by evidence is the use of orals to make final pass/fail decisions for borderline candidates taking written tests. It is not rational to use an oral, one of the most unreliable assessment tools, to make a crucial pass/fail decision on a test that in actuality has much higher reliability. Fortunately, that practice is gradually changing. To address the intrinsic difficulties, orals (which many still believe to hold high validity in assessing professional behaviour) can be more reliable if short standardised questions and more examiners are used. Even then, achieving the level of reliability for high-stakes tests is not feasible, and linguistic disadvantage introduces unacceptable bias.

The assessment of 'shows how'

Long and short cases

The use of unstandardised real patients as 'long' or 'short' cases to test clinical skills was abandoned many years ago in North America. Change has been relatively slow elsewhere although the authenticity and reliability of this test format has been increasingly challenged. Traditionally, a single long case, where the candidate interviewed a patient for 30–60 minutes and then presented the case to examiners, was unobserved. Ironically, this actually assessed at a 'knows how' rather than 'shows how' level. In addition, given the context specificity of clinical skills, it is unacceptable to use a single case for a summative assessment. Yet, little published psychometric research on long cases has been published. Initial data (Figure 14.3) suggested that test length is again the key to increasing reliability (Wass et al, 2001a). Attempts have been made to improve the long case format. Observing interaction with patients, perhaps predictably, improves both its validity and the provision of feedback (Wass and Jolly, 2001). More structured long case formats have been developed. The Objective Structured Long Examination Record (OSLER) (Gleeson, 1994) and the Leicester Assessment package (Fraser et al, 1994) both include some direct assessor observation of candidates interviewing patients. Unless the format of long and short cases is improved by viewing candidate–patient interactions and test length is extended to include more cases, the unreliability of this traditional format does not justify its use as a summative tool. An unreliable test cannot be valid.

Objective structured clinical examinations

New methodology was needed. Harden and Gleeson (1979) conceptualised the OSCE in 1979. Candidates rotate through a series of 'stations' based on clinical competencies applied across a range of contexts. Skills can be integrated to different degrees within stations. Thus, OSCEs can be adapted as learners advance in their training. The format has become the mainstay of assessment at the level of 'shows how' in both undergraduate and postgraduate settings. It offers the capacity to modify both station length and complexity of task according to the level of expertise required. The wider sampling of cases and structured assessment format increase reliability. OSCEs are popular because they improve the balance between validity and reliability. They present a solution to measuring the complexity and integration of clinical competence at a 'shows how', rather than 'knows how', level. In terms of utility, however, there are drawbacks. The validity of OSCEs is open to challenge (Hodges, 2003). Firstly, with the demise of the long case, real patients have been increasingly replaced by standardised role players who simulate patients. Howley (2004) offers a review of the literature on their use. Learners interact with standardised patients (SP) previously trained to simulate a realistic clinical scenario with a predetermined emotional state. The assessee's performance is evaluated by the SP, or an observer, or both against the blueprinted competencies. Simulations are the norm in North America, where SPs are extensively trained to carry out the dual role of patient and assessor. This ensures the consistency and reproducibility of scenarios needed to achieve the level of reliability required by North American licensing tests (Colliver et al, 1989). For high-stakes examinations, the costs of training can be justified within the utility equation. This is arguably at the expense of validity. These highly trained 'assessor SPs' tend to become 'professional' rather than 'real' patients. Simulation of physical signs, such as skin rashes or hepatomegaly, is impossible. Real patients can be used where available. In the Western world, the logistics of doing that are becoming increasingly challenging (Sayer et al, 2002).

A second concern about the validity of OSCEs is that reducing integrated skills to checklist items on a mark sheet can impact on both assessees and assessors. Validity may be lost as complex skills, requiring an integrated professional judgement, become fragmented by the relatively short station length (generally 5–10 minutes). Candidate performance, if guided by rote learning rather than practice, can become unrealistic (Talbot, 2004). Experts, as discussed above, develop global pattern recognition. Examiners can find it difficult to work with itemised tasks (Hodges et al, 1999). Scoring against a checklist of items is not as objective as originally supposed. There is increasing evidence that global ratings, particularly by physicians, are as reliable as checklist formats (Regehr et al, 1998). Neither global nor checklist ratings offer a true 'gold standard' of judging performance. While checklists may not capture all aspects of physician–patient interactions, global ratings may be subject to other rater biases. Clinicians internalise different standards and approaches to practice. Extensive rater training is required to ensure consistency. An alternative approach excludes the assessor by using written information collected at 'post-encounter' stations. Candidates spend 5–7 minutes recording their findings from the SP encounter. It has been argued (Williams et al, 1999) that this approach yields similar data at both the item and test level and minimises some shortcomings of checklists. At some expense to validity, OSCEs have withstood the test of time and sufficiently balanced the challenges of utility at a 'shows how' assessment level. The setting, though, remains apart from the real world. As discussed above, assessment of competence at this simulated level does not necessarily predict actual performance. In an attempt to overcome this, there is a significant shift towards assessment in workplaces.

The assessment of 'does'

There have been significant advances over the last decade in workplace-based assessment (WBA) (Norcini and Burch, 2007), a change with potential for significant educational advantage. Increased curriculum integration encourages more contact with patients from the start of medical school. A patient-centred approach to care can improve health outcomes (Beck et al, 2002; Little et al, 2001). It makes sense to design test methodology to drive patient-centred learning and increase holistic understanding of patients' needs. To achieve this, assessment must emulate the reality of a patient's journey through the health services. We need to know how learners perform in the working world and not in a pre-planned controlled environment. At the same time, there is compelling evidence that giving formative feedback to learners, while assessing them in workplaces, can ultimately improve achievement (Norcini and Burch, 2007). Intrinsic to WBA is the need to embed multiple assessment tools in the curriculum and ensure that learners are assessed at the appropriate level of Miller's model. As the concept of in-training assessment programmes has evolved (van der Vleuten and Schuwirth, 2005), there has been reluctance in some arenas to conceptualise assessment instruments as part of an overall programme. Moving from individual assessment instruments to programmes has created new challenges that are only just beginning to be explored (Davies et al, 2009).

Interestingly, modifications of more traditional methods are coming to the fore. Assessment of clinical competencies in the UK Foundation postgraduation 2-year residency programme is entirely workplace-based. The methods used are, essentially, adaptations of the observed long case (*mini-CEX*), OSCE stations (*direct observation of procedures (DOPs)*), and an oral (*case-based discussion*) (Modernising Medical Careers, 2008). In a sense, there is a swing away from OSCEs back to more traditional methods modified to address context specificity, the issue which originally led to their demise. Most knowledge tests can be improved to test at the 'knows how' rather than 'knows' level within a traditional written paper format. It remains difficult, though, to assess synthesis and evaluation (Figure 14.1). WBAs, such as audit projects and portfolios, may well prove the answer to assessing a trainee's ability to apply knowledge at those higher levels of Bloom's hierarchy. With adequate sampling to cover a range of contexts, assessors, and methods, workplace assessment should theoretically be able to realise adequate reliability. Given the difficulties of standardising content and training assessors, it remains to be seen whether these methods can ever achieve more than medium-stakes reliability. Other biases such as score inflation due to the formative nature of the assessment are of concern (Govaerts et al, 2007).

Workplace-based assessment: methods

Norcini and Burch (2007) have reviewed current methodology. The mini-Clinical Evaluation Exercise (mini-CEX) provides feedback on clinical skills by observing part of an actual clinical encounter (Norcini et al, 2003). By taking a 'snapshot', it provides a window into a real consultation. The strength of the mini-CEX lies in its OSCE-style approach. Mini assessments should take place on different days with different assessors and in different contexts. That allows good case sampling and integrates short observation into normal working activities. Direct observation of procedural skills (DOPS) adopts a similar approach for the assessment of skills (Wilkinson et al, 2008). Case-based discussions, or chart-stimulated recall, assess doctors on patient records for whom they have been directly responsible. These are modified orals designed to assess clinical decision-making and patient management. Similar instruments are being developed, based on the same principle of direct observation in clinical settings; wards, outpatient clinics, or operating theatres. This is a time of development. The real challenges lie in combining the tools to achieve reliability while at the same time ensuring that the learners receive constructive formative feedback. In actuality, relative unstandardised approaches, failure to train assessors, and time restraints imposed by clinical practice impact on both (Wilkinson et al, 2008). An innovative approach and exploration of different methodologies is essential.

Direct observation has drawbacks. Observing learners may influence their performance (the Hawthorne effect). It is not a true assessment of actual performance (Hays et al, 2002). One logical step is to remove the rater from the room. That can be done covertly in the workplace to simulate performance (Gorter et al, 2001). Videoing events may offer advantages over direct assessment because both doctors and patients learn to ignore video equipment (Ram et al, 1999a). Video clips offer the additional benefit of creating examples of performance isolated from the event, which can be used to train assessors or rate the interaction independently. Learners can review their performance. Although widely adopted in primary care settings (Campbell and Murray, 1996; Ram et al, 1999a), logistics can be prohibitive (Hays et al, 2002).

Assessment of professionalism

Assessing professional behaviour has gained increasing attention in recent years (Ginsburg et al, 2000). Papadakis's et al (2005) research highlighted the importance of adding this dimension (Figure 14.5); she demonstrated that unprofessional behaviour as a medical student may predict subsequent poor performance in independent practice. David Stern's book *Measuring Medical Professionalism* (see Further reading) reviews the complexity of this area of assessment extensively. In the workplace, multi-source feedback (MSF) methodology, derived from the literature on organisations (Bracken et al, 2001), is now extensively employed. Direct feedback of an individual's professional behaviour is gained from colleagues. Its popularity arises from the belief that MSF is one of the few methods to assess professionalism and psycho-social skills. Online administration makes it relatively easy to administer. The collation of colleagues' views provides a reliable series of scores across a number of domains, which can be compared with self-assessment (Archer et al, 2005).

Patient feedback

Another approach centres on the direct involvement of patients. When assessing clinicians, it seems logical to include patients' views. Patient satisfaction surveys must not be confused with patient feedback. In the latter, patients are asked to comment on a series of high-level competencies, such as clinical care and professionalism. These methods are increasingly used around the world, often in high-stakes situations. The evidence for their robustness is mixed. Patients' scores correlate poorly with ratings on professional behaviour obtained from work colleagues. They rarely highlight dissatisfaction with their doctors (Crossley et al, 2008) even though colleagues have raised serious concerns (Archer and McAvoy, 2009). Patients may assess professionalism differently from clinical colleagues, although, given the strong similarities of the questions being asked of both, this seems unlikely (Campbell et al, 2008). Politically, it is hard to argue that patients should be excluded from assessing their own doctors. Current methodologies suggest they are either being asked the wrong questions or are not empowered to answer honestly.

Self-assessment and self-monitoring

Most studies define self-assessment as an individual's ability to identify their own strengths and weaknesses compared to those perceived by others. It has long been hypothesised that engaging the learner in self-assessment places them at the centre of the process. More reliance on self-assessment should theoretically increase the educational impact. Yet, evidence suggests the process is poor (Ward et al, 2002). It is

informed by culture and gender rather than a shared reality. Self-assessment appears to be methodologically flawed (Eva and Regehr, 2005). Social psychologists view our behaviour and performance as shaped by our unconscious minds (Bargh, 1999). These are self-serving, primarily focusing on self-preservation. For example, when learners are given negative feedback, they blame external factors and distance themselves from any personal responsibility (Alimo-Metcalfe, 1998). Self-assessment must currently be viewed with caution as an assessment tool.

Self-assessment should not be confused with self-monitoring and reflection. Self-monitoring is the ability to respond to situations shaped by our own capability in a particular context. Reflection, often used interchangeably with self-assessment, represents a very different and important concept. It is a conscious and deliberate process focusing on understanding events and processes to bring about self-improvement (Mann et al, 2009), discussed in more detail in Chapter 2. Reflection is clearly important and may be part of self-monitoring (Eva and Regehr, 2005). Yet, although intuitive, there is little evidence that we achieve a better understanding of ourselves through reflection (Mann et al, 2009). Learners should seek the views of others external to themselves (Eva and Regehr, 2007), which places even greater emphasis on delivering high-quality assessments to ensure valid and reliable feedback is delivered and learners are appropriately supported (Archer, 2010).

These important concepts remain central to our ability to learn from external feedback on assessment performance. Eva and Regehr argue that the 'health professional community should predominantly be concerned with identifying contextual factors that influence self monitoring behaviours in the moment of action rather than worrying about the accuracy of generic and broader self assessments of ability' (Eva and Regehr, 2007). This is not to say all individuals respond to feedback in the same way. Individual receptiveness is complex and related to self-awareness, demographic similarity, and acquaintance, and it appears to fall with age (Archer, 2010). A better understanding of these concepts is required if we are to harness successfully the formative feedback, which external assessment offers learners.

Portfolios

One approach to self-monitoring within assessment programmes has been the introduction of portfolios. Broadly defined as a tool for gathering evidence and a vehicle for reflective practice, a wider understanding is developing of portfolios' potential use in assessment. Portfolios include documentation of, and reflection on, a learner's personal professional journey. Validity is added to formative assessment. This must be weighed against reliability for summative purposes (Driessen et al, 2005). A recent literature review suggests that these difficulties may not be insuperable (Driessen et al, 2007). The learning portfolio for the UK Foundation Programme provides an interesting example (Modernising Medical Careers, 2008). We need more evidence of its efficacy as an assessment tool. Portfolios have the potential to support reflection. They provide a unique source of evidence to help us understand learners. For portfolios to be effective, though, mentoring is essential to ensure learners reflect constructively on their experience. Without that, the formative role of a portfolio is threatened. The topic of portfolio learning, reflection, and mentoring is also discussed in Chapter 13.

Evaluating assessments: quality assurance

Any attempt at assessing performance has to balance validity and reliability, which makes compromise inevitable. Decisions need to be carefully weighed in relation to the purpose and context of both individual assessments and the assessment programme as a whole. One may, for example, choose a method with lower reliability to accentuate the effect on learning or perhaps even because stakeholders find it acceptable. That may be defensible if the method chosen is only a small part of a total assessment programme. Other, more reliable tests should also be included. The overall programme may contain any method, whether traditional or modern, depending on its stated purpose. This must meet a range of quality criteria in addition to those mentioned in the utility formula (Baartman et al, 2006). Table 14.4 summarises the steps intrinsic to quality assuring

Table 14.4 Ten principle steps for the design and quality assurance of an assessment programme

	Principle	Step
1	Define the purpose of the test	Clarity and transparency of purpose from the start are essential. Use assessment to 'mirror' and 'drive' the educational outcomes of the training programme
2	Select the overarching competency structure	Define the learning outcomes you aim to assess over the training period. At which level: knowledge, competence, or performance?
3	Define the longitudinal novice-to-expert pathway	The programme design should include longitudinal assessment elements and acknowledge the development of expertise across training. At what level on the novice-to-expert scale are you testing?
4	Design a blueprint	Map the competencies being tested against the curriculum: blueprint to ensure the design is comprehensive and reflects the philosophy of the curriculum
5	Balance formative and summative feedback	A balance is essential between formative and summative assessment. We need more evidence on how to achieve this within assessment programmes
6	Choose appropriate tools	Apply the 'utility equation' (see text) to determine which tests to use and when
7	Involve stakeholders	Ensure stakeholders (trainers, trainees, managers, patients) are actively involved in designing and evaluating the programme
8	Aggregation/triangulation	Judgements of overall performance must be based on aggregated multiple sources of information and triangulation of findings
9	Programme evaluation	There must be systematic attention to feedback, both quantitative and qualitative
10	Quality assurance (of test design and administration)	The assessment programme must be continuously monitored and adjusted to ensure constructive alignment with the curriculum and its impact on learning

Modified from Baartman et al (2006).

assessment programmes (Wass and van der Vleuten, 2006).

Even in well-constructed assessment packages, there are still compromises to be made (van der Vleuten and Schuwirth, 2005). Robust programmes cannot be constructed if they contain poor component parts that fail to stand up to individual scrutiny. Combining the performance of individual components to estimate overall composite reliability, as with the battery of tests used in the past for clinical examinations (Wass et al, 2001b), presents a psychometric challenge as yet unanswered (Davies et al, 2009). One approach is to screen for poor performance and only offer additional assessment methods to struggling trainees. The alternative is a comprehensive assessment programme for all. Each approach has the same important principle at its core. To gain a true reflection of an individual's ability, sampling across performance in terms of domains, contexts, timelines, and methods is fundamental to success.

Setting standards

Quality inferences about, and expectations of, levels of performance are critical to any assessment. Well-defined and transparent procedures must be set in place to achieve that. When assessment is used for summative purposes, a defensible pass/fail level must be agreed. In reality, there are no hard and fast scientific parameters for achieving one. It is essential that people setting standards are well acquainted with the learners and the expectations of the curriculum. At the same time, learners must fully understand what is expected of them. Various methods are available to support the process. It has to be acknowledged that there are no gold standards. The standard setting process should be viewed as a triangulation of methodologies to justify and defend the parameters being set. It cannot occur in isolation. Final decisions are inevitably informed partly by prior knowledge of the programme and learners and, unavoidably at times, by political influences. We offer guidelines for the methods available.

Criterion referencing

Comparison of performance with peers – that is, *norm referencing* – is used in examination procedures where a specified number of candidates are required to pass. Performance is described relative to the positions of other candidates. A fixed percentage, for example, all candidates one standard deviation below the mean, always fails. Any variation in difficulty of the test is compensated for. In contrast, variations in the ability of cohorts sitting the test are not accounted for. If the group is above average in ability, those who might have passed in a poorer cohort will fail. This is clearly unacceptable for clinical competency licensing tests, which aim to ensure that candidates are safe to practise. If all trainees meet the standard, then a pass rate of 100% should be achievable. A clear standard, below which doctors would not be considered 'fit to practise' needs to be defined. Such standards are set by *criterion referencing*, where the minimum standard acceptable is agreed. The reverse problem now faces assessors. Although differences in candidate ability are accounted for, variation in test difficulty becomes the key issue. Standards should be set for each test, item by item. Various methods have been developed to do this: 'Angoff', 'Ebel', 'Hofstee', and 'Contrasting method'. Cusimano (1996), Norcini (2003), and Champlain (2004) offer comprehensive reviews of these methodologies, which can be time consuming but are essential. They permit the setting of a pass/fail cut score prior to and independent of the actual test results. The outcome can then be cross-referenced with this standard and adjustments made (see below) for measurement error. A final decision on the pass/fail score is then reached. The process enables a group of stakeholders (not just assessors) to participate. Lay people can be involved in the setting of standards for health care, a principle that increasingly mirrors the educational philosophy of patient-centred practice (Southgate and Grant, 2004).

More recently, methodology has been introduced using the examiner cohort itself to set the standard during assessments. Examiners, after assessing a candidate, indicate which students they judge to be borderline. The mean mark across all examiners (and there is invariably a range) is taken as the pass/fail cut off (Wilkinson et al, 2001). The robustness of this method across different cohort of examiners remains to be seen (Downing et al, 2003c). Recently, this borderline method has been extended to more reliable regression techniques that are very suitable for application to OSCEs (Kramer et al, 2003). This method is proving useful. Inevitably, as examiner cohorts change, conceptions of borderline will change too. It is important to train assessors before standard setting procedures to achieve consensus on borderline 'just competent' performance. The concept can be difficult to internalise but, unless this is achieved, borderline standards may vary with different assessor groups. Selection of methodology will depend on available resources, the consequences of misclassifying examinees, and decisions involving stakeholders. Standard setting is best viewed as an art rather than a science. Using more than one method triangulates opinions and informs final decisions. Unfortunately, learners do not fall neatly into competent and incompetent groups. The pass/fail score has to be agreed within a continuum of performance. The standard setting process inevitably involves error and uncertainty. That makes it even more crucial to create a transparent process, which ensures that the final decision is accountable and defensible. It must not be capricious.

Measuring validity

As discussed above, validity is a complex and fluid concept. Assessment methods are never valid or invalid. Assessors must collate evidence and build a case for validity. Traditionally, to help build a framework for achieving this, a range of 'facets' was identified (Table 14.2). These acknowledge that appraising the validity of a test requires multiple sources of evidence (Wass and van der Vleuten, 2006). Many educators still refer to these. 'Face' validity represents an overview of the assessment measuring whether the educational intentions have been honoured. 'Content' validity requires analysis of whether subject matter has been comprehensively covered. It is also important to evaluate whether the test was appropriate to learners' level of expertise. That is termed 'construct validity'. These three facets of validity are relatively easy to evaluate. 'Predictive validity' is more challenging. This requires longitudinal follow-up to measure whether trainees' subsequent clinical performance correlates positively with their previous assessment grades: that is, do the top scoring candidates on knowledge tests subsequently do best in the health care arena? There is some evidence, for example, that UK school 'A' level grades are the best predictors of subsequent postgraduate performance (McManus et al, 2003). Finally, to ensure emphasis is placed on the educational impact of assessment, the consequences of the test, 'consequential validity', should be appraised (Wass and van der Vleuten, 2006). 'Does the test produce the desired educational outcome?' is an important question to ask of any assessment.

This initial, rather pragmatist view of validity has changed. In its contemporary conceptualisation, one unitary concept, 'construct validity', is offered (Downing, 2003b). We believe that this redefining of validity is essential to the development of new assessment methodology. The single term embraces the multiple sources of evidence (Table 14.5) needed

Table 14.5 Sources of evidence for measuring validity

Source of evidence	Type of evidence	Conclusions sought
Content	Map the assessment against the test specification or blueprint	Have the intended learning outcomes been adequately covered in sufficient contexts?
Response process	Scrutinise the integrity of the data: evaluate test material, accuracy of judgements, quality of simulation, etc.	Have all the sources of error associated with the test administration been controlled or eliminated as far as is possible?
Internal structure	Assess available statistical or psychometric evidence	How well did the examination questions perform: discrimination, reproducibility, and generalisability? Did items intended to measure the same variables within the test correlate well or not?
Relationship to other variables	Seek confirmatory evidence to prove the test is measuring what was intended by comparing with previous assessments?	How do the results converge or diverge with performance on other tests? Positive correlations confirm similar and negatives ones different abilities
Consequences	Investigate the consequences of the test	What evidence is there that the outcomes of the test benefited or harmed the candidate?

Adapted form Downing (2003b).

to evaluate and interpret the outcomes of an assessment. It enables us to move away from the traditional individual descriptive 'facets' outlined above and focus more on the sources of evidence needed to validate an assessment process. Five sources of evidence have been identified (Downing, 2003b), which can be used to support or refute the validity of assessment outcomes (Table 14.5). By weighing evidence from both score measurements and quality assurance processes, a more logical, theoretically based, and defensible conclusion can be drawn about whether the original 'hypothetical' intentions have been met or not. The context of an assessment, that is, whether it is a 'high-stakes' summative or a 'low-stakes' more formative process, is also integral to any final conclusions on test validity. Scrutinising assessments against this framework (Table 14.5) offers a useful approach to evaluating validity. Intrinsic to this lies the reality, emphasised above, that quality data are needed to evaluate validity. The integrity of the results (response process), performance of test items (internal structure), and correlations with other test outcomes are all concrete measurements that should be robust. The process loses all value if the test data itself has not reliably ranked candidate performance. A test cannot be valid unless it is also reliable.

Measuring reliability

Reliability has been defined as the reproducibility of assessment data or scores, over time or occasions (Downing, 2004). We have chosen briefly to outline three approaches to measuring test reproducibility: internal consistency, classical theory, and generalisability (G) theory. References are given for further detailed reading. A plea for different psychometric approaches, which depend less on these rather reductionist measurement of reliability and validity, has been made (Schuwirth and van der Vleuten, 2006). Currently, though, generalisability theory remains the gold standard (Brennan, 2001).

Internal consistency

Internal consistency is based on the concept of 'test–retesting'. This assumes an ideal situation where a repeat test offered to the same group of learners results in 100% reproducibility; that is, candidate performance on the two tests correlates with a coefficient of 1.0. As already discussed, that is never achieved. There are inevitable sources of variance. Cronbach

and Shavelson (2004) developed a statistical method to measure internal consistency within a single test: 'Cronbach alpha'. Statistically, the test is split into two and candidate ranking across the two halves are analysed. The method is dependent on the homogeneity of the test material. Both halves of the test should be measuring identical clinical constructs. All candidates must have answered the same questions to ensure that significant sources of variance are eliminated. Cronbach's alpha can be used to measure consistency within items, agreement between raters, internal agreement of rating scales, and the stability of scores on multiple occasions. It is of limited value in more complex assessments where inter-case and inter-rater consistencies present a significant source of error variance.

Classical test theory

Classical test theory assumes that each learner has a true score ('the signal') that would be obtained if there were no errors in measurement attributable to external factors ('the noise'). In reality, as discussed, there is always some variance or 'noise' attributable to examiner performance, conditions of testing, etc. A true score is a learner's average score if measured an infinitely large number of times, when all measurements are independent and stable across different observers and situations. The difference between the observed score and the learner's true score is the measurement error. The candidate score on any test inevitably does not totally reflect their true ability. The difference between the true score and the observed score is the result of errors in measurement.

$$\text{Observed score} = \text{True score} + \text{Error}$$

Classical test theory can only estimate reliability by evaluating one source of potential error at a time. It rests on a 'crossed test' design. Learners' scores are measured against a single source of error; for example, 'the test item'. The learners must all take identical test items. This has significant limitations:

Case specificity

As already discussed, competency is context-specific. One case does not generalise to another. Classical test theory cannot be applied to tests, such as traditional vivas or long cases, where the cohort of candidates have not been assessed on the same questions under the same conditions. Even when identical cases are used, as in OSCEs, failure to standardise patients or role play to ensure identical conditions can result in significant error variance.

Inter-rater reliability

Observers often vary in their interpretation of an assessment even when assessing a learner simultaneously. Inter-rater differences can cause significant error variance. Assessor performance needs to be monitored and training is essential. It helps to build a common understanding of the process and the standard expected. However, there is limited evidence that training assessors effectively reduces inter-rater variance (van der Vleuten and Swanson, 1990).

Intra-rater reliability

Assessors do not necessarily rate consistently. Checklists have evolved in an attempt to reduce this error although evidence now shows that global ratings may be more reliable than checklists (Reznick et al, 1998). Reliability is expressed as a coefficient that represents the proportion of true to error variance:

$$\text{Reliability}(R) = \text{True variance}/(\text{True variance} + \text{Error variance})$$

An example of a fully crossed design is when all candidates take the same written paper, which is marked by the same examiner. There are two potential sources of error: (1) test items; (2) examiner ratings. Only two facets are calculable using classical test theory; candidate ability (true variance) and examination items (error variance) In reality, the additional error of examiner inconsistency (*intra-rater error*) cannot be measured (Figure 14.6).

Standard error of the measurement

Reliability, the probability that an identical pass/fail decision will be made on retesting, is reported in these studies as a coefficient between 0 and 1. A coefficient of 1 represents 100% reliability; in reality, never achieved. The level to aim for is debatable

(Downing, 2004). In 'high-stakes' testing, where important progression decisions need to be made, setting robust reliability is essential to achieve defensible pass/fail decisions on assessment scores. At a minimum, coefficients of 0.8–0.89 should be aimed for (Downing, 2004). If the stakes are less high, then lower levels are acceptable although less confident and subsequently less defensible. It is increasingly accepted that the precision of measurement – that is, 95% confidence limits – must be defined by applying the standard error of measurement (SEM) at the cut score. The square root of the measurement error ($\sqrt{\text{measurement error}}$) constitutes the SEM. Ninety-five percent confidence intervals are determined by the SEM multiplied by 1.96. Cronbach and Shavelson (2004) ultimately argued that reliability coefficients are more honestly and usefully expressed as confidence limits. When using test–retest theory, this requires a correction for the spread of scores:

$$\text{SEM} = \text{Standard deviation of scores}\sqrt{1 - \text{Cronbach alpha}}$$

By applying confidence limits to pass/fail scores, as determined by standard setting procedures, decisions become more defensible. Raising the agreed cutoff scores by two standard errors of measurement assures 95% confidence that all passing candidates would still be judged competent if retested. The pass/fail score can be adjusted according to the level of confidence required. Using standard errors of measurement, learners can be evaluated in terms of their proximity to the pass mark. Those approaching the pass score will increasingly have confidence intervals that cross it. There is uncertainty about their accurate placement on the one side or the other of the pass mark. More data on their performance needs to be accrued. This is good educational practice. Identifying and understanding the needs of individuals who are potentially struggling is clearly beneficial.

Generalisability (G) theory

Generalisability (G) theory is an extension of classical test theory designed to overcome these limitations in measuring error variance. It enables several sources of variance error within a test; for example, cases, assessors, and candidates to be quantified individually (Brennan, 2001). A 'nested' rather than 'crossed' assessment design is used. The candidate score is taken as the main facet and analysed individually against each potential source of variance. A single OSCE case can be 'nested' within a rater who sits

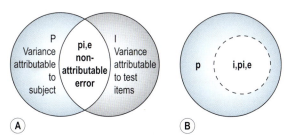

Figure 14.6 • A. Variance in crossed design, p = true variance, i = item variance, pi,e = un-attributable (error). B. Variance in nested design, p = true variance, i,pi,e = un-attributable (error).

at one OSCE station throughout the examination. By maintaining the rater and the station as a constant, the variance attributable to the candidate can be estimated. All other variance remains as unattributable error. To assess variance due to assessor ratings, two assessors would need to be nested within a single OSCE station throughout the examination. By keeping the item constant, the impact on candidate score of assessor ratings (inter-rater error) can be estimated. From the variance components, a G coefficient can be calculated, using the same classical test formula:

$$\text{Reliability}(R) = \text{True variance}/(\text{True variance} + \text{each error variance source})$$

Generalisability theory integrates the discriminating ability of the test and the reproducibility of the result. The coefficient will always be lower than with the classical approach as it takes into account all possible sources of error simultaneously.

Decision (D) studies

The generalisability coefficient is an estimate based on the actual assessment data from which it is formulated. It is also possible to predict test reliability if one of the facets were to be theoretically changed; for example, if the number of cases or number of raters (or indeed both) were to be increased. Decision studies use statistical modelling to modify assessment designs to improve reliability. Generalisability theory was employed in this way, for example, to predict OSCE reliability for a varying number of stations and raters in the example offered previously in this chapter (Figure 14.3). Such predictions can be used to inform the design of future assessments modifying test length, number of items or assessors to identify combinations that achieve acceptable levels of reliability. Although generalisability and decision studies are powerful, prediction does not replace measurement. Decision studies rely on the data presented to them. Modelling assumes that any new sample of subjects, assessors, and items is identical. It is always good practice to re-evaluate reliability.

Item response theory

Classical and generalisability test theories are sample-dependent. They centre on candidate scores. Assessment of item performance is always confounded by the characteristics of subjects taking the items at that point in time. Yet, for test design, it is important to isolate the performance of items *per se*, for example, level of difficulty, to both understand their individual properties and apply items independently of a particular cohort of examinees. This theoretical approach allows error variance due to candidate cohort ability to be excluded. Only then can items stand alone. A constant independent measurement scale for items can be generated. This permits both scaling of difficulty and legitimate comparison of performance; for example, of changes in student ability if they take the item sequentially over time. Three common item response theory models exist and are reviewed by Downing (2003a). Although technically difficult to apply, awareness of this model is important to understand computer-adaptive testing where the candidate follows a testing pathway determined by their personal capability. The theory can also be used for adjusting rater error in clinical performance assessments.

Future challenges in assessment: implications for practice

The tensions between an educationally formative approach to assessment and the summative stance needed to protect the public from doctors who are unfit to practise continue to dominate the assessment of clinical learners. There are several domains in which assessment is in its infancy and remains a challenge for development and improvement. Setting national standards through a National Licensing Examination is established practice in North America but remains a continuing source of debate elsewhere (Archer, 2009). With increasing globalisation and movement of the medical workforce, international standards should, arguably, be considered to ease migration. Yet, there are concerns in the United Kingdom that, where there is no national licensing system, standards at graduation may differ across medical schools within a single country alone (Boursicot et al, 2006). Opponents argue that standardising exit assessment from medical schools leads to a lack of diversity in curricula and their delivery, preventing innovation. Because of the limitations of assessment methodology, a national examination will focus on lower levels of Miller's triangle. Doctors and medical schools may be ranked unfairly as actual performance will not be addressed. North American experience, on the other hand, demonstrates that a national licensing test can predict poor performance (Tamblyn et al, 2007). The debate continues, dominated by a concern that a summative end point to medical education will stifle formative development.

Workplace-based assessment remains in its infancy. We are still searching for effective measures of attitudinal behaviours. Experts find it difficult to agree on the definition of professionalism, let alone how to measure it. Of the numerous scales designed to rate communication, there is little evidence that any one is better than another. Patient ratings of professionalism can differ considerably from those given by experts. Quality of care and patient safety depend on effective inter-professional teamwork. There is no validated method of assessing this. There is some early evidence that MSF can identify poor performance. Patient feedback, though, does not appear to discriminate. At the same time, research is focusing on the complexities of self versus peer assessment. The use of multiple methods of assessment can overcome many of the limitations of individual test formats. We need a better understanding of how learners and assessors achieve their professional judgements. The difficulties intrinsic to the imposition of summative progression decisions on a formative process remain unresolved.

Longitudinal assessment avoids excessive testing at any one point in time. It serves as a foundation for monitoring professional development. The collation of results into a portfolio resembles the art of diagnosis; it demands that learners synthesise a varied range of information to establish an overall picture. This is ideal for appraisal, but as discussed, raises important concerns if used for revalidation. We need a better understanding of the emerging evidence that knowledge *per se* can deteriorate as expertise develops. Clinical expertise implies practical wisdom. Experience enables doctors to manage ambiguous unstructured problems, balance competing explanations, avoid premature closure, and note exceptions to rules and principles. Even under stress, they have the skills to risk decisions that are acceptable but imperfect. Testing either inductive or deductive thinking in situations where there is no consensus on the correct answer presents formidable psychometric challenges. New approaches to combining qualitative and quantitative data on expertise are required if portfolio assessments are to be widely applied and withstand the test of time. Proposals to base revalidation on appraisal lack evidence for its efficacy as a summative tool. Whether formative confidential processes can effectively and fairly assume the summative function of licensing to practise is highly debatable, an issue as yet unresolved.

The direction of travel is, we believe, justified. Assessment must adopt a more formative educational approach. At the same time, new methods and programmes must demonstrate reliability as well as validity. Critics argue that WBA performance judgements lack the robustness needed to make decisions on progression. Yet it is logical to identify trainees in difficulty early to offer more formative support and ensure they progress. A change in the culture of assessment is essential to instil a new assessment ethos in educational supervision. Inevitably, that will take time. A greater understanding of the psychometrics of these novel assessment programmes must be the focus of future research.

References

Alimo-Metcalfe B: Professional forum: 360° feedback and leadership development, *Int J Select Assess* 6:35–42, 1998.

Archer JC: European licensing examinations – the only way forward, *Med Teacher* 31:215–216, 2009.

Archer JC: State of the science in health professional education: effective feedback, *Med Educ* 44:101–108, 2010.

Archer J, McAvoy P: Multi source feedback in high stakes assessment. International physicians assessment coalition, Quebec, Canada, Abstract only. Available at: http://www.ozzawa13.com/OZZAWA%20Abstracts%20and%20Posters.pdf. Accessed December, 2009.

Archer JC, Norcini J, Davies HA: Use of SPRAT for peer review of paediatricians in training, *BMJ* 330:1251–1253, 2005.

Baartman LKJ, Bastiaens TJ, Kirschner PA, et al: The wheel of competency assessment: presenting quality criteria for competency assessment programmes, *Stud Educ Eval* 32:153–177, 2006.

Bargh JA: The unbearable automaticity of being, *Am Psych* 54:462–479, 1999.

Beck RS, Daughtridge R, Sloane PD: Physician–patient communication in the primary care office: a systematic review, *J Am Board Fam Pract* 15:25–38, 2002.

Bloom BS: *Taxonomy of educational objectives*, London, 1965, Longman.

Boursicot KM, Roberts TE, Pell G: Standard setting for clinical competence at graduation from medical school: a comparison of passing scores across five medical schools, *Adv Health Sci Educ* 11:173–183, 2006.

Boursicot KAM, Roberts TE, Burdick WP: *Structured assessments of clinical competence*, Edinburgh, 2007, ASME Education.

Bracken DW, Timmreck CW, Church AH: *The handbook of multisource feedback: The comprehensive resource for designing and implementing MSF processes*, San Francisco, CA, 2001, Jossey-Bass.

Brailovsky C, Charlin B, Beausoleil S, et al: Measurement of clinical reflective capacity early in training as a predictor of clinical reasoning performance at the end of residency: an experimental study on the script concordance test, *Med Educ* 35:430–436, 2001.

Brennan RL: *Generalizability theory*, New York, 2001, Springer-Verlag.

Campbell LM, Murray TM: The effects of the introduction of a system of mandatory formative assessment for general practice trainees, *Med Educ* 30:60–64, 1996.

Campbell JL, Richards SH, Dickens A, et al: Assessing the professional performance of UK doctors: an evaluation of the utility of the General Medical Council patient and colleague questionnaires, *Qual Safe Health Care* 17:187–193, 2008.

Cantillon P, Irish B, Sales D: Using computers for assessment in medicine, *BMJ* 329:606–609, 2004.

Champlain de A: Ensuring the competent are truly competent: an overview of common methods and procedures used to set standards on high stakes examinations, *J Vet Med Educ* 31:62–66, 2004.

Charlin B, van der Vleuten CPM: Standardised assessment of reasoning in contexts of uncertainty: the Script Concordance Approach, *Eval Health Prof* 27:304–319, 2004.

Choudhry NK, Fletcher RH, Soumerai SB: Systematic review: the relationship between clinical experience and the quality of health care, *Ann Int Med* 142:260–273, 2005.

Colliver JA, Verhulst SJ, Williams RG, et al: Reliability of performance on standardised patient cases: a comparison of consistency measures based on generalizability theory, *Teach Learn Med* 1:31–37, 1989.

Cronbach LSR, Shavelson RJ: My current thoughts on coefficient alpha and successor procedures, *Educ Psychol Meas* 64:391–418, 2004.

Crossley J, Davies H, Cooper C, et al: A district hospital assessing its doctors for re-licensure: can it work? *Med Educ* 42:359–363, 2008.

Cusimano MD: Standard setting in medical education, *Acad Med* 71 (Suppl):S112–S120, 1996.

Davis M, Karunathilake I: The place of the oral examination in today's assessment systems, *Med Teach* 27:294–297, 2005.

Davies H, Archer J, Southgate L, et al: Initial evaluation of the first year of the Foundation Assessment Programme, *Med Educ* 43:74–81, 2009.

Downing SM: Item response theory: applications of modern test theory in medical education, *Med Educ* 37:739–745, 2003a.

Downing SM: Validity: on the meaningful interpretation of assessment data, *Med Educ* 37:830–837, 2003b.

Downing SM: Reliability: on the reproducibility of assessment data, *Med Educ* 38:1006–1012, 2004.

Downing SM, Lieska GN, Raible MD: Establishing passing standards for classroom achievement tests in medical education: a comparative study of four methods, *Acad Med* 78: S85–S87, 2003.

Dreyfus HL, Dreyfus SE: Putting computers in their proper place: analysis versus intuition in the classroom. In Sloan D, editor: *The computer in education: a critical perspective*, Columbia, NY, 1984, Teachers' College Press.

Dreyfus HL, Dreyfus SE: *The power of human intuition and expertise in the era of the computer*, New York, 1986, Free Press.

Dreyfus SE: Four models v human situational understanding: inherent limitations on the modelling of business expertise USAF, *Office Sci Res*, 1981, ref F49620-79-C-63.

Driessen EW, Tartwijk van J, Overeem K, et al: Conditions for successful reflective use of portfolios in undergraduate, *Med Educ* 39:1221–1229, 2005.

Driessen E, Tartwijk J, van der Vleuten CPM, et al: Portfolios in

medical education: why do they meet with mixed success? A systematic review, *Med Educ* 41:1224–1233, 2007.

Epstein RM: Assessment in medical education, *N Eng J Med* 356:387–396, 2007.

Eraut M: *Developing professional knowledge and competence*, London, 1994, Falmer.

Eva KW, Regehr G: Self assessment in the health professions: a reformulation and research agenda, *Acad Med* 80:S46–S54, 2005.

Eva KW, Regehr G: Knowing when to look it up: a new conception of self-assessment ability, *Acad Med* 82 (S10):S81–S84, 2007.

Farmer EA, Page G: A practical guide to assessing clinical decision-making skills using the key features approach, *Med Educ* 39:1188–1194, 2005.

Flexner A: *Medical education in the United States and Canada*, New York, 1910, Carnegie Foundation for the Advancement of Teaching.

Fraser R, McKinley R, Mulholland H: Consultation competence in general practice: establishing the face validity of prioritised criteria in the Leicester assessment package, *Br J Gen Pract* 44:109–113, 1994.

Frijns PHAM, van der Vleuten CPM, Verwijnen GM, et al: The effect of structure in scoring methods on the reproducibility of tests using open ended questions. In Bender W, Hiemstra RJ, Scherbier AJJA, Zwierstra RP, editors: *Teaching and assessing clinical competence*, Gromingen, 1990, Boekwerk, pp 466–471.

Ginsburg S, Regehr G, Hatala R, et al: Context, conflict, and resolution: a new conceptual framework for evaluating professionalism, *Acad Med* 75(10 Suppl):S6–S11, 2000.

Gleeson F: The effect of immediate feedback on clinical skills using the OSLER. In Rothman AI, Cohen R, editors: *Proceedings of the Sixth Ottawa Conference of Medical Education*, Toronto, 1994, University of Toronto Bookstore Custom Publishing, pp 412–415.

Gorter SL, Rethans JJ, Scherpbier AJJA, et al: How to introduce incognito standardized patients into outpatient clinics of specialists in rheumatology, *Med Teach* 23:138–144, 2001.

Govaerts MJ, van der Vleuten CPM, Schuwirth LW, et al: Broadening perspectives on clinical performance assessment: rethinking the nature of in-training assessment, *Adv Health Sci Educ Theory Pract* 12:239–260, 2007.

Harden RM, Gleeson FA: Assessment of medical competence using an objective structured clinical examination (OSCE), *J Med Educ* 13:41–54, 1979.

Hays RB, Davies HA, Beard JD, et al: Selecting performance assessment methods for experienced physicians, *Med Educ* 36:910–917, 2002.

Hodges B: Validity and the OSCE, *Med Teach* 25:250–254, 2003.

Hodges B: Medical education and the maintenance of incompetence, *Med Teach* 28:690–696, 2006.

Hodges B, Regehr G, McNaughton N, et al: OSCE lists do not capture increasing levels of expertise, *Acad Med* 74:1129–1134, 1999.

Howley LD: Performance assessment in medical education: where we've been and where we're going, *Eval Health Prof* 27:285–303, 2004.

Jamtvedt G, Young JM, Kristoffersen DT, et al: Audit and feedback: effects on professional practice on health care outcomes, *Cochrane Libr* 1–31, 2003.

Kramer A, Muijtjens A, Jansen K, et al: Comparison of a rational and an empirical standard setting procedure for an OSCE. Objective structured clinical examinations, *Med Educ* 37:132–139, 2003.

Lave J, Wenger E: *Situated learning. Legitimate peripheral participation*, Cambridge, 1991, Cambridge University Press, 1991.

Little P, Everitt H, Williamson I, et al: Observational study of effect of patient centeredness and positive approach on outcomes of general practice consultations, *BMJ* 323:908–911, 2001.

McManus IC, Smithers E, Partridge P, et al: A levels and intelligence as predictors of medical careers in UK doctors: 20 year prospective study, *BMJ* 327:139–142, 2003.

Mann K, Gordon J, Macleod A: Reflection and reflective practice in health professions education: systematic review, *Adv Health Sci Educ* 14:595–621, 2009.

Memon MA, Joughin GR, Memon B: Oral assessment and postgraduate medical examinations: establishing conditions for validity, reliability and fairness, *Adv Health Sci Educ*, 2009 doi:10.1007/s10459-008-9111-9.

Messick S: Validity. In Linn RL, editor: *Educational measurement*, ed 3, Washington, DC, 1989, American Council on Education Macmillan, pp 13–104.

Miller GE: The assessment of clinical skills/competence/performance, *Acad Med* 65:S63–S67, 1990.

Modernising Medical Careers: 2008, Available at: http://www. foundationprogramme.nhs.uk/pages/ home/training-and-assessment. Accessed December 2009.

Muijtjens AM, Hoogenboom RJ, Verwijnen GM, et al: Relative or absolute standards in assessing medical knowledge using progress tests, *Adv Health Sci Educ* 3:81–87, 1998.

Newble DI, Swanson DB: Psychometric characteristics of the objective structured clinical examination, *Med Educ* 22:325–334, 1996.

Norcini JJ: Setting standards on educational tests, *Med Educ* 37:464–469, 2003.

Norcini JJ, Burch V: Workplace-based assessment as an educational tool. AMEE Guide No. 31, *Med Teach* 29:855–871, 2007.

Norcini JJ, Swanson DB, Grosso LJ, et al: Reliability, validity and efficiency of multiple choice questions and patient management problem items formats in the assessment of physician competence, *Med Educ* 19:238–247, 1985.

Norcini JJ, Lipner RS, Kimball HR: Certifying examination performance and patient outcomes following acute myocardial infarction, *Med Educ* 36:853–859, 2002.

Norcini JJ, et al: The mini-CEX: a method for assessing clinical skills, *Ann Int Med* 138(6):476–481, 2003.

Papadakis MA, Teherani A, Banach MA, et al: Disciplinary action by medical boards and prior behavior in medical school, *N Engl J Med* 353:2673–2682, 2005.

Ram P, Grol R, Rethans JJ, et al: Assessment of general practitioners by video observation of communicative and medical performance in daily practice: issues of validity, reliability and feasibility, *Med Educ* 33:447–454, 1999a.

Ram P, van der Vleuten CPM, Rethans J, et al: Assessment in general practice: the predictive value of written-knowledge tests and a multiple-station examination for actual medical performance in daily practice, *Med Educ* 33:197–203, 1999b.

Ramsey PG, Carline JD, Inui TS, et al: Predictive validity of certification by the American Board of Internal Medicine, *Ann Int Med* 110: 719–726, 1989.

Regehr G, MacRae H, Reznick R, et al: Comparing the psychometric properties of checklists and global rating scales for assessing performance on an OSCE-format examination, *Acad Med* 73:993–997, 1998.

Rethans JJ, Sturmans F, Drop R, et al: Does competence of general practitioners predict their performance? Comparison between examination setting and actual practice, *BMJ* 303:1377–1380, 1991.

Rethans JJ, Norcini JJ, Baron-Maldonado M, et al: The relationship between competence and performance: implications for assessing practice performance, *Med Educ* 36:901–909, 2002.

Reznick RK, Regehr G, Yee G, et al: Process-rating forms versus task-specific checklists in an OSCE for medical licensure. Medical Council of Canada, *Acad Med* 73:S97–S99, 1998.

Roberts C, Sarangi S, Southgate L, et al: Oral examinations, equal opportunities and ethnicity: fairness issues in the MRCGP, *BMJ* 320:370–374, 2000.

Rowntree D: *Assessing students – how shall we know them?* London, 1987, Kogan.

Royal College of Physicians UK: *Doctors in society: medical professionalism in a changing world*, 2005. Available at: www.rcplondon.ac.uk/pubs/books/ docinsoc. Accessed December 2009.

Rughani A: *Assessment blueprint of general practice*, 2007. Available at: http://www.pmetb.org.uk/index. php?id=968. Accessed December 2009.

Rust C, O'Donovan BO, Price M: A social constructivist assessment process model: how the research literature shows us this could be best practice, *Assess Eval Higher Educ* 30:231–240, 2008.

Sayer M, Bowman D, Evans D, et al: Use of patients in professional medical examinations: current UK practice and the ethico-legal implications for medical education, *BMJ* 324:404–407, 2002.

Schmidt HG, Norman GR: How expertise develops in medicine: knowledge encapsulation and illness script formation, *Med Educ* 41:1133–1139, 2007.

Schuwirth LWT, van der Vleuten CPM: ABC of learning and teaching in medicine: written assessment, *BMJ* 326:643–645, 2003.

Schuwirth LWT, van der Vleuten CPM: Different written assessment methods: what can be said about their strengths and weaknesses? *Med Educ* 38:974–979, 2004.

Schuwirth LWT, van der Vleuten CPM: A plea for new psychometric models in educational assessment, *Med Educ* 40:296–300, 2006.

Shepard LA: The role of assessment in a learning culture, *Educ Res* 29:4–14, 2000.

Southgate L, Grant J: *Principles for an assessment system for postgraduate training*, 2004, Postgraduate Medical Training Board. Available at: http://www.pmetb.org.uk/fileadmin/user/QA/Assessment/Principles_for_an_assessment_system_v3.pdf. Accessed December 2009.

Southgate L, Campbell M, Cox J, et al: The General Medical Council's Performance Procedures: the development and implementation of tests of competence with examples from general practice, *Med Educ* 35 (Suppl 1):20–28, 2001.

Stalenhoef-Halling BF, van der Vleuten CPM, Jaspers TAM, et al: The feasibility, acceptability and reliability of open-ended questions in a problem based learning curriculum. In Bender W, Hiemstra RJ, Scherpbier AJJA, et al, editors: *Teaching and assessing clinical competence*, Boekwerk, 1990, Groningen, pp 1020–1031.

Swanson DB: A measurement framework for performance based tests. In Hart IR, Harden RM, editors: *Further developments in assessing clinical competence*, Can-Heal, 1987, Montreal, pp 13–45.

Swanson DB, Norman GR, Linn RL: Performance-based assessment: lessons from the health professions, *Educ Res* 24:5–35, 1995.

Swanson DB, Clauser BE, Case SM: Clinical skills assessment with standardized patients in high-stakes tests: a framework for thinking about score precision, equating and security, *Adv Health Sci Educ* 4:67–106, 1999.

Talbot M: Monkey see, monkey do: a critique of the competency model in graduate medical education, *Med Educ* 38:587–592, 2004.

Tamblyn R, Abrahamowicz M, Dauphinee D, et al: Physician scores on a national clinical skills examination as predictors of complaints to medical regulatory authorities, *JAMA* 298:993–1100, 2007.

Tombeson P, Fox RA, Dacre JA: Defining the content for the objective structured clinical examination component of the Professional and Linguistic Assessment Board examination: development of a blueprint, *Med Educ* 34:566–572, 2000.

van der Vleuten CPM: The assessment of professional competence: developments, research and practical implications, *Adv Health Sci Educ* 1:41–67, 1996.

van der Vleuten CPM, Schuwirth LWT: Assessing professional competence: from methods to programmes, *Med Educ* 39:309–317, 2005.

Van der Vleuten CPM, Swanson DB: Assessment of clinical skills with standardised patients: state of the art, *Teach Learn Med* 2:58–76, 1990.

Vygotsky LS: *Mind and society: the development of higher psychological processes*, Cambridge, MA, 1978, Harvard University Press.

Ward M, Gruppen L, Regehr G: Research in self-assessment: current state of the art, *Adv Health Sci Educ* 7:63–80, 2002.

Wass V, Jolly B: Does observation add to the validity of the long case? *Med Educ* 35:729–734, 2001.

Wass V, van der Vleuten CPM: Assessment in medical education and training. In Carter Y, Jackson N, editors: *A guide to medical education and training*, Oxford, 2006, Oxford University Press, pp 105–128.

Wass V, Jones R, van der Vleuten CPM: Standardised or real patients to test clinical competence? The long case revisited, *Med Educ* 35:321–325, 2001a.

Wass V, McGibbon D, van der Vleuten CPM: Composite undergraduate clinical examinations: how should the components be combined to maximise reliability? *Med Educ* 35:326–330, 2001b.

Wass V, van der Vleuten CPM, Shatzer J, et al: Assessment of clinical competence, *Lancet* 357:945–949, 2001c.

Wass V, Roberts C, Hoogenboom R, et al: Effect of ethnicity on performance in a final objective structured clinical examination: qualitative and quantitative study, *BMJ* 326:800–803, 2003a.

Wass V, Wakeford R, Neighbour R, et al: Achieving acceptable reliability in oral examinations: an analysis of the Royal College of General Practitioner's Membership Examination's oral component, *Med Educ* 37:126–131, 2003b.

Williams RG, McLaughlin MA, Eulenberg B, et al: The patient findings questionnaire: one solution to an important standardized patient examination problem, *Acad Med* 74:1118–1124, 1999.

Wilkinson TJ, Newble DI, Frampton CM: Standard setting in an objective structured clinical examination: use of global ratings of borderline performance to determine the passing score, *Med Educ* 35:1043–1049, 2001.

Wilkinson J, Crossley J, Wragg A, et al: Implementing workplace-based assessment across the medical specialties in the United Kingdom, *Med Educ* 42:364–373, 2008.

Further reading

Downing SM, Haladyna TM: *Handbook of test development*, Mahwah, 2006, Erlbaum Associates.

Jackson N, Jamieson A, Khan A: *Assessment in medical education and training*, Oxford, 2007, Radcliffe Publishing Ltd.

Stern DT: *Measuring medical professionalism*, Oxford, 2004, Oxford University Press.

Streiner DL, Norman GR: *Health measurement scales. A practical guide to their development and use*, Oxford, 2005, Oxford University Press.

Quality assurance of teaching and learning: enhancing the quality culture

15

Diana Dolmans   Renée Stalmeijer
Henk van Berkel   Ineke Wolfhagen

CHAPTER CONTENTS

ABC

Glossary

Internal quality assurance Activities undertaken within a school to monitor and improve educational quality.

Quality assurance A system to enhance the use of evaluative data for monitoring and improving educational quality.

Quality control A system to monitor whether a minimum set of predefined standards is reached.

Quality culture A culture or organisational mind-set in which staff members are motivated and empowered continuously to deliver high-quality education.

Total Quality Management; see, also, quality improvement See main Glossary, p. 343.

Outline

Quality assurance of teaching and learning in higher education has gained more and more attention over the years. This chapter focuses on different concepts behind quality and quality assurance. It describes principles that should be taken into account when measuring educational quality, interpreting evaluative data, and continuously improving education. It argues that quality assurance requires more than introducing evaluation instruments and creating structures or systems. Quality assurance requires commitment, ownership, and involvement on the part of learners and teachers, and the creation of a quality culture; otherwise, it will not result in continuous improvement of teaching and learning.

© 2011, Elsevier Ltd.
DOI: 10.1016/B978-0-7020-3522-7.00015-2

Introduction

In order to prepare future professionals adequately to deliver high-quality health care, our medical and health sciences training programmes should be of a high quality. Quality assurance of teaching and learning is important since it is aimed at continuously improving the quality of medical and health sciences training programmes. We explain how quality assurance has evolved over the years.

Reasons behind the growth in importance of quality assurance

There is increased interest for several reasons. One is that the number of learners has increased over the years, which has led to more money being spent and more attention being paid to efficiency. Another reason is a growing climate of accountability, which is forcing higher education institutes to demonstrate that their educational programmes are of high quality (Spencer-Matthews, 2001).

Different opinions about the concept "quality"

Measuring quality is not easy since it is a concept that has multiple meanings in an educational context. Harvey and Green (1993) stress that quality is a relative concept; it is stakeholder-relative. So, for example, employers and learners may have different opinions about the quality of an educational programme. Employers will use criteria different from those used by learners to judge quality. Employers may focus on the competencies acquired by learners, whilst learners focus on the quality of the teachers. Quality can be viewed from different perspectives: for example, exceptional, as perfection, as fitness for purpose, as value for money, or as being transformative (Harvey and Green, 1993). Exceptional means that quality is something special or unique; the standard is very high. Perfection is achieving a faultless result. Although the concepts of being exceptional and perfect are closely related, the emphasis in quality as perfection is on being "perfect", not "special". Furthermore, perfection also embodies prevention. Quality as fitness for purpose focuses on whether a product or service meets customers' needs or the mission of the institute. Fitness

for purpose also implies an orientation towards improvement. Quality as value for money stresses efficiency, effectiveness, and accountability. Quality as being transformative emphasises enhancing and empowering participants; it focuses on the process of changing the customer. It also stresses the importance of the value-added component of an educational programme in terms of the difference between input and output and improvements in learners' self-awareness (Harvey and Green, 1993). The value-added approach tries to correct for differences in quality of learner input (Tam, 2001). In sum, quality is a relative concept and different stakeholders might have different perspectives on what constitutes quality in an educational programme. As a consequence, different stakeholders should be involved in measuring educational quality, an issue that is explored later in this chapter.

From control to continuous improvement

Different terms are used in the literature to describe the process of determining the quality of an educational programme, including quality control, quality assurance, and Total Quality Management (Sallis, 2002). Quality control is one of the oldest, from which perspective quality is aimed mainly at detecting or eliminating products that are not up to standard (Sallis, 2002). Quality control is a system to check whether products or processes provided have reached predefined standards (Tam, 2001). It focuses on compliance with standards (EUA, 2006). The emphasis is on detection. Later, the term quality assurance was introduced. The focus here is not only on detecting but also on preventing errors or mistakes. Furthermore, this concept makes quality the responsibility not just of an external inspector, but of an organisation's workforce. It stresses not only the importance of proving quality but also of improving it. Nowadays, the term Total Quality Management (TQM) is often used. TQM is about creating a quality culture where the aim of every member of the staff is to delight their customers, and where the structure of the organisation allows them to do so (Sallis, 2002). TQM implies an organisational culture that is aimed at continuously improving the quality, in the case of an educational programme, of teaching and learning. The term quality culture refers to an organisational culture in which, on the one hand, individual staff members enhance quality through holding shared values, beliefs, and commitments whilst, on the other, management at the institutional level enhances quality and coordinates individual efforts to bring about permanent improvements (EUA, 2006). So, nowadays, there is an emphasis on having a higher education culture that continuously enhances educational quality.

Internal versus external quality assurance

A distinction is often made between internal and external quality assurance. Internal quality assurance concerns the activities undertaken by a school to evaluate and improve the quality of its educational programmes; it focuses mainly on improvement. External quality assurance means activities undertaken by external bodies – accreditation committees, for example – to control educational quality. The main aim of external quality assurance is to identify whether a programme complies with a set of minimum standards. The focus within this chapter is on internal quality assurance: activities undertaken by medical or health science schools continuously to improve the quality of their programmes.

Aims of internal quality assurance

Although continuous improvement should be at the very heart of quality processes (Bowden and Marton, 2000), quality assurance in most of today's educational institutes is aimed at controlling as well as improving educational quality. A growing climate of accountability is forcing educational institutes to show that they deliver quality. When quality assurance is aimed at improvement, it should provide faculties with feedback on the quality of their curriculum on which decisions for change can be based. It should look at input, process, and output. Improvement implies that quality assurance is aimed at diagnosing weaknesses in the curriculum. When quality assurance is aimed at controlling educational quality, the emphasis is more on providing policy makers or directors with information as to whether a product or a process has quality. It deals more with proving and controlling than improving. It is important to define clearly what the aim of internal quality assurance is, since this determines which methods should be chosen. That issue will be discussed next.

A cyclical process of continuous improvement

To ensure that quality assurance results in continuous improvement, it should be a cyclical process with three steps: (1) measuring, (2) judging, and (3) improving (Dolmans et al, 2003). In the first step, educational quality is measured. In the second step, the data collected are compared with standards to make decisions about strengths and weaknesses. In the third step, priorities and plans for improvement are set. After carrying out the changes, the three steps are repeated to measure whether changes have resulted in improvements. During each step, several principles should be taken into account. These principles, discussed below, are ordered around the three steps of measurement, judgement, and improvement.

How to measure quality

The first step in quality assurance is to make measurements; see (Box 15.1). Many higher education institutes collect a lot of data about the quality of their educational programmes. When measuring educational quality, several principles need to be taken into account. One is that measurement instruments should be based on theories. Another is that different stakeholders should be involved. A third one is that a

Box 15.1

Steps in quality assurance in teaching and learning

Measure
- Base instruments on theories about effective teaching
- Include different stakeholders
- Use mixed methods
- Use reliable and valid instruments
- Ensure periodic measurements

Judge
- Define standards before collecting evaluative data
- Organise dialogues about the data

Improve
- Define who is responsible for monitoring improvements
- Build a culture of continuous improvement; develop a sense of ownership, commitment, and involvement among learners and staff members

mixture of valid and reliable measurement instruments should be used. These principles are explained and illustrated below.

From theories to measurement instruments

When measuring educational quality, it is important to define first which key aspects of an educational programme determine it. Defining those key educational aspects is not easy. They can be derived from theories on human learning or can be based on the literature of effective teaching. For example, when measuring the quality of tutors in a problem-based curriculum, Maastricht University decided to focus on theoretical notions underlying problem-based learning. Those notions included active learning, self-directed learning, contextual learning, and constructive learning. They imply that tutors should stimulate learners to be actively involved in their own learning and to acquire a deep understanding of the subject. Tutors should also stimulate learners towards self-directed learning, towards applying the knowledge acquired to different contexts or problems, and towards collaborative discussions and interactions in their groups. The items of a questionnaire that was then developed and tested for its reliability and validity were based on those theoretical notions (Dolmans and Ginns, 2005). In conclusion, the items included in measurement instruments should be derived from what has been shown in the literature to determine the quality of an educational programme. In other words, the instrument is based on evidence about effective learning and teaching. All too often, measurement instruments consist of a list of items with no underlying theoretical notions or framework and which give no clear indication what aspects need improvement.

From one stakeholder to different stakeholders

Another issue that needs to be considered is which stakeholders should be involved. Those stakeholders may include learners, teachers, alumni, and policy makers. It is preferable to involve more than one stakeholder group in determining quality because it is a stakeholder-relative concept. As explained earlier, different stakeholders may have different opinions about what constitutes high-quality learning

and teaching. It is, of course, very important to involve learners, because they are the primary customers or clients. Teachers are also important because they are also internal customers who develop, deliver, and improve educational programmes. Both learners and teachers will have their own opinions about the concept of quality, what determines it, and how teaching can best influence learning. Alumni working in professional practice are also important stakeholders, since they can judge the relevance of the educational programme to their professional activities. Finally, policy makers can be involved as stakeholders although they mostly use information collected for other stakeholders to manage and organise curricula.

From one method to mixed methods

Many different types of instruments can be used to measure educational quality, including questionnaires, rating scales, interviews, observations, and focus groups (Braskamp and Ory, 1994). Which instrument is most suitable depends on the aim of the individual quality assurance activity. Evaluation processes useful for *improvement* must yield rich, descriptive, and qualitative information that illuminates sources of difficulty in order to bring about change. Evaluation processes most suited to *accountability* or control purposes must yield fairly objective, standardised, and externally defensible information (Dolmans et al, 2003). Although those aims and the instruments associated with them are not mutually exclusive, an emphasis on one may limit the pursuit of another. Rating scales mainly provide reliable and valid information that can be used to prove quality, whereas interviews and focus groups mainly provide rich information that can be used to improve quality. Since quality assurance often aims both to improve and to prove or control education quality, it is preferable to use not one but multiple sources of data (Cashin, 1999). When evaluating the performance of a teacher, for example, it is preferable to use several different instruments such as learner ratings, colleagues' peer ratings, and educational products designed by the teacher to obtain a broad picture of their performance. In some universities, teachers are encouraged to develop a teaching portfolio that can be used to evaluate their teaching performance. Teaching portfolios of that sort are enriched by including a variety of different sources of information.

From unreliable and non-valid to reliable and valid measurements

It is important to ensure that evaluative data are valid (Does the instrument measure what it is intended to measure?) and reliable (Does the instrument reveal consistent results?), especially when those data are used for accountability purposes. As an example, a rating scale filled out by learners to evaluate the performance of tutors in a problem-based curriculum has to provide reliable and valid data when they are used for promotion and tenure decisions. The tutor rating scale used at the Faculty of Health Medicine and Life Sciences at Maastricht University has been validated (Dolmans and Ginns, 2005) in terms of its content and construct validity. Content validity was ensured by basing development of the questionnaire on the theoretical notions of effective tutoring explained above. Construct validity was tested by means of a confirmatory factor analysis, in which the theoretical notions behind the instrument were tested against the data. Furthermore, we investigated how many learner responses per tutor were needed to make reliable judgements about the tutor's performance during any one period of tutoring; six out of ten learner responses were needed to make reliable or generalisable judgements (Dolmans and Ginns, 2005). Although most teachers enjoy being rated by learners, some argue that learner ratings of teaching behaviour are not valid because they are biased by the grades they give (giving lenient grades results in better learner ratings) or their popularity (Cashin, 1999). Reviews focusing on the validity and reliability of learner ratings, on the contrary, tend to show that learner ratings are statistically reliable, valid for most uses, relatively unaffected by biases such as grading leniency, useful to improve teaching, and able to support decisions, particularly when they include data from a variety of sources (Cashin, 1999; Marsh and Roche, 2000). Finally, although it is *generally* safe to assume that learner ratings are reliable and valid, it is important to test the reliability and validity of *specific* instruments, especially when ratings are used to inform high-stakes decisions.

From *ad hoc* measurements to periodic measurements

Evaluation activities should be carried out at regular and appropriate intervals, because carrying them out on an *ad hoc* basis reduces stakeholder involvement.

Furthermore, erratic measurement makes it difficult to measure whether changes result in improvement. It is difficult, however, to define the optimal frequency of measurement, because it depends on the situation. If a course occurs over many weeks, it is perhaps necessary to conduct a mid-term evaluation. This information can be used to carry out improvements during the latter part of the course. A course might be evaluated each year or only once in 2 years. If the evaluative data are positive, if very few changes are carried out in between evaluations, or if sources for conducting evaluation activities are limited, the frequency could be once every 2 years. However, evaluation activities should be carried out frequently enough to measure whether changes result in improvements.

How to judge or interpret evaluative data

The second step in quality assurance is to judge or interpret evaluative data. Two principles need to be considered during this step.

From absolute standards to relative standards

It is important to define standards before reporting data to avoid disagreement about how to interpret them later on. When defining standards, a distinction can be made between an absolute standard and a relative standard. For example, if a five-point rating scale is used, with 1 representing "strongly disagree" and 5 meaning "strongly agree", a score of 3.0 could be considered the absolute minimum standard. If a tutor scores below 3, the tutor's performance is insufficient and needs to improve considerably. Absolute standards are difficult to define, because in most cases no gold standard is available, and it is also difficult to define realistic ones. Relative standards are based on reference data, for example, by comparing courses over years or different courses within a year. Relative standards can be used only when comparative data are available. Furthermore, it is important to keep in mind that a relative standard could result in a low standard if the reference data are low. When evaluating the performance of tutors in a problem-based course by means of a rating scale filled out by learners, one could use a relative standard in combination with an absolute standard.

The average score of an individual tutor could, for example, be compared with the average scores of all tutors in the course and a minimum standard of 3.0 chosen. A tutor with an overall score of 3.3 does not have an insufficient score from an absolute point of view. If the average score of all tutors is 3.8, however, a tutor with a score of 3.3 scores below the average of all tutors or below the relative standard, which means that improvements are needed.

From reporting towards a dialogue

Institutes of higher education typically gather a great deal of data and produce many reports in which data are reported about the quality of their educational programmes. But all too often those reports are not used to improve quality. The main reason is poor communication of the results within the organisation. When evaluation reports are sent around and there is no dialogue or discussion about the results, those evaluation reports will not be used to improve quality. Thus, in order to engender real involvement with quality assurance and develop a quality culture, dialogue is crucial. It is important to have dialogue about the results at various levels within the organisation. Furthermore, it is important to keep in mind that different bodies within the organisation may need different reports and dialogue about the reports may need to be organised at different levels within the organisation. Individual tutor ratings and feedback from learners, for example, should be sent to individual tutors. A tutor with a poor score should be offered chances to reflect on the data and receive further coaching or training (Martens and Prosser, 1998). Specific feedback given by learners is very valuable for tutors but the chair of the department in which a tutor works needs only an overall score, which can be used during annual review sessions between the teacher and the department chair. The director of the educational institute does not need specific information per tutor, but needs information at an aggregate level such as the percentage of tutors in each discipline that are scoring poorly. This information can be used by the director during annual review meetings with the chairs of different departments. Thus, it is important to set up dialogue about evaluative data at different levels of an organisation and think carefully which information should be sent to whom and at what level. Dialogue is crucial to make sure that results are actually used for continuous improvement.

How to continuously improve education

The ultimate aim of educational quality assurance is continuous improvement and it is improvement that is the most difficult step. Two issues are very important: first, a clear definition of responsibilities, and second, an organisational culture in which every member cares about continuously improving educational quality. These two issues are now explained.

Towards defining responsibilities

It is often not clearly defined who is responsible for which aspect of a quality assurance system in higher education institutes. In order to ensure that evaluative data are used to carry out improvements, responsibilities have to be defined. It is necessary to define who is responsible for constructing the instruments, interpreting and reporting results, and carrying out improvements. At our Faculty of Health, Medicine, and Life Sciences, staff members have been appointed to a task force on quality assurance. This task force is responsible for the construction of the evaluation instruments, interpretation, and reporting of data. It is also responsible for ensuring the reliability and validity of data. The task force, consisting of experts on quality assurance, is not responsible for the collection of the data, which is the responsibility of coordinators of the different courses. The coordinators are also responsible for formulating plans for improvement based on the evaluative data. The director of the educational institute is responsible for monitoring whether the evaluative data have resulted in actions for continuous improvement of educational quality. When a tutor has a low score (at or below the minimum standard), for example, the coordinator of the course should first have a conversation with the tutor about the poor score. If the problem persists, the director of the educational institute will have a dialogue during their annual review meeting with the head of the department in which the tutor works. The head of department will also discuss their performance scores with his staff members during annual review meetings. The taskforce on quality assurance is available to give advice, but is not responsible for using tutor evaluation data in promotion and tenure decisions. In other words, responsibilities should be clearly defined.

Towards a culture of continuous improvement

Defining responsibilities and clear procedures within an educational organisation are prerequisites for successful quality assurance. But even when responsibilities and procedures have been defined, members of the organisation do not always act according to them. In other words, quality assurance can appear to be well integrated into the organisational structure, but is not in fact well integrated because it is not yet a full part of the organisational culture. In many institutes, quality assurance activities have been introduced but they do not result in continuous improvement of education because the cultural change that is needed for continuous improvement has not taken place. Quality assurance often leads to a system that looks good on paper but is not, in reality, owned by people; as a result, there is no change (Spencer-Matthews, 2001). A lot of evaluation instruments are introduced, a lot of data are collected, and a lot of reports are written, but these actions result only in marginal improvement. Quality cultures are fragile and very sensitive to over-bureaucratisation (EAU, 2006). The cultural change that is needed to ensure that evaluation activities result in continuous improvement is much more difficult to achieve. Changes in attitudes, values, and beliefs are necessary to ensure that quality assurance results in continuous improvement; and changing attitudes requires a long-term effort and strong human resource management (Cruickshank, 2003).

Although much is yet to be known about how to achieve a quality culture, ownership, commitment, and involvement in quality assurance from participants within the organisation are crucial. The introduction of a quality culture requires an appropriate balance of bottom-up and top-down aspects: a balance in involvement, communication, and commitment from individual staff members on the one hand and management at the institutional level on the other (EUA, 2006). Creating a quality culture takes time; it is a long-term effort to enhance quality permanently.

Implications for practice

Quality is a stakeholder-relative concept, which means that different stakeholders have different opinions about the concept of educational quality. It is important to include those different stakeholders, use mixed methods, organise dialogues, and define responsibilities clearly. Continuous improvement of quality should be at the very heart of a higher education institute. But that requires more than clear procedures and responsibilities. It requires an organisational mind-set with a customer-oriented culture or a culture in which staff members are motivated and empowered to deliver high-quality education (Sallis, 2002). Establishing a quality culture within a school requires commitment and involvement from all stakeholders within the school and is a long-term effort.

References

Bowden J, Marton F: *The university of learning*, UK, 2000, Kogan Page.

Braskamp LA, Ory JC: *Assessing faculty work. Enhancing individual and institutional performance.* San Francisco, 1994, Jossey-Bass.

Cashin WE: Learner ratings of teaching: uses and misuses. In Seldin P, editor: *Changing practices in evaluating teaching*, Bolton, 1999, Anker, pp 25–44.

Cruickshank M: Total quality management in the higher education sector: a literature review from an international and Australian perspective, *TQM Bus Excellence* 14(10):1159–1167, 2003.

Dolmans DHJM, Ginns P: A short questionnaire to evaluate the effectiveness of tutors in PBL: validity and reliability, *Med Teach* 27 (6):534–538, 2005.

Dolmans DHJM, Wolfhagen HAP, Scherpbier AJJA: From quality assurance to total quality management: How can quality assurance result in continuous improvement in health professions education? *Educ Health* 16 (2):210–217, 2003.

EUA: *Quality culture in European universities: a bottom-up approach*, Belgium, Brussels, 2006, European University Association (EUA) publication.

Harvey L, Green D: Defining quality, *Assess Eval Higher Educ* 18(1):9–34, 1993.

Marsh HW, Roche LA: Effects of grading leniency and low workload on learners' evaluations of teaching. Popular myths, bias, validity or innocent bystanders? *J Educ Psychol* 92(1):202–238, 2000.

Martens E, Prosser M: What constitutes high quality teaching and learning and how to assure it, *Qual Assur Edu* 6(1):28–36, 1998.

Sallis E: *Total Quality Management in education*, UK, 2002, Kogan Page.

Spencer-Matthews S: Enforced cultural change in academe. A practical case study: implementing quality management systems in higher education, *Assess Eval Higher Educ* 26(1):51–59, 2001.

Tam M: Measuring quality and performance in higher education, *Qual Higher Educ* 7(1):47–54, 2001.

Further reading

Cashin WE: Learner ratings of teaching: uses and misuses. In: Seldin P, editor: *Changing practices in evaluating teaching*. Bolton, 1999, Anker, pp 25–44.

Sallis E: *Total Quality Management in education*, UK, 2002, Kogan Page.

Developing learning resources

16

Rachel H. Ellaway

CHAPTER CONTENTS

ABC

Glossary

Affordances The things an artifact can or might be perceived to do irrespective of whether it was intended to serve those purposes.

Agency The extent to which an individual has control over their situation. Simulation involves more learner agency than a lecture does.

Blended learning environment A learning environment combining physical and embodied resources with electronic and online resources.

Chunking The reductionist principle of breaking a large or complex body of information into simpler, hopefully more digestible, parts.

Communication system Any networked set of tools that supports communication between multiple individuals. This can include text messaging, email, discussion boards, as well as more esoteric forms such as Twitter.

Copyright The legal right to control how any material or tangible idea is reproduced and who benefits from such reproduction.

Creative Commons A licensing model for content that defines conditions of use somewhere between full copyright and public domain.

Expertise reversal When an educational intervention reduces or inhibits learning rather than enhancing or enriching it.

Granularity The amount of detail or specificity (or the lack thereof) in a system, artifact, or process.

Haptic device A machine that simulates the touch and force feedback of physical objects.

Hardware Any physical device or infrastructure that supports or is controlled by software.

Immersion The extent to which an individual is focused on a particular task in terms of how unaware they are of other events in their environment.

In silico A Latinism indicating the existence of something running in software, intended to be equivalent in concept to *in vivo* and *in vitro* descriptions in the biomedical sciences.

Continued

© 2011, Elsevier Ltd.
DOI: 10.1016/B978-0-7020-3522-7.00016-4

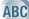

Glossary (continued)

Knowledgebase Any organised and structured body of knowledge. For instance a textbook, a library or a reference resource like Wikipedia or Medpedia.

Learning resource Any kind of artifact or tool designed, built, or employed for the purpose of supporting teaching, learning, or assessment and used by learners, teachers, or other participants in support of educational activities.

Lifecycle The various stages in the development, use, and disposal of an artifact or process.

Narrative Account of the world told from a human perspective containing temporal sequence, personality, motive, causality, and consequence.

Picture Archiving and Communication System (PACS) PACS is mostly used for managing imaging resources such as X-rays, MRIs, CTs, angiograms, and ultrasound recordings.

Palimpsest Originally a medieval document written on animal skin where a text was scraped off and another added in its place. Used in technical terms to reflect the presence of earlier and related forms on the design and use of tools and systems.

Part task trainer Any physical simulation or training device that is designed for a particular skill and may represent a section of a human body in lesser or greater fidelity. Examples include individual plastic arms used for venepuncture training and suture pads.

Personal learning environment A more or less integrated set of software tools assembled by a learner for their own use in their educational activities.

Podcast A compound term of 'broadcast' and iPod (representative of a music player) and used to denote syndicated audio files available over the web.

PowerPoint A near-ubiquitous computer-based slide and presentation tool from Microsoft.

Requirements Structured exposition of the required functions and behaviours of a system (physical and/or computer-based) used as the basis for constructing or adapting the system to meet the requirements

Sequencing The ordering, connectivity, and interdependence of different aspects of a common process or system.

Serious gaming The use of games or aspects of games for purposes other than entertainment; typically education, assessment, and training.

Software Any code or content running on a computer system – software is in part defined as that which runs on hardware.

Standards and specifications In technical terms, a specification is a recommendation, whereas a standard is a mandated set of rules. Both establish one or more shared patterns for organising activities and information.

Synchronous At the same time (as opposed to asynchronous). Participation in a live concert is synchronous; viewing a recording of the concert is asynchronous.

Syndicated content Any material created by one party and placed at a single location for multiple subscribing parties to access and use. Examples include news feeds, podcasts, and vodcasts.

Total cost of ownership (TCO) An economic model that considers all costs, both hidden and overt, associated with employing a technology, system or other intervention. TCO includes the costs associated with training, staffing, and facilities, as well as costs associated with disposal and replacement.

Virtual learning environment An integrated software system, typically web-based, made up of multiple and discrete course or program containers providing content, communication, assessment and tracking.

Virtual patient An interactive computer simulation of a real-life clinical scenario for the purpose of medical education, or assessment.

Virtual world Any software and hardware combination that allows its users to work or interact in a space through an avatar and that approximates to the real world. Also called a synthetic world.

Vodcast A variant on the term 'podcast' that involves video rather than audio.

Wetware A term for humans (and other animals) involved in a system that also involves software and or hardware components. The use of the term emphasises the integration and interaction of the person as a system component.

Outline

This chapter is concerned with the variety of resources that can be used in medical education, the ways in which they can be used, and any implications for practice. This chapter will start with some definitions and a typology of learning resources, it will then review many of the key underlying concepts in resource provision and use and consider learning resource lifecycles and the economics of their use. The chapter concludes with a review of some of the emerging factors that impact on the kinds of resources we may use in the future and their implications for practitioners in the years to come.

Scope

There are examples of learning resources in medical education going as far back as Persian, Egyptian, Greek, and Roman times (Loechel, 1960). Indeed, the use of artifacts and tools to support and enhance learning is one of the defining aspects of 'education'. Because so many kinds of learning resources are used in contemporary medical education, let us define the term 'learning resource':

> A learning resource is any kind of artifact or tool designed, built or employed for the purpose of supporting teaching, learning or assessment and used by learners, teachers or any other participants in one or more educational undertaking.

To further clarify the concept, it is helpful to consider borderline examples. For instance, an integrated curriculum that employs many learning resources may itself be considered a learning resource, because learners and teachers use the curriculum as an artifact through which they can contextualise their past, current, and future activities. Similarly, assessment items may or may not be considered learning resources, depending on the context in which they are used. An exam question may be considered a learning resource when it is used as a group problem in a classroom setting. The same question would not be regarded as a learning resource if it were used for purely summative assessment purposes. Clearly, the context of use defines (or redefines) a learning resource as much as any of its intrinsic properties.

Causality and context

The use of a learning resource is never causal. Simply making learning resources available to learners will not guarantee any kind of result. At best we can consider a probabilistic model of learning affected or catalysed by the use of a learning resource. Not only does this reflect the reality of learning but it also helps us understand the importance of design (that is, design of the resource itself and/or design of the activity context in which it is used). Essentially, a learning activity should be designed to effect its intended learning objectives for as high a percentage of its target learners as also demonstrates importance of context, typically in the form of an educational activity with associated learning objectives and target learners.

Clearly, almost anything can, in the right context, be used as a learning resource. A resource becomes a *learning* resource when it is incorporated into some kind of educational activity. Educational intent is therefore the defining factor that in turn is typically expressed in terms of learning objectives. While the design and application of learning objectives is a much wider topic than can be adequately covered in this chapter, the use of objectives is an important step in using any resource for learning.

The next consideration is who the intended learners are supposed to be. One way of answering this question is to view any group of learners as being made up of, say, quartiles, ordered on the basis of their learning abilities (with regard to specific topics). The top quartile (that typically uses every opportunity afforded to them and always excel), the bottom quartile (that often fails to use the opportunities afforded to them and always struggles), and lower and higher middle quartiles – see Figure 16.1. It is rare that resources would be targeted only at the higher quartiles (C and D in Figure 16.1) as they need little additional help to do well; most learning resources are typically targeted at the lower two quartiles (A and B). This model may of course not reflect a global assessment of learners' abilities; it is simply a means of identifying (for instance from exam performance) what topics and concepts are particularly problematic for learners. Resources and the activities that employ them can therefore be more readily targeted at addressing the less tractable or accessible parts of the curriculum. For example, pre-clinical topics such as partial pressures or statistics often prove particularly challenging to learners.

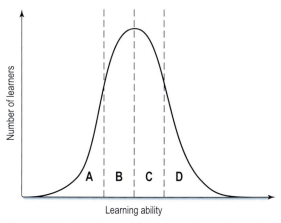

Figure 16.1 • Quartile model of learners in any given class or cohort.

Additional information or activities can always be provided for the brighter or more industrious learners so as to create a more inclusive range of experiences. A key consideration with this model is whether the goal is to reduce the difference between the top and bottom quartiles (such as additional support, remediation) or to highlight these differences more clearly (such as in formative or summative assessment).

Context clearly has a determining impact on the efficacy of any learning resource including the abilities of the instructor using a resource or how well aligned it is to the curriculum. In part, this reflects the probabilistic relationship between exposure to educational interventions and learning taking place, but it also highlights the importance of teachers (and their support staff) having sufficient facility and understanding of how to use resources as well as there being good alignment between any such use and the wider curriculum context.

A typology of learning resources

Having established a conceptual space for thinking about learning resources, the next step is to consider a more focused typology of learning resources in medical education.

Type A: Information and knowledge resources

These are typically text-based materials such as books, articles, and websites supported with diagrams, illustrations, photographs, audio, video, or animations. Notable forms in medical education include:

- *Textbooks:* systematically organised, canonical, and relatively context-free texts on single domains or topics intended for learners (rather than for an expert or lay audience). The material is typically structured so as to support a learning process. The format is largely text-based with diagrams, illustrations, and other more visual material supporting the text. Traditionally, programmes or courses identify a few key textbooks that are referenced. Other non-key texts are referenced but less often. Health care subjects (and in particular medicine) also make significant use of key reference materials including clinical

handbooks (such as the *Oxford Handbook* series), pharmacopoeia (such as the *British National Formulary*), and expert opinion-based resources (such as UpToDate).

- *Study guides and materials:* specific to a course or subject context. Study guides are descriptive resources that are about both the organisation of a learning context as well as supporting learning itself (although this varies between institutions and cultures). Study materials on the other hand are issued in support of a particular activity and typically mix instructions to learners and tutors with course content. Study materials can take a number of different forms including lecture notes, problem-based learning (PBL) cases, and activity briefings such as for a simulated patient (SP) session. Typically, tutors or course organisers create their own study guides and materials, although some limited use is made of third-party resources.

- *Presentations:* typically take the form of lecture slides and notes, which are either computer based, such as PowerPoint, or older forms, such as overhead projector materials or 35 mm slides. Although PowerPoint has been around for several decades, it is only recently that it has become the *de facto* format for giving presentations. At present, preparing to give a lecture or talk is primarily about writing a PowerPoint presentation, while the talk itself is framed by the data projector's glare and the susurration of its fan.

Once created, the next issue is how to make presentations available to learners. In addition to projection in a live lecture, presentations may also be webcast or recorded for subsequent viewing and review. Many teachers just give their learners the slide deck but should it be before the event, during the event, or after the event? Opinions vary, especially given the ways this is seen as affecting attendance and attention at lectures. Learning resource issues do not end with giving the presentation; they can also involve the provision of slides in other formats such as handouts. One other consideration regards how much sense a slide deck makes outside the context in which it was given. There are many who consider themselves adept at e-teaching, because they place their slides online even though they have little or no idea whether doing so is useful or effective, particularly in the absence of a presenter to create meaning around their presentation.

- *Syndicated content:* serially published resources that are streamed or downloaded from a common point to subscribing client systems. There are several common forms:

– *Feeds* are primarily text and image based and they underpin the world's news websites, blogs, and other online information providers. The main uses of feeds in medical education are to keep abreast of new developments, to follow educational blogs, and to receive news and updates on a course (if they are provided in a feed format).

– Audio-only *podcasts* are perhaps the most widely used syndicated materials in medical education with a great many institutions now publishing their lectures in a podcast format. Subscribing to a podcast means that each time a new edition is put online, it is flagged as such to subscribers and they can then download the file for listening as and when they want. The proliferation of music players (such as the iPod) has made this particularly well aligned to contemporary learner lifestyles. For instance, Apple's iTunes platform has a whole section dedicated to iTunesU (see Figure 16.2)

including a great many health care education offerings, all of which are free and open to use. Vodcasts are essentially the same as podcasts except they use video rather than audio. While podcasts are like serial on-demand radio broadcasts, vodcasts are more like on-demand television.

• *Primary sources:* typically research papers are a key part of educational activity designs such as PBL and the development of skills in evidence-based medicine (EBM). Sources may also include 'grey' literature such as government reports, strategy papers, and other non-peer reviewed materials. The role of the institutional library is key in using primary sources both in terms of developing literature searching and appraisal skills and in terms of ensuring technical access to sources both online and physical.

• *Knowledgebases:* aggregate websites, wikis, and databases of resources and information such as clinical guidelines. Wikipedia is perhaps the best known and most used online knowledgebase and in many ways the most contentious. Wikipedia can be more comprehensive and up to date than more

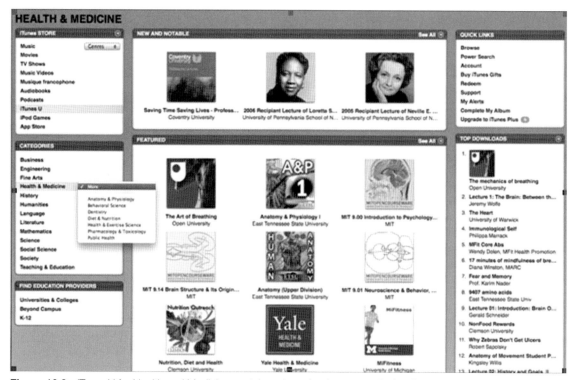

Figure 16.2 • iTunesU for Health and Medicine contains a large (and ever-growing) collection of podcasts and vodcasts on a range of medical and health care topics.

traditional sources by making all of its information open to public editing and alteration. Some celebrate the 'wisdom of crowds', while others bemoan the 'cult of the amateur' in this approach (Keen, 2007). Increasingly limited specialist community knowledgebases such as Medpedia (http://www.medpedia.com) are emerging, which limit edit access to acknowledged subject specialists as a way of harnessing the power of collaborative and dynamic publishing while retaining significant editorial control.

- *Instructional software:* this was, at least for a while, the main focus of the educational technology movement. Computer-assisted learning packages (CALs) proliferated with CD-ROM (and more recently DVD-ROM) or web-based instructional multimedia titles proliferated in the 1990s and early 2000s covering a great many subjects. While many of these titles still exist (such as the A.D.A.M., PathCAL and CLIVE series), the economics of creating these packages means that they largely serve the niche markets that are able to sustain them. One of the predominant areas that make use of instructional software is continuing medical education (CME) with substantial instructional multimedia offerings from providers such as BMJ Learning. Software resources do not have to be whole compiled packages; it is increasingly common for smaller components and individual files to be made available as reusable learning objects, including games, puzzles, and videoclips.

As a whole, type A resources tend to be passive (no change in state in response to a user's input) or at best active (responding to input but not changing), but low in interactivity (changing in dynamic ways). The dominant instructional model is therefore primarily one of knowledge transfer or just-in-time reference.

Type B: Environments that contain or provide the context for educational activities

Type B resources include systems, activity designs, and workflows. Key type B designs in medical education include:

- *Virtual learning environments* (VLEs, also called learning management systems – LMS): integrated software systems, typically web-based, made up of multiple and discrete course or programme containers providing content, communication, and other activities such as assessment and tracking. VLE systems have tended to take the form of large commercial systems such as Blackboard or Desire2Learn, open sources such as Moodle or Sakai, more specialised tools such as LAMS or Janison or any number of locally developed systems. Most off-the-shelf VLEs are based on multiple course containers, each of which has a range of tools that can be configured by the tutor, with the boundaries between course instances being particularly strong, thereby limiting access to the current members of a course instance and thereby excluding the extended programme community. Locally developed systems, on the other hand, tend to follow tightly integrated single programme approaches that reflect the culture and dynamics of the cultures that built them. Because courses run many times, VLEs need to be able to track and isolate different instances of the same course as well as manage access and permissions to materials and tools in the different course containers. They also need to be able to track individuals and groups regarding what they do, and when they do it. This panoptic quality is one of the defining aspects of a VLE and strangely one of its less well-considered properties, although there is growing concern as to the extent and use of tracking and monitoring in educational technologies (Land and Bayne, 2005). VLEs can be learning resources at three levels: as a resource in their own right, as a context and container for resources, and as an environment within which resources can be developed.

- *Personal learning environments:* a more recent phenomenon where web-based collaboration and management tools are adapted for learners to create their own personal or shared spaces. Typically built around generic platforms (such as Facebook, Google, Flickr, YouTube), these personal learning environments shift the focus away from institutional systems and tend to intertwine social and educational activities and identities. The longer-term effects of such activity taking place beyond institutional oversight and control has yet to be fully understood.

- *Portfolios:* these involve the management of collections of materials, reflections, or other items that are intended to represent a learner over time, typically although not always based on their progress towards one or more educational or professional objectives. Paper-based portfolios are being superseded by online systems that may combine functions of blogs, repositories, and assessment tools. This is both their strength and their weakness; there are all sorts of portfolio designs and models, many of which are incompatible. For instance, there are significant differences between systems that are about demonstrating the 'best of me' and 'all of me', between learner and tutor control, between formative and summative assessment (or no assessment at all), between submitted items being fixed or editable, or between periodic or open-ended events and submissions. As with many new technologies, language and shared understanding have yet to catch up with the possible and actual practices using such systems.

- *Communication systems:* systems such as email, instant messaging, and texting are still the main way for learners to communicate amongst themselves (other than Facebook). However, audio and video conferencing systems underpin any learning environment where learners and tutors are not permanently collocated. These range from room-based videoconferencing (requiring dedicated equipment and rooms) to desktop or web conferencing using systems such as Connect, Illuminate or Wimba or simple voice or video tools such as Skype.

- *Assessment systems:* are increasingly being used in medical education. Although these are not primarily used as learning resources, they can be configured to provide banks of formative and self-assessment tests and quizzes as resources for learning. The other main application of assessment in providing learning resources is in adaptive hypermedia. These are systems that adapt their content and activities in response to learner requirements. For instance, activities may get increasingly difficult for a successful learner, while a less able one may receive more help and mentoring.

- *Gaming:* the term 'serious gaming' follows the commercial success and social impact of computer games and platforms. Educational games can take all sorts of forms, following common patterns such as card or board games, TV gameshows, or video games. Virtual worlds such as Second Life appear very gamelike but differ from games, particularly because they have no fixed purpose (you either bring purpose in with you or create it within the world for others) (Castronova, 2005). Although the concept of a 'game' has overtones of juvenilia

or distraction from more serious matters, there is a growing body of evidence for its efficacy and ability to engage both learners and their teachers in highly effective (and often enjoyable) ways (Aldrich, 2005).

- *Physical spaces:* places such as classrooms, laboratories, and libraries can also be considered to be type B learning resources. It is interesting that at a time when online modalities make up more and more of the education environment, face-to-face learning and the creative use of physical space are also undergoing a renaissance.

- *Social and cultural resources:* the communities in which learners are working (such as in electives or clinical placements) can also be valuable learning resources. This is particularly the case when considering the many professions that interact with medicine and when learning about minority and socially distinct communities. For example, the author's own institution, Northern Ontario School of Medicine, makes significant use of its communities as resources for its learners placed across the million square kilometers of the northern province (see http://www.nosm.ca).

Type C: Tools that act on the world or on other resources or artifacts

Not only can type C artifacts be considered resources in their own right but also they are notable in being able to be used to generate other learning resources. Type C resources can be grouped into two basic categories:

- *Software:* such as personal information management applications (calendars, contacts), word processors, databases, and spreadsheets can also be learning resources, both as tools that allow learners to manage and manipulate information and as the subject of learning when teaching them how to use these tools. This is also the case for more specialised applications such as bibliographic and citation tools.

- *Hardware:* there are a great many devices that can be used as learning resources, including computers (desktops, laptops, notebooks), PDAs and smartphones, smartboards, cameras, microphones, projectors, and audience response systems ('clickers').

Although type C resources can be found in almost every part of health care education, these are major topics in their own right and we will not be expanding on this particular area in this chapter.

Type D: Simulations of artifacts, places or people

Simulation bridges the knowledge and affective and psychomotor aspects of learner development while providing a safe and controlled environment whose primary purpose is to support the learning process rather than patient care. Simulation can therefore be seen as an essential step between didactic learning and bedside practice – the amount of simulation used at the start of a learning episode and how much remains in practice depend on the needs of the subject, the profession, and the learners involved (Issenberg, 2006).

The other side of simulation is virtuality – the representation of real-world processes or equivalents in software (or, as it is increasingly described, *in silico*). Virtuality would seem to be a modern phenomenon, arising primarily from the multimedia, simulation, and gaming capabilities of computers and associated devices (Box 16.1). However, the unreal, the simulated,

---

Box 16.1

Virtual patients

A virtual patient is 'an interactive computer simulation of real-life clinical scenarios for the purpose of medical training, education, or assessment' (Ellaway et al, 2006b). There are lots of virtual patient designs such as linear (the path is predefined), schema (moving through a linear set of explorations), branching (making choices, developing strategies, and exploring consequences), and world (spatial control and social interactions). Learners may take different roles (physician, patient); designs may be for exploration, experience, and formative or summative assessment, and may involve plain text narratives or complex multimedia.

There are three dominant themes in virtual patient design: narrative, simulation, and gaming. Narrative is critical to the way virtual patients allow learners to explore different roles and motives, which evolve over time. Simulation is important because of the essential basis in real-world problems and settings. Gaming reflects the ways that virtual patients allow learners to try different strategies to solve the case within a well-defined set of rules.

New virtual patient designs and applications are being developed all the time with a growing number of tools (free and commercial) to help teachers build or adapt virtual patients – see www.virtualpatients.eu for more information and examples.

---

and the intangible are not new in medical education. We can more properly consider embodied physical resources with mechanical properties and non-embodied virtual resources with properties arising from software abstractions. Even the most virtual resource requires some embodiment, not least because we as users are intrinsically embodied. Whether this is in the form of user interfaces, controllers or input and output devices such as cameras, monitors, and printers, or more esoteric forms such as goggles or haptic devices, the virtual and the physical are intrinsically connected. New technologies such as electronic paper, wearable computers, and sophisticated mobile devices are blurring this divide even more.

Although simulators have much in common with other types of resources, they have many distinct and essential qualities:

- Simulation is dependent on consensual pretence and illusion; learners know and even depend on knowing that simulation is not real. It is more precise therefore to call this dissimulation than simulation, the intent of the latter being to truly deceive (Baudrillard, 1994).

- There is a fundamental alignment to and reflection of the practice domain in simulation. This can include appearance, sound, touch, symbols and language, procedures, and social norms.

- Simulation supports the phenomenon of the psychosocial moratorium; that is, through dissimulation relative to their everyday life it allows learners to step out of their existing identities to explore and develop new identities (for instance, as health care professionals).

Type D resources include:

- *Mannequins:* whole-body human models that allow learners to treat and otherwise interact with them and respond appropriately.

- *Part task trainers:* these may range from simple suturing pads through disembodied arms for phlebotomy training to video-driven laparoscopic simulators.

- *Informatics trainers:* these are versions of systems used in health care, such as electronic health records and picture archiving and communication system (PACS).

- *Equipment simulators:* such as anaesthetics machines.

- *Wetware:* humans (and other animals) can also be used as learning resources, in particular real patients in bedside teaching or SPs in more controlled simulation settings.

Key concepts

The list of different types and forms of learning resources given in the last section is far from exhaustive. Exploring each of these areas could consume many volumes, so, for the purposes of this chapter, we will consider a number of key and common concepts and themes that unite them and point to ongoing innovation and development in this area:

- *Diversity of application:* teaching, learning, and assessment resources differ from one another; they are used by individuals and groups undertaking different roles to support different kinds of actions and processes. For instance, while a learning resource may be selected or exclusively used by a learner, a teaching resource is designed to be used by a teacher working with one or more learners. The processes and instructional models used in learning resources and in teaching resources can therefore differ quite considerably (Ellaway, 2009a).
- *Diversity of method:* there are many educational models and approaches, such as knowledge transfer, sequencing, chunking, scaffolding, schema building, testing, and practice, that can be (and are) applied to learning resources. All artifacts embody the perspectives, values, and worldviews of the people who created them, and it is not particularly hard to recognise behaviourist, constructivist, pedagogical (youth), andragogical (adult), and even heutagogical (self-directed) models that are intrinsic to a resource or the activity in which it is used. Recognising and making explicit the intrinsic philosophies in learning resource design allows for better selection and evaluation of resources and minimises tacit coercion towards predefined educational practices.
- *Fluidity of medium:* the binary distinction between electronic and paper forms is fading and the 'blended learning environment' is rapidly becoming the norm. Although they are used in all sorts of combinations, different media have particular boundaries, both paper-based forms and digital forms such as text, image, audio, animation, video, and 3D. For instance, search is almost entirely limited to text and a scan or photograph of text may appear the same as real text but behave quite differently. While multimedia as a topic is almost entirely about visuals and audio, there are other less common modalities that work with other senses such as touch (haptics). Boundaries are being continually challenged and blurred through the use of multimodal and multimedia mashups (*ad hoc* combinations of different modes and media) to create new tools and services.
- *Affordances:* a resource does not just do what it is supposed to do; it usually does or enables a range of other actions and perspectives. The things that a resource can do or might do are called its 'affordances'. For instance, the affordances of a textbook include providing authoritative factual information, representing the preemptive choices of what its authors think as important (and by omission unimportant), costing money, and being fixed in time and place. The affordances of a PowerPoint presentation, on the other hand, include presenting ideas sequentially, combining text, images, videos and animations, packaging all these as a single file, and being able to run them as a presentation. They also include enforcing sequentiality, controlling pacing based on what can be put on a slide, strong templating, and handling the financial burden of acquiring the software and updates. Considering the affordances of a resource not only helps us to identify the ways in which learners may use or misuse a resource but also allows for a fuller evaluation of their efficacy and impact.
- *Cognitive affordances:* frame the learning relationship between the resource and the learner. Resources may be passive (the resource stays the same, irrespective of what the user does – such as a paper PBL case), active (the resource responds to input but does not change – such as a multimedia package), or interactive (the resource changes in dynamic ways – such as a mannequin or SP). Interestingly, while books may seem fairly passive, they afford written annotations and many learners seek out secondhand textbooks with good annotations from their previous owners. Two other related and possibly even more critical cognitive affordances are agency (how much direct control the learner has over the learning experience – for instance, a game has a lot more agency than a book) and immersion (how much the internal reality of a resource dominates a learner's attention relative to other foci of attention – for instance, narratives are typically more immersive than a scientific report).
- *Instructional design:* has developed out of behaviourist philosophies of education and is predicated on two principles – (a) there are objectively good ways of design learning

experiences and (b) these can be codified as a set of rules and guidelines for practitioners. One of the main themes in instructional design is the concept of 'cognitive load', a model of instructional design that considers a resource or activity to impose three kinds of load on the learner (Sweller, 1988):

- *Intrinsic* – the load caused by the inherent difficulty of what is being taught
- *Germane* – the load caused by the method of instruction and the form of learning
- *Extraneous* – the load caused by anything that is not intrinsic or germane

Simply put, cognitive load theory suggests that any resource or activity design can be enhanced by removing all extraneous load (unnecessary graphics, details, and inappropriate media choices – such as trying to describe a square using only words rather than just showing an image) and adjusting germane load to best suit the learners' abilities. Intrinsic load cannot be changed, but it can be ameliorated by creating subsets of a complex topic and then carefully re-integrating them to achieve understanding of the larger topic. Other cognitive phenomena include scaffolding (providing lots of support at first but then removing assistance as the learner develops mastery) and expertise reversal (learning is stalled or even driven down by using resources that are too easy) (Kalyuga et al, 2003).

- *Ethics:* learning resource design, use, and support involves a number of ethical dimensions, particularly where learning resources change the balance of equity in a learning environment. For instance, learners are increasingly expected to buy computers and pay for their own printing where previously the equivalent resources would have been provided for free by their educational institution. There are also ethical concerns over accessibility, and not just for those with a physical or cognitive disability; it is a professional responsibility for teachers to make their work as accessible to their learners as possible. Although this may seem obvious, there are regrettably few teachers who make the effort to check their work for understandability and ease of use. The last major ethical concern is with respect to access. Not everyone will have the same level of access to resources (whether they are physical or online). This is a particular concern for institutions running programmes across multiple sites (a growing number worldwide), particularly where equivalence of opportunity is an accreditation requirement. Taking a lowest common denominator approach is not necessarily the most educationally effective way of responding to such challenges. Powerful learning resources do not have to be complex, just effective.

- *Creativity:* although technical skills (both electronic and traditional) are important for the effective use of learning resources, the role of instructor and learner creativity remains an essential part of creating or reusing learning materials (Ellaway et al, 2005). This may involve creativity in terms of new materials or new kinds of materials, new uses of existing materials, or completely new approaches that challenge previous practice and thinking. A particularly good example of such innovation is how artifacts from the arts (such as novels, poems, paintings, music, and movies) can be used in medical education (Powley and Higson, 2005).

Lifecycle

Learning resources clearly come from somewhere; they exist somewhere while they are being used and they eventually go somewhere else once their time is done. We can consider a lifecycle model as following a number of stages:

- *Identify needs and requirements:* first of all an educational need, problem, or opportunity is identified and then formalised by developing a set of requirements for the proposed learning resource. These requirements should state the learning objectives, level of learner, possible strategies, and contextual considerations, and set out the material to be covered.

- *Review existing options:* although there is always a temptation to create something anew, the next step should be to evaluate whether there is any existing (and readily available) resource that can meet the identified requirements. This may go one of three ways:

  - If there is a resource that meets the requirements, then the resource can be acquired, possibly involving buying, borrowing, or taking a copy of the existing material. This inevitably means entering into some relationship with the resource's originators or owners, usually expressed as a licence or as a set of terms and conditions. It is important that there is some agreement as to what each party can and cannot do, and what their responsibilities are.

- If the requirements are similar to what an existing resource can provide, then it may make more sense to repurpose or customise it to meet the identified needs. This depends on such adaptation being possible technically (whether the resource be changed at all), legally (within the terms of the licence or other conditions of use), and practically (within the resources – time, skills, cost – available). See economics section on reusable learning objects (RLOs).

- If there is nothing that can directly meet the identified requirements, then the resource must be created. In order to do this, the requirements are transformed into one or more outline designs that may involve storyboarding or some other structured representation. The resource is then constructed along the lines of the design. Construction should involve testing and evaluation to make sure that it matches the identified needs and satisfies its users.

• *Deployment:* once the resource exists, it then needs to be deployed for teachers and learners to use. Deployment may involve a number of different steps and levels. For instance, we have already identified curriculum integration as a critical success factor. Another important consideration is to what extent the resource is core or an augmentation to a core set of activities. Returning to the earlier model of cohort quartiles, the top quartile will probably use a learning resource even if it is non-core, while the lower quartile may very well not – clearly not a good outcome if the lower quartile is the target group! There are also more practical issues such as how the resource is to be accessed. For instance, the resource may be placed into the programme or course VLE or made available through the library or as a set of physical course materials. No matter what way it is published, it should be easy to find and discover. One of the advantages of using online material is that it can be linked and cross-linked to and from anywhere. Framing is an important consideration in constructing the utility of a learning resource. Although it includes the extent and form of curriculum integration, framing also reflects the ways in which the teacher presents and discusses the resource and the

opinions and ratings of other learners. This social construction or reconstruction of a resource is often overlooked but can make all the difference in its uptake.

• *Evaluation:* once a resource is being used, it should be evaluated and improvements or changes made, based on the results of the evaluation. There are several key dimensions:

- Decide what it is that is being evaluated; although most evaluations concentrate on educational effectiveness, there are other key factors such as alignment, economics (return on investment, total cost of ownership, TCO), hidden curricula factors, and displacement or diffusion of effort.

- Educational effectiveness should be considered as one important factor among many others, particularly as the over all benefits and drawbacks arising from using a resource may not be identified if only the educational dimensions are considered. Figure 16.3 illustrates a framework based on seven factors that can change as a result of an educational intervention (Ellaway, 2009b). These are pedagogy (educational effectiveness) and resources (cost, time, skill required), interaction (communication, understanding), freedom (individuality, autonomy), granularity (detail, diversity), politics (power, control), and distal (external perspectives). Each factor can involve both positive and negative impact. An intervention may have an equally positive and negative impact on pedagogy but other factors may be more or less advantageous, which changes the overall effectiveness or

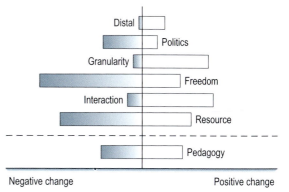

Figure 16.3 • A visual representation of the AIDA framework. There are seven factors (pedagogy, resource, interaction, freedom, granularity, politics, distal) – about here.

utility (see Figure 16.3). Evaluation data can be used to improve the resource itself, to change the activities in which it is used, the way it is presented or to rethink the learning objectives and the wider educational context of use.

- *Sustainability:* over time any resource gradually becomes a legacy item representing older and possibly redundant practices or knowledge. Sustaining it may involve a wide range of tasks and responsibilities:
  - Technical sustainability has been a particular challenge for electronic materials, as continually changing computer technologies prevent older materials running on newer machines. Compared with books, which may be tens or even hundreds of years old and still useful, many electronic resources do not remain technically viable much past 10 years and often a lot less than that. The adoption of technical interoperability standards is intended to help address this problem but the lifetimes of digital media (CD/DVD-ROM, tape, disc) are also quite short. One result has been that learning resources have in effect become more ephemeral, with their original substance relocated to the activities in which they are used.
  - Medical knowledge is constantly in flux. Any learning resource that contains factual knowledge will almost inevitably become increasingly out of date as the knowledgebase advances (although anatomy and other less dynamic disciplines are less prone to this issue). Sustaining the factual accuracy of learning materials may involve purchasing a newer edition of a resource, changing the resource directly, or adding addenda highlighting the changes.
  - The educational model may also go out of date. Educational practice involves a mix of evidence-based practices and social and cultural constructs that change over time. Furthermore, different teachers often have different takes on what is taught and how it is taught; the resources used by one teacher may therefore be rejected by the successor. While some materials may have little intrinsic activity built into them (textbooks), others will have a strong internal activity model (such as simulations and games). Changing the educational model can be complicated, although the use of new technical specifications (like IMS Learning Design) that provide an abstract but explicit model of an instructional

activity and tools that implement it (such as LAMS – http://www.lamsfoundation.org) make it possibly less challenging.
  - Terms of use may also change over time. For instance, access to third-party resources may be granted on a lease rather than ownership basis, ownership may change and in doing so change the rights of users, permissions may be withdrawn, and even the legal status of an organisation or its teachers and learners may change.

- Sooner or later a resource will become unwanted or unusable. This raises issues around whether it is to be archived or disposed of and how the environment will work in its absence.

The whole learning resource lifecycle can be considered as a single cyclic model (see Figure 16.4).

Unfortunately, but perhaps predictably, real life rarely conforms to such a rational and planned model as we have set out here. Resources can be created out of curiosity, and requirements and purposeful design may be omitted in favour of trial and error and there may be no evaluation, sustainability, or disposability model in place. This somewhat *ad hoc* approach is now increasingly challenged by evidence-based practice. The principles set out in Table 16.1, although basic in nature, establish an empirical basis for learning resource design and set a standard for future practice and development.

Lifecycle also involves contextual, cognitive, cultural, and educational dimensions. Some additional factors for consideration include:

- *Alignment:* resources are designed; they represent the preemptive choices and philosophies of those that design them. Their subsequent users (teachers and learners) may or may not be sympathetic to these imposed forms, which may in turn be more or less aligned to a programme's model or philosophy. Resources with more of an activity component tend to be more susceptible to

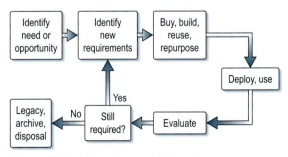

Figure 16.4 • Lifecycle model for learning resources.

Table 16.1 Colvin Clark and Mayer's evidence-based principles for designing and using learning resources ordered by effect size (multimedia has the highest effect, redundancy the lowest) (Clark and Mayer, 2008)

Principle	Description
Multimedia	Use words and graphics rather than words alone
Coherence	Additional interesting material can disrupt learning
Personalisation	Use conversational style and narrative guidance
Pretraining	Make sure that learners are trained and prepared to use the material
Contiguity	Integrate words and graphics
Segmenting	Manage complexity by breaking a lesson into parts
Modality	Present words as audio narration rather than text
Redundancy	Explain visuals with words in audio or text but not both

these kinds of problems although style, language, and selection of content can also be problematic. Wherever possible, resources should either be designed as close as possible to the context of use or be built so as to be easily adapted and realigned to different contexts of use.

- *Roles:* 'designer' is just one of the many roles involved in creating and using learning resources. Others include end users (teachers, learners), meta-professionals (learning technologists and instructional designers), editors, evaluators, librarians, publishers, and so on. Each role involves different perspectives and responsibilities and this reemphasises the subjectivity and cultural construction of significance and value of learning resources. It is also important to note the considerable variance in role, status, and authority between institutions and cultures; what happens in one context may be organised very differently in another.
- *Palimpsests:* new resources typically follow older patterns, not least because including familiar elements makes the less familiar aspects more accessible. Something truly and completely new can be quite inaccessible and incomprehensible

without familiar clues, metaphors, and models to work with. Less useful forms can get incorporated at the same time as more useful older patterns are employed. For instance, using a page metaphor in a learning object may help orient a learner to the way material is presented but it can also impose (materially or in the learner's mind) linearity, typographic constraint, and a passive relationship to the material being presented.

- *Aggregation:* learning resources may be used quite independently of each other or in clusters or collections. Simpler resources are often grouped (such as image banks) with descriptive metadata supporting user discrimination between them. Inter-resource relationships may be asynchronous (interoperability – sharing the same formats and wrappers for interchange or exchange) or synchronous (integrated – sharing data or some other runtime aspect).
- *Making as learning:* the educational benefits of learning resources do not just arise from their use; they can also be gained through their creation. Not only do the learners have to undertake the research to support the design but also they need to consider the best way to present the material and support the desired learning outcomes. This is in part related to the 'knows', 'knows how', 'shows how', and 'does' model of developing clinical competence (Miller, 1990) with resource authoring being a strong bridge between 'knows how' and 'shows how'.

Economics

A learning resource clearly represents an investment of time and money, not just to create it but also to sustain it over time. Although economic factors are often played down in favour of cognitive and professional factors in the literature, real-world practice is determined as much by what is fiscally possible as by what is desirable.

As an illustration of why this is a critical topic, let us consider the many initiatives during the 1990s to create courseware as a response to the new opportunities in teaching and learning afforded by increasingly cheap and ubiquitous personal computers in the learning environment. A huge commitment was made to creating materials individually, institutionally, and even at national and international levels. A reflection of Mao's doctrine of 'let a hundred flowers blossom'

Table 16.2 A total cost of ownership (TCO) model for learning resources

Lifecycle	Direct costs	Indirect costs
Requirements	Time spent (salaries, diversion)	Acquiring skills in requirements gathering and analysis
Buy	Cost of purchase or licence	Finance and contracts support
Build	Salaries of developers, time taken to develop	Training, accommodation, support for developers
Adapt	Cost of purchase or licence, salaries of developers, time taken to develop	Finance and contracts support, training, accommodation, support for developers
Deploy	Time, resource-specific infrastructure (systems, servers, buildings), training, documentation	Client hardware, power, context infrastructure (network, power, support, security), orientation, and framing
Evaluate	Time spent (salaries, diversion), costs of upgrading, adapting or changing	Impact on educational context (method, course, programme) of information and change
Sustain	Depreciation (based on lifetime and replacement costs), time spent making changes and maintaining resource	Warranty and maintenance, context infrastructure (network, power, support, security), costs associated with resource failure
Dispose	Replacement and migration costs, disposal or archiving investment	Archivists and systems

dominated; certainly capacity was built, knowledge gained, and the field advanced. However, almost all of these resources are now lost to technological and cultural change. The investment might have been worth it in terms of developing practice in using educational multimedia, but that is almost all that remains. An equivalent investment in paper-based resources would have left a far more permanent legacy in terms of extant learning resources.

A TCO model allows us to consider both direct and indirect costs at every stage of the resource lifecycle (as outlined in the previous section), the key dimension being those costs not immediately associated with the resource but still essential to its creation, deployment, and operation. An outline of such costs is given in Table 16.2.

A greater part of the costs associated with any intervention or technology are indirect and often go unnoticed; for instance, one model estimated that only 23% of the cost of technology is the technology itself; 21% is direct labour and 56% indirect labour (Kaestner, 2008). Although this model was developed in the context of primary and secondary schools, the importance of TCO is clearly shown; unless all costs are evaluated, the true value and impact of any resource or intervention can not be fully understood or appreciated.

There are a number of developments and initiatives that are looking to address issues of cost and flexibility in educational resources:

- The idea of 'reusable learning objects' was developed in part as a response to the high rate of technical attrition and in part as a way to get better return on investment for educational materials. It was also framed by the Internet model of discrete but combined and discoverable content (text, images, etc.). Although there are many definitions for RLOs (some very broad, others very narrow), perhaps the simplest is that an RLO is 'any digital resource that can be reused to support learning' (Wiley, 2000, p 7). Reusable learning objects offer a granular approach with each object addressing a single discrete topic or learning objective, a focus on education and instruction and the ability to function meaningfully in different contexts of use. There are now a great many published RLOs in repositories such as MedEdPortal, HeAL, and JorumOpen but their utility and uptake has been less than might have been expected, partly through teacher inertia and partly because there are more pressing problems in education than providing content.

- Educational technology standards and specifications are increasingly important in assuring longevity, reusability, and efficiency in production and sustainability of all educational systems and resources (see Box 16.2). Groups like the IEEE, IMS Global, ADL, and MedBiquitous have all published common reference models

Box 16.2

Cornucopia?

There is a common misconception that whatever material you want or need can be found online. However, things online are only what someone has put there; there is no systematic programme to ensure that the web represents all human knowledge. In fact not only are there many gaps but also much of the material is contradictory, subjective, and in many cases incorrect and even dangerous. So what learning resources are 'out there'?

There are several specialised health care education collections like MedEdPortal, HeAL, and CHEC-CESC and there are many resources in media collections like Flickr (images) and YouTube (videos) that are appropriate or even targeted at educational use. Many of these sites allow for the creation of dedicated channels such as those for Clinical Skills Online or Pocketsnips. Other image sources include Wikimedia Commons, Public Health Image Library, and MedPedia. Of particular note is the Open Courseware movement where whole institutions post their learning materials online for free use and reuse. So far only a few medical schools (such as Tufts) have followed this route. One of the main advances of Open Courseware is a clear demonstration of the benefits of making materials widely available, while the real value is still based on presence and participation in a programme of study.

Resources may also be tools. There are many free tools available online, many of which are open source (this means that they can be freely adapted as well as reused). Notable open source educational tools include Moodle, Sakai, Joomla, LAMS, and OpenLabyrinth.

Remember to make sure that you check the terms of use before downloading and using any resource.

for institutions and manufacturers to make their products interoperable with each other. This allows materials to be moved laterally from different systems or longitudinally from predecessor to successor systems. Standards and specifications can also represent a collaborative expert model of what might in business circles be called 'best practice' and can thereby simplify and extend the learning environment for the learner and teacher (even though their implementation may be problematic for the developers) (Smothers et al, 2008).

The other side of economics is to do with liabilities, rights, and licences. A learning resource is not a neutral artifact; it informs and guides learners in ways that may or may not be correct or even safe. It is usual practice therefore to include some kind of declaration regarding liability (who is responsible) and warranty (what happens when there is a problem). These are important concerns even if the resource is never going to be used outside the context in which it was created.

As soon as something is created, intellectual property (IP) comes into play. Unless otherwise contracted, the rights of a substantial innovation belong to the individual(s) who created it. However, the things employees create during or as part of their contracted work typically belong to the organisation they work for. Intellectual property is a concept larger than copyright but in the area of learning resources copyright is by far the main concern and this is complicated by there being no common model for defining rights for educational resource creation and use.

There is a continuum between full copyright and public domain: the former meaning that all rights are reserved and permission must be given to make legal use of a resource, the latter waiving rights altogether and allowing for any kind of use without requiring any kind of permissions from their authors. Creative Commons is one of a number of licensing models that sits between copyright and public domain, reserving some rights and giving others away. Creative Commons is particularly noteworthy both because it is particularly focused on content (as opposed to software for instance) and because it has proved very popular with individuals and institutions alike and has been translated into many different legal jurisdictions worldwide. A Creative Commons licence can be applied to a resource by its author(s) to specify to subsequent users whether:

- the authors must be identified as such with the work (attribution)
- changes, extractions, and incorporations can be made (derivatives)
- commercial use can be made of the resource or its derivatives
- the same conditions pertaining to the original are passed on to any derivatives (share alike)

By clearly stating the terms of its use, a resource can be safely published and reused. Without any such declaration the assumption must be one of full copyright and no use can be made without permission from its owners. There are some circumstances where limited reuse and copying are allowed, such as in libraries or under the terms of fair use agreements. But even this should be undertaken with care and consideration, not just for the copyright owners but also as an exemplar to the learners. Far too many teachers use copyrighted materials without permissions and this sends inappropriate messages to learners about what they can and should do with other people's intellectual property.

The other main legal concern regarding learning resources, particularly in health care, is around confidentiality and privacy, primarily (but not exclusively) on behalf of patients. Health care institutions typically have consent policies and processes for recordings (images, videos, etc.) of patients while they are in a condition of care. However, if the terms of consent are not passed on with the resource, then subsequent uses may break the terms of consent, creating legal as well as professional liabilities for all concerned. It is good practice to make sure that any material that identifies patients is anonymised as far as possible (without losing utility) and properly consented with the terms of that consent appended or otherwise attached to the resource to ensure that subsequent use follows the wishes of the patient involved (Ellaway et al, 2006a).

Future developments

All future-gazing is doomed to ridicule and often what seemed like the future turned out to be the present in disguise. However, we can fairly safely predict that the Internet will continue to grow and change and research will improve our understanding and use of learning materials. At the same time, innovation and social, political, and cultural change will continue to confuse and distract faster than we can build sound evidence-based practice to manage this change. Cost will continue to be a major driver but new advances will change the economic distribution and the focus of where these costs fall. Institutional boundaries will be challenged as learners and faculty become increasingly nomadic within the broader infosphere and in such a world the idea of a learning resource may be altogether transformed and diversified. Of course it will be interesting to see whether any of this comes to pass.

Implications for practice

There is clearly more to designing and using learning resources than preparing handouts and slides. New technologies provide an ever-growing repertoire of tools and designs for learning and we are still coming up with new and innovative forms. This diversity presents significant challenges to teachers in keeping up with new developments and in deciding how and whether they should incorporate them into their practice. This chapter has set out the need for critical reflection on and discourse about the nature, application, and effects of learning resources on learners, teachers, institutions, and professions. If this chapter has introduced more complexity to your work, I apologise, but I hope you have also developed a greater appreciation of how to handle that complexity and make it work for rather than against you.

References

Aldrich C: *Learning by doing,* San Francisco, CA, 2005, Pfeiffer.

Baudrillard J: *Simulacra and simulation,* Ann Arbor, MI, 1994, University of Michigan Press.

Castronova E: *Synthetic worlds: the business and culture of online games,* Chicago, IL, 2005, University of Chicago Press.

Clark RC, Nguyen F, Sweller J, et al: *Efficiency in learning,* San Francisco, CA, 2006, Pfeiffer.

Ellaway RH: e-Learning and e-teaching. In Dent JA, Harden RM, editors: *A practical guide for medical teachers,* Edinburgh, UK, 2009a, Churchill Livingstone, pp 229–237.

Ellaway RH: eMedical teacher: optics on assessment, *Med Teach* 31 (6):571–573, 2009b.

Ellaway R, Dewhurst D, Quentin M, et al: *ACETS: assemble, catalogue, exemplify, test and share (Internet),* 2005. Available from http://www.acets.ac.uk/resources/acetspub.pdf. Accessed November 25, 2009.

Ellaway R, Cameron H, Ross M, et al: Clinical recordings for academic non-clinical settings: CHERRI Project Report (Internet), 2006a. Available from http://www.cherri.mvm.ed.ac.uk/cherri.pdf. Accessed November 25, 2009.

Ellaway R, Candler C, Greene P, et al: *An architectural model for MedBiquitous*

virtual patients, Baltimore, MD, 2006b, MedBiquitous.

Issenberg SB: The scope of simulation-based healthcare education, Simulation in Healthcare: *The Journal of the Society for Simulation in Healthcare* 1(4):203–208, 2006.

Kaestner R: A holistic view of the total cost of technology, *School Business Affairs* 74(10):21–22, 2008.

Kalyuga S, Ayres P, Chandler P, et al: The expertise reversal effect, *Educ Psychol* 38(1):23–31, 2003.

Keen A: *The cult of the amateur,* London, UK, 2007, Nicholas Brealey Publishing.

Land R, Bayne S: Screen or monitor? Surveillance and disciplinary power in online learning environments. In Land R, Bayne S, editors: *Education in cyberspace*, London, UK, 2005, Routledge Falmer.

Loechel WE: The history of medical illustration, *Bull Med Libr Assoc* 48 (2):168–171, 1960.

Miller G: The assessment of clinical skills/competence/performance, *Acad Med* 65:563–567, 1990.

Powley E, Higson R: *The arts in medical education: a practical guide*, Abingdon, UK, 2005, Radcliffe.

Smothers V, Greene P, Ellaway R, et al: Sharing innovation: the case for technology standards in health professions education, *Med Teach* 30 (2):150–154, 2008.

Sweller J: Cognitive load during problem solving: effects on learning, *Cogn Sci* 12(2):257–285, 1988.

Wiley DA: *The instructional use of learning objects (Internet)*, 2000. Available from http://www.reusability.org Accessed November 25, 2009.

Further reading

Clark RC, Mayer RE: *e-Learning and the science of instruction*, San Francisco, CA, 2008, Pfeiffer.

Ellaway R, Masters K: AMEE Guide 32: e-learning in medical education, *Med Teach* 30(5):455–489, 2008.

Horton W: *e-Learning by design*, San Francisco, CA, 2006, Pfeiffer.

Mayer RE, editor: *The Cambridge handbook of multimedia learning*, New York, 2005, Cambridge University Press.

Selecting for medicine

17

Harold Reiter   Kevin W. Eva

CHAPTER CONTENTS

ABC

Glossary

Accreditation Council for Graduate Medical Education (ACGME) competencies A compendium of competencies expected to be mastered by graduate-level medical trainees (residents) in the United States.

CanMEDS roles in Canada A compendium of roles expected to be mastered by graduate-level medical trainees (residents); as its name suggests, this compendium originated in Canada, but it has been widely accepted internationally.

Computer-based Assessment for Sampling Personal Characteristics (CASPer) Developed in Canada 2003–2010, this method of assessment (largely dependent upon video-based situational judgement) purports to measure softer skills domains of professionalism and personal qualities.

CDAMS Report Indigenous Health Curriculum Development Project – National Audit & Consultations Report produced in 2004, on behalf of the Australian Government Department of Health and Ageing – Office for Aboriginal & Torres Strait Islander Health.

Emotional Intelligence (EI) Model This model suggests a self-perceived ability to identify, assess, and manage the emotions of oneself, of others, and of groups.

Educational Testing Service (ETS) Founded in 1947, near Princeton, New Jersey; develops and administers many different types of tests, including aptitude tests.

Five Factor Model (Big Five) A model of personality traits obtained through factor analysis of all personality traits described prior to 1990; these five traits are defined as Openness to experience, Neuroticism, Extraversion, Conscientiousness, and Agreeableness; Five Factor Model testing is used extensively in the field of human resources.

Continued

© 2011, Elsevier Ltd.
DOI: 10.1016/B978-0-7020-3522-7.00017-6

Glossary (continued)

Good Medical Practice A compendium of principles and values of health care provision, produced by the General Medical Council in the United Kingdom.

Graduate Australian Medical School Admissions Test (GAMSAT) An aptitude test, conducted primarily for postsecondary educational-level applicants to Australian medical schools.

Grade Point Average (GPA) A measure of academic achievement used extensively in Canada, Australia, and the United States.

Institute for International Medical Education (IIME) Compendium of requirements expected to be mastered by medical school graduates internationally.

Myers–Briggs Type Indicator (MBTI) A personality test first developed in 1962, intended to measure preferences between countervailing personality types as defined by the four dichotomies related to introversion, intuition, thinking, and perceiving.

Medical College Admissions Test (MCAT) An aptitude test, conducted in conjunction with the Association of American Medical Colleges (see Glossary, Chapter 19), which developed through several iterations from initial medical school applicant aptitude testing in 1928. It is widely required by Anglophone medical schools in North America.

Medical Council of Canada Qualifying Examination (MCCQE) The national licensure test in Canada.

Multiple Mini-Interview (MMI) A series of short interviews (often 10), conducted as a bell-ringer examination in a continuous circuit on multiple applicants at one time.

Minnesota Multiphasic Personality Inventory (MMPI) A personality test initially developed in the 1930s, with primary use related to testing mental health.

Revised Neuroticism–Extroversion–Openness Personality Inventory (NEO–PI–R) A commonly used instrument for Big Five Factor personality testing.

Reliability See main Glossary, p 340.

Scholastic Aptitude Test (SAT) An aptitude test, used primarily for entry after high school into postsecondary educational institutions in the United States, taken by over 2 million secondary school students annually.

University of Cambridge Local Examinations Syndicate (UCLES) Europe's largest assessment centre; this was established in 1858, some 66 years after Cambridge was the site of the first recorded written examinations in Europe.

United Kingdom Clinical Aptitude Test (UKCAT) Aptitude test conducted for applicants to UK medical schools, first run in 2006.

Unified Mark Scheme (UMS) A points system used as a measure of academic achievement in the United Kingdom.

Validity See main Glossary, p 341.

Outline

The last century has witnessed dramatic changes in how we view the science and art of selecting medical students, and in the tools available to achieve the task. Many of today's challenges in learner selection were cited in the Carnegie Foundation's Flexner Report 100 years ago. In recognition of the visionary nature of that report, this chapter tells the story of the last century's changes through its lens. The years preceding the report were characterised by ignorance, real or feigned, of the science of selection, dubbed the 'age of ignorance'. The years following the report, sparked by it, were marked by steady advances in the assessment of candidates' cognitive abilities, hence the 'age of cognitive advancement'. More recent advances in assessment of candidates' professional and personal qualities have marked an 'age of professional advancement'. All those advances have made candidate selection a less random process, constraining the space in which 'other considerations' – often reflecting particular societal values – could thrive. While the evidence base pertaining to admission decisions has grown to a point where decision-making in the absence of data has become less defensible, there are still important societal needs to be addressed. As a result, the 'age of balance' is now upon us. This chapter describes the challenges of selecting learners 'fairly'. It identifies where progress has been made over the last 100 years, discusses the relative advantages and disadvantages of available assessment tools, reflects on the difficulty of balancing the merits of candidates against societal needs, and speculates on future directions for research on how to select medical learners.

Introduction

Post-secondary health education institutions are charged with producing societies' future health care providers. Priorities for health professions education have evolved over many years, reflected in and directed by the ways trainees have been selected. Admissions protocols are clearly the most important determinant of who will practice medicine; arguably, they are also the most important determinant of how medicine will be taught and how the profession will be shaped. As a result, the history of admissions is the history of medical education over the last 100 years. The accelerated pace of emerging knowledge and the increasing demand for practitioners to be accountable to society have been mirrored by changes in selection practices. In the eighteenth century, an apprenticeship model dominated education; mastery of knowledge was not consistently achievable because admissions processes and curricular conditions were variable. The selection of health care providers was more often related to extraneous factors like money, family, and caste than to individuals' personal traits or intellects. Much has since changed, and changed for the better but there is not, nor should there be, an end to this story so long as we strive continually to improve selection.

The centenary of the Flexner Report provides a historic lens through which to witness those changes, not only because so much has changed over the 100 years but also because so much of that change was presaged in it. This chapter cites the Report liberally, not just to honour it on its centenary, but because many issues it addressed are timeless.

> Practically the medical school is a public service corporation. It is chartered by the state; it utilizes public hospitals on the ground of the social nature of its service. The medical school cannot then escape social criticism and regulation. It was left to itself while society knew no better. But civilization consists in the legal registration of gains won by science and experience; and science and experience have together established the terms upon which medicine can be most useful.
>
> (Flexner, 1910, p 154)

Moments of transformation arise from gains won by science and experience; changing political, social, and cultural imperatives; the vision and talent of galvanising individuals; and, some believe, the divine hand of God. Evaluating the relative contribution of each is best left to historians, biographers, and theologians. This chapter deals, instead, with several moments of transformation in chronological order. They are made most visible by contrasting the age that preceded a transformative moment with the age that followed it. Before the Flexner Report, there was an 'age of ignorance' of principles of assessment. After Flexner, reliable and valid assessment tools of cognitive ability were developed and applied, which led to an 'age of cognitive advancement'. As concerns over cognitive ability receded, lack of professional 'soft skills' became more central. Only recently, reliable and valid assessment tools of those domains have begun to bear fruit, sparking a shift into the 'age of professional advancement'. As one concern falls to the march of progress, another arises to take its place. Just as cognition was replaced by professionalism, professionalism is now being replaced by a more

insidious challenge, as we stand on the doorstep of an 'age of balance'.

The First Age – pre-1910: the age of ignorance

> "Men get in, not because the country needs the doctors, but because the schools need the money." "What is your honest opinion of your own enrolment?" a professor in a Philadelphia school was asked. "Well, the most I would claim," he answered, "is that nobody who is absolutely worthless gets in"!
>
> (Flexner, 1910, p 35)

It would be overkind to attribute the widespread ignorance about selecting learners in pre-Flexnerian America to lack of scientific method; it would also be inaccurate. In 520 BCE, under the leadership of Ezra and Nehemiah, a host of Jews returned to the land of Israel 70 years after the Babylonian exile and destruction of the First Holy Temple. In the interregnum, the intricate laws of sacrifice and defilement had been forgotten to a great extent so the priestly caste was required to undergo assessment of that knowledge, which was critical to their duties in the newly built Second Holy Temple. The Old Testament (Haggai 2, 10–13) introduces the concept of enhancing test reliability by using multiple questions (Babylonian Talmud) over 2400 years before Flexner. More recently, the University of Cambridge Local Examinations Syndicate (UCLES), Europe's largest assessment centre, was established in 1858 (52 years before the Flexner Report), Cambridge having also been the site of the first recorded written examinations in Europe some 66 years earlier (Stray, 2005). A way of assessing medical school applicants was thus available for those institutions that chose to use them. What was understood then is understood now: multiple questions of knowledge provide a more accurate assessment than a single sample. Just because someone knows one thing about a subject does not mean that they know the subject well.

Despite that knowledge, the selection of learners for medical school (and postgraduate training, such as it existed at the time) was remarkable for its lack of standards and accountability. The measurement of skills in 1910 was a poor cousin of what it is now but it was well enough developed to cast a dim shadow on medical schools that willfully chose to ignore it or, worse, professed to uphold it, but responded to bribes. As Flexner describes:

Indeed, the advertising methods of the commercially successful schools are amazing. Not infrequently advertising costs more than laboratories. The school catalogues abound in exaggeration, misstatements, and half-truths. The deans of these institutions occasionally know more about modern advertising than about modern medical teaching. They may be uncertain about the relation of the clinical laboratory to bedside instruction; but they have calculated to a nicety which "medium" brings the largest "return."

(Flexner, 1910, p 19)

Nor did poor performance in medical school provide a barrier to future practice. As described of many nineteenth-century American medical schools:

No applicant for instruction who could pay his fees or sign his note was turned down. State boards were not as yet in existence. The school diploma was itself a license to practice. The examinations, brief, oral, and secret, plucked almost none at all. . . The man who had settled his tuition bill was thus practically assured of his degree, whether he had regularly attended lectures or not.

(Flexner, 1910, p 7)

The advent of standard setting

The twentieth century brought little improvement. Three methods of standard setting for admission became commonly used – high school graduation, an 'equivalent' entrance exam, or the approval of an appointed 'medical examiner'. Beneath that gloss, admission to most medical schools continued to depend not so much on the content of one's mind or soul as the content of one's wallet.

To get at the real admission standard, then, of these medical schools, one must make straight for the "equivalent". On the methods of ascertaining and enforcing that, the issue hangs. Now the "equivalent" may be defined as a device that concedes the necessity of a standard which it forthwith proceeds to evade. . .If the standard were enforced, the candidates in question, not offering a graduation diploma from an accredited high school, would be compelled to enter by written examination. But the examination is, as things stand, only another method of evasion. Neither in extent nor in difficulty do the written examinations, in the relatively rare cases in which they are given, even approximate the high school standard. Nor are they meant to do so. . . There remains a third method of cutting below an actual high school standard, – the method indeed that provides much the most capacious loophole for the admission of unqualified students under the cloak of nominal compliance with the high school standard. The agent in the transactions about to be described is the medical examiner, appointed in some places by voluntary agreement

between the schools, elsewhere delegated by the state board, or by the superintendent of public instruction acting in its behalf, for the purpose of dealing with students who present written evidence other than the diploma of an accredited high school. It is intended and expected that this official shall enforce a high school standard. In few states is this standard achieved. . . The schools do not want the rule enforced, and the boards are either not strong enough or not conscientious enough to withstand them. Formerly, written examinations were used in part; but they were given up "because almost everybody failed."

(Flexner, 1910, pp 30–33)

If you are not yet completely disheartened by the admissions processes of the era, Flexner drives one further stake into the heart of the matter.

There is no protection against fraud or forgery. . . In visits to medical colleges certificates were found from non-existent schools as well as from non-existent places.

(Flexner, 1910, p 36)

Institutions, whose existence was driven more by producing high-quality physicians and less by producing high-quantity bank statements, began to change the age of ignorance:

The credit for the actual initiative belongs fairly to the institutions that had the courage and the virtue to make the start. The first of these was the Chicago school, which is now the medical department of Northwestern University, and which in 1859 initiated a three-year graded course. Early in the seventies the new president of Harvard College startled the bewildered faculty of its medical school into the first of a series of reforms that began with the grading of the existing course and ended in 1901 with the requirement of an academic degree for admission. . . Towards this consummation President Eliot had aimed from the start; but he was destined to be anticipated by the establishment in 1893 of the Johns Hopkins Medical School on the basis of a bachelor's degree, from which, with quite unprecedented academic virtue, no single exception has ever been made.

(Flexner, 1910, pp 11–12)

An increasing number of medical schools followed that lead, which provided fertile ground for the Flexner Report.

The Second Age – 1910–1990: the age of cognitive advancement

What safeguards may society and the law throw about admission to a profession like that of law or of medicine in order that a sufficient number of men may be induced to enter it and yet the unfit and the undesirable may be excluded? – (Flexner, 1910 – Introduction by Henry S. Pritchett, President of the Carnegie Foundation, p xiv)

Cognitive assessment

The use of cognitive assessments has become ubiquitous over the last century, and research and development have enhanced once-simple tools in sophisticated ways. Measures come in two main types – academic achievement and aptitude tests. The former are reported in different ways in different countries including Unified Mark Scheme (UMS) points in the United Kingdom and Grade Point Average (GPA) in Canada, Australia, and the United States. For much of the world, that means coursework grades at either the secondary school (e.g. UMS in the United Kingdom and GPA in Australia) or post-secondary school (e.g. GPA in Canada and the United States) level. Because they use serial measurements, records of academic achievement predict future performance in medical school quite well (Kreiter and Kreiter, 2007). The greater the number of measurements, the greater the accuracy. There seem to be diminishing returns if grades from more than ten courses are used. That said, the usefulness of academic records can sometimes be lessened by additional factors.

In some parts of the world, grading schemes are set such that no discrimination can be made between top candidates, all of them simply receiving 'A-levels' or 'Pass' as their summative record of achievement. In others, there is potential for 'grade inflation' both before (Rojstaczer, 2009) and during medical training (Speer et al, 2000). While an applicant's field of study has been suggested as a major source of inequity in GPAs, it seems to have less effect than the applicant's institution of origin (Trail et al, 2006), though the nature and size of that bias are unclear. There has been no shortage of evidence-based attempts to equate academic achievement across institutions. National accrediting bodies, where they exist, would seem to be the natural entities to do so but, sadly, they have not played a major role. Some academics have taken up the challenge with limited success. All attempts have involved connecting the scores of institutions of origin to a gold standard. In one attempt, GPA was adjusted based on aptitude test scores to promising effect when national certification examination results were treated as the outcome measure against which the influence of this adjustment was compared (Didier et al, 2006). The use of aptitude tests as a gold standard is understandable, as a well-conducted aptitude test can provide even better validity than academic scores.

Aptitude tests

The Scholastic Aptitude Test (SAT) is now used by over 2 million secondary school students annually in the United States when applying to post-secondary educational programmes. The origins of general aptitude tests preceded Flexner but aptitude tests specific to medical school admission came later. The reformation of American medical education that followed Flexner increased accountability, which meant higher attrition rates from medical schools. In response, the 'SAT for medical students' was born in 1928 which, after many iterations, came to be known as the Medical College Admission Test (MCAT). All but one of the 139 Anglophone medical schools in the United States and Canada (as of this writing) include MCAT in their admission requirements. Efforts to produce medical school admissions aptitude tests elsewhere are, relative to the MCAT, still in their infancy. The United Kingdom Clinical Aptitude Test (UKCAT) was first run in 2006, too recently for predictive validity data to be available (UKCAT Annual Report, 2006). Preliminary predictive validity data for the Graduate Australian Medical School Admissions Test (Wilkinson et al, 2008) do not yet compare favourably with MCAT. The various tests used in other countries include aptitude tests (e.g. the Undergraduate Medicine and Health Sciences Admission Test in Australia and New Zealand and the Psychometric Entrance Test in Israel) and tests falling midway between testing secondary school curriculum material and aptitude (the A-levels, or Advanced Levels of the General Certificate of Education in the United Kingdom with similar variants in many Commonwealth countries, including India, Pakistan, Hong Kong, and South Africa). The most recent MCAT format, which began in 1991, includes multiple choice question sections on verbal reasoning, biological sciences, and physical sciences as well as an essay 'writing sample' section. The MCAT shifted to computer-based testing in 2007, and faces its next major overhaul in 2013. It is now a better predictor of the final step to national licensure ($r = 0.49$ without correction for disattenuation) than GPA ($r = 0.29$), the combination of the two predicting slightly better still, at a rate of $r = 0.52$ (Julian, 2005). The verbal reasoning component of MCAT is less affected by the passage of time from admission than other MCAT sections and academic records (Siu and Reiter, 2009) and correlates strongly with clinical decision-making and patient interaction endpoints on national licensure examinations (Donnon et al, 2007).

Like all assessment measures, however, aptitude tests have detractors. Average MCAT scores are lower for African-Americans and Hispanic Americans than for Caucasians and Asian-Americans (MCAT Report, 1999). Yet if a bias exists, it is more prevalent in the GPA, which tends to undervalue African-American candidates, even relative to MCAT (Koenig et al, 1998). The applicant must pay to take the test (albeit with financial support for American MCAT-takers), which is prodigiously long. It has also been suggested that, notwithstanding the strong correlation of aptitude test scores with national licensure results, they are poor markers of future performance in practice. That last belief is, however, unsupportable. Candidate results on national licensure examinations do predict salient outcomes. Appropriate use of diagnostic tests and prescription practices, for example, were more common in people who scored higher on the Quebec Family Medicine Certification Examination or on the Medical Council of Canada Qualifying Examination (Tamblyn et al, 2002). Peer estimates of clinical ability correlate strongly with scores on American Board of Internal Medicine certification examination scores (Ramsey et al, 1989). There are fewer complaints against physicians who score higher in communication skills and clinical decision-making components of the Medical Council of Canada Qualifying Examination (Tamblyn et al, 2007). Survival rates following heart attacks are higher in patients of physicians who score higher on American Board of Internal Medicine certification examinations (Norcini et al, 2002).

Those findings are very important, given that the long time between medical school application and post-training medical practice stands in the way of assessing the relationship between admission variables and long-term outcome variables; it introduces all sorts of confounding variables and makes it hard to track individuals as they move from one level of training to another. National licensure examinations, therefore, represent an important surrogate measure of real practice. Thus, despite the various criticisms that can be launched towards MCAT or GPA, Flexner's demand for stricter standards and diligent accountability has improved patient care. Measures have been enhanced so it is possible to select medical students who will perform better on national licensing examinations and, ultimately, provide better patient care. Yet, the story is not over.

The Third Age – 1990–2010: the age of professional advancement

It is necessary to install a doorkeeper who will, by critical scrutiny, ascertain the fitness of the applicant; a necessity suggested in the first place by consideration for the candidate, whose time and talents will serve him better in some other vocation, if he be unfit for this; and in the second, by consideration for a public entitled to protection from those whom the very boldness of modern medical strategy equips with instruments that, tremendously effective for good when rightly used, are all the more terrible for harm if ignorantly or incompetently employed.

(Flexner, 1910, p 22)

Professional as well as cognitive attributes

Perhaps it is sufficient to provide patients with physicians they need as opposed to physicians they want. So long as the correct prophylaxis to ill health is recommended, the correct diagnosis made, the correct dosage of the correct drugs or the correct procedure provided, and the correct follow-up maintained, a practitioner with a surly disposition will do as well as a practitioner with a sunny one on many measures of competence. That stance, together with the relationships between test performance and practice success outlined above, might suggest that it is not worth selecting for bedside manner. More than 90% of complaints to American state boards, however, are on the basis of professional, rather than cognitive skills (Papadakis et al, 2005). That might be because cognitively weak medical school applicants have been weeded out by the judicious use of GPA and aptitude tests. Further, the finding might be engendered by patients and family members having the ability, or willingness, to judge physicians on the basis of professional comportment, and not on the basis of clinical acumen. The latter interpretation is supported by a report on the categorisation of complaints in the District of Columbia in 1952, a time when GPA was less trustworthy and aptitude tests were not yet in use ubiquitously (Stokes, 1952). Then, as now, most complaints were about doctors' professionalism. Patients may not know when their physicians lack sufficient knowledge, but they can certainly detect lack of communication skills.

There has been greater scepticism in the last few decades about the argument that medical knowledge is enough for good medical practice. The medical community and society have come to believe that the physician's attributes that are 'tremendously effective for good when rightly used', and 'all the more terrible for harm if ignorantly or incompetently employed' (Flexner, 1910, p 22), are not merely cognitive ones. Specification of the CanMEDS roles in Canada (Frank and Danoff, 2007), ACGME competencies in the United States, Good Medical Practice principles and values of the General Medical Council in the United Kingdom, and IIME global minimal essential requirements internationally all speak to the importance of professionalism. The community has come to consider the active listener, caring hand, and considerate soul to be valid, and at times critical, attributes of physicians, and that is presumably why fewer complaints are lodged against physicians scoring more highly in communication skills (Tamblyn et al, 2007). To provide for the needs of patients and respond to the unique characteristics of all clinical situations, something more than an extensive knowledge base is required. Given that historical context, it is only natural that greater emphasis would be placed upon developing reliable and valid admissions instruments that tap into various 'non-cognitive qualities' (an unfortunate term that is commonly used to differentiate academic performance from the dozens of other characteristics valued in physicians). Defining qualities as 'non-cognitive', 'soft skills', or 'professionalism' suggests a sharp divide between those qualities and cognitive abilities. That divide is patently artificial. Health care providers need compound abilities that flow seamlessly between cognitive and 'non-cognitive' ones if they are to understand the needs of patients and help them understand health care options. Nevertheless, the discussion of a health care provider as a professional is more easily conveyed through emphasising unique 'non-cognitive', 'soft skills'; and an ability to assess those skills is at hand after faltering beginnings.

Personality testing

Personality testing, using the Minnesota Multiphasic Personality Inventory, or the Myers–Briggs Type Indicator, has been used for workforce placement decisions, but without supportive evidence about its predictive validity (Boyle, 1996). Better predictive validity has emerged from the Big Five Factor Model of personality, which presents five dimensions of personality as descriptors – openness, conscientiousness, extraversion, agreeableness, and neuroticism. Of the five, only conscientiousness has shown incremental benefit for future job performance in meta-analysis of human resource studies (Barrick and Mount, 1991). The validity of conscientiousness for selecting medical students has not been confirmed, and the positive correlation found between it and GPA (Ferguson et al, 2003) suggests that it might be superfluous. Further, medical school applicants are quite a homogeneous population and benefit, therefore, from a fine measurement tool that can maintain high reliability. Some medical schools (Ferguson et al, 2003; Lievens et al, 2002; Luh et al, 2007; Lumsden et al, 2005) and some dental schools (Chamberlain et al, 2005; Poole et al, 2007; Smithers et al, 2004) have found personality testing useful, but never in a consistent or convincing manner (Kulasegaram et al, 2009).

Emotional intelligence

Support for the use of emotional intelligence measures is even less defensible. The Emotional Intelligence Model concerns a self-perceived ability to identify, assess, and manage the emotions of one's self, of others, and of groups (Bradberry and Greaves, 2009). Claims of validity are highly questionable, both in medical education (Lewis et al, 2005) and in the general literature (Landy, 2005). Like personality testing, measures of emotional intelligence are uncomfortably dependent upon self-assessment, scores of which are often internally consistent – but consistently inaccurate (Eva and Regehr, 2007). Whereas there is one commonly used construct for personality testing (Big Five Personality Testing) and one commonly used instrument to measure it (Revised Neuroticism–Extroversion–Openness Personality Inventory, or NEO–PI–R), there is no common construct, measure, or way to interpret the results of disparate studies of emotional intelligence, and so no common sense in using it at the present time.

References

Nor is there much evidence that reference letters or personal statements, which rarely indict candidates and in which even weaknesses are portrayed as hidden strengths, are valid. No wonder that no predictive validity for these measures has been found in meta-analyses of either medical schools (Albanese et al, 2003) or health care professional schools (Salvatori, 2001).

Interviews

All this has led to interviews being the road most travelled. The interview began its doorkeeper role most inauspiciously: as a way to get the desirable (moneyed) applicants in and keep undesirable (racially identified) applicants out. For early twentieth-century commercial American medical schools with paying students unable to meet any reasonable non-pecuniary standard for admission, Flexner states that *"the written examination has been transformed into an informal after-dinner conversation between candidate and examiner"* (Flexner, 1910, p 32). A medical examiner assigned the task of interviewing led an unenviable life.

> [T]he examiners lack time, machinery, and encouragement for the proper performance of their ostensible office. They are busy men: here, a county official; there, a school principal; elsewhere, a high school professor. A single individual, after his regular day's work is over, without assistance of any kind, is thus expected to perform a task much more complicated than that for which Harvard, Columbia, and the University of Michigan maintain costly establishments. There is no set time when candidates must appear. They drop in as they please, separately: now, before the medical school opens, again, long after; sometimes with their credentials, sometimes without them. There is no definite procedure. At times, the examiner concludes from the face of the papers; at times from the face of the candidate.
>
> (Flexner, 1910, pp 32–33)

The face of the candidates would, a generation later, become the reason for interviewing at Ivy League medical schools. An interview, together with asking prospective applicants whether they had ever changed their last name, proved helpful at Harvard in reducing the percentage of Jewish matriculants from 25% to the 15% found to be more palatable by the deanery (Karabel, 2005).

Even in an age when interviews are not used with malevolent intent, admissions processes worldwide still have to contend with the inherent limitations of interviews for assessing soft skills. It has been shown time and again that interview scores do not predict future job performance (Albanese et al, 2003; Salvatori, 2001) and an applicant's score on one interview is a poor predictor of the same applicant's score on another interview (Kreiter et al, 2004). Such inconsistencies make the interview an inherently unreliable measure. An admissions office would never offer admission based on a single cognitive assessment because of the unreliability of the test yet the same office will make an offer based on a single interview. False comfort is obtained by having multiple raters, yet the variability between two interview performances far exceeds the variability between two rater scores on a single performance (Axelson and Kreiter, 2009). Intuition tells us that we can discern good interviews from poor ones, and perhaps we can, but of what use is that discernment if the applicant can be expected to perform differently in the next interview.

Multiple interviews

The potential for enhancing reliability and hence validity through multiple interviews seems to have been stumbled upon almost by accident in 1982 (Meredith et al, 1982), during an admissions process where each applicant had four independent interviews. Another 20 years were to pass before the multiple interview method was used intentionally to enhance reliability and predictive validity (Eva et al, 2004a). The chief advantage of increasing the number of independent interviews is to dilute out those interview scores less reflective of a particular individual's ability. We have all experienced interviews in which we did well, and others in which we did poorly. That variation is not so much due to changes in our skill as the change in context from interview to interview. Indeed, compared to the changing context from interview to interview (test–retest reliability of 0.18), changing interviewer is a minimal concern (inter-rater reliability of 0.64) (Eva et al, 2004b). What this means is that a more accurate assessment of candidates can be achieved by single raters in each of three interviews than by a panel of three raters in one interview. Intuitively, we know this to be true. If we had three scouts to send to a football match to assess a striker, we would not send all three scouts to one game, but rather one scout to each of three games, as the varying conditions of the game (state of field, injuries to team-mates and opponents, weather conditions, score) create different contexts in which to assess the striker more accurately. Empirically, schools worldwide have now reported interview reliabilities robustly above 0.7 when 12 mini-interviews are used, a much more satisfactory result than the test–retest reliabilities <0.2 typically found on two interviews. Such improvements in reliability have enabled better prediction of later clinical performance and national licensure scores independent of, and complementary to, that predicted by cognitive measures (Eva et al, 2009; Reiter et al, 2007).

Whether the domains measured reflect non-cognitive skills (Eva et al, 2004a), critical thinking (Roberts et al, 2009), or some other aspect of ability, the incremental value in predicting national licensure results (Eva et al, 2009; Hofmeister et al, 2009) make multiple interviews valuable. Whether variability in performance should be attributable to context specificity, rater differences, measurement error, or some other factor remains to be pinned down conclusively (Kreiter et al, 2004). The value of this research was that it opened eyes to the instability of performance and the need to sample performance in non-cognitive domains, findings that are consistent with contemporary views of the state versus trait debate of human behaviour (Eva, 2003) and professionalism (Ginsburg et al, 2000).

Computer assessment

While an increasing number of medical schools worldwide shift to the Multiple Mini-Interview (MMI), most have a far larger number of applicants than they can possibly accommodate in interviews of any format. That leaves the challenge of determining how to test professional skills reliably and remotely for very large numbers of candidates. At least three groups have taken on the challenge, all using video clips to set scenarios to which applicants have to respond. The Educational Testing Service (ETS) in the United States, in conjunction with MCAT, produced a communications module (Kylonnen, 2005), which unfortunately suffered from the need to match the modern MCAT computer-based testing format and from setting too low an expectation level of applicant performance. In Belgium, an approach that correlated with subsequent grades in softer skill medical school courses (Lievens et al, 2005) was brought to an abrupt end by the overseeing national body, which vetoed

further implementation due to concerns over test cost and technical feasibility (Lievens and Sackett, 2006). There were even more promising results in Canada with a Computer-based Assessment for Sampling Personal Characteristics (CASPer) (Dore et al, 2009). Unlike ETS, the McMaster group had the advantage of being able to compare different test formats empirically. In the transition from MMI to a computer-based format, there were a few unwelcome surprises, each directing further research and development along a narrower path. An hour of CASPer testing time provided overall test generalisability even higher (0.82) than 2 hours of MMI testing time (0.75). Yet correlations between the two tests, both meant to reflect the same domain, and often based upon the same scenarios, was only 0.15 when CASPer responses were audio-recorded. When responses were provided in written short answer format, the correlation jumped to 0.51, without disattenuation, a figure repeated on subsequent study with other endpoints (Dore et al, 2009). That correlation was higher when the responses were based on film-clip challenges and lower for written challenges, a finding reflected by results from the Belgian group (Lievens and Sackett, 2006). Those results suggest that, at the very least, a screening test of professional skills is possible. Whether any of those endeavours will eventually come to fruition is not known. What is no longer open to question is that something will fill the need for widespread testing of professional skills. If we have learnt nothing else since Flexner, we have confirmed that necessity is the mother of invention. Once the assessment need has been identified, be it cognitive or professional, a way will be found to address that need.

As for those methodologies that, despite reasonable attempts, have failed to show predictive validity, what is their role? Whither the traditional interview? Whither the reference letter? Whither the personal statement? Whither personality testing? Whither emotional intelligence testing? As more data accumulate, it becomes harder to ignore the temptation to allow them all to wither.

The Fourth Age – 2010 and beyond: the age of balance

Widening access

To this point, the story of selecting learners has been relatively straightforward. At the cognitive end of the (artificial) cognitive to non-cognitive continuum, aptitude tests and course grades provide sufficient information (though there are contextual variables that must be considered). At the non-cognitive end, MMIs and (potentially at least) computer-based testing are currently the preferred instruments, though local circumstances will have a strong influence on the final choice. Important though local contexts may be, tailoring admissions efforts to the broader societal values and their shifts across place and time are a far greater challenge. There is, in the words of the United States Supreme Court (Grutter v. Bollinger, 2003) a compelling interest in enhancing African-American and Hispanic-American presence in US medical schools; there is interest in providing reasonable access to applicants from lower socio-economic strata in the United Kingdom (Powis et al, 2007); and there is interest in enhancing Aboriginal presence in Australia (CDAMS, 2004), New Zealand, and Canada (2020 Vision, 2004). There is a compelling interest in many jurisdictions in producing a higher generalist/specialist ratio. Additionally, individual schools may have mandates to promote rural practitioners or certain languages. Such needs strain both those who have to devise admissions policies and those who defend them in public. That is true worldwide and means inevitable attempts to strike the best balance in admissions protocols and decisions made about individual candidates. Two examples follow, which show the complexity of the processes.

'Tailoring' admissions

The first example is on the generalist/specialist front, where progress has been made in increasing the popularity of generalist careers, albeit more due to changes in curriculum than in admissions processes (Rabinowitz et al, 2008). Literature reviews have consistently identified older age and female sex as factors that predict choice of a generalist career (Bland et al, 1995; Lawson and Hoban, 2003). Unfortunately, older graduates complete fewer years of service before retirement and women more commonly work part-time (Boerma and van den Brink-Muinen, 2000). Moreover, at least some jurisdictions would deem it a punishable human rights offence to admit candidates preferentially on the grounds of age or sex. The second example concerns race-related policies in the United States, which provide a more sophisticated illustration of

discrimination based on demographic variables. Selecting on the basis of race alone (dubbed 'broad tailoring' in Supreme Court decisions; Gratz v. Bollinger, 2003; Grutter v. Bollinger, 2003) has been defined as inappropriate discrimination, which runs afoul of the American Constitution. Using race as one factor among many ('narrow tailoring'), however, has been deemed allowable, but only within certain limits. Such decisions are predicated on the only acceptable compelling interest, as defined by Supreme Court Justice Powell (Regents of the University of California v. Bakke, 1978), which is 'obtaining the educational benefits that flow from an ethnically diverse student body'. That poses several problems. There are few hard data to show that a greater presence of under-represented minorities significantly enhances the educational experience of the student body and probably even less need for it now compared to 1978 simply because current diversity levels are higher than those of a generation ago. Even more fundamentally, however, the 'compelling interest' identified in Justice Powell's decision explicitly ruled out an educational institution skewing its admissions policies on the contention that increasing the number of under-represented minority physicians would result in better health care coverage for underserved communities from the same minority group.

Committee-based decision making

Accepting for the moment that there are compelling reasons to admit certain groups preferentially, every admissions committee needs to determine how it will use the data it collects during admissions processes. On the one hand, it could be argued that the most fair and objective way of admitting students is to use mechanical, algorithmic strategies (often referred to as actuarial methods) to combine data, letting the rank ordering determine who will be offered admission. Opponents of such strategies argue that judgemental, holistic decisions (often referred to as committee-based) are more appropriate as one needs to consider each individual's situation to give everyone a fair chance. The Supreme Court (Gratz v. Bollinger, 2003) opened the door wider for holistic, non-mechanical assessment methods, recognising that they tend to advantage applicants from under-represented minority groups who traditionally have fared less well on course grades and aptitude tests. Ostensibly, the assumption is that file review by experienced admissions personnel provides added value.

Unfortunately, the truth seems to lie elsewhere. In the only study of its kind, the University of Minnesota Medical School (Schofield and Garrard, 1975) followed two cohorts of medical students in the same class. One-third had been selected solely on objective measures – course grades and aptitude test scores combined in a mechanical way. The other two-thirds were selected by committee after extensive file review. Despite considerably more human resource input, the committee-selected group functioned no better than the mechanically selected group on intramural testing, national licensure examinations, or postgraduate training placement. This is not a finding unique to medical schools. A retrospective review of the files of 3000 parolees in the State of Illinois in 1928 (Burgess, 1968) identified 21 predictor variables for subsequent parole violations; the mechanistic approach to parole decisions was a better predictor of future violations than a holistic, traditional method of file review by expert parole board members. More recently, a literature review (Grove and Meehl, 1996) identified 136 studies directly comparing mechanistic with holistic methods of selection. Only 8 studies showed the holistic approach to have better predictive validity, the other 128 studies being evenly split between showing no advantage and detriment for the holistic approach. Despite the imprimatur of the United States Supreme Court and the intuitive attraction of allowing committees to debate the relative merits of applicants and weight particularly important variables in an individual-by-individual manner, the holistic approach has been largely discredited (McGaghie and Kreiter, 2005).

Striking a balance

Again, however, using actuarial methods creates a challenge when society seeks to represent a subset of the population better. One extreme is to say that only subgroup applicants who outperform other applicants on the selected admissions tools should gain entry. Another extreme is to set the level of competition for most applicants based on merit, but admit all members of a subgroup who meet some minimally sufficient lower threshold. Between the two extremes, compromise can be found, even while maintaining a mechanistic approach. While the details are beyond the scope of this chapter, Kreiter has shown that it is possible to use constraint optimisation processes, which entail setting one absolute value (e.g. the number of applicants from low

socio-economic status to be admitted) and then optimising all other variables (i.e. objective scores like aptitude test scores) in the applicant pool to meet that single absolute constraint (Kreiter, 2002). Alternatively, using compromise methods of cut point scoring (Reiter and MacCoon, 2007), the relative perceived importance of individual merit and the compelling interest can both be defined as the arbiter of how many from the 'compelling interest group' are admitted. Any of these approaches is problematic when an insufficient proportion of the subgroup of interest meets the level of sufficiency, because then individuals in that subgroup benefit at the expense of the society they are selected to serve.

How, then, can a compelling interest be met given the very real possibility of insufficient numbers? Demographic data in the United States suggest that there are insufficient proportions of African-Americans and Hispanic-Americans competing at the post-secondary educational level (Sleeth and Mishell, 1977) to fill their share of medical school seats (Kane, 1976) without running awry of the Supreme Court's admonition to use race only in a narrowly tailored fashion. These concerns are true, if less well documented, in other jurisdictions around the globe. They lead us to conclude that, while much attention has been devoted to the 'shape of the river' in post-secondary educational systems, the source of the problem lies in the confluence of the headwaters of primary/secondary education and differing social/cultural educational values. So, there is a need for substantial policy change to support members of disadvantaged subgroups before they are old enough to be considered for medical school admission.

The cost of compromise

As assessment tools of cognitive and professional skills have evolved and selection has become a more scientific process, the power of expert selectors has been challenged by weight of numbers. Admissions offices, moreover, are having to compromise to improve access for 'the poor boy' (Flexner, 1910), to assuage the racial divide, and to realise the imperfectly defined educational benefits of diversity. But when compromise occurs, what ultimately suffers is patient health. It is incumbent upon Flexner's medical schools to produce the best physicians and upon society at large to address dangerous inequalities of primary and secondary education and unfair access based upon socio-economic status. Doing so will make it unnecessary to compromise meritocratic decisions for the sake of political whims. Therefore, we come not to praise compromise but to bury it. A century after Flexner, what we need is a lot more health consumer entitlement and a lot less social enlightenment. What we need is a lot more Flexner and a lot less flexibility. What we need is to be spared well-intentioned compromise that nevertheless may produce suboptimal health care. For reasons of posterity, Abraham Flexner gets the last word on the subject:

> We have no right, it is urged, to set up standards which will close the profession to "poor boys." What are the merits of this contention? The medical profession is a social organ, created not for the purpose of gratifying the inclinations or preferences of certain individuals, but as a means of promoting health, physical vigor, happiness – and the economic independence and efficiency immediately connected with these factors. Whether most men support themselves or become charges on the community depends on their keeping well, or if ill, promptly getting well. Now, can anyone seriously contend that in the midst of abundant educational resources, a congenial or profitable career in medicine is to be made for an individual regardless of his capacity to satisfy the purpose for which the profession exists? It is right to sympathize with those who lack only opportunity; still better to assist them in surmounting obstacles; but not at the price of certain injury to the common weal. Commiseration for the hand-spinner was not suffered for one moment to defeat the general economic advantage procurable through machine-made cloth. Yet the hand-spinner had a sort of vested right: society had tacitly induced him to enter the trade; he had grown up in it on that assurance; and he was now good for nothing else. Your "poor boy" has no right, natural, indefeasible, or acquired, to enter upon the practice of medicine unless it is best for society that he should.

Flexner Report, pp 42–43

Implications for practice

A century of change in the selection of learners has taught many lessons on the ground and in the sky. On the ground, the chief lesson is a simple one – use only reliable and valid assessment tools. There are few tools that meet those criteria – academic achievement (grades), aptitude test scores, and psychometrically robust variants of the MMI technique. Applying the lesson can be hard and each institution must mould the tools to match its peculiar set of challenges – resource constraints, local mission statements, and characteristics of the applicant pool. Applying the lesson may be further limited by what is acceptable to an admissions office, as a purely data-driven process often fails to reflect stakeholders' biases, be it conscious or unconscious, benign or malignant, reflective or independent of compelling societal need. In the sky, the lessons are more opaque. Change is being driven by rapid changes in technology. As access to the entire world shrinks into laptop and handheld computers, distance education proliferates and academic achievement becomes a more heterogeneous construct. The shift may deservedly move towards aptitude tests, which will need to be developed and implemented on a large scale. Changes in what makes computers tick may nevertheless carry less impact than changes in what makes admissions stakeholders tick. While outcomes-driven research in the selection of learners is nothing new, there seems to be a heightening awareness of its power. That power derives from more than one source. The generally high level of competitiveness for medical school seats ensures that there are large databanks to explore. Further, as the previously small number of reliable predictor and outcome variables increases, the potential number of cross-correlations increases exponentially. It is entirely possible, that for all the changes we have seen over the last one hundred years, *we ain't seen nothing yet.*

References

2020 Vision: Moving Forward with a Good Mind. Report from the 28–29 September, 2004. Symposium, held at Six Nations of Grand River, co-hosted by Six Nations and McMaster University, co-chaired by the Honourable Roy J. Romanow and Chief Roberta Jamieson.

Albanese MA, Snow MH, Skochelak SE, et al: Assessing personal qualities in medical school admissions, *Acad Med* 78(3):313–321, 2003.

Axelson R, Kreiter C: Rater and occasion impacts on expected preadmission interview reliability, *Med Educ* 43(12): 2009.

Babylonian Talmud: Tractate Pesachim, pp 16b–17a.

Barrick MR, Mount MK: The big five personality dimensions and job performance: a meta-analysis, *Per Psy* 44:1–26, 1991.

Bland CJ, Meurer LN, Maldonado G: Determinants of primary care specialty choice: a non-statistical meta-analysis of the literature, *Acad Med* 70:620–641, 1995.

Boerma WG, van den Brink-Muinen A: Gender-related differences in the organization and provision of services among general practitioners in Europe: a signal to health care planners, *Med Care* 38(10): 993–1002, 2000.

Boyle GJ: Myers-Briggs Type Indicator (MBTI): Some psychometric limitations, *Austr Psychol* 30(1): 71–74, 1996.

Bradberry T, Greaves J: *Emotional Intelligence 2.0*, San Francisco, 2009, Publishers Group West.

Burgess EW: Factors determining success or failure on parole. In Bruce AA, editor: *The workings of the indeterminate sentence law and the parole system in Illinois, Springfield IL: Illinois Committee on Indeterminate Sentence Law and Parole*, 1968, pp 205–249 (originally published 1928).

CDAMS Indigenous Health Curriculum Development Project – National Audit & Consultations Report, VicHealth Koori Health Research & Community Development Unit, Discussion Paper 11 August 2004, from the Australian Government Department of Health and Ageing – Office for Aboriginal & Torres Strait Islander Health.

Chamberlain TC, Catano VM, Cunningham DP: Personality as a predictor of professional behaviour in dental school: comparisons with dental practitioners, *J Dent Educ* 69:1222–1236, 2005.

Didier T, Kreiter CD, Buri R, et al: Investigating the utility of a GPA institutional adjustment index, *Adv Health Sci Educ Theory Pract* 11(2): 145–153, 2006.

Donnon T, Paolucci EO, Violato C: The predictive validity of the MCAT for medical school performance and medical board licensing examinations: a meta-analysis of the published research, *Acad Med* 82(1):100–106, 2007.

Dore KL, Reiter HI, Eva KW, et al: Extending the interview to all medical school applicants – computer-based multiple sampling evaluation of non-cognitive skills (CMSENS), *Acad Med* 84(10 Suppl.):s9–s12, 2009.

Eva KW: On the generality of specificity, *Med Educ* 37:587–588, 2003.

Eva KW, Regehr G: Knowing when to look it up: a new conception of self-assessment ability, *Acad Med* 82(10 Suppl):s81–s84, 2007.

Eva KW, Rosenfeld J, Reiter HI, et al: An admissions OSCE: the multiple mini-interview, *Med Educ* 38(3):314–326, 2004a.

Eva KW, Reiter HI, Rosenfeld J, et al: The relationship between interviewers' characteristics and ratings assigned during a multiple mini-interview, *Acad Med* 79(6): 602–609, 2004b.

Eva KW, Reiter HI, Trinh K, et al: Predictive validity of the multiple mini-interview for selecting medical trainees, *Med Educ* 43(8):767–775, 2009.

Ferguson E, James D, O'Hehir F, et al: Pilot study of the roles of personality references, and personal statements in relation to performance over the five years of a medical degrees, *Br Med J* 326:428–431, 2003.

Flexner A: *Medical education in the United States and Canada bulletin number four (the Flexner report)*, New York, 1910, The Carnegie Foundation for the Advancement of Teaching.

Frank JR, Danoff D: The CanMEDS initiative: implementing an outcomes-based framework of physician competencies, *Med Teach* 29(7):642–647, 2007.

Ginsburg S, Regehr G, Hatala R, et al: Context, conflict, and resolution: a new conceptual framework for evaluating professionalism, *Acad Med* 75(10 Suppl):S6–S11, 2000.

Gratz v.et al: Bollingeret al: *539 U.S. 244*, 2003.

Grove WM, Meehl PE: Comparative efficiency of informal (subjective, impressionistic) and formal (mechanical, algorithmic) prediction procedures: the clinical-statistical controversy, *Psychol Public Policy Law* 2:293–323, 1996.

Grutter v. Bollinger et al: 539 U.S. 306:123, 2003.

Haggai: Old Testament, Chapter 2, Verses 10–13.

Hofmeister M, Lockyer J, Crutcher R: The multiple mini-interview for selection of international medical graduates into family medicine residency education, *Med Educ* 43(6):573–579, 2009.

Julian ER: Validity of the Medical College Admission Test for predicting medical school performance, *Acad Med* 80(10):910–917, 2005.

Kane TJ: National education longitudinal study racial and ethnic preferences in college admission. In Jencks C, Phillips M, editors: *The black-white test score gap*, Washington, DC, 1976, Brookings Institution Press.

Karabel J: *The chosen: the hidden history of admission and exclusion at Harvard, Yale and Princeton*, New York, 2005, First Mariner Books.

Koenig JA, Sireci SG, Wiley A: Evaluating the predictive validity of MCAT scores across diverse applicant groups, *Acad Med* 73(10): 1095–1106, 1998.

Kreiter CD: The use of constrained optimization to facilitate admission decisions, *Acad Med* 77(2):148–151, 2002.

Kreiter CD, Kreiter Y: A validity generalization perspective on the ability of undergraduate GPA and the medical college admission test to predict important outcomes, *Teach Learn Med* 19(2):95–100, 2007.

Kreiter CD, Yin P, Solow C, et al: Investigating the reliability of the medical school admissions interview, *Adv Health Sci Educ Theory Pract* 9(2):147–159, 2004.

Kulasegaram K, Reiter H, Hackett R, et al: 2009, Non-association between NEO-5 personality tests and multiple mini-interview, *Adv Health Sci Educ Theory Pract* 2009 Dec 15 [Epub ahead of print].

Kylonnen P: *Educational Testing Service. Video-based communication skills test for use in medical college. Presented within session 29.040, Assessment of non-cognitive factors in student selection for medical schools, 2005 Annual Meeting, American Educational Research Association, Montreal, April 12, 2005.*

Landy FJ: Some historical and scientific issues related to research on emotional intelligence, *J Organ Behav* 26:411–424, 2005.

Lawson SR, Hoban JD: Predicting career decisions in primary care medicine: a theoretical analysis, *J Contin Educ Health Prof* 23:68–80, 2003.

Lewis NJ, Rees CE, Hudson JN, et al: Emotional intelligence in medical education: measuring the unmeasurable? *Adv Health Sci Educ Theory Pract* 10:339–355, 2005.

Lievens F, Sackett PR: Video-based versus written situational judgment tests: a comparison in terms of predictive validity, *J Appl Psychol* 91(5):181–1188, 2006.

Lievens F, Coetsier P, De Fruyt F, et al: Medical students' personality characteristics and academic performance: a five-factor model perspective, *Med Educ* 36: 1050–1056, 2002.

Lievens F, Buyse T, Sackett PR: The operational validity of a video-based situational judgment test for medical college admissions: illustrating the importance of matching predictor and criterion construct domains, *J Appl Psychol* 90(3):442–452, 2005.

Luh SP, Yu MN, Lin YR, et al: A study on the personal traits and knowledge base of Taiwanese medical students following problem-based learning instructions, *Ann Acad Med Singapore* 36:743–750, 2007.

Lumsden MA, Bore M, Millar K, et al: Assessment of personal qualities in relation to admission to medical school, *Med Educ* 39:258–265, 2005.

McGaghie WC, Kreiter CD: Holistic versus actuarial student selection, *Teach Learn Med* 17(1):89–91, 2005.

MCAT Report: *Characteristics of the 1999 MCAT Examinees.Report of the association of American Medical Colleges*, 1999. www.aamc.org/mcat. Accessed December 2008.

Meredith KE, Dunlap MR, Baker HH: Subjective and objective admissions factors as predictors of clinical clerkship performance, *J Med Educ* 57(10 Pt 1):743–751, 1982.

Norcini JJ, Lipner RS, Kimball HR: Certifying examination performance and patient outcomes following acute myocardial infarction, *Med Educ* 36(9):853–859, 2002.

Papadakis MA, Teherani A, Banach MA, et al: Disciplinary action by medical boards and prior behavior in medical school, *N Engl J Med* 353(25): 2673–2682, 2005.

Poole A, Catano VM, Cunningham DP: Predicting performance in Canadian dental schools: the new CDA structured interview, a new personality test, and the DAT, *J Dent Educ* 71:664–676, 2007.

Powis D, James D, Ferguson E: Demographic and socio-economic associations with academic attainment (UCAS tariff scores) in applicants to medical school, *Med Educ* 41(3):242–249, 2007.

Rabinowitz HK, Diamond JJ, Markham FW, et al: Medical school programs to increase the rural physician supply: a systematic review and projected impact of widespread replication, *Acad Med* 83(3): 235–243, 2008.

Ramsey PG, Carline JD, Inui TS, et al: Predictive validity of certification by the American Board of Internal Medicine, *Ann Int Med* 110(9): 719–726, 1989.

Regents of University of California v. Bakke: *438 U.S.* 265, 1978.

Reiter H, MacCoon K: A compromise method to facilitate under-represented minority admissions to medical school, *Adv Health Sci Educ Theory Pract* 12(2):223–237, 2007.

Reiter HI, Eva KW, Rosenfeld J, et al: Multiple mini-interviews predict clerkship and licensing examination performance, *Med Educ* 41(4): 378–384, 2007.

Roberts C, Zoanetti N, Rothnie I: Validating a multiple mini-interview question bank assessing entry-level reasoning skills in candidates for graduate-entry medicine and dentistry programmes, *Med Educ* 43(4):350–359, 2009.

Rojstaczer S: *Grade inflation at American Colleges and Universities*, 2009. http://www.gradeinflation.com. Accessed September 22, 2009.

Salvatori P: Reliability and validity of admissions tools used to select students for the health professions, *Adv Health Sci Educ Theory Pract* 6(2):159–175, 2001.

Schofield W, Garrard J: Longitudinal study of medical students selected for admission to medical school by actuarial and committee methods, *Br J Med Educ* 9:86–90, 1975.

Siu E, Reiter HI: Overview: what's worked and what hasn't as a guide towards predictive admissions tool development, *Adv Health Sci Educ Theory Pract* 14(5):759–775, 2009.

Sleeth BC, Mishell RI: Black under-representation in United States medical schools, *N Engl J Med* 297(21):1146–1148, 1977.

Smithers S, Catano VM, Cunninghman DP: What predicts performance in Canadian dental schools? *J Dent Educ* 68:598–613, 2004.

Speer AJ, Solomon DJ, Fincher RM: Grade inflation in internal medicine clerkships: results of a national survey, *Teach Learn Med* 12(3): 112–116, 2000.

Stokes W: The complaints that reach our grievance committee, *Med Ann Dist Columbia* 21(3):157–158, 1952.

Stray C: From oral to written examinations: Cambridge, Oxford and Dublin 1700–1914, *History Univ.* 20(2):94–95, 2005.

Tamblyn R, Abrahamowicz M, Dauphinee WD, et al: Association between licensure examination scores and practice in primary care, *JAMA* 288(23):3019–3026, 2002.

Tamblyn R, Abrahamowicz M, Dauphinee D, et al: Physician scores on a national clinical skills examination as predictors of complaints to medical regulatory authorities, *JAMA* 298(9):993–1001, 2007.

Trail C, Reiter HI, Bridge M, et al: Impact of field of study, college and year on calculation of cumulative grade point average, *Adv Health Sci Educ Theory Pract* 13(3):253–261, 2008.

UKCAT Annual Report, 2006, Available at: http://www.ukcat.ac.uk/pdf/UKCAT%20Annual%20. Accessed September 18, 2009.

Wilkinson D, Zhang J, Byrne GJ, et al: Medical school selection criteria and the prediction of academic performance, *Med J Aust* 188(6): 349–354, 2008.

Further reading

Reiter HI, Eva KW: Reflecting the relative values of community, faculty, and students in the admission tools of medical school, *Teach Learn Med* 17(1):4–8, 2005.

Sackett PR, Borneman MJ, Connelly BS: High-stakes testing in the higher education and employment – appraising the evidence for validity and fairness, *Am Psycho* 63(4): 215–227, 2008.

Predicting and guiding career success in medicine

18

Katherine Woolf   Chris McManus

CHAPTER CONTENTS

> **ABC**
>
> ## Glossary
>
> **Personality; Agreeableness** One of the 'Big Five' personality traits. Agreeableness, or its opposite tough-mindedness, refers to the degree to which an individual is generally cooperative and compliant to the wishes of others. Agreeable individuals tend to be likeable and straightforward. Tough-mindedness is however, when making essential but unpopular decisions.
>
> **Personality; Conscientiousness** One of the 'Big Five' personality traits. Conscientiousness refers to the amount that a person is generally organised, tidy, and methodical, pays attention to detail, and is achievement-motivated. Low C individuals are often more imaginative and artistic, and find it easier to see the bigger picture or take imaginative risks.
>
> **Contest mobility** Sociological view of success in which all individuals are perceived as having the potential to achieve and compete with one another in open and equal contest for success. Particularly favours hard work.
>
> **Personality; Extraversion** One of the 'Big Five' personality traits. Extraversion and its opposite, introversion, refer to the amount that a person generally enjoys stimulation from the environment. Extraverts tend to be sociable and enjoy exciting activities. Introverts tend to prefer their own company and enjoy quieter activities.
>
> **Career success; Extrinsic** Objective aspects of career success, for example salary increases, promotion.
>
> **Generalised self-efficacy** The belief in one's overall ability to achieve across a variety of situations.

Continued

© 2011, Elsevier Ltd.
DOI: 10.1016/B978-0-7020-3522-7.00018-8

ABC

Glossary (continued)

Holland's typology Psychological theory of career choice and success which outlines 6 types of interest and 6 corresponding types of career. These are Realistic, Investigative, Artistic, Social, Enterprising, and Conventional (often abbreviated to RIASEC). The more congruence between a person's interests and their career type, the more satisfied that person is hypothesised to be.

Human capital Sociological concept of the skills, experience, and knowledge that an individual acquires, and which increases a person's economic value and chances of success at the workplace.

Individual differences psychology The study of how individuals differ from one another in terms of factors that influence success or failure. Particularly concerned with personality and intelligence.

Career success; Intrinsic Subjective psychological aspects of career success; for example, job satisfaction.

Locus of control Psychological trait or state describing the amount of control individuals believe they have over outcomes affecting them. Individuals with Internal LOC tend to believe that their actions determine outcomes, whereas those with External LOC tend to believe that outcomes are determined mainly by the actions of others. Some measures also include a third form, known as Fate or Chance, which is completely out of anyone's control.

Motivation; extrinsic See main Glossary, p 339.

Motivation; intrinsic See main Glossary, p 339.

Personality; Neuroticism One of the 'Big Five' personality traits. Neuroticism, and its opposite, Emotional Stability, refer to a person's typical level of anxiety. High Neuroticism is associated with anxiousness, depression, and self-consciousness. Moderate levels of anxiety have, however, evolved to be adaptive and low N individuals often take unnecessary risks without considering their consequences.

Personality; Openness to experience One of the 'Big Five' personality traits. Openness to Experience refers to the amount that a person is generally interested in theories and ideas. High O individuals tend to be intellectual and artistic. Low O individuals tend to prefer the concrete to the abstract, are less good at fantasising, and are more conservative politically and morally.

Organisational sponsorship Opportunities for career progression offered by organisations to their employees.

Outcome expectations From social cognitive career theory; the belief that a particular behaviour or course of action will lead to specific outcomes.

Personality: the Big 5 Modern trait personality theories generally recognise five important dimensions of personality, consisting of: Agreeableness;

ABC

Glossary (continued)

Conscientiousness; Extraversion; Neuroticism; and Openness to Experience, which are described separately. Together they account for much of the important variations in personality.

Socio-cognitive career theory (SCCT) Lent and Brown's application of Bandura's Social Cognitive Theory to career success. It emphasises the importance of outcome expectations, goal setting, and self-efficacy on career outcomes.

Self-determination theory (SDT) Psychological theory of motivation and behaviour from Edward Deci and Richard Ryan. Particularly concerned with the influences on self-determined (i.e. autonomous, self-regulated) behaviour. Distinguishes between intrinsic and extrinsic motivation.

Self-efficacy See main Glossary, p 340.

Social cognitive theory; see also self-efficacy See main Glossary, p 340.

Sponsored mobility Sociological view of success in which individuals are singled out early on as having potential and given specific help and advantages in order to help them reach that potential.

Vocational psychology Study of the work-related experiences and behaviours of individuals. Particularly concerned with theories of career choice, motivation, and satisfaction.

'Each of them – as is often the way with men who have selected careers of different kinds – though in discussion he would even justify the other's career, in his heart despised it.'

Leo Tolstoy (1877, *Anna Karenina*)

Overview

This chapter provides information, first on which doctors can base the career advice they give to other doctors, second which can help them reflect on and gain insight into their own careers, and third to assess the extent to which general theoretical principles can inform an understanding of medical careers. We examine various psychological theories of career success and apply the findings to medicine. They enable us to understand what it means to have a successful medical career, and whether we can predict which doctors will be successful and under which circumstances. If the chapter contains one key message, it is that 'people differ'; or as it was put so much more elegantly by Kluckhohn (1953):

'Every man is in certain respects a) like all other men, b) like some other men, c) like no other men.'

Any understanding of careers has to acknowledge those three levels, of invariance, similarity, and individuality.

A good career

What is a good or a successful career? Such a seemingly simple question has no obvious answer, for the crucial reason that not only do careers differ so very much but so also do the people having them. As therefore was the case for Tolstoy's Levin and Oblonsky, 'one man's meat is another man's poison'. The point would seem trivially obvious were it not that medicine has a long tradition of looking for simple, one-size-fits all, solutions to complex problems. When new drugs are introduced, the typical question is, 'Does it work?', but less commonly is it asked, 'For whom does it work, why, and how would we know?' Career guidance for UK medical students and doctors is likewise often based on a similar model of a single method, applied to all, and intended to help all. Many years ago, clinical psychology adopted a very different approach to managing the problems of patients, there being no single off-the-peg treatment for most psychological conditions, because people and their symptoms differ so much. So, instead, there are general principles, and most cognitive and behavioural therapies are bespoke treatments, tailored to the specific circumstances of individual patients.

Parsons (1909) recognised the importance of choosing the right career in the opening words of his book, *Choosing a vocation*, published in 1909:

> No step in life, unless it may be the choice of a husband or wife, is more important than the choice of a vocation. The wise selection of the business, profession, trade or occupation to which one's life is to be devoted and the development of full efficiency in the chosen field are matters of the deepest moment.

It is worth re-emphasising Parsons' point that it is not only career choice that matters but also career development.

Careers and specialities differ in many of their working conditions, but there is at least as much variation in the ways that different people experience any particular working condition. The psychological literature is rich with theories about how and why different individuals choose and enjoy their careers, and likewise, why they do not enjoy their careers.

Career counsellors and vocational psychologists, whose primary interests are in how individuals choose careers, and what determines success in those careers, respectively, are interested in how individual and environmental factors influence career choice and outcomes. They are interested in how insight into the values, beliefs, personality, and aptitudes of individuals, typically determined by psychometric test results, relates to success. Career success is viewed not only in the objective terms of financial reward, promotion, responsibility or productivity but also as individuals' experiences, satisfaction, sense of personal achievement, opportunities, and life-satisfaction.

Within the broad remit of career counselling, 'medicine' is often treated as a single entity, with little consideration given to the vast range of its specialities. Early medical training is indeed fairly uniform. In the United Kingdom, the General Medical Council oversees curriculum standards for undergraduate education and the majority of graduates are employed in the National Health Service (NHS), which has a nationally standard set of career structures. That apparent homogeneity masks the differences in training approaches and day-to-day experiences of, for instance, a neurosurgeon, a part-time GP in a remote rural practice, an inner-city GP, a full-time medical school dean, a clinical oncologist, a forensic psychiatrist, and a molecular biology researcher. Although all underwent a broadly equivalent undergraduate education, each needs different knowledge, skills, and abilities; they need to update those skills continually in different ways; they gain differing types and amounts of recognition for their work; and they differ in the satisfaction and stress they get from their careers. They also differ in their sense of perspective, not only on their careers but also on those for whom they are caring, as was nicely described by Helman (2006):

> On the one hand is family medicine with its slow revelation to the doctor of a life pattern, or a pattern of disease, in an individual or a family. On the other is the image of a person revealed instantaneously in a hospital clinic by the technology of scientific medicine: X-rays, scans, blood tests – and often in a rushed consultation between two strangers. It's the fundamental difference between the briefest glimpse and a lengthy narrative. Between a snapshot and a long novel.

The lessons learnt from vocational psychology and career counselling provide a challenge for doctors when thinking about their own careers and also when guiding other doctors in making successful career choices.

Career success

Career success can be defined as the positive work-related and positive psychological outcomes of an individual's experiences over the course of their working life (Judge et al, 1994; Seibert and Kraimer, 2001). It can be extrinsic, measured objectively in terms of material rewards such as pay and promotion to high-status and prestigious jobs. It can also be intrinsic, measured subjectively in terms of the psychological rewards received such as inherent enjoyment of one's work, attainment of personal goals, and satisfaction of personal values (Judge et al, 1999; Ng et al, 2005; Pachulicz et al, 2008). Extrinsic and intrinsic career success are conceptually different and only moderately correlated, just as job performance (the degree to which people accomplish objectively measurable tasks) is only moderately correlated ($r = 0.3$) with subjective job satisfaction (Judge et al, 2001). Understanding how and why intrinsic and extrinsic outcomes differ is therefore a vital part of making informed and successful career choices.

Intrinsic versus extrinsic outcomes: self-determination theory

The intrinsic–extrinsic distinction came to prominence with Richard Ryan and Edward Deci's self-determination theory (SDT: cf. Deci and Ryan, 2008). SDT is concerned with why people are motivated to make particular choices in their lives, such as taking exercise or studying hard, and what effect those choices have on their well-being and life satisfaction. It identifies three universal human psychological needs of autonomy (having choice), relatedness (being close to other people), and competence (believing one is good at what one does). It argues that the more opportunity we have to fulfil those needs, the more motivated and more happy we are likely to be. Indeed, a recent study showed that adults with a mean age of 75 who felt they had attained their life's intrinsic goals by, for example contributing to their community, aspiring to personal development, and building up meaningful relationships, had greater psychological need satisfaction, and were less anxious about and more accepting of their own death than those who had attained extrinsic goals of financial success, power, physical appeal, and social recognition (Van Heil and Vansteenkiste, 2009).

Intrinsic motivation

Intrinsically motivated behaviours are those which, by their nature, fulfil the need for autonomy. They are performed simply because it is enjoyable to perform them. If you are lucky enough to have a job which you would do regardless of extrinsic rewards such as pay or recognition, you are likely to be motivated to continue in that job and work hard. Intrinsic motivation is a feature of early life: babies tend to be motivated to do things they find intrinsically enjoyable. Unfortunately, as responsibilities grow, there are fewer and fewer chances to engage in intrinsically motivated behaviours and one has to rely instead on extrinsic rewards and punishments for motivation. Some extrinsically motivated behaviours, doing the ironing to avoid being nagged for example, can be unfulfilling and unsatisfying, and it is difficult to summon up the motivation to perform them, and perform them well. However, other extrinsically motivated behaviours can lead to considerable satisfaction.

Extrinsic motivation

The key difference between unsatisfying and satisfying extrinsically motivated behaviours is, according to SDT, the amount of autonomy one has in deciding to perform the behaviour, as well as the competence and relatedness the behaviour affords. If you had little say in whether or not you did the ironing (low autonomy), and you are not very good at it (low competence), and you do it alone (low relatedness), you will probably avoid doing it again, except to avoid the extrinsically motivating punishment of being nagged. However, if you feel that it is important to dress neatly for work and make your own decision to do the ironing (high autonomy), and then you find you are actually an efficient ironer (high competence), and your partner chats to you as they hang the clothes after you have ironed them (high relatedness), you will probably feel a greater sense of satisfaction from doing it and will be motivated to continue (e.g. Richer et al, 2002). In that situation, the level of autonomous motivation you felt was determined by the amount you had internalised the importance of looking neat at work. That is still extrinsic (you are not ironing for the love of it), yet it is motivating.

Autonomy

Extrinsic motivation can therefore be strong and persistent if it is autonomous. Autonomous motivation (whether intrinsic or extrinsic) is a predictor of success in terms of job satisfaction, job commitment (Lam and Gurland, 2008; Richer et al, 2002), persistence in academic contexts, and good grades (Burton et al, 2006; Vansteenkiste et al, 2004). It also leads to effective performance, particularly on complex tasks that require creativity and problem solving (Deci and Ryan, 2008). In doctors, autonomy positively predicts job satisfaction, job commitment, and higher publication rates for clinical academics, and negatively predicts burnout. In medical students, autonomous motivation predicts greater academic attainment and increased persistence with medical studies (Barnett et al, 1998; Freeborn, 2000; Hoff et al, 2002; Sobral, 2004). Self-determination theorists would suggest choosing careers that mostly involve tasks you would just love doing (intrinsic autonomous motivation) or consider very important (extrinsic autonomous motivation), whilst avoiding those that consist of pointless tasks you would be forced to do (extrinsic controlled motivation).

Reward

This may seem obvious, but the rewards a job offers can sometimes tempt people to ignore the need for autonomy. Indeed, the intrinsic or extrinsic nature of rewards and career goals are themselves predictors of success. A longitudinal study of German graduates showed that those with extrinsic career goals at graduation were less likely to be satisfied with their careers after 7 years, despite having achieved greater salary and status (Abele and Spurk, 2009). This may be because the participants' expectations were unrealistically high and therefore remained unfulfilled, or because the pursuit of extrinsic goals is associated with the attainment of extrinsic rewards of status and money rather than the intrinsically rewarding job satisfaction. Similarly, a study from the United States found that workers who had a particular desire for the extrinsic goal of promotion were less likely to be satisfied (Wayne et al, 2001). In medicine, a study of 165 US medical students found that the intrinsic goals and rewards of 'a balanced work and professional life', 'being a good communicator with patients' and 'professional and intellectual growth', were rated as the most important determinants of satisfaction (Reed et al, 2004) above extrinsic factors of 'financial security' and 'respect from colleagues and the community'

According to SDT, a job or career that rewards you by allowing you to be with the people who are important to you at home or at work, that makes you feel like you are good at what you do, and that gives you the chance to make your own decisions is more likely to lead to job satisfaction than one that only affords financial rewards and status. There is even evidence from numerous studies that extrinsic rewards such as material wealth, outward physical beauty, and social status can undermine intrinsic motivation (Deci et al, 1999), reduce creativity, and inhibit complex problem-solving ability (Gagne and Deci, 2005), and thus lead to less needs satisfaction. It has, however, been argued that it is not whether the reward is extrinsic, but how the reward is presented that is important. A study of 947 primary care physicians in the United States showed that job satisfaction was negatively associated with financial incentives for productivity, but positively associated with financial incentives for quality assessed by audit (Grumbach et al, 1998). So, it is worth considering whether the rewards on offer for a job are likely to make the job seem trivial, because this will probably decrease intrinsic motivation, or whether they convey the job's personal or social significance, as this is thought to increase intrinsic motivation.

Importantly, autonomous motivation is not inborn or static, but can be nurtured in medical students by clinical teachers (Williams et al, 1997). Doctors wanting to support career development could therefore consider making the learning and/or working environments of doctors in training more autonomous and supportive. That can be achieved by listening to the needs of students and trainees, understanding their points of view, encouraging them to make their own choices, and giving them sufficient information to make those choices.

Individual and environmental predictors of career success

Motivation and rewards influence career success, but what about other predictors? As with almost all aspects of human life, influences on career success arise both from within individuals and from the environment, and often interact to determine outcomes. For example, a study of 1435 UK junior doctors found that doctors' ratings of job quality were mostly related to the particular team, hospital, or trust in which they worked. In contrast, reported stress levels in the same doctors related almost entirely to individual differences in personality and other attributes, rather than to job characteristics. In fact the stress levels of two doctors working in identical posts were no more similar than those of two doctors chosen at random and working in different teams, in different hospitals, in different trusts, overseen by different deaneries (McManus et al, 2002). The individual and environmental variables commonly explored in vocational and occupational psychology include self-efficacy, human capital, organisational sponsorship, personality, locus of control, and demographics. An overview of research evaluating the impact of these factors on career success is given, and also discussed in the context of medicine.

Self-efficacy and socio-cognitive career theory

The concept of self-efficacy, the belief that one has the motivation and ability to perform a specific task, was made famous by Albert Bandura's Socio-Cognitive Theory of Behaviour (Bandura, 1977; also discussed in Chapter 2), which emphasises the reciprocal influences of behaviour and thoughts on each other. For example, if medical students believe they are able to take blood effectively because they know they have practised in the clinical skills lab ('thoughts'), the first time they take blood in real life, their hands are less likely to shake, they are more likely to remember the steps to take, and they are more likely to be successful ('behaviour'). Their success then feeds back to influence how they feel about themselves as someone who takes blood ('thoughts') and how likely they think it is they will be able to successfully take blood from patients in the future ('thoughts'), which then influences how successful their subsequent attempts actually are ('behaviour'). SCT therefore focuses on the ways in which people act, or in psychological terms, behave, to change specific situations and thus change their beliefs, thoughts, feelings, and subsequent behaviours in similar situations. Within the SCT cycle of behaviour change, self-efficacy determines choice of action, persistence, and emotional reactions to obstructions. Self-efficacy has been found to be positively related to task performance across a variety of occupations (Judge et al, 2007; Stajkovic and Luthans 1998) and, in the context of SCT, self-efficacy is considered to be situation-specific and amenable to change.

Social cognitive career theory

Robert W. Lent's social cognitive career theory (SCCT: Lent et al, 1994) applies Bandura's ideas to a career setting. Self-efficacy is central to the theory, as are outcome expectations and goals. Outcome expectations are personal beliefs about the consequences of one's actions: for example, a person might believe that 'if I decide to become a doctor (action) then I will help sick people recover/never be out of a job/be respected by society (consequences)'. Personal success, seeing other people succeeding in similar situations, being encouraged verbally by others, and feeling positive whilst engaging in tasks are all theorised to improve both self-efficacy and positive outcome expectations. Self-efficacy and positive outcome expectation encourage people to set positive career goals, which improve career success by organising and guiding behaviour, and encouraging persistence in the face of setbacks.

According to SCCT, doctors wanting to improve their trainees' career success should try to improve trainees' self-efficacy, manage their outcome expectations, and help them set positive and achievable goals. That can be achieved by creating positive environments in which trainees can practise their skills, receive constructive feedback and encouragement, and encounter people who are role models of good professional clinical practice.

Generalised self-efficacy

It should be pointed out that psychologists have also postulated the existence of an individual differences trait called generalised self-efficacy (GSE), which is the *general* self-perception that people have of themselves as more or less capable in most situations (Eden and Zuk, 1995). GSE is relatively stable across situations and is conceptually and psychometrically distinct from state self-efficacy (Stajkovic and Luthans, 1998). In some ways, it is conceptually closer to personality than Bandura's version of self-efficacy. GSE is a potentially important predictor of job satisfaction: a meta-analysis of studies from between 1967 and 1997 found that GSE had a corrected correlation of 0.45 with job satisfaction, explaining 9% of the variance in that variable (Judge and Bono, 2001), and a more recent study found that GSE measured at graduation positively predicted career satisfaction in medicine and other jobs 7 years later, both directly and indirectly via increasing salary and status (Abele and Spurk, 2009).

Human capital and organisational sponsorship

SCCT explains how person variables (self-efficacy, outcome expectancies, goals, and socio-demographic variables) interact with environmental variables and behaviour in a reciprocal fashion. The environmental variables important in SCCT include objective factors such as amount and quality of educational experiences available and financial support for training. That is what sociologists call organisational sponsorship. SCCT also highlights the interaction between person and environmental variables and in particular the amount of investment people put into their own resources, such as education. That is what sociologists refer to as human capital (Becker, 1964).

Sponsored mobility

The sociological concepts of organisation sponsorship and human capital originated in the sponsored mobility and contest mobility perspectives of career progression and success. In the sponsored mobility approach, those with potential are identified early-on by the elite, and because resources are finite, only they are given support to progress (Coleman, 1988). Thus, in the sponsored mobility approach, organisational sponsorship and mentoring are vital to success.

Contest mobility

By contrast, the contest mobility approach is based on the belief that anyone can progress in a career as long as they show themselves to perform well in their job and be useful to the organisation in which they work. It is considered to be the foundation of the 'American dream'; the lowliest individual can achieve the highest rewards, as long as they work hard enough. An example is Sonia Sotomayor, the first Hispanic Latin appointment to the US Supreme Court, who said

> [my mother] taught [my brother and myself] that the key to success in America is a good education. And she set the example, studying alongside my brother and me at our kitchen table so that she could become a registered nurse. We worked hard. I [...went on to] Yale Law School, while my brother went on to medical school.
>
> Crombie (2009)

In the contest mobility approach, individual motivation, self-efficacy, and human capital are considered keys to success.

Organisational sponsorship, human capital, and career success

Organisational sponsorship and human capital have varying and even additive effects on career success. Wayne et al (2001) studied several hundred workers at a large US manufacturing organisation. Their regression analysis showed that workers who had positive relationships with their superiors (organisational sponsorship) had higher salary increases over an 18-month period (beta = 0.20), were more likely to be rated as worthy of promotion (beta = 0.30), and also had higher job satisfaction (beta = 0.12). The link between human capital and success was less clear; workers with more education were no more likely to be promoted, have pay increases, or be satisfied than their less-educated colleagues, but having the opportunity for greater training whilst employed was linked to higher job satisfaction (beta = 0.24). A meta-analysis by Ng et al (2005) also found that workers who had greater organisational sponsorship in terms of supervisor support, career sponsorship, and training and skills development opportunities were more likely to be satisfied (mean $r = 0.43$) and also had higher salaries (mean $r = 0.23$). However, in contrast to Wayne et al, Ng et al also found that salary was positively correlated with the human capital variables of hours worked, work experience, educational level, and political skills and knowledge (mean $r = 0.27$).

Mentoring

Mentoring is a form of organisational sponsorship that has attracted much attention. It can vary in formality, and mentors can be from within or without the protégé's field. Eby et al (2008) conducted a meta-analysis of youth, academic, and workplace mentoring. Outcomes were measures of behaviours, health, relations, motivation, attitudes, and extrinsic and intrinsic career outcomes. The results showed a small but statistically significant effect of mentoring on extrinsic career success ($r = 0.05$) and a larger effect on job skills development: that is, increases in human capital ($r = 0.11$). The largest effects of mentoring were on satisfaction ($r = 0.16$) and positive attitudes ($r = 0.14$), but even these were relatively small.

It can be difficult to know what aspect of mentoring improves success; for example, does the psychological support from a mentor improve a worker's confidence and self-efficacy? Or is it that a mentor can introduce the worker to powerful people? A meta-analysis by Kammeyer-Mueller and Judge (2008) explored how the differing functions of mentors influenced success. Having a mentor, increased job satisfaction (beta = 0.25), even after taking into account human capital (e.g. education) and self-evaluations, and this was due to practical rather than psychological aspects of mentor support. However, in terms of salary, human capital (beta = 0.26) and demographics (beta = 0.10) had more influence than mentorship.

The question of who gets a mentor is also important. Is it the more proactive, motivated, well-educated, well-connected workers who seek out and get mentors? And if so, is it these factors rather than the mentoring per se that influence success? Singh et al (2009b) attempted to disentangle the effects of mentoring from human capital, engagement in proactive career behaviours, and the creation of career-related social networks. They used a powerful longitudinal design to determine whether having an informal mentor impacted on the extrinsic and intrinsic career success of 236 Australian public and private sector employees, when controlling for those other factors. The results showed that people with an informal mentor were more likely to be promoted over a 2-year period (beta = 1.15) but were no more likely to have an increase in salary. Salary increase was instead predicted by human capital: that is, training (beta = 0.17) and education (beta = 0.16). Protégés were also more likely to expect to get promotion (beta = 0.77) and less likely to want to change careers (beta = −0.33) but were no more likely to be satisfied with their careers. Career satisfaction was instead predicted by perceptions that work was challenging (beta = 0.11). In an accompanying study, Singh et al (2009a) looked at who gets a mentor, showing that 'rising stars' – those who had previously been more likely to be promoted, who expected to get promoted, and who developed their skills and engaged in career progression activities – were more likely to get mentors, which does indeed suggest that underlying individual factors are an important confounder.

Mentoring in medical career development

A systematic review of the effects of mentoring on career progression in academic medicine showed that mentors were generally perceived by participants to be an important part of their training experience, particularly in terms of career satisfaction, although the studies showed wide variation in the proportion of medical students and doctors who reported having a mentor (Sambunjak et al, 2006). Unfortunately, 87% of the studies in the review were cross-sectional, and the authors report that the poor quality of many of them as well as diverse outcome measures made it impossible to calculate an effect size for mentoring in medicine.

To summarise, organisational support, including mentoring, appears to have a positive effect on workers' career satisfaction and retention as well as on extrinsic measures such as promotion and salary. Much of the research within medicine however involves small-scale cross-sectional research projects, which make it difficult to assess the size of the effects of these factors on doctors' progression, and few studies control for personality variables, which we will see, can be a key influence on career outcomes.

Personality

SDT and SCCT explain how motivations, goals, and outcome expectancies influence attainment and satisfaction. Sociological career theories explain how human capital and organisational sponsorship affect career progression and success, and predict that demographic variables will also exert a key influence. But what explains how people react differently in the same situation? Although much of psychology examines what people have in common (e.g. how we perceive objects, how we learn to use language, and how we remember facts), there are also many studies looking at how each person differs from other people, which is known as the study of individual differences. Personality is a key area of individual differences research and, because it is a major influence on motivations, attitudes, behaviours, and career outcomes, it is also important in career research.

The idea that there are different personality traits which influence human thought and behaviour is an ancient one, and the English language is full of words used to describe different human dispositions and aspects of character. Over the course of the twentieth century, researchers came to a consensus that personality traits influence behaviour, and that these traits are generally stable over time (Matthews and Deary, 1998). So, although people's reactions will differ in different situations, people who are worriers will tend to be anxious, those who like talking to people will seek out opportunities to interact with others, and so on. There are many competing theories of personality, and factors such as GSE (see earlier) and locus of control (see later) are sometimes considered facets of personality. In the early 1990s, however, the Five Factor Model (FFM) of personality became predominant.

The FFM of personality

The Big Five personality traits are Neuroticism (N), Extraversion (E), Openness to Experience (O), Agreeableness (A), and Conscientiousness (C). They have been found in both men and women across many different cultures (McCrae and Costa, 1997). High N is associated with anxiety, hostility, depression, self-consciousness, impulsivity, and vulnerability. Neurotic individuals tend to worry and have low mood, whereas Low N (stable) individuals are calm, poised, and emotionally stable. High E is associated with gregariousness, assertiveness, activity, excitement seeking, and positive emotions, so extraverted individuals enjoy high-energy situations involving others, whereas Low E (introverted) individuals prefer their own company and avoid risk. High O is associated with creativity, appreciating aesthetics, and thinking about feelings, actions, ideas, and values, so open individuals tend to be intellectual, whereas Low O individuals favour the concrete over the abstract. High A is associated with being trustworthy, straightforward, altruistic, compliant, modest, and tender-minded. Agreeable individuals tend to be kind, likeable, and person-oriented, whereas low A individuals tend to be perceived as arrogant, aloof, and uncaring. High C is associated with self-discipline, achievement-striving, order, deliberation, and competence. Conscientious individuals tend to work hard, whereas Low C individuals tend to be non-conformist and disorganised.

Although it is tempting to assume that some personality types are intrinsically better (it seems a no-brainer to ask who would not want to employ agreeable, conscientious, stable individuals?), it must be remembered that modern societies have many and varied roles, and all personality types probably have niches in which they are particularly effective. Creative individuals, for instance, such as research scientists or art students, are often less agreeable and less conscientious than others, in large part because they need to create a space in which they can follow their own ideas, rather than satisfy the immediate needs of the society around them. About a half of the variance in personality is probably due to genes, which suggests that it may well be variance itself that has been selected for. Intermediate levels of anxiety or neuroticism are probably optimal so that, to use a cartoon-strip analogy, all of us are descendants of those Palaeolithic ancestors who were neither so free of anxiety that they were rapidly eaten by sabre-toothed tigers, nor so obsessed with personal safety that they never left their caves for fear of being eaten and died of starvation as a result. Society does need some people who are very anxious (disasters happen and we need people who worry about the future), and it also needs people who are not anxious in high-risk situations and get on with the job in hand (soldiers, surgeons, and so on).

Personality and career outcomes

Personality predicts career outcomes. A meta-analytic review across various professions showed that conscientiousness was significantly related to job proficiency (corrected $r(rc) = 0.23$) in many different occupational groups (Barrick and Mount, 1991) and another study by the same authors showed that the link between C and job performance was particularly high in jobs with higher levels of autonomy (Barrick and Mount, 1993). A longitudinal paper from the United States showed C positively predicted extrinsic career success ($r = 0.50$; Judge, et al, 1999) and a meta-analysis by Ng et al (2005) showed C positively predicted salary ($r_c = 0.07$), promotion ($r_c = 0.06$), and satisfaction ($r_c = 0.14$). It should be remembered, however, that most of these and other studies have mainly looked at jobs which are extrinsically rewarded and where the outcomes are clearly defined rather than open-ended and creative. Part of the reason conscientiousness predicts extrinsic career outcomes is that it also predicts the human capital factor of academic success. In particular, C positively predicts attainment at medical and dental school (Ferguson et al, 2002).

Just as conscientiousness positively predicts outcomes, so neuroticism is often found to be a negative predictor of both extrinsic and intrinsic success (Judge et al, 1999; Ng et al, 2005), whereas the relationships of extraversion, openness, and agreeableness with job outcomes are less clear. The most recent meta-analysis by Ng et al (2005) showed that E and O were both positively correlated with satisfaction, salary, and promotions, whereas A was positively related to satisfaction but negatively correlated with salary. A US study of nearly 500 university students and graduates tested whether the type of occupation mediated the effect of personality on career success, finding that for individuals in people-oriented occupations, A was negatively related to salary, which suggests that agreeable individuals want to work in people-oriented occupations even when they do not receive financial rewards for it (Seibert and Kraimer, 2001). A study of 1668 UK doctors (McManus et al, 2004) showed that personality influenced stress levels, approaches to work, and perceptions of the workplace. Neurotic doctors were more stressed and perceived they had higher workloads as well as lower autonomy in their work. By contrast, extraverted doctors were less stressed, and agreeable doctors perceived their workplace to be supportive with help available as needed, possibly because they were better at getting on with other members of their teams. Conscientious doctors tended to feel they had lower workloads, which is probably partly because conscientious doctors were more organised than the neurotic doctors.

How can we interpret these research findings in practice? Personality traits are stable and enduring, but that does not mean that the unconscientious neurotics amongst us are doomed to a life of failure. Just as it has been said that 'genes are not destiny', nor is personality. Personality does influence the way humans react in many situations, but humans can choose to behave contrary to their innate personality. Encouraging individuals to have an insight into their own strengths and weaknesses by knowing and understanding their personality traits, and recognising how they might behave, think, and feel differently in situations to the ways that other people do, are probably helpful in a range of situations. For example, understanding that one is not, say, terribly conscientious can help someone make a particular effort to be organised; or knowing that one is more neurotic than others can help in making special efforts to learn to cope with stressful situations. Insight can also help in choosing certain jobs that particularly suit one's personality. Indeed, a meta-analysis found that personality predicted satisfaction, but that the effect was mediated by environmental factors, the suggestion being that people self-select into particular jobs in which they feel suited (Dormann and Zapf, 2001).

Locus of control

Individual differences help explain how people differ in the ways they interpret what may objectively seem like very similar situations. According to SCCT, a person's beliefs about their own abilities and their outcome expectations are key determinants of behaviour, actual outcomes, and subsequent thoughts and beliefs. However, some people appear pessimistic in the face of success and others appear to be unfazed by failure (Rotter, 1990). This behaviour is considered by some to be a function of people's beliefs about how much their behaviour influences their experiences, which in psychology is called locus of control (LOC). People who believe they can influence their own fate have internal LOC. They tend to be alert, take action, and believe that their actions and behaviours have specific consequences. Those who believe that their fate is out of their hands have external LOC. They tend to attribute events in their lives to luck, misfortune, or the actions of powerful others. Some researchers believe that LOC is a personality trait which, although similar to neuroticism, is additional to the Big Five. Thus, they believe it to be relatively stable (Ng et al, 2006). Timothy Judge and colleagues consider that internal LOC, along with self-efficacy, high self-esteem, and low neuroticism, is a key component of self-regard or self-evaluation (Judge and Bono, 2001). It is not clear, however, that LOC is the same across all situations and therefore care should be taken in considering it to be a stable personality trait like the Big Five.

Locus of control and career development

Internal LOC (the belief that one can control one's environment) is related to psychological well-being (Judge et al, 1998), which fits with the SDT idea that autonomy (the opportunity to exert control over one's actions and environment) is a basic psychological need which leads to well-being if satisfied. And, as with autonomy, LOC has been found to correlate with both intrinsic and extrinsic career success. A meta-analysis of 222 studies showed that people with internal LOC had higher job satisfaction ($r_c = 0.33$) and were more committed to their jobs ($r_c = 0.24$). They were more intrinsically motivated ($r_c = 0.18$) and of higher self-efficacy ($r_c = 0.28$). They experienced their jobs more positively in terms of autonomy ($r_c = 0.24$), found their jobs challenging ($r_c = 0.26$), and were less likely to burn out ($r_c = -0.27$), feel overloaded, have work–family conflict, or be stressed. They also had more extrinsic success. They were more likely to be highly rated by others ($r_c = 0.17$) and themselves ($r_c = 0.12$) and had higher salaries ($r_c = 0.16$) (Ng et al, 2006). Another meta-analysis of the predictors of extrinsic and intrinsic career satisfaction by the same group found that locus of control was one of the variables that correlated most closely with career satisfaction ($r_c = 0.47$) (Ng et al, 2005).

Socio-demographic variables

As well as the psychological factors of motivation, self-efficacy, and personality, and the sociological variables of organisational sponsorship and human capital, two key influences on career outcomes are the demographic variables of gender and ethnicity. These are discussed in relation to medical careers.

Gender and career outcomes

Overall, fewer women than men are registered to practice medicine in the United Kingdom; however, the proportion varies between specialities, general practice, and paediatrics having the highest proportion of women and surgery having the lowest. The male to female ratio in the United Kingdom mirrors that in many countries around the world, including the United States, Norway, Russia, Sweden, Finland, Australia, and Canada (Elton, 2009; Kilminster et al, 2007). The proportion of women entering medical school in the United Kingdom however is now slightly higher than the proportion of men. This has stirred up interest and debate about the career choices, progression, and success of women medical students and doctors, and how they may affect patient outcomes and workforce planning in the NHS and elsewhere. As an aside, it is important to note that the absolute number of men entering medicine in the United Kingdom has been stable for some time (Elton, 2009). This section concentrates on research which has investigated how being male or female impacts on extrinsic and intrinsic career success in medicine.

Gender and extrinsic success

Women medical students are generally more extrinsically successful than men (Ferguson et al, 2002; Kilminster et al, 2007) as is mostly the case across higher education (although; gender differences are less predictable in UK Royal College membership examinations (British Medical Association, 2006; Dewhurst et al, 2007)). It is unclear why males underperform in some undergraduate examinations, although there is some evidence that female medical

students are more conscientious, which positively predicts academic performance (Woolf, 2009). It has been suggested that differences are due to consultation style, particularly as women doctors tend to achieve higher marks in practical clinical examinations than men. Differences between the genders in communication are however probably smaller than the differences within the genders (Cameron, 2009) and reported gender differences in communication style may be partly due to stereotypical views of and expectations on women (Kilminster et al, 2007).

In domains other than assessment, female medics tend to be *less* extrinsically successful than males. A study of 13,844 Norwegian doctors showed that men were much more likely to hold a position of leadership, even when the results were stratified by age, thus allowing for cohort effects (Kværner et al, 1999). A study of 235,776 US medical school graduates from 1979 to 1993 showed that, although women doctors were more likely to enter academic medicine than men, they were less likely to progress to associate or full professor (Nonnemaker, 2000). In the United Kingdom, women are less likely to achieve consultant or GP principal status compared to men and, if they do achieve it, it takes them longer, mainly because they are more likely to work part-time or take career breaks than men (Taylor et al, 2009). Unsurprisingly, women doctors earn less over the course of their careers than men, as is also the case outside medicine (Elton, 2009).

Gender and intrinsic success

Are women doctors less intrinsically successful than men? A study of 2584 Canadian doctors, 10% of whom were female, showed that women were more stressed at work than men but did not report less global job satisfaction (Richardsen and Burke, 1991); but a more recent study of nearly 400 Canadian psychiatrists and surgeons found that women in both specialities were less satisfied with their careers than men (Lepnurm et al, 2006). Environmental factors may be important in determining gender differences in doctors' career satisfaction. In a study of nearly 2000 US medical school faculty members, women with children were more likely to take on the majority of child-related responsibilities and were less likely than men with children to be satisfied with their careers, whereas men and women without children were equally satisfied (Carr et al, 1998). Another US study of 4501 female doctors found that approximately 80% of participants were satisfied with their careers (as is generally found across occupations; Furnham, 2008); however, nearly a third of the female doctors surveyed said they might not choose medicine if they had their time again, and having children was again related to job dissatisfaction (Frank et al, 1999).

Ethnicity and career outcomes

First, it is important to point out that ethnicity is a complex variable, which has different interpretations and meanings in different situations (Malik, 2008). To lessen confusion, the following research findings relate mainly to the United Kingdom and 'ethnic minority' is used to describe people from non-white groups.

The number of ethnic minority doctors practising medicine in the United Kingdom has increased (Goldacre et al, 2004) and is likely to continue to do so because ethnic minorities are well-represented at medical school (British Medical Association, 2004). This partly reflects the fact that ethnic minorities are more likely to enter higher education generally than their white counterparts (Connor et al, 2004). Modood (2005) has commented on the desire that South Asians have for their children to gain qualifications and thus attain 'upward mobility'. It is unclear exactly how these factors affect the motivations and goals. There is, however, a stereotype that Asian medical students and doctors are more likely to have been coerced into medicine by pushy parents (Woolf et al, 2008), and there is a danger that applying this stereotype to individuals will have detrimental affects on their self-efficacy and performance (Steele, 1997).

Ethnicity and extrinsic and intrinsic success

Once at medical school, UK ethnic minority medical students are more likely to fail or perform poorly in undergraduate examinations (Ferguson et al, 2002; Woolf, 2009). This does not appear to be due to any significant differences in socio-economic status or learning styles (Woolf, 2009) and reflects patterns found elsewhere in higher education (Richardson, 2008). Furthermore, as a group, ethnic minority doctors, including those trained in the United Kingdom, are in many ways less extrinsically successful than white doctors. They are more likely to be referred to the General Medical Council (Esmail and Abel, 2006), they are at greater risk from discrimination in job applications (Esmail and Everington, 1993), are less likely to be selected for GP training (Brown

et al, 2001), and are more likely to fail membership examinations of many of the Royal Colleges (British Medical Association, 2006; Dewhurst et al, 2007). In terms of intrinsic success, doctors from ethnic minorities on the whole have less job satisfaction, and are more likely to want to leave patient-facing jobs (Sibbald et al, 2003; Simoens et al, 2002). Ethnic minority doctors are less likely to view the NHS as an equal opportunities employer, feel less supported by nursing staff, and be gloomier about their career prospects (Lambert et al, 2000). Doctors and medical students from ethnic minorities are, however, somewhat less likely to report stress and burnout (Prosser et al, 1999).

It is clear that further steps need to be taken to explore and ensure gender and ethnic equality in the medical profession.

Choice and career success

Many of the antecedents of career success discussed earlier – gender, ethnicity, socio-economic factors influencing education and personality, for example – are originally determined by chance or, to put it differently, by genetics. However, most people also have choices in their careers (although, as we have seen, people differ as to how much choice they perceive they have). We have discussed the SDT view of choice, which considers autonomy to be fundamental to well-being and intrinsic success, but there are plenty of other theories that examine the career choices people make. One of us has written elsewhere about theories of career choice applied to medicine (McManus and Goldacre, 2008), in particular Holland's typology. Briefly, Holland's theory seeks to predict career success by the degree to which people's interests and their personality match the characteristics of their jobs, called congruence (Holland, 1996). According to Holland, people and their jobs can be categorised as realistic (conservative, practical, and seeks tangible rewards), investigative (analytical, intellectual, and enjoys deep learning), artistic (innovative, unconventional, and creative), social (empathetic, enjoys interacting with others and helping others), enterprising (persuading, gregarious, and seeks material rewards) or conventional (orderly, technical, and careful). These categories are arranged in a hexagon shape, some types being closer than others. Medics are often thought to be investigative (e.g. surgeon, anaesthetist), artistic (e.g. hospital physician), and social (e.g. psychiatrist) types (Borges et al, 2004; Petrides and McManus, 2004).

Intrinsic career success is a key component of Holland's theory, according to which person–environment congruence should lead to satisfaction. Meta-analyses have yielded mixed support. The most recent one at the time of writing is by Tsabari et al (2005). They found a correlation of $r = 0.16$ between congruence and satisfaction but there was also significant variation in the studies analysed, part of which seems to be due to different measurement instruments. Congruence, however, does appear to predict other pertinent outcomes. Tracey and Robbins (2006) conducted a study of 80,574 students at 87 US universities, which showed that subject and interests congruence predicted academic success and persistence over and above entry qualifications, and that congruence was particularly important if those with low interest at entry were to persist with their studies. Few studies have examined the impact of congruence in different medical careers, presumably because medicine is often seen as a single career, rather than embracing many different types of career.

Modelling the predictors of career success

We have seen the person and environmental variables suggested by various career theorists affect extrinsic and intrinsic job success, but do those factors affect one another and can we combine them to more powerfully predict career success? In this section, we provide a summary of a longitudinal study by Pachulicz et al (2008), which examined the predictors of extrinsic and intrinsic career success in a group of 1269 emergency physicians in the United States. It provides a good overview of the various types of factors that predict the different types of outcomes that make a good medical career.

Pachulicz and colleagues administered 38-page questionnaires at three time points, measuring human capital, organisational sponsorship, socio-demographics, and individual differences. Extrinsic career success was measured as the number of academic leads, the number of emergency medicine (EM) leads, and salary change from time 1 to time 3. Intrinsic career success was measured as career satisfaction and meeting of expectations. There were also three outcome measures of staff turnover:

retirement, thinking of leaving EM, and thinking of leaving medicine. In addition to gaining longitudinal information about participants over three time points, new participants were added at each time point to the total sample to maintain sample sizes. Over 80% of the respondents were male, about 90% were white, over 80% were married, and nearly 80% had children living with them.

The authors conducted three analyses: one for men, one for women, and one for men and women combined. A diagram of the latter is shown in Figure 18.1. Doctors who had high career satisfaction and the greatest increases in salary were most likely to intend to stay in EM or in another field within medicine, and were least likely to intend to retire within 5 years. Career satisfaction was driven by the nature of the work: those who perceived it as challenging, who had organisational support, and whose work did not interfere with other commitments were most satisfied. Individual differences also played their part. Doctors with higher self–efficacy, and interestingly those who were less social, were most satisfied. In terms of extrinsic success, doctors who worked longer hours were more likely to be promoted to leadership positions and have salary increases, and were more likely to intend to stay in EM. Older doctors and those who had spent the longest time in EM had the smallest increases in salary and were most likely to retire or leave EM. Pachulicz et al speculated that a lack of an increase in salary drove doctors to retire; however, an alternative explanation is that older doctors were more likely to be earning high salaries at the start of the study and thus their salaries did not increase as much as younger doctors over the course of the study, and they were more likely to retire due to their age.

The other two analyses showed some gender differences. For women, having more qualifications was negatively related to salary, whereas there was no effect for men. Conversely, the negative effect of age on salary was only significant for men. There was a significant interaction between ethnicity and gender on salary, with white females achieving greater salary increases than non-white females, but white males achieving smaller increases than non-white males. In terms of career satisfaction, women's career satisfaction was positively predicted by self-efficacy. Less clear were the reasons why satisfaction was, for women, negatively predicted by the 'social' individual differences variable. For men, work excitement and organisational support were the most important predictors of career satisfaction.

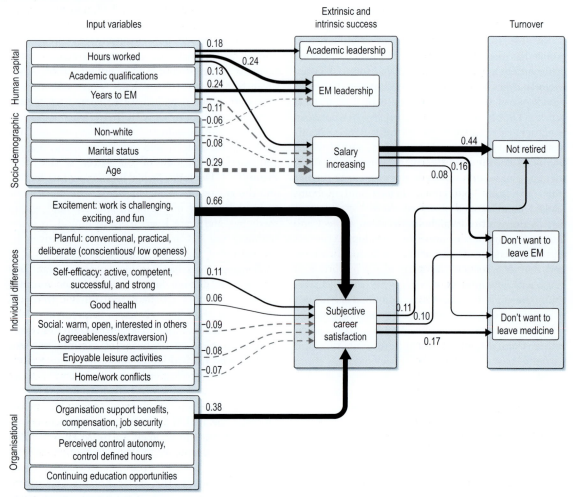

Figure 18.1 • Standardised estimates of the relationship of extrinsic success (promotions and salary increases) with human capital and socio-demographics; and of intrinsic success (career satisfaction) with individual differences and organisational variables. Relationships of extrinsic and intrinsic success with turnover (retirement, desire to leave emergency medicine (EM), and desire to leave medicine) also shown. Data from Pachulicz et al's longitudinal study of 1269 EM physicians in the United States. Black arrows show positive relationships and grey broken arrows show negative relationships. Variables to the left are theorised to predict variables to the right. Correlations between input variables were not calculated, neither were relationships between intrinsic and extrinsic success factors.

Career counselling and success

Having given an overview of predictors of career success, the next step is to examine how trainees are guided into successful careers. The national restructuring of UK doctors' careers in 2005 means they now have to make decisions about their specialities approximately 18 months after graduation; however, little formal career counselling is built into UK medical training. Medical schools may run a few sessions on speciality choice, and once qualified, doctors can refer to online resources or an educational supervisor to help them choose specialities. Doctors in difficulty can be referred to a career counselling service via their postgraduate deanery. But, in general, medics rarely come into contact with trained career counsellors or partake in official career interventions.

Career intervention and choice

Could career interventions help doctors make more successful career choices? There is evidence from outside medicine that career interventions can be effective, at least when the outcome variables are related to certainty and/or satisfaction with choice. Less clear is how career interventions lead to extrinsic or intrinsic career success. Brown et al (2003) and Richard (2005) have reviewed the evidence surrounding the 'active ingredients' of career interventions and put forward suggestions for effective interventions. Brown et al (2003) combined their review with evidence from the broader psychological literature to formulate 15 hypotheses around which future career interventions could be built. These fall into four main categories. First, successful interventions should include written goal setting and planning. Second, this planning should be conducted in conjunction with individualised feedback and advice from counsellors based, for example on a participant's completion of a computer-guided intervention, and taking account of special or unusual circumstances. Third, career interventions should encourage participants to use resources that provide information about occupations. Fourth, interventions should include some career-related disclosures by seniors about difficulties they have overcome, thus providing modelling opportunities.

Richard (2005) takes a broader view of career interventions, encompassing their content and process as well as the infrastructure required to deliver them in practice. In terms of content, Richard suggests that interventions should enable participants to synthesise self-knowledge about their values, interests, personality, and skills with knowledge about organisations, occupations, and educational requirements. Interventions should equip participants with the ability to plan and make decisions. In terms of process, Richard reiterates Brown et al's suggestions in relation to written goal setting and so on. In addition, Richard advocates the use of a variety of delivery modes to reach people from disparate groups: the collaboration, articulation, and communication of goals and plans to family and friends; the integration of interventions in existing educational programmes; and stringent intervention evaluations. In terms of infrastructure, Richard suggests that effective interventions require qualified and committed leadership and staff as well as institutional support in the form of adequate facilities, materials, and resources. Peer advisory services or alumni shadowing services are recommended to increase participant acceptance, collaboration, and communication of goals and plans. Finally, Richard takes a broader view, extolling the virtues of a 'lifelong career guidance services' to improve the productivity and economic viability of entire countries.

This chapter has mainly been concerned with early medical careers and the decisions taken then. There is perhaps a case for integrating lifelong career support for doctors with existing professional development programmes. Medical schools are well placed to start the delivery of career interventions, which should be evidence-based, stringently evaluated, and could be used to test hypotheses and refine career theory, as well as of course, increase doctors' extrinsic and intrinsic career success.

Chapter summary

At the start of this chapter, we said it is difficult to know what a good career is, let alone how to predict who will have one and why. That is because career success is, in many ways, subjective and, as with all complex human phenomena, depends on the interplay between a multitude of individual and environmental variables. Bearing that in mind, we have overviewed some key psychological theories to illuminate the predictors of intrinsic and extrinsic career success.

According to SDT, autonomy is one of the underpinnings of psychological well-being in human beings and many, although not all, studies have shown that it influences both intrinsic and extrinsic career success. When making career choices, then, it may be useful for individuals to evaluate their own motivations and ensure that they are as autonomous as possible. Encouraging people to follow their intrinsic rather than their extrinsic goals may also help them achieve greater overall well-being. SCCT states that high self-efficacy leads to career success, both extrinsic and intrinsic. Whilst some researchers believe that self-efficacy is a personality-type trait which is generalisable across situations, its original socio-cognitive conceptualisation emphasises that an individual's feelings of self-efficacy depend on the situation and can change with feedback from their own actions as well as from others. Doctors can therefore make efforts to bolster their students' and trainees' self-efficacy and self-confidence by providing feedback in a manner which is constructive and designed to improve performance; and those responsible for organising doctors' training programmes can help provide the space and development opportunities which will enable this to happen in practice. Indeed, research into the organisational support and human capital influences on careers shows that supervisors' actions and the way organisations are structured in terms of providing training opportunities can have a crucial influence on individual trainees' career success. Opportunity for skills development and support from supervisors can be effective in promoting career satisfaction (and thus reducing turnover) and also, to an extent, in helping employees achieve promotions and salary increases. When choosing a career, it is therefore important to establish whether it will provide these types of support and opportunities.

Other individual variables – personality, gender, and ethnicity – are also predictive of success. Individuals high in neuroticism and low in conscientiousness, as well as females and ethnic minorities, are less likely to achieve many types of extrinsic and intrinsic career successes. So what can be done about this? In terms of personality, self-knowledge is the key to adapting positively to a situation. Knowing a person's preferences, strengths, and weakness can help them make choices based on their values, motivations, and knowledge of how they are likely to react and feel in different situations. There is also some evidence that a match between interests and job characteristics is likely to lead to employee satisfaction. In the case of gender and ethnicity, the responsibility is also with employers to acknowledge and better understand group differences and make appropriate changes to ensure equality and fairness.

To sum up, then, the key requirements for making and guiding successful career choices are, first, knowledge of oneself and about the details of jobs and career path, and second, an ability to reflect on and plan around that knowledge. This chapter has outlined some important areas to consider when making those plans; however, it cannot be a substitute for career guidance interventions, more of which should be given to doctors throughout their training. Most of the studies we have cited come from the psychological rather than the medical education literature and many of the best were conducted in the United States with largely non-medical samples. The relative homogeneity of medical education and postgraduate medical employment in the United Kingdom provides an ideal environment for conducting high-quality research. We need to take this opportunity to conduct longitudinal studies, grounded in theory, with large samples. We also need to ensure career counselling and interventions with doctors are evidence-based and stringently evaluated. Only then will we really understand how best to predict and guide doctors' careers.

Implications for practice

A good career means different things to different people. Individuals should reflect on their own work-related motivations, preferences, and strengths and weaknesses, and make decisions in the light of those reflections. Supervisors can help their trainees' career progression by encouraging them to reflect in that way, and by tailoring the advice they provide to individuals accordingly.

Motivation is a driver of career success. Supervisors can encourage autonomous, self-determined motivation by listening to students and trainees, trying to understand their points of view, and encouraging them to make their own work-related choices by giving them sufficient information, skills, and opportunities.

Bolstering self-efficacy, managing outcome expectations, and setting positive and achievable goals can positively influence career success. Supervisors can do so by creating positive environments in which students and trainees can practice their skills; and by giving constructive feedback and encouragement. Superiors should also be aware that they are role models and act accordingly.

Support from senior staff, including mentoring, can improve career outcomes. Trainees should make efforts to foster good relationships with their supervisors, particularly early in their careers. Supervisors can take on formal or informal mentoring roles.

Some psychological factors that influence career success (e.g. GSE, locus of control, personality) are partly genetically determined, but that does not mean that they cannot be altered. Humans have large frontal lobes, whose function, in large part, is to provide voluntary control over more primitive instinctual impulses. Supervisors can encourage individuals to have insight into their own strengths and weaknesses by knowing and understanding their personality traits, and recognising how they might behave, think, and feel differently from other people.

Gender and ethnicity influence career success. The ethnic differences remain difficult to explain. Wide-ranging, high-quality research is required to understand them, which should include trials of interventions with careful monitoring of outcomes. Gender differences in career progression seem to be at least partly related to the higher proportion of women with greater family commitments. Changes to working environments and the working culture to allow more flexibility may facilitate gender equality at the medical workplace.

Formalised, evidence-based career counselling could start at the medical school and continue throughout professional development. Medical schools are well placed to start the delivery of career interventions, which should be evidence-based and stringently evaluated. They could be used to test hypotheses and refine career theory, as well as increase doctors' perceived career success.

References

Abele AE, Spurk D: The longitudinal impact of self-efficacy and career goals on objective and subjective career success, *J Vocat Behav* 74:53–62, 2009.

Bandura A: Self-efficacy: toward a unifying theory of behavioral change, *Psychol Rev* 84:191–215, 1977.

Barnett RC, Carr PL, Boisnier AD, et al: Relationships of gender and career motivation to medical faculty members' production of academic publications, *Acad Med* 73:180–186, 1998.

Barrick MR, Mount MK: The big five personality dimensions and job performance: a meta-analysis, *Pers Psychol* 44:1–26, 1991.

Barrick MR, Mount MK: Autonomy as a moderator of the relationships between the big five personality dimensions and job performance, *J Appl Psychol* 78:111–118, 1993.

Becker GS: *Human capital: a theoretical and empirical analysis, with special reference to education*, New York, 1964, National Bureau of Economic Research.

Borges NJ, Savickas ML, Jones BJ: Holland's theory applied to medical specialty choice, *J Career Assess* 12:188–206, 2004.

British Medical Association: *Demography of medical schools – a discussion paper*, London, 2004, British Medical Association.

British Medical Association: *Examining equality: a survey of Royal College examinations*, London, 2006, British Medical Association.

Brown CA, Wakefield SE, Bullock AD: The selection of GP trainees in the West Midlands: audit of assessment centre scores by ethnicity and country of qualification, *Med Teach* 23:605–609, 2001.

Brown SD, Ryan Krane NE, Brecheisen J, et al: Critical ingredients of career choice interventions: more analyses and new hypotheses, *J Vocat Behav* 62:411–428, 2003.

Burton KD, Lydon JE, D'Alessandro DU, et al: The differential effects of intrinsic and identified motivation on well-being and performance: prospective, experimental, and implicit approaches to self-determination theory, *J Pers Soc Psychol* 91:750–762, 2006.

Cameron D: A language in common, *Psychologist* 22(7):578–581, 2009.

Carr PL, Ash AS, Friedman RH, et al: Relation of family responsibilities and gender to the productivity and career satisfaction of medical faculty, *Ann Intern Med* 129:532–538, 1998.

Coleman JS: Social capital in the creation of human capital, *Am J Sociol* 94: S95–S120, 1988.

Connor H, Tyres C, Modood T, et al: Why the difference? A closer look at higher education minority ethnic students and graduates, Department for Education and Skills. RR552, 2004.

Crombie N: Sotomayor pledges impartial justice if confirmed, *The Oregonian* 13 July, 2009.

Deci EL, Ryan RM: Facilitating optimal motivation and psychological well-being across life's domains, *Can Psychol* 49:14–23, 2008.

Deci EL, Koestner R, Ryan RM: A meta-analytic review of experiments examining the effects of extrinsic rewards on intrinsic motivation, *Psychol Bull* 125:627–668, 1999.

Dewhurst N, McManus IC, Mollon J, et al: Performance in the MRCP(UK) examination 2003–4: analysis of pass rates of UK graduates in relation to self-declared ethnicity and gender, *BMC Med Educ* 5(1):8, 2007.

Dormann C, Zapf D: Job satisfaction: a meta-analysis of stabilities, *J Organ Behav* 22:483–504, 2001.

Eby LT, Allen TD, Evans SC, et al: Does mentoring matter? A multidisciplinary meta-analysis comparing mentored and non-mentored individuals, *J Vocat Behav* 72:254–267, 2008.

Eden D, Zuk Y: Seasickness as a self-fulfilling prophecy: raising self-efficacy to boost performance at sea, *J Appl Psychol* 80:628–635, 1995.

Elton MA: *Women and medicine: the future*, London, 2009, Royal College of Physicians.

Esmail A, Abel P: The impact of ethnicity and diversity on doctors' performance and appraisal, *Br J Health Care Manag* 12:303–307, 2006.

Esmail A, Everington S: Racial discrimination against doctors from ethnic minorities, *BMJ* 306:691–692, 1993.

Ferguson E, James D, Madeley L: Factors associated with success in medical school: systematic review of the literature, *BMJ* 324:952–957, 2002.

Frank E, McMurray JE, Linzer M, et al: For the Society of General Internal Medicine Career Satisfaction Study Group. Career satisfaction of US women physicians: results from the Women Physicians' Health Study, *Arch Intern Med* 159:1417–1426, 1999.

Freeborn DK: Satisfaction, commitment, and psychological well-being among HMO physicians, *West J Med* 174:13–18, 2000.

Furnham A: *The psychology of behaviour at work: the individual and the organization*, ed 2, Hove, 2008, Psychology Press.

Gagne M, Deci ED: Self-determination theory and work motivation, *J Organ Behav* 26:331–362, 2005.

Goldacre MJ, Davidson JM, Lambert TW: Country of training and ethnic origin of UK doctors: database and survey studies, *BMJ* 329:597–600, 2004.

Grumbach K, Osmond D, Vranizan K, et al: Primary care physicians' experience of financial incentives in managed-care systems, *N Engl J Med* 339:1516–1521, 1998.

Helman C: *Suburban Shaman: tales from medicine's frontline*, London, 2006, Hammersmith Press.

Hoff T, Whitcomb WF, Nelson JR: Thriving and surviving in a new medical career: the case of hospitalist physicians, *J Health Soc Behav* 43:72–91, 2002.

Holland JL: Exploring careers with a typology, *Am Psychol* 51:397–406, 1996.

Judge TA, Bono JE: Relationship of core self-evaluations traits – self-esteem, generalized self-efficacy, locus of control, and emotional stability – with job satisfaction and job performance: a meta-analysis, *J Appl Psychol* 86:80–92, 2001.

Judge TA, Cable DM, Boudreau JW, et al: An empirical investigation of the predictors of executive career success, Working Paper 9 4 – 0 8. Center for Advanced Human Resource Studies (CAHRS) Cornell University ILR School, 1994.

Judge TA, Locke EA, Durham CC, et al: Dispositional effects on job and life satisfaction: the role of core evaluations, *J Appl Psychol* 83:17–34, 1998.

Judge TA, Higgins CA, Thoresen CJ, et al: The big five personality traits, general mental ability, and career success across the life span, *Pers Psychol* 52:621–652, 1999.

Judge TA, Thoresen CJ, Bono JE, et al: The job satisfaction–job performance relationship: a qualitative and quantitative review, *Psychol Bull* 127:376–407, 2001.

Judge TA, Jackson CL, Shaw JC, et al: Self-efficacy and work – related performance: the integral role of individual differences, *J Appl Psychol* 92:107–127, 2007.

Kammeyer-Mueller JD, Judge TA: A quantitative review of mentoring research: test of a model, *J Vocat Behav* 72:269–283, 2008.

Kilminster S, Downes J, Gough B, et al: Women in medicine – is there a problem? A literature review of the changing gender composition, structures and occupational cultures in medicine, *Med Educ* 41:39–49, 2007.

Kluckhohn C: *Personality in nature, society, and culture*, New York, 1953, Knopf.

Kværner KJ, Aasland OG, Botten GS: Female medical leadership: cross sectional study, *BMJ* 318:91–94, 1999.

Lam CF, Gurland ST: Self-determined work motivation predicts job outcomes, but what predicts self-determined work motivation? *J Res Pers* 42:1109–1115, 2008.

Lambert TW, Goldacre MJ, Evans J: Views of junior doctors about their work: survey of qualifiers of 1993 and 1996 from United Kingdom medical schools, *Med Educ* 34:348–354, 2000.

Lent RW, Brown SD, Hackett G: Toward a unifying social cognitive theory of career and academic interest, choice, and performance, *J Vocat Behav* 45:79–122, 1994.

Lepnurm R, Dobson R, Backman A, et al: Factors explaining career satisfaction among psychiatrists and surgeons in Canada, *Can J Psychol* 51:243–255, 2006.

McCrae RR, Costa PTJ: Personality trait structure as a human universal, *Am Psychol* 52:509–516, 1997.

McManus IC, Goldacre MJ: Predicting career destinations. In Carter Y, Jackson N, editors: *Medical education and training: from theory to delivery*, Oxford, 2008, Oxford University Press, pp 59–78.

McManus IC, Winder B, Paice E: How consultants, hospitals, trusts and deaneries affect pre-registration house officer posts: a multilevel model, *Med Educ* 36:35–44, 2002.

McManus IC, Keeling A, Paice E: Stress, burnout and doctors' attitudes to work are determined by personality and learning style: a twelve year longitudinal study of UK medical graduates, *BMC Med* 2:29, 2004.

Malik K: *Strange fruit: why both sides are wrong in the race debate*, Oxford, 2008, Oneworld Publications.

Matthews G, Deary IJ: *Personality traits*, Cambridge, 1998, Cambridge University Press.

Modood T: *Multicultural politics: racism, ethnicity and muslims in Britain*, Minnesota, 2005, University of Minnesota Press.

Ng T, Eby LT, Sorensen KL, et al: Predictors of objective and subjective career success: a meta-analysis, *Pers Psychol* 58:367–408, 2005.

Ng T, Sorensen KL, Eby LT: Locus of control at work: a meta-analysis, *J Organ Behav* 27:1087, 2006.

Nonnemaker L: Women physicians in academic medicine – new insights from cohort studies, *N Engl J Med* 342:399–405, 2000.

Pachulicz S, Schmitt N, Kuljanin G: A model of career success: a longitudinal study of emergency physicians, *J Vocat Behav* 73:242–253, 2008.

Parsons F: *Choosing a vocation*, Boston, 1909, Houghton Mifflin.

Petrides KV, McManus IC: Mapping medical careers: questionnaire assessment of career preferences in medical school applicants and final-year students, *BMC Med Educ* 4(18):2004.

Prosser D, Johnson S, Kuipers E, et al: Mental health, burnout and job satisfaction in a longitudinal study of mental health staff, *Soc Psychiatry Psychiatr Epidemiol* 34:295–300, 1999.

Reed VA, Jernstedt GC, McCormick TR: A longitudinal study of determinants of career satisfaction in medical students, *Med Educ Online* 9:11, 2004.

Richard GV: International best practices in career development: review of the literature, *Int J Educ Vocat Guid* 5:189–201, 2005.

Richardsen AM, Burke RJ: Occupational stress and job satisfaction among physicians: sex differences, *Soc Sci Med* 33:1179–1187, 1991.

Richardson JTE: The attainment of ethnic minority students in UK higher education, *Stud High Educ* 33:33–48, 2008.

Richer S, Blanchard C, Vallerand RJ: A motivational model of work turnover, *J Appl Soc Psychol* 32:2089–2113, 2002.

Rotter JB: Internal versus external control of reinforcement: a case history of a variable, *Am Psychol* 45:489–493, 1990.

Sambunjak D, Straus SE, Marusic A: Mentoring in academic medicine: a systematic review, *JAMA* 296:1103–1115, 2006.

Seibert SE, Kraimer ML: The five-factor model of personality and career success, *J Vocat Behav* 58:1–21, 2001.

Sibbald B, Bojke C, Gravelle H: National survey of job satisfaction and retirement intentions among general practitioners in England, *BMJ* 326 (7379):22, 2003.

Simoens S, Scott A, Sibbald B: Job-satisfaction, work-related stress and intentions to quit of Scottish GPs, *Scott Med J* 47:80–86, 2002.

Singh R, Ragins BR, Tharenou P: Who gets a mentor? A longitudinal assessment of the rising star hypothesis, *J Vocat Behav* 74:11–17, 2009a.

Singh R, Ragins BR, Tharenou P: What matters most? The relative role of mentoring and career capital in career success, *J Vocat Behav* 75:56–67, 2009b.

Sobral DT: What kind of motivation drives medical students' learning quests? *Med Educ* 38:950–957, 2004.

Stajkovic AD, Luthans F: Self-efficacy and work-related performance: a meta-analysis, *Psychol Bull* 124:240–261, 1998.

Steele CM: A threat in the air: how stereotypes shape intellectual identity and performance, *Am Psychol* 52:613–629, 1997.

Taylor KS, Lambert TW, Goldacre MJ: Career progression and destinations, comparing men and women in the NHS: postal questionnaire surveys, *BMJ* 338:b1735, 2009.

Tolstoy LK: Anna Karenina, 1887. Available from http://www.readprint.com/work-1431/AnnaKarenina-Leo-Tolstoy. Accessed November 26, 2009.

Tracey TJG, Robbins SB: The interest-major congruence and college success relation: a longitudinal study, *J Vocat Behav* 69:64–89, 2006.

Tsabari O, Tziner A, Meir EI: Updated meta-analysis on the relationship between congruence and satisfaction, *J Career Assess* 13:216–232, 2005.

Van Heil A, Vansteenkiste M: Ambitions fulfilled? The effects of intrinsic and extrinsic goal attainment on older adults' ego-integrity and death attitudes, *Int J Aging Hum Dev* 68:27–51, 2009.

Vansteenkiste M, Simons J, Lens W, et al: Motivating learning, performance, and persistence: the synergistic effects of intrinsic goal contents and autonomy-supportive contexts, [Miscellaneous Article], *J Pers Soc Psychol* 87:246–260, 2004.

Wayne SJ, Liden RC, Kraimer ML, et al: The role of human capital, motivation and supervisor sponsorship in predicting career success, *J Organ Behav* 20:577–595, 2001.

Williams GC, Saizow R, Ross L, et al: Motivation underlying career choice for internal medicine and surgery, *Soc Sci Med* 45:1705–1713, 1997.

Woolf K: *The academic under-performance of medical students from ethnic minorities*, PhD thesis, 2009, University of London.

Woolf K, Cave J, Greenhalgh T, et al: Ethnic stereotypes and the underachievement of UK medical students from ethnic minorities: qualitative study, *BMJ* 337:a1220, 2008.

Further reading

Arthur MB, Hall DT, Lawrence BS: *Handbook of career theory*. Port Chester, 1989, Cambridge University Press.

Holland JL: *Making vocational choices: a theory of vocational personalities and work environments*, 3rd ed, Odessa, FL, 1997, Psychological Assessment Resources.

Developing teachers and developing learners

19

LuAnn Wilkerson   Lawrence Hy Doyle

ABC

Glossary

Association of American Medical Colleges (AAMC)
The organisation represents all 131 accredited US and 17
accredited Canadian medical schools; approximately
400 major teaching hospitals and health systems; and
nearly 90 academic and scientific societies. Through its
many programmes and services, the AAMC supports the
entire spectrum of education, research, and patient care
activities conducted by our member institutions.

Aboriginal Term related to indigenous peoples, used
here in relations with people in Australia and Canada.

Academy of educators A new organisational structure
in medical schools directly tied to the support of the
educational mission of the institution.

Attention-deficit/hyperactive disorder (ADHD)
Chronic condition often associated with inattention and
impulsive behaviour. Treatment is usually associated
with counselling and/or medications.

**Association for the Study of Medical Education
(ASME)** A UK-based organisation with international
membership, which 'seeks to improve the quality of
medical education by bringing together individuals and
organisations with interests and responsibilities in
medical and health care education'.

Attending Faculty physician responsible for the care of
patients while supervising care given to patients by
postgraduate trainees and/or medical students (USA).

**Best Evidence Medical Education (BEME)
collaboration** A group of individuals or institutions who

Continued

DOI: 10.1016/B978-0-7020-3522-7.00019-X

ABC

Glossary (continued)

are committed to the promotion of Best Evidence Medical Education.

Consultant See main Glossary, p 338.

Faculty development Programme designed to improve the skills of faculty members, usually in areas related to education, such as lecturing skills, curriculum development, or assessment design.

Faculty member A person, generally with a terminal degree, who is often expected to be successful in clinical work, research, teaching, and community service.

Foundation for the Advancement of International Medical Education and Research (FAIMER) A non-profit component of the Educational Commission for Foreign Medical Graduates (ECFMG) devoted to providing "educational opportunities and research and data resources that inform health care policies and create sustainable improvements in health outcomes." It is best known for its maintenance of *The International Medical Education Directory* and provision of International Fellowships in Medical Education.

Family medicine Specialty of medicine in the United States related to primary care of adults and children, often including obstetrics. Similar to general practice in the United Kingdom.

Foundation Doctor or Foundation Trainee See main Glossary, p 340.

General practice; see also family medicine Specialty of medicine in the United Kingdom, similar to a family medicine practitioner in the United States, serving as the first line of health care and treatment within the UK system.

General Medical Council (GMC) See main Glossary, p 341.

Higher education Education after secondary school, at a university, college, or professional school, in a discipline such as Medicine or Law.

Imposter syndrome Also known as the imposter phenomenon, in which a student or professional, more often a woman, has an internal experience of being an imposter rather than fully qualified for her or his earned academic or professional station.

Intern See main Glossary, p 339.

Liaison Committee on Medical Education (LCME) The nationally recognised accrediting authority for medical school programmes, leading to the MD degree in the US and Canadian medical schools.

Learner development An academic approach that focuses on building learning skills, attitudes, knowledge, and meta-cognition through targeted programming, directed practice, peer-tutoring, and individual counselling.

ABC

Glossary (continued)

Medical Education Unit Office at many medical schools around the world focusing on the support and study of education. Such offices may include curriculum development, faculty development, evaluation, and educational research.

Mission-based budgeting A financial model that aims to identify the flow of funds in a medical school so that each goal or mission of the institution is the recipient of funds in relation to the amount of work, often titrated by quality indicators, required to uphold that goal or mission.

Medical Schools Council (MSC) Organisation that represents the interests and ambitions of UK Medical Schools as they relate to the generation of national health, wealth, and knowledge through biomedical research and the profession of medicine.

One Minute Preceptor A widely accepted teaching model that summarises important tasks or "microskills" for clinical teaching. The model begins with the diagnosis of the learner's needs and results in focused teaching and feedback. The teaching steps include: ask for a commitment; probe for supporting evidence; teach a general rule; tell the learner what s/he did right and the effect it had; and correct mistakes.

Pastoral counselling Pastoral counselling moves beyond the support or encouragement a religious community can offer, by providing psychologically sound therapy that weaves in the religious and spiritual dimension. From aapc.org

Postgraduate trainee See main Glossary, p 339.

Sami The Sami (also spelled Saami) are the 100,000 Indigenous inhabitants of Norway, Sweden, Finland, and the Russian Kola Peninsula.

Specialist trainee See main Glossary, p 341.

Student Affairs Office Student support office at many US medical schools that may include registrar, financial aid, academic support, academic scheduling, career advising, and general well-being programmes.

World Federation for Medical Education (WFME) A global organisation concerned with education of medical doctors at all levels. It serves as an umbrella organisation for six regional medical education associations. It is active in the promotion of guidelines and standards for worldwide use in the accreditation and continuous improvement of medical schools.

World Health Organisation (WHO) The directing and coordinating authority for health within the United Nations system, which is responsible for leadership on global health, from research to policy, and monitoring and assessing health trends.

Outline

The greatest investment of any educational institution is in its teachers, and the reason for that investment is its learners. Teachers develop; learners develop; the institution grows as well. In this chapter, we will consider the types of programmes needed to create and sustain a learning community of teachers and learners. The first section of the chapter describes a range of programmes useful in assisting faculty members in developing their skills as teachers and the organisational structures needed to support such programmes. The second section addresses: the needs of learners, from students to postgraduate trainees; the design of learning skill development programmes; and typical activities and skills included in such programmes. The section ends with a discussion of the need to extend such programming in order to better prepare the wider range of learners trying for entry into medical school.

Introduction

Educational institutions that invest in the development of their teachers and learners can be called learning organisations according to Senge (1990). Such organisations, capable of continuous adaptation and growth, demonstrate a commitment to five broad principles, which can be used as a lens through which to view the work of medical schools and health care institutions in creating and sustaining faculty and learner development programmes:

- Continuous personal mastery
- Common mental models
- Shared vision
- Team-learning
- Systems thinking

The learning organisation is committed to *personal mastery*. Individuals within such a community, both faculty and learners, never stop learning. It is the journey itself that is important. While individual learning by itself does not necessarily translate into organisational learning, without individual learning, there can be no organisational or community learning.

The members of a learning organisation share a common *mental model* of desirable actions. In order for the organisation to move in a chosen direction, all members of that organisation must have access to and ability to influence the strategic plan or conceptual model that will guide future actions. Such a model is the product of community members working together: in our case, teachers and learners.

The learning organisation actively works to engage all of its members in developing a sense of the possible, *a shared vision*. Mutual and regular feedback is a key requisite for elaborating on the vision and refining it to meet the needs of the various community constituencies.

The organisation changes by reflecting on its successes and challenges. Time and resources are committed to building a *team-learning* environment in which members of the organisation learn from and with one another. Working together, teachers and learners develop a trust and a commitment to continuous improvement based on mutually understood needs.

The learning organisation is committed to *systems thinking* as opposed to governance from the top down. A learning community is most likely to develop when the organisation understands its existence within the system which encompasses it as well as the microsystems of which it is composed. Medical education institutions include multiple microsystems – central administration, individual academic departments, health care delivery service lines, curricular systems, learners at varying levels, and staff essential to the work product of each constituency. It is incumbent on the learning organisation to develop in response to the varying needs of each group of which it is composed.

Faculty and learner development programmes can serve as the engine that drives the development of a learning organisation. Such programmes instil a commitment to excellence, develop shared models of desirable behaviour, create a common vision, instil a team-learning spirit, and facilitate systems thinking.

Developing teachers

Until the mid 1960s, university faculty members, including those in medical schools, were considered fully prepared for their role as teachers (Sorcinelli, 2006). An advanced degree in their specialty was all that was required since effective teaching was defined as demonstrating expertise in the specified content area through publications and research grants. Faculty development was synonymous with sabbaticals, research opportunities, and travel to professional meetings. Beyond content expertise, good teachers were born, not made. In 1955, George

Miller, a faculty member at the University of Buffalo School of Medicine, USA, and Steve Abrahamson, a faculty member in the School of Education, acquired funding to establish a partnership between the two schools called the Project in Medical Education. The goal of the Project was to explore how to apply the growing body of research and theory in education to medical education. A young medical student, Hilliard Jason, who had been extremely vocal about problems in medical school teaching, was invited to join the Project. Jason subsequently became a founder of teaching improvement programmes in medical education (Wilkerson and Anderson, 2004).

In higher education, the growing demand by university students during the 1960s for better teaching led to increased use of teaching evaluations and pressure on university professors to consider the existence of actual skills of teaching – similar to those required of pre-college teachers – that could be learnt and developed. Guided by the work of Berquist and Phillips, Gaff, and Centra, the field of faculty development emerged in higher education in the 1970s (Sorcinelli, 2006). The improvement of teaching skills became a central focus of the field, although Berquist and Phillips also advocated the need for attention to organisational structures that support teaching, and development of the faculty member both as a person and a professional.

Current definitions of faculty development largely focus on the skills of the individual teacher, including teaching skills, scholarship, and well-being issues. However, faculty development also includes goals related to the improvement of individual courses, the broader curriculum, and student learning, and a focus on organisational development to improve the policies and practices of the institution to better support the teaching and learning environment. In this chapter, we focus on aspects of faculty development related to the improvement of teaching and learning.

Teacher training, historically a part of preparing school teachers, extended from the United States (Jason and Westberg, 1982) to the wider world through the World Health Organisation (WHO) and its teacher training programmes (Guilbert, 1981). During this same period in the United Kingdom, general practitioners were taking on specialist training and programmes arose to develop the skills of such GPs as teachers. Yet 30 years later, many medical schools and training programmes still provide limited opportunities for faculty members to develop their skills as teachers. Faculty members

continue to report a lack of opportunity to learn how to teach. They feel unsupported in their work as teachers. Almost every recent report on medical education worldwide includes a call for more attention to preparing faculty members for their roles as teachers, including establishing adequate rewards for their teaching contributions (Cohen, 2009; GMC, 2009). Accreditation standards for medical schools in the United States (www.lcme.org/standard. htm) and the United Kingdom (GMC, 2009) require the development of faculty and residents as teachers.

Designing a comprehensive faculty development programme

Three features are central to the development of a comprehensive faculty development programme designed to support the educational mission of a medical education centre: (1) an organisational structure to support the work of teaching and teachers, (2) a variety of faculty development activities and resources targeted at the differing educational roles and individual needs of teachers, and (3) a reward system that values excellence in the various educational roles needed in the institution (Wilkerson and Irby, 1998). These features require an ongoing investment of capital and cannot be sustained without a commitment from the highest level of the organisational unit involved, whether that is a department, a medical school, an academic medical center, a centre of postgraduate medical education, or an entire health care system.

Organisational structure to support teaching and teachers

As educational programmes have increased in complexity, teachers have found themselves confronting teaching situations unlike any that they experienced themselves. Thus, the time-honoured way of learning to teach in medicine – copying one's own teachers – is no longer adequate. Problem-based learning (PBL), mannequin-based simulations, e-learning platforms, and multimedia smart classrooms were not part of most teachers' experiences as learners. Even clinical experiences have changed, now employing novel learning experiences within multi-professional teams, service-learning, community immersions, hand-held computing, and outcome-oriented patient care. Several organisational structures have emerged over the past 50 years to support the teaching responsibilities of faculty members and their development as teachers: medical education units and 'academies' of educators.

Medical education units

Academic departments are rarely set up in such a way as to provide assistance to faculty members in developing their skills as teachers. General practice, or family medicine, is an exception, both in the United Kingdom and the United States, with the presence of behavioural scientists or educationalists who can help both trainees and faculty grow as educators. More commonly, medical schools have developed medical education units charged with faculty development, sometimes coupled with other educational responsibilities, such as programme evaluation, educational technology, curriculum support, and educational scholarship. In a 2001 WHO survey of medical schools around the world, Boelen and Boyer (2001) found that 58% of the 895 medical schools that responded in a survey had medical education units. Amin et al (2005) profiled 30 Asian medical schools, 72% of which had medical offices. Albanese et al (2001) reported that 50% of North American medical schools had such units although all have an officer at dean level who oversees medical student education and may bear some responsibility for faculty development.

The academy movement

For the past century, the educational mission of medical schools has continued to be subservient to the clinical and research activities of faculty members (Bloom, 1989), which are organised around departmental structures. A mission that extends across departments, such as the education of medical students, may be without the resources, faculty, and political strength needed to accomplish it. A new organisational structure is beginning to emerge directly tied to the support of the educational mission of medical schools and postgraduate training programmes. Known as academies, these structures are designed as a geographical 'commons' for skilled teachers (Huber and Hutchings, 2005), through which they can gather to share ideas about teaching and learning as part of their ongoing professional development. Through academies, such educators can be rewarded, encouraged to innovate, provided with faculty development, assisted in developing a scholarly approach to teaching, and nurtured as educational scholars (Irby et al, 2004). In a 2003 survey of medical schools in the United States (Dewey et al,

2005), 21% reported the recent establishment of such an academy as a formal school-wide organisation with a mission to support the work of faculty as teachers with dedicated resources for faculty development, scholarship in education, and innovation. Membership is usually composed of distinguished educators selected via peer review. In the United Kingdom, a national Institute for Teaching and Learning was established in the late 1990s, then renamed the Higher Education Academy, which has similar aims but with a mission to serve faculty development needs across the whole higher education sector. Each subject area or grouping of cognate areas has a national Subject Centre (located in a host university) to act as a resource and foster collaboration and cross-fertilisation in all aspects of UK higher education. The Medicine, Dentistry, and Veterinary Medicine Subject Centre, based in the Faculty of Medical Sciences, Newcastle University, provides support to all UK medical, dental, and veterinary schools (see http://www.medev.ac.uk/). More recently, a national Academy of Medical Educators has been established to focus on the needs of faculty across medical schools and residency training sites (see http://www.medicaleducators.org/).

A range of teaching improvement programmes targeted to needs

Over the past 15 years, evidence on the effectiveness of continuing professional development activities in changing physician behaviour has continued to grow. Mazmanian and Davis (2002) conclude that three key features have been consistently identified as essential: (1) education based on assessment of needs, (2) opportunities for interaction with peers and practice of the skills to be learnt, and (3) longitudinal, sequenced multi-method activities. Although their review is focussed on changes in clinical practice and patient outcomes, the findings mirror those from studies on changing teacher behaviours and learner outcomes (Steinert et al, 2006; Wilkerson and Irby, 1998).

In teaching improvement, needs assessment has often taken the form of surveys of faculty members to determine their interest or self-assessed competency in a variety of teaching skills. While this strategy can be useful, it does not cover the broad range of skills needed by faculty members as educators. Taking institutional need as the defining issue, there are faculty who are: new to the institution who want to understand career expectations and develop basic skills in teaching; experienced teachers who carry the greatest teaching load and may be expected to implement new learning modalities or to improve their performance in clinical or classroom teaching; teachers appointed to serve as educational leaders of courses, clerkships, residency training programmes, and continuing professional development activities; and those teachers who wish to make education the focus of their scholarship. Each of these groups operates within an organisational structure that needs to nurture their accomplishments in order to create, sustain, and constantly improve the educational programmes of the institution.

Needs of new faculty as teachers

Each year medical schools, academic medical centres, and academic community practice groups experience an influx of new teachers, who may be foundation trainees, first-year residents, or specialist trainees. Medical schools may also employ new faculty members, especially those who are expected to provide patient care, or identify new community-based trainers who will teach medical students or postgraduate trainees. Benor and Mahler (1987) stress the need to orient these new teachers to the core values that underlie the teaching programmes of the institution in order to prepare them to participate fully in its educational mission. Before assuming teaching responsibilities, whether formally in the classroom and clinical settings or informally during clinical work, new teachers need to know the norms and expectations for teaching and be able to identify opportunities to teach. For example, new foundation trainees or residents may believe they do not have time to teach, usually meaning that there are no conference-room seminars for which they are responsible. However, residents have innumerable opportunities to teach when supervising medical students or junior trainees on ward rounds, in the operating theatre, and late at night on call.

Many medical schools provide an orientation for new faculty. Orientation sessions typically focus on academic expectations, promotion criteria, and career advancement. Such sessions may also provide a chance for new faculty to connect with more senior faculty for purposes of career mentoring and research collaboration. A typical new faculty orientation lasts a half or full day and includes presentations on various institutional resources and guidance on the academic promotion process. However, there are a number of innovative models, which include the use of online virtual orientation modules (Walling and Chinn,

2002), an informal welcoming reception with key administrators and information booths, and a small group mentoring programme (Pololi et al, 2002). New faculty members who will become a part of the teaching faculty, however, also need an introduction to the prevailing educational mission of the institution, information about expectations and opportunities to teach, and some beginning teaching skills. At UCLA, we have expanded a more traditional orientation day on resources and promotion processes to include a choice of teaching skill workshops, an informal buffet lunch hosted by the faculty development office, and a panel discussion on teaching opportunities and resources.

New groups of postgraduate trainees enter our institutions each year, creating an unending group of new teachers who need to understand our expectations for teaching and how to fulfil them. In the 1960s, special programmes for residents as teachers began to appear but did not become a significant part of faculty development programmes until the 1980s (Bensinger et al, 2005). In a review of resident-as-teachers programme evaluation studies from 1975 to 2008, Post and colleagues (Post et al, 2009) identified 47 articles, of which 24 provided outcome data for the programmes described. Programmes included lectures, practice sessions (such as 'microteaching'), and retreats, often based on the 'One Minute Preceptor' model (Neher et al, 1992), and ranged in length from 1 to 15 hours. Using a variety of outcomes measures, the studies demonstrated changes in teaching behaviour, self-reported confidence, and learner evaluations of residents' teaching. Based on their review, the authors recommend interventions, such as exploration of the One Minute Preceptor, which should be of 3 hours or longer in duration.

Needs of effective teachers

A growing body of research has demonstrated the effects of excellent clinical teachers on medical students' knowledge, clinical skills, and specialty choice (Griffith et al, 2000; Wimmers et al, 2006). This work underlines how important it is to provide opportunities for faculty members to develop strong teaching skills, at least in the clinical setting. A 1998 review by Wilkerson and Irby described the changing view of teaching improvement approaches over time, as the predominant educational theories guiding faculty development shifted from behavioural to cognitive, and then to social constructivist, in line with wider changes in the epistemology of medical education described in Chapter 2. Effective interventions across models included workshops of 2 days or more, teaching evaluations coupled with individual consultation, and longitudinal fellowships or courses. In a Best Evidence Medical Education (BEME) review on faculty development initiatives to improve teaching, Steinert et al (2006) identified almost 3000 articles from 1988 to 2002 describing teaching improvement programmes in medical education. The majority of programmes were workshops or seminars focusing on classroom and clinical teaching, which included topics such as lecturing, facilitating group discussion, teaching during patient care, providing effective feedback, and evaluating learner performance. More recently, basic skill workshops have also included teaching with simulations and educational technology.

The BEME review highlights a number of issues that continue to require study and innovation in relation to teaching improvement interventions, first considering the issue of participation. Should basic teaching skill training be a mandatory requirement of medical school teachers as it is for teachers of younger learners? In voluntary programmes, it is often the best teachers who understand the importance of continuous improvement and make the time to participate. Several medical schools have required participation in basic teaching skills training or produced incentives tied to promotion for participation in order to reach more teachers. In the United Kingdom, GP vocational training sites require trainers to participate in some manner of teacher training course.

A second consideration is the question of context. To what degree should basic teaching skills workshops be linked to specific courses or rotations? This linkage strategy produces a targeted audience, the opportunity to identify very specific needs, a context from which to draw examples for experiential components, and more identifiable scheduling possibilities.

A third consideration is how much faculty development is needed by an individual instructor. Reviews have consistently identified the need for numerous interventions over time. One strategy for increasing the impact of single workshops is to link them together to produce more extended engagement. To maximise flexibility and choice, The Center for Faculty Development at St. Michael's Hospital, University of Toronto, has developed a 'Stepping Stones' programme. Participants can earn a Certificate in Teaching by participating in 26 hours of workshops and 17 hours of more theoretically focused medical education journal club sessions

over a 2-year period (see: http://www.cfd.med.utoronto.ca/programmes/stepping-stones.html).

Fourth is the issue of delivery modalities. To date, most teaching improvement interventions have been delivered in face-to-face sessions with an emphasis on peer interaction and collaborative learning. The use of online multimedia materials on teaching has the potential to increase participation, especially in a distributed education system. For example, to support clinical teachers across the entire state affiliated with a health professions training programme, the North Carolina Area Health Education programme offers web-based multi-media, interactive modules on clinical teaching skills, the Expert Preceptor Interactive Curriculum (EPIC), which is linked to a centrally monitored online discussion forum at: http://www.ncahec.net/hcprofessionals/preceptor.htm.

To further maximise access and meet individual preferences, the programme also offers each teaching improvement module as a printed manual, a single-page 'thumbnail sketch' for quick review, a web-based self-instructional module, or a 1-hour seminar scheduled to meet the preferences of teachers in a specific community. Participation is encouraged by rewarding it with continuing professional development credit. Other modalities that require exploration include peer coaching, mentoring, reflective writing and discussion, communities of practice, and pay-for-performance. Critical to the effectiveness of teaching improvement interventions of any type are the use of multi-faceted learning methods, opportunities for practice with feedback, the involvement of supportive colleagues, and repeated involvement over time (Steinert et al, 2006).

The BEME review also emphasises the need for more high-quality programme evaluation studies to further increase understanding of the features and outcomes of faculty development (Steinert et al, 2006).

Needs of educational leaders and innovators

Educational programmes require faculty members who are prepared to design and implement them based on a sound understanding of what is known about how people learn and the evidence supporting various educational approaches. In a period of ever-changing curricula, these faculty members need to understand issues in organisational change and possess the leadership skills needed to guide that change. These faculty members determine the selection criteria and admissions processes for students, postgraduates, and faculty; they design and set the standards for competency assessment; they create outcome measures to meet accountability and accreditation standards; they recognise and respond to new challenges in medicine by leading curricular changes that address those challenges, e.g. increased demands for clinical productivity, changes in health care delivery systems, changing community demographics. Preparation for educational leadership and innovation requires faculty development interventions that go beyond the acquisition of basic teaching skills.

The medical education literature is rich in descriptions of longitudinal faculty development programmes for a select cohort of faculty members in the form of certificate, fellowship, and degree programmes designed specifically to grow educational leaders and innovators. A survey of medical education deans in North America by Searle et al (2006) identified 42 educational fellowship programmes. A special issue of *Academic Medicine* (November 2006) included articles on nine of these medical education fellowship programmes. The content of the fellowships emphasised both an understanding of current theories of learning and the implications for curriculum design and evaluation, approaches to curriculum design, and issues in organisational change including leadership. Gruppen et al (2006) summarised the 'Common Themes and Overarching Issues' in a final article in the issue:

> Each of the nine schools has incorporated best practices in education to prepare faculty to lead, develop, teach, and evaluate educational initiatives. Furthermore, framing these efforts as forms of scholarship consistent with the academic advancement of participating faculty fostered the expansion of expertise on which the programmes could draw … All nine schools completed some form of institutional, departmental, and/or individual faculty needs assessment, resulting in clearly defined programme goals and objectives for their fellowship programmes. These goals and objectives then led to the selection of a programme structure and specific instructional methods, informed by the literature on faculty development, adult learning, leadership, and other sources from the behavioral and social sciences. The programmes were implemented and then evaluated to determine the degree to which the objectives were met. On the basis of this evaluation, each of the programmes was then revised.
>
> (pp 990–991)

Internationally, the Foundation for Advancement of International Medical Education & Research (FAIMER) provides similar longitudinal opportunities for 'international health professions educators who have the potential to play a key role in improving health professions education at their schools' (www.faimer.org/education/institute/index.html). FAIMER offers a 2-year faculty development programme that includes sessions on curriculum development, education methods, leadership, and professional networking conducted via two residential sessions and an online discussion forum (Norcini et al 2005). The UK-based Association for the Study of Medical Education (ASME) offers an annual programme on Developing Leaders in Healthcare Education (http://www.asme.org.uk/conferences-a-courses/) as does the US Harvard Macy Institute (www.harvardmacy.org/) on which the former is based.

Needs of educational scholars

Finally, some faculty members choose to focus their academic scholarship on medical education. Through research and writing, they seek to develop new knowledge about learning in medicine, synthesise existing studies to produce 'best evidence', apply best evidence to teaching practices, test its efficacy in producing intended learner outcomes, and publish and disseminate innovations with evidence of effectiveness. Skills required include: accessing and appraising the relevant literature in psychology, education, and health professions education; designing educational research and evaluation studies; collecting and analysing data; writing and presenting results; and developing networks of professionals with similar interests.

Some faculty members come more easily to these skills, building on prior work in scientific research or biostatistics. Most require some additional study to translate their medical research experience into the specific skills and understanding needed for more applied social science and/or qualitative research. As in the domain of biomedical research, preparation for a career as a medical education scholar usually requires hours of study and mentored scholarly activity, such as that provided through participation in a medical education research fellowship or degree programme in medical education. Some of the medical education fellowships described above also include an in-depth research component with mentored scholarship. A good example is the Medical Education Scholars programme at the University of Michigan, USA. This year-long fellowship includes a seminar on study design and completion of a mentored educational research study. As of 2003, the 35 graduates of the Scholars programme had published

9 peer-reviewed papers, delivered 21 oral presentations at national meetings, and submitted 16 educational grants (Gruppen et al, 2003).

A search of the internet (July 2009) turned up articles and information on 40 master's degree programmes in medical education around the world, many including online components, with the largest number of programmes in the United Kingdom. The development of research skills in any domain requires an intensity of involvement that may be difficult for the typical medical school faculty member to sustain. For this reason, faculty development programmes in educational scholarship require a commitment of institutional resources, protected time for faculty participants, and the involvement of doctoral-level trained educational researchers, especially when a formal degree is provided, to ensure an appropriate level of quality (Pugsley et al, 2008).

Interventions designed to meet the needs of individual teachers range from short workshops to intensive, longitudinal courses or even degree programmes. In the BEME review of teaching skill programme outcomes referred to earlier, the authors identified 53 articles from 1980 to 2002 that met their inclusion criteria (Steinert et al, 2006). The majority of these studies evaluated participants' satisfaction; a smaller number included evidence of change in knowledge or behaviour. Only three studies provided evidence of change in students or residents being taught by participants. Effective programmes were characterised by the following:

- Opportunities to practice new teaching skills
- Feedback, both on its own, and in association with practice
- A collegial atmosphere with opportunities for peer learning
- Application of educational principles in programme design and delivery
- A mixture of learning modalities

More recent studies provide examples of the types of well-designed evaluation studies called for in the BEME review, while including a greater focus on learner outcomes (Gozu et al, 2008; Notzer and Abramowitz, 2008; Branch et al, 2009).

A reward system that values excellence in education

Building organisational structures to support education and providing a range of faculty development programmes related to teacher needs are insufficient to sustain the educational mission of a medical school. The organisational vitality of any school depends on the system of recognition and rewards provided in support of its educational mission (Bland et al, 2002). A vibrant learning organisation values inquiry, innovation, scholarly teaching, and educational scholarship. It promotes and rewards continuous quality improvement and empowers individuals by providing visible credit for their accomplishments as teachers. Essential policies and procedures needed to support the educational mission include a clear statement by leadership that quality teaching is required and funded, a visible programme for reporting and evaluating teaching for promotion, a variety of awards for excellence in multiple aspects of teaching, recognition of the value of scholarship related to teaching, and a budget structure that encourages, rather than discourages, educational innovation.

As an interesting exercise, examine the mission statement of any medical school or academic medical centre. Does the word 'education' appear in the statement? The University of Pittsburgh School of Medicine, USA, offers a view of a clear statement of the importance of education in the institution. Its mission is simply stated: 'A different kind of medical school. A different kind of medicine'. The web page of the School of Medicine opens with a description of that difference. The Dean's State of the School Address linked from that page reinforces this institutional vision by opening with an update on medical student education and a description of several innovations, including a new requirement for a scholarly project, the initiation of mini-electives for first- and second-year students, and the growth of an Academy of Master Educators.

A clear role for evidence of teaching quantity and quality as part of promotion provides another indicator of an institution's commitment to its educational mission. The recommendations of a consensus conference hosted by the Association of American Medical Colleges' (AAMC) Group on Educational Affairs (Simpson et al, 2007) distinguished between effective teaching, scholarly teaching, and educational scholarship. All three are important to the educational mission but the latter two constitute evidence of quality beyond learner evaluations. Scholarly teaching is based on educational theory and best practices and requires an awareness of changing evidence about what works to maximise learning. Classroom and clinical teaching, advising and mentoring, and contributions to learner assessment should all be valued.

Evidence supporting the quality of scholarly teaching may include:

- 'Learners' confidential evaluations of instructors' teaching using standardised forms with open-ended comments ...
- Peer evaluation of teaching using a standardised format and process, ...
- A list of teaching awards and honours accompanied by descriptions of their selection process and criteria, ...
- Evidence of learning, including pre- and post-content, with an eye toward objectives, format, organisation, and innovation (p 11) (Simpson et al, 2007).

Educational scholarship is work done to contribute to the body of theory and practice in medical education that is publicly shared, open for others to build on, and peer-reviewed. Curriculum development and leadership of significant educational components are often included along with more traditional publications and presentations to the larger community of medical educators. Some medical schools have adopted Boyer's definition of scholarship (Boyer, 1990) and/or Rice's expanded version (Rice, 2005) to include the scholarship of teaching: *discovery* of new knowledge about learning, *application* of existing knowledge to new educational problems, *synthesis* of existing studies in teaching and learning, and *scholarly teaching* that demonstrates sound principles of education. Under this expanded definition, the production of instructional materials, textbooks and chapters, and innovative course designs are considered appropriate types of scholarship. The majority of North American medical schools have established separate promotion tracks for clinician educators to which this broader definition of scholarship has been applied. However, there remains a concern about equality in status for such tracks (Fleming et al, 2005).

Educational accomplishments can be documented in a teaching portfolio in which both quantity and evidence of quality are presented in tandem. In a survey of US medical schools in 2002 (Simpson et al, 2004), 64% reported using a teaching portfolio that included at least three of the following components:

- Personal statement, e.g. philosophy, goals
- Teaching activities – course, role
- Advising and mentoring activities
- Curriculum development products
- Honours/Awards related to teaching

- Teaching evaluations from students, residents, and/or peers
- Evidence of dissemination of educational innovations
- Faculty development activities
- Reports of learner outcomes

In addition to the use of a portfolio, institutional policies that clearly state a requirement for teaching, particularly medical student teaching, and expectations for the quality of that teaching are important in providing a clear message that education is a priority. Until the promotion committee or dean refuses to review a promotion dossier lacking evidence of teaching, or insists on improvements in teaching quality as a standard for promotion, stated policy related to a requirement for teaching may not be interpreted as serious.

Awards and honours for the wide variety of educational activities in which faculty members engage provide another means of rewarding the educational contributions of faculty. While teaching awards from students or residents (e.g. 'Lecturer of the year') are highly prized by faculty, it is important for the institution to recognise other types of educational contributions that go beyond outstanding teaching. Peer nominations can result in awards for curricular innovation, educational leadership, mentoring, or clinical performance assessment. Membership in the type of academy described earlier is another form of educational recognition by one's peers. A broad range of awards with many, rather than a few, being recognised can serve as an incentive for attracting and retaining faculty members in key educational roles within the department or across the institution. Such honours and awards can be enriched when the selection process is transparent and well documented.

A final ingredient in the organisation of a learning-oriented organisation is a clearly identified budget for education, often referred to as mission-based budgeting. The concept is a simple one: to align the institutional budget with its educational mission while stimulating quality improvement (Ridley et al, 2002; Watson and Romell, 1999). Issues to be addressed include decisions on the scope of funds to be included in the mission-based aspect of the institutional budget, alignment of funds and missions, metrics of allocation to account for quantity and quality, and tools for measuring both.

A vibrant medical education organisation requires attention to the organisational features in place to support that community. Faculty development can help create a collegial learning community that shares a vision for personal excellence, continuous learning, and scholarship in teaching; promotes continuous quality improvement through collaborative reflection and action; and makes the contributions of scholarly teachers and educational scholars visible and rewarded. Creating and sustaining organisational vitality requires the empowerment of both personal and corporate leadership to lobby for the very best educational programme delivered by scholarly teachers and informed by the work of educational scholarship to maximise the learning of those entrusted into our care.

Developing learners

One of the significant changes in medical education in the new millennium is a commitment to help learners improve their skills and potential in regards to the learning experience in medical school and residencies. In the past, ill-prepared learners were left to fail. Some schools admitted all applicants with an expectation that a significant number would fail out. The ethos instilled from day one of medical school was embodied in a common saying: 'Look to your left; look to your right; one of you will not be here at graduation.' Today, in countries with populations as large as that of the United States and small as that of Mozambique, the learners who are admitted represent a valuable asset of that country. Investing in their success academically and personally makes economic sense, given the cost and time required to train a physician. A failure to complete a medical education degree is expensive for the individual and the country since it reduces the number of physicians prepared to meet the needs of that country's citizens.

As increasingly heterogeneous groups of learners enter the medical education pipeline, it becomes incumbent on medical schools and residencies to develop a vision of, and programmes for, academic success for everyone. In socioeconomically disadvantaged communities, few high school students may graduate prepared for the demands of medical school. During medical school, students may encounter personal and academic difficulties. Even some residents continue to struggle with the assessments required to maintain progress toward full licensure. The cost to society of any of these learners dropping out of the physician 'pipeline' is significantly higher than the cost of helping to develop their academic skills for success.

Establishing a learner development programme

Accreditation standards for medical schools in the United States (www.lcme.org/standard.htm) and the United Kingdom (GMC, 2009), as well as the quality improvement standards of the World Federation for Medical Education (WFME, 2003), include a requirement for academic support or retention programmes, along with personal counselling, for medical students. Medical students and residents themselves recognise the need for learning skills development. One of the authors (Lawrence Doyle) has worked as a learning skills specialist for 30 years with learners from high school through to medical residencies. When he has visited medical schools in other countries, students have approached him to discuss study and test-taking skills relevant to their particular curriculum. At Universidad Eduardo Mondelane in Maputo, Mozambique, for example, first-year medical students arranged a late Friday afternoon session, identifying a student to translate, and then working together to learn from a presenter who did not speak their language. At Esculela de Latino Medicina in Havana, students from many different countries were eager to talk about study skills, particularly those for whom Spanish was a second language. At the National University of Singapore, medical students, on viewing a poster about study skills as the 'missing element' in a medical school curriculum, stopped for a quick discussion with the author about the types and levels of skills appropriate for medical students and subsequently recruited their colleagues to continue the discussion later in the day.

In designing programmes to develop medical students and residents as learners, a series of issues need to be addressed:

1. Who should be the target of programme activities?
2. What knowledge, skills, and attitudes do the targeted learners need to succeed academically and personally?
3. How can the programme be best integrated with existing curricular and clinical requirements?
4. What types of activities and services should be included?

The first question in planning a learning development programme concerns the target audience. Should the focus be on learners in academic difficulty, all learners, or some balance of the two? This is a good question best answered by the fact that since even elite athletes use a coach, it seems important to extend learning skills activities to all learners, especially for those skills required for lifelong learning as a physician.

A needs assessment will provide guidance in setting programmatic goals and designing services. Existing learners, recent graduates, faculty members, professional educators, staff in a student affairs office, and community practitioners can reflect on the challenges that they have faced as learners in the classroom and clinical setting to provide a broad perspective for planning (Uijtdehaage et al, 2007b). Once a programme is implemented, the needs assessment results can be used as a measure of programme effectiveness and a guide for continuous improvement (Uijtdehaage et al, 2007a).

The next decision in building a learning development programme is whether learning skills should be taught in a separate course, embedded across the curriculum, or only addressed through individual counselling. Although there is little evidence to support one approach over the other, it is clear that learning skills must be explicitly addressed rather than just implicitly modelled if all learners are expected to develop them (Perkins, 2009). If embedded in an existing course or clinical attachment, students or residents will need to receive feedback on their successful demonstration of learning habits, suggesting that faculty development and learner development actually go hand in hand.

It is important for a learner development programme to provide a number of services. Several of these could be linked to other units within the institution: for example, offices of student affairs or medical education. Attachment to offices of medical education may, in fact, strengthen learner development activities by tying them more closely to academic components of the institution. The following services are those most commonly provided.

Individual learning skills counselling

Individual counselling may include discussion of particulars related to learner performance, time management practices, sleep schedules, or moving from a surface learning approach to one more conducive to deeper understanding. It may also include individual assessments related to study skills, reading level, problem-solving skills, or referrals to other professionals for psychiatric problems or learning differences/disabilities. An individualised learning contract is a useful device for structuring activities and identifying the particular goals for each learner.

Workshops

Group sessions on particular learning skills or strategies can help to communicate the importance of personal and academic development to all learners. Topics such as analysing examination performance, scheduling study time, and preparing for licensing exams prove quite popular, particularly when the sessions provide an opportunity to practice newly learnt skills with feedback from peers and faculty. Additional learners, beyond those in academic difficulty, will often attend such workshops to gain insights or 'secrets', helping to destigmatise the development programme as being applicable only to those in academic difficulty.

Peer-tutoring

Peer-tutoring provides an opportunity for learners to learn from more advanced learners who have already successfully completed particular courses, mastered clinical skills, and/or demonstrated effective study strategies. The training of peer-tutors is important in that the simple mastery of the material is necessary, but not sufficient for a tutor. In addition, some screening and selection is required, as not all students will be suited to the role of peer-tutor. It is also important that the peer-tutors learn to serve as facilitators of learning rather than merely re-lecturing the targeted content. Helping peer-tutors learn about open-ended questioning, reflective listening, and modelling of learning behaviours can enhance their effectiveness.

One form of peer-tutoring, supplemental instruction (SI), integrates lessons on memorisation, problem solving, time management, and concept mapping into content review sessions for a targeted course (Hurley et al, 2003). A Medical Scholars Programme is another peer-tutoring model based on the work of Triesman (Osborn and Fullilove, 1993; Triesman, 1993). Peer-tutors meet weekly for 2 hours with groups of 20–25 learners to collectively answer questions in anatomy, biochemistry, and physiology framed in such a way as to relate basic science to clinical conditions. Studies have shown that medical students enrolled in such programmes perform better on subsequent basic science tests and licensing examinations than might be predicted by their admissions data.

Personalised assessment

Individual assessments of learning skills can be helpful for learners at all levels, but basic skills inventories such as the following, which are well studied in the literature, are particularly useful in the context of medical education:

- Learning and Study Skills Inventory (www. hhpublishing.com/_assessments/LASSI/)
- Approaches to Learning and Studying Inventory (Mattick et al, 2004)
- Approaches and Study Skills Inventory for Students (ASSIST) from Enhancing Teaching and Learning Environments, University of Edinburgh (www.etl.tla.ed.ac.uk/questionnaires/ASSIST. pdf)
- Nelson–Denny Reading Test (www.riverpub. com/products/ndrt/index.html)
- Cognitive Behaviour Survey (Mitchell, 1994; Mitchell et al, 2009)
- Whimbey Analytical Skills Inventory (Whimbey and Lochhead, 1999)

One of the authors (Lawrence Doyle) has used these instruments to provide individual learners from pre-medical students, through to residents with a personalised assessment of their readiness for the challenges of continuous and self-directed learning. Such assessments, and discussions of a particular learner's performance, can illustrate for the individual whether the mix of study and test-taking habits adopted over years of previous success as a learner are helping or hindering performance in the current setting. Repeated studies have shown that surface learning is the least successful strategy for medical students. Most medical students adopt a strategic approach in which they shift their study skills, from memorising to working for a deeper understanding, based on the nature of the examinations they are preparing to take.

Practice tests and formative assessments

Accurate assessment of one's knowledge and skills is an essential aspect of lifelong learning (Davis et al, 2006). Skills in self-monitoring and self-assessment can be promoted through the use of practice tests and formative assessments coupled with reflection and feedback. For example, weekly formative assessments are part of the medical student curriculum at UCLA with the goal of promoting students' accurate assessment of their level of understanding on factual recall, application, and interpretation questions related to content of the previous week or assigned readings (Krasne et al, 2006). The results of formative assessments or practice tests of any type can

assist faculty, academic support professionals, or peer-tutors, as they guide students in reflecting on current personal results by asking them to identify their depth of understanding, specific knowledge gaps, and projected levels of performance. Faculty feedback on student insight and accuracy is an important aspect of this reflective process (see also Chapter 13).

Well-being counselling and referrals for fitness appraisal

Accreditation standards for medical schools often include the need for personal support systems to assist students in productively managing the physical and emotional demands of medical school. These are not necessarily psychiatric services, although the assessment of learning disabilities may be important to provide. Instead, a well-being programme can teach successful coping mechanisms by linking learners with more advanced learners and faculty members who have successfully navigated similar experiences, by providing a comfortable place for informal learner gatherings, and by offering a friendly listener when learners just need to talk. Formal support groups can be created to address topics such as family issues, professional identity, career choice, death and dying, body image, substance abuse, gender roles, and cultural differences. Learning support professionals can provide referrals to other professionals for in-depth assessment of learning disabilities such as dyslexia or attention-deficit/hyperactivity disorder (ADHD), or for psychological or pastoral counselling for issues such as the 'imposter phenomenon' in which students come to view their acceptance to or continuance in medical school as a sham that will soon be dispelled (Clance and Imes, 1978).

Evaluation and curriculum development

Curricular evaluation and development responsibilities are not typically embedded in a student affairs office, but located in other parts of the institution. However, access to such resources can significantly affect success of a student development programme. Assistance in designing, conducting, and analysing needs assessment surveys and programme evaluation studies can be extremely valuable in developing, improving, or sustaining a learning support programme. Summative evaluations of a particular iteration of programming can identify features associated with programmatic success. Well-developed formative assessments can be used for continuous quality improvement.

Establishing a culture of learning

Learning to learn is a critical skill that must be deliberately practised if it is to develop. Thus, programmes for learner development should be integrated with the curriculum planning and evaluation processes for the institution. A culture of learning needs to permeate the curriculum, and the entire institution, if students and postgraduate trainees are to value the development of their skills as learners.

Structured with this goal in mind, the format of classroom sessions and clinical rotations can provide learners with opportunities to engage in guided self-assessment, to set their own learning goals, and to access the resources needed to direct their own learning. For example, in PBL, learners learn to draw on their prior knowledge, ask questions about issues raised in a problem that they do not personally understand, and educate themselves and one another through subsequent self-study. The problems create a level of 'desirable difficulty' where challenge motivates without overwhelming (Bjork, 1994). Team-based learning (Searle et al, 2003) reinforces the value of self-quizzing and peer teaching. Being assigned the responsibility to care for a patient in a clinical placement can stimulate the learner to search out and critically appraise the current evidence on treatment options. These skills need to be made a part of the assessment of learner performance as well, if the message about their importance is to be clearly communicated to students or residents.

Faculty development is critical to the success of a learning culture so that the intended curriculum is implemented in a way that reinforces learning skills and engages learners in using the type of study habits described above. John Hattie, New Zealand author of *Visible Learning* (Hattie, 2009), in a published interview, described the effects of what teachers do on learning outcomes based on his review of meta-analyses relating teaching to achievement (Shaughnessy and Moore, 2008):

> What teachers do matters; and what certain teachers do matters in a most positive manner. The most powerful influences on students come from those who know their subject matter and who are trained in the proficiencies of 'teaching in a most deliberate and visible manner' with a particular emphasis on teaching learning strategies in the context of the subject being taught. Strategic thinking and the skills needed to deal with the challenge of the unfamiliar are the keys to teaching and learning.
>
> (p 240)

Creating a viable learning community outside class is also important in developing a learning culture. In teaching calculus to college students, Triesman and his colleagues (Triesman, 1993) observed strong social influences on the academic performance of different groups of students, largely along ethnic and racial lines. In seeking an explanation, Triesman considered differences in performance motivation, prior education, family support, and socio-economic status, but none of these variables seemed to matter. He then designed a case study to interview and videotape the students as they studied the material outside class. What he found was that the social interactions and focus of the two groups were extremely different. The college students who did poorly tended to study alone, did not take advantage of other students or faculty as resources, and tended to separate the educational and social parts of their lives. The students who were successful did study alone at times, but a regular part of their study was an interaction with other students in which they talked about education and their future careers, critiqued each others' problem solving and use of language, practised on old tests, and sought the support of acquaintances or older siblings who had completed the coursework. The underperforming group did not use any of these strategies. However, when the underperforming group of students was taught to work together, and to interact about their education and future careers, their academic performance improved. The learning community programme was so successful that it continues to be replicated, successfully, at colleges, universities, and medical schools around the world (Osborn and Fullilove, 1993).

Barriers to implementation

Few learning skills counsellors are available, particularly at the medical school level where skills counselling might include work on advanced science materials, preparation for licensing examinations, study strategies for mastering an ever-expanding body of scientific knowledge, and skills for succeeding in the unstructured learning environment during clinical rotations. Few courses of study exist for the development of learning skills counsellors who are familiar with the special demands of medical education. Although graduate courses in education and psychology are numerous, most focus on younger learners, rather than adults, or on research rather than application. Some medical schools have drawn on the expertise of professional medical educators with expertise in cognition and learning. Alternatively, faculty members from the basic or clinical sciences with experiences in the various learning environments in medical education can develop the skills and knowledge relevant to providing learner development services through a review of the relevant literature on learning, both in general and in medicine, and discussions with established medical education learning skills professionals at other institutions. The fellowships in medical education discussed earlier in this chapter could be helpful to a basic science or clinical teacher interested in making this transition to learning specialist.

Learning to learn strategies

A review of research on learning conducted by a panel of experts for the US National Academies of Science from a variety of fields, from neuroscience to education, identified three key principles in successful learning, presented in the report *How People Learn* (Council, 2000). They bear a striking resemblance to the cognitive principles of learning, described in Chapter 2:

- Pre-existing knowledge is the basis of new understanding.
- Deep understanding involves developing a conceptual framework that can enhance memory and facilitate transfer to new situations.
- Active engagement in learning requires making continual decisions about what and how to learn and monitoring one's own thinking.

The goal of learner development programmes is to help learners of any age understand the process of learning and develop the attitudes, knowledge, and skills needed to maximise that process. Topics generally include strategies for reading, note-taking, memorisation, deep understanding, test-taking, time management, physical readiness, self-quizzing, and behaviour modification. The following suggestions have been particularly valuable over the years for medical students and residents with whom we have worked.

Reading

The simple act of reading daily for periods of an hour or more can increase one's reading comprehension and enlarge vocabulary. Initially skimming over material prior to a closer reading and, some time later,

employing a post-reading process can help learners develop a deeper understanding of the material studied as well as a better overall memory of factual detail through purposeful repetition. Active self-questioning during reading, in which learners, after a page or two, ask themselves what are the key concepts here, how do they relate to things they already know, and how might the concepts apply to a real-life situation, can strengthen both retention and comprehension. Reciprocal reading, developed by Ann Brown and Anne Marie Sullivan Palinscar for use with school-age children, engages two students in questioning, summarising, clarifying, and predicting by alternating 'teacher' and 'learner' roles using a text that both have read. These active reading strategies are not often used by less well-prepared learners, who tend to simply re-read the text, with the second reading simply being done more quickly. Given the amount of reading expected in medical school, students need to be able to read for understanding the first time round, and to increase their reading speed without the loss of comprehension. Active reading strategies can reduce the time spent on re-reading and move the learner beyond 'rote' memorisation to the development of a deeper conceptual framework into which subsequent facts can be integrated.

Note-taking

The major point in any discussion of note-taking strategies with learners is the importance of active engagement throughout a lecture or reading session. With the advent of Podcasts and easy access to digital files of lecture slides, learners no longer have to attempt to write down every word in a lecture. Instead, they can engage in constant decision-making about the relative importance of concepts and details that can then be reflected in their written notes taken as they listen. For example, learners should determine the importance of a concept delivered by the lecturer and vary their note-taking format to reflect relative importance by varying indentation from the left margin or marking with differently coloured pens. These strategies keep learners involved while providing an organisation to their notes that is useful for subsequent review. Since more than half the information in a lecture is forgotten within the next 24 hours, one of the most important study skill activities is simply to review materials the same day they were presented rather than waiting until the weekend. Lecture notes, like other texts, can be approached with the same active reading strategies discussed above.

Lectures that are recorded and archived or broadcast as Podcasts have the advantage of linking the words of the lecture to the slide being shown at that point in the lecture. Rather than simply listening to the entire lecture again, the learner can decide what portion of a lecture he or she needs to review and jump immediately to that linked slide and presentation.

Memory

Mnemonics for learning medicine have been passed down from generation to generation of medical students, such as OLDCART or SOCRATES for assessment of pain (i.e. Onset–Location–Duration–Characteristics–Aggravating Factors–Relief–Treatment – or – Signs and symptoms–Onset–Character–Radiation–Alleviating Factors–Timing–Exacerbating Factors–Severity), ROYGBIV (Red–Orange–Yellow–Green–Blue–Indigo–Violet for the colours of the visible portion of the electromagnetic spectrum or of the rainbow), and OILRIG (Oxidation Is a Loss of electrons while Reduction Is a Gain of electrons) from general chemistry. A certain amount of sheer memory continues to be important in medicine. In the early stages of learning, the mnemonic provides scaffolding for disparate ideas that do not yet make 'logical sense' or for linking the unfamiliar with something familiar. While such mnemonics lose their power as understanding deepens, they can remain important in areas where use of that understanding is called upon infrequently. A mnemonic later provides a safety net checklist so that essential aspects of the concept or procedure are not inadvertently forgotten due to infrequent use. Useful mnemonics can be visual or verbal, original or inherited, graphic or textual. The only criterion is that they must be compelling enough to be remembered by the user (Whimbey and Lochhead, 1999)!

Test-taking

A critical tool in improving test-taking skill is error analysis from actual or practice examinations. *Problem Solving & Comprehension*, 6th Edition (Whimbey and Lochhead, 1999) provides an excellent practice test for identifying and analysing non-content-related errors, such as misreading, making unsupported inferences, failing to consider all of the options, not following through on ones' own logic, or frequently changing answers. An error analysis of actual examination questions allows for identification of content-related errors as well. Content errors might be due to learners mistakenly failing to cover the material at all during study or purposefully ignoring some material judged to be unimportant. A second type of content error occurs when the learner is not able to apply known material to a new situation. This could be a problem with transfer, not seeing the similarity between the test item and the learnt material, or it could be a problem of having memorised the material rather than using active reading methods to reach a deeper understanding. Content mistakes can be reduced by learners applying active reading and note-taking strategies. Anxiety can be a third cause of examination difficulties. Under stress, learners may not read the questions carefully, block on answers that they would otherwise know under non-test conditions, have difficulty in apportioning their time, or engage in second-guessing themselves. Test anxiety may require psychological counselling if it persists after the problem has been identified and the learner has worked on addressing it. Finally, some persistent difficulties may be the result of actual learning disabilities that require formal assessment. If clinically identifiable learning disabilities are found, the learner may require modified testing conditions such as extended time or isolation to avoid distractions.

Time management

The amount of material to be learnt or clinical work to be accomplished in a typical medical school curriculum may require new time management skills for students, especially when entering a new phase of responsibility. Students can be encouraged to create a personal schedule of appointments, classes, and study times and construct an active to-do list. A schedule helps the student break a task down into manageable portions that can be accomplished within a particular day or study session, thereby making the entire task easier to complete. To-do lists can help the student to make appropriate decisions for a given bit of free time. With the extensive scheduling and notes programmes available on smart phones and other handheld devises, these personal planning activities are easier to implement than ever before and have the added benefit of ever-present message alert systems.

Deliberate practice

Drawing on decades of work on expertise in fields as diverse as chess and music, Ericsson and his colleagues (Ericsson, 2004; Ericsson et al, 1993) have identified the characteristics of deliberate practice associated with reproducible skilled performance. Such practice is distinguished from mere experience by four features: (1) a targeted goal, (2) a motivation to improve, (3) frequent feedback, and (4) opportunities for repetition with increasing levels of challenge. Deliberate practice can be helpful as learners seek to develop new learning skills or master new concepts or clinical skills. Learners can be taught how to structure their study periods to include practice tests with items selected to demonstrate accomplishment of a clearly defined, relatively narrow goal. Feedback needs to be available from a coach, although studies continue to refine what type of feedback is most helpful. Mastery requires a study schedule that includes returning to one's learning goal from time to time with new contexts or examples embedded in subsequent practice tests. The role of the learning skills specialist is to assist the learner in setting a manageable goal, given the time and resources available, securing mechanisms for feedback, and developing a study plan that includes spaced practice and re-testing.

Peak performance skills

Academic performance can be greatly affected by a person's psychological readiness. This is a regular part of athletic training but less commonly applied to improving academic performance. Strategies from the fields of Sports Psychology or Peak Performance (Jarvis, 2000) can help learners maximise their psychological readiness for academic tasks such as studying, attending lectures, taking examinations, or even managing difficult interactions with colleagues, faculty, or patients.

Psychological readiness means that the level of stress associated with performance is experienced as challenging but not overwhelming. The Yerkes–Dodson curve shown in Figure 19.1 (Jarvis, 2000) shows that one's performance is often related to the level of underlying stress produced by the event or resulting from unrelated life situations. Performance actually rises to a peak with increasing stress before dropping off as the stress reaches overwhelming levels. Learners need to understand the difference between good stress and bad stress, between productive challenges and debilitating anxiety. They need to recognise the onset of negative stressors and use relaxation exercises to lower stress levels. Relaxation exercises provide one means of managing stress so that the learner avoids or delays a negative level of stress.

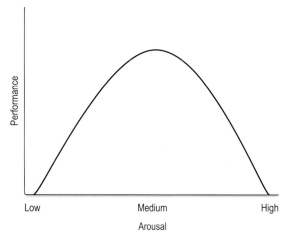

Figure 19.1 • The Yerkes–Dodson curve.

Controlled breathing is one form of relaxation exercise. Taking slow deep breaths tends to increase the oxygen content of the blood, increase blood flow to the brain, and loosen and expand chest muscles. Breathing practice begins by simply filling and emptying ones lungs to a slow, consistent count of four. Repeating this slow cycle has a calming effect that is brought on more readily with regular practice. Adding a four-count hold between inhaling and exhaling tends to help focus on the breath rather than the coming performance. A second relaxation strategy involves releasing muscle tension by first tensing a group of muscles, holding it tense, and then relaxing it. Progressive relaxation involves repeating the strategy on sequential muscle groups over the entire body. If the count of the cycle is extended until the muscle group tires, this exercise can help learners fall sleep more effectively after a period of intense concentration. With enough practice, the relaxation response can become an almost automatic response to situations that the participant finds stressful.

Psychological readiness may also mean that the person is primed for an upcoming action. The process of visualisation is a powerful tool for priming. It may also have some of the same practice effects as actually performing that same action. Research on a special type of neuron in the brain, the mirror neuron, suggests that when a person observes or visualises an action, the neural pathway that is activated in his or her brain is similar to that used during actual performance of that action (Gallese et al, 2004). For example, an Olympic athlete getting ready to compete in an event would find it quite natural to envision him or herself completing the course, making the ski jump, swimming the required laps. For students or residents preparing to take an examination, such visualisation can involve imagining the types of questions that they will be able to answer after studying specific content or what a positive performance on a patient encounter to be observed by a faculty member will look like. The more vivid and multi-sensorial the image becomes, the more effective it can be in priming the learner for a particular performance.

A third area of psychological readiness requires developing self-confidence. Athletes turn to self-talk to build confidence and increase persistence while preparing for challenging performances. When learners constantly tell themselves that they have difficulty on standardised tests or cannot perform well in mathematics, they may produce a self-fulfilling prophecy (Aronson and Steele, 2005). Without self-confidence, learners may fail to persist in the face of difficulty, lose confidence in what they know during an examination, or even decide not to pursue medicine after experiencing one failure. Self-talk can be supplemented by positive messages from faculty members and counsellors about high expectations for success.

Even concentration can be practised. Focussing visually on a particular object, a candle for instance, and practicing staying focussed on that object for expanded periods of time can help one learn how to narrow focus. In the same concentration exercise, by attempting to widen and narrow the visual field, the learner can experience the ability to control concentration. Similar strategies in terms of focusing on one's hearing, or other sensory input, then expanding and narrowing awareness of that stimulus, can help the learner to later control the distractions that are so much a part of modern life.

Psychological readiness includes physical readiness as well, e.g. nutrition, sleep, exercise, and caffeine. The timing and content of meals are as important to learners as to athletes. Complex carbohydrates, protein, and limited amounts of fat can all affect a learner's ability to pay attention during a long day of classroom or clinical work. Eating a suitable breakfast has been associated with improvements in academic performance. Caffeine, which can be helpful to learning in small doses, has been shown, in larger doses, to limit a learner's ability to assimilate new information or to make new associations with previously learnt information. Ingestion of refined

sugars can lead to a drop in blood sugar, which may hinder concentration.

Sleep is a central issue for discussion with learners as well. Humans tend to need 8 hours of sleep. Recent studies suggest that 90-minute REM cycles provide time for consolidating information and that missing a cycle can inhibit recall (Axmacher et al, 2009). Students may believe that the way to master the enormous amount of material in a medical school curriculum is to study long into the night, day after day. Sleep deprivation is a common complaint among post-graduate trainees and at the heart of policies designed to control the pattern and amount of work permitted for residents. In addition to concerns about patient safety, this lack of sleep may actually decrease learning effectiveness. While recommendation from an instructor or learning skills specialist that more sleep might be appropriate is oftentimes met with disbelief, after such a simple modification of behaviour, performance generally improves. Exercise, stretching, and cardiovascular activities can help the learner to stay healthy and provide a counterpoint to the intense concentration involved in studying.

A learner who understands these simple exercises for psychological readiness will learn that responses to stress, time management, concentration, and persistence are under his or her personal control and not dictated by life or academic situations. Combined with healthy lifestyle habits that promote physical readiness for learning, the learner is ready for peak performance. A learning skills counsellor can address these strategies in individual coaching sessions or workshops when particularly challenging academic activities are upcoming or completed.

Action–reflection–action cycle

Learning from immersion in clinical care responsibilities can be maximised, for students and residents, if the learner is taught to use an action–reflection–action approach to generate useful, personal knowledge (Boshuizen, 2004). Students often see clinical work as unplanned and spontaneous. However, as even the most urgent situation can benefit from planned action, the first critical skill is creating a prepared mind. Gut intuition is insufficient unless that intuition is informed by extensive knowledge and experience. However, learners with little actual experience in caring for a patient with a given complaint can prepare for the patient encounter by learning to visualise the rhythm and routine (the algorithm) of the presenting complaint, and subsequently predicting the desirable consequences. Preparation, when time permits, can also include background reading or asking questions of experienced peers or teachers. Such preparation helps the learner to create an interpretive frame within which effective, rapid decision-making can occur. A second critical skill, often missed in the process, is reflective analysis, raising questions such as whether the desired outcome was achieved. And if not, why not? Or if so, why so? Such reflection can be either an individual or a team activity. In order to use this newly generated knowledge successfully in subsequent patient care situations, the learner then must create conditional knowledge in the form of 'if-then' linkages between complex knowledge and desirable actions and outcomes, or at a more advanced level, illness scripts. These more generalised knowledge structures avoid over-contextualisation of learning and assist in retrieval for subsequent application in new clinical situations.

Widening participation: preparing a pipeline to medicine

Beyond improving the learning skills and performance of current medical students or residents, an increasingly important reason to build learning development programmes is the emphasis on widening participation in the medical workforce. As Garlick and Brown (2008) note, in discussing the development of the Extended Medical Degree Programme in the United Kingdom:

> Today's prevailing view is that tomorrow's doctors should reflect the social and ethnic diversity of the countries in which they practise. To this end, initiatives to widen participation have been started in medical schools in several countries.
>
> (p 111)

Such an expanded focus can be seen worldwide, from a programme for Aboriginal Medical and Dental Health at the University of Western Australia to the new Northern Ontario School of Medicine in Canada, where faculty are working to increase the numbers of Aboriginal students enrolled. In the universities of Bergen and Tromsø in Norway, special admissions programmes have worked for over 40 years to increase the numbers of Sami people who matriculate in medical school. A new standard for medical school accreditation in the United States

requires that 'each medical school must develop programmes or partnerships aimed at broadening diversity among qualified applicants for medical school admission' (www.lcme.org/standard.htm). In the United States, having a diverse student body in medical school has been shown to be associated with a greater commitment on the part of graduating physicians to social justice and a readiness to care for patients unlike themselves (Saha et al, 2008). Studies in the USA have also shown that physicians from underserved populations are more likely to serve those populations, thus improving access to care (Saha and Shipman, 2008).

In reaching out to new student populations, medical schools will need to draw from groups that have not traditionally been competitive for, or even interested in, pursuing a career in medicine. A significant portion of such students come from disadvantaged educational and/or economic backgrounds and have academic records that are weak when compared with their demonstrated record of commitment to, and experience with, medically underserved communities. It is incumbent on medical schools to provide leadership to outreach and pipeline programmes that begin early in students' educational lives, to strengthen confidence, and build academic skills in order to create a competitive diverse applicant pool for medicine.

Pipeline programmes in the United States, in existence since the mid-1970s, have traditionally focused on high school and college students, often providing summer residential programmes on a university medical school campus so that participants have a chance to experience the medical school environment. Such programmes are typically six to eight weeks in duration and designed to provide participants with exposure to science and mathematics prerequisites for medical school. These programmes usually include some clinical experience or the opportunity to shadow a health care professional. The Robert Wood Johnson Foundation's Summer Medical and Dental Education Programme (SMDEP, www.smdep.org/) coordinated by the AAMC and the American Dental Education Association is for college students who are 2 years away from applying to medical school. While the majority of SMDEP programmes re-teach basic maths and science competencies, at UCLA the programme includes a large amount of learning skills development and curricular activities focused on practising those skills. Students learn the skills of asking questions about scientific and clinical phenomena, locating sources to answer those questions, and explaining what they have learnt to a peer in PBL tutorials. Working in other small groups led by medical students, who are often themselves from disadvantaged backgrounds, learners search the internet to learn about a common health disparity or the features of a community lacking access to health care. After collecting information to define the problem, learners explore what is currently being done to address the selected issue and recommend changes in health policy, the design of health care systems, community engagement, or even medical education to help resolve the problem. They collaborate as a group in creating a presentation on their recommendations for the faculty and other students enrolled in the programme. Learners also spend time in personal choice reading to work on speed and vocabulary. Participating learners have demonstrated a move from a surface to a deeper approach to learning, improved reading skills, higher scores on practice examinations on science materials, a broader range of problem solving strategies, and an increased commitment to pursuing a career in medicine or dentistry (Doyle, unpublished data).

Conclusion

Faculty members develop. Learners develop. The environment for teaching and learning continuously improves. That is the rhythm of a learning organisation. Resources committed to faculty and learner development should be seen as investments in

creating, sustaining, and enhancing the vitality of a medical school or academic health care institution, preparing these institutions to productively respond to the educational implications of the constantly changing demands of scientific discovery and the health care needs of our communities.

Implications for practice

A vibrant learning organisation requires attention being given to the policies and programmes in place in medical schools and other medical education institutions to support the educational mission. Faculty development can help create a collegial learning community that shares a vision for personal excellence, continuous learning, and scholarship in teaching; promotes continuous quality improvement through collaborative reflection and action; and makes the contributions of scholarly teachers and educational scholars visible and rewarded. Learner development can provide the personal and professional skills needed to maximise learning during the long educational process of developing medical expertise. Creating and sustaining organisational vitality requires the empowerment of both personal and corporate leadership to lobby for the very best educational programmes delivered by scholarly teachers and informed by the work of educational scholarship to maximise the learning of those entrusted into our care.

References

Albanese MA, Dottl S, Nowacek GA: Offices of research in medical education: accomplishments and added value contributions, *Teach Learn Med* 13:258–267, 2001.

Amin Z, Hoon Eng K, Gwee M, et al: Medical education in Southeast Asia: emerging issues, challenges and opportunities, *Med Educ* 39:829–832, 2005.

Aronson J, Steele C: Stereotypes and the fragility of academic competence, motivation and self concept. In Elliot A, Dweck C, editors: *Handbook of competence and motivation*, New York, 2005, The Guilford Press, pp 436–456.

Axmacher N, Draguhn A, Elger C, et al: Memory processes during sleep: beyond the standard consolidation

theory, *Cell Mol Life Sci* 66:2285–2297, 2009.

Benor DE, Mahler S: Teacher training and faculty development in medical education, *Isr J Med Sci* 23:976–982, 1987.

Bensinger L, Meah Y, Smith L: Resident as teacher: the Mount Sinai experience and a review of the literature, *Mt Sinai J Med* 72 (5):307–311, 2005.

Bjork RA: Memory and metamemory considerations in the training of human beings. In Metcalfe J, Shimamura AP, editors: *Metacognition: knowing about knowing*, Cambridge, MA, 1994, MIT Press, pp 185–205.

Bland CJ, Seaquist E, Pacala JT, et al: One school's strategy to assess

and improve the vitality of its faculty, *Acad Med* 77:368–376, 2002.

Bloom S: The medical school as a social organization: the sources of resistance to change, *Med Educ* 23:228–241, 1989.

Boelen C, Boyer MH: *A view of the world's medical schools: defining new roles*, Geneva, 2001, World Health Organisation.

Boshuizen HPA: Does practice make perfect? A slow and discontinuous process. In Boshuizen HPA, Bromme R, Gruber H, editors: *Professional learning: gaps and transitions on the way from novice to expert*, Dordrecht, 2004, Kluwer Academic Publishers.

Boyer EL: *Scholarship reconsidered: priorities of the professoriate*,

Princeton, NJ, 1990, Princeton University Press.

Branch WT, Frankel R, Gracey CF, et al: A good clinician and a caring person: longitudinal faculty development and the enhancement of the human dimensions of care, *Acad Med* 84:117–125, 2009.

Clance P, Imes S: The imposter phenomenon in high achieving women: dynamics and therapeutic intervention, *Psychother Theory Res Pract* 16:231–247, 1978.

Cohen JJ: *Revisiting the medical school education mission at a time of expansion*, New York, NY, 2009, Josiah Macy, Jr. Foundation.

Council NR: *How people learn: brain, mind, experience, and school: expanded edition*, Washington, DC, 2000, National Academies Press.

Davis DA, Mazmanian PE, Fordis M, et al: Accuracy of physician self-assessment compared with observed measures of competence: a systematic review, *JAMA* 296 (9):1094–1102, 2006.

Dewey CM, Friedland JA, Richards BF, et al: The emergence of academies of educational excellence: a survey of US medical schools, *Acad Med* 80 (4):358–365, 2005.

Ericsson KA: Deliberate practice and the acquisition and maintenance of expert performance in medicine and related domains, *Acad Med* 79(10 Suppl):S70–S81, 2004.

Ericsson KA, Krampe RTh, Tesch-Romer C: The role of deliberate practice in the acquisition of expert performance, *Psychol Rev* 100:363–406, 1993.

Fleming VM, Schindler N, Martin GJ, et al: Separate and equitable promotion tracks for clinician-educators, *JAMA* 294:1101–1104, 2005.

Gallese V, Keysers C, Rizzolati G: A unifying view of the basis of social cognition, *Trends Cogn Sci* 8 (9):396–403, 2004.

Garlick PB, Brown G: Widening participation in medicine, *Br Med J* 336:1111–1113, 2008.

GMC: *Tomorrow's doctors*, London, 2009, General Medical Council.

Gozu A, Windish DM, Knight AM, et al: Long term follow-up of a 10-month programme in curriculum development for medical educators: a

cohort study, *Med Educ* 42(7): 684–692, 2008.

Griffith CH, Georgesen JC, Wilson JE: Six-year documentation of the association between excellent clinical teaching and improved students' examination performances, *Acad Med* 75(10 Suppl):S62–S64, 2000.

Gruppen LD, Frohna AZ, Anderson RM, et al: Faculty development for educational leadership and scholarship, *Acad Med* 73:137–141, 2003.

Gruppen LD, Simpson D, Searle NS, et al: Educational fellowship programs: common themes and overarching issues, *Acad Med* 81:990–994, 2006.

Guilbert JJ: *Educational handbook for health personnel*, Geneva, 1981, World Health Organisation.

Hattie JAC: *Visible learning: a synthesis of eight hundred meta-analyses related to achievement*, New York, 2009, Routledge.

Huber M, Hutchings P: *The advancement of learning: building the teaching commons*, San Francisco, CA, 2005, Jossey-Bass.

Hurley KF, McKay DW, Scott TM, et al: The supplemental instruction project: peer-devised and delivered tutorials, *Med Teach* 25(4):404–407, 2003.

Irby D, Cooke M, Lowenstein D, et al: The academy movement: a structural approach to reinvigorating the educational mission, *Acad Med* 79:729–736, 2004.

Jarvis M: *Sport psychology*, London, 2000, Taylor & Francis.

Jason H, Westberg J: *Teachers and teaching in US medical schools*, Norwalk, CT, 1982, Appleton-Century-Crofts.

Krasne S, Wimmers PF, Relan A, et al: Differential effects of two types of formative assessment in predicting performance of first-year medical students, *Adv Health Sci Educ* 11:155–171, 2006.

Mattick K, Dennis I, Bligh J: Approaches to learning and studying in medical students: validation of a revised inventory and its relation to student characteristics and performance, *Med Educ* 38:535–543, 2004.

Mazmanian PE, Davis DA: Continuing medical education and the physician as a learner: guide to the evidence, *JAMA* 288(9):1057–1060, 2002.

Mitchell R: The development of the cognitive behavior survey to assess medical student learning, *Teach Learn Med* 7:233–240, 1994.

Mitchell R, Regan-Smith M, Fisher M, et al: A new measure of the cognitive, metacognitive, and experiential aspects of residents' learning, *Acad Med* 84:918–926, 2009.

Neher JO, Gordon KC, Meyer B, et al: A five-step 'microskills' model of clinical teaching, *J Am Board Fam Med* 5:419–424, 1992.

Norcini JJ, Burdick W, Morahan PS: The FAIMER Institute: creating international networks of medical educators, *Med Teach* 27:214–218, 2005.

Notzer N, Abramowitz R: Can brief workshops improve clinical instruction? *Med Educ* 42:152–156, 2008.

Osborn E, Fullilove M: *Lessons learned from FIPSE projects II*, San Francisco, 1993, University of California The Medical Scholars Program. Washington, DC, Office of Post Secondary Education.

Perkins DN: *Making learning whole: how seven principles of teaching can transform education*, San Francisco, CA, 2009, Jossey-Bass.

Pololi L, Knight SM, Dennis K, et al: Helping medical school faculty realize their dreams: an innovative, collaborative mentoring program, *Acad Med* 77(5):377–384, 2002.

Post RE, Quattlebaum RG, Benich JJ: Residents-as-teachers curricula: a critical review, *Acad Med* 84: 374–380, 2009.

Pugsley L, Brigley S, Allery L, et al: Counting quality because quality counts: differing standards in master's in medical education programmes, *Med Teach* 30:80–85, 2008.

Rice E: Scholarship reconsidered: history and context. In O'Meara K, Rice RE, editors: *Faculty priorities reconsidered: rewarding multiple forms of scholarship*, San Francisco, CA, 2005, Jossey-Bass, pp 17–31.

Ridley GT, Skochelak SE, Farrell PM: Mission aligned management and allocation: a successfully implemented model of mission-based budgeting, *Acad Med* 77:124–129, 2002.

Saha S, Shipman SA: Race-neutral versus race-conscious workforce policy to improve access to care, *Health Aff (Millwood)* 27:234–245, 2008.

Saha S, Guiton G, Wimmers PF, et al: Student body racial and ethnic composition and diversity-related outcomes in US medical schools, *JAMA* 300(10):1135–1145, 2008.

Searle NS, Haidet P, Kelly PA, et al: Team learning in medical education: initial experiences at ten institutions, *Acad Med* 78(10 Suppl):S55–S58, 2003.

Searle NS, Hatem CJ, Perkowski L, et al: Why invest in an educational fellowship program? *Acad Med* 81:936–940, 2006.

Senge P: *The fifth discipline: the art and practice of the learning organization,* New York, 1990, Doubleday.

Shaughnessy M, Moore T: A reflective conversation with John Hattie, *North Am J Psychol* 10:239–248, 2008.

Simpson D, Hafler JP, Brown D, et al: Documentation systems for educators eeking academic promotion in US medical schools, *Acad Med* 79:783–790, 2004.

Simpson D, Fincher RME, Hafler JP, et al: *Advancing educators and education: defining the components and evidence of educational scholarship,* Washington, DC, 2007, Association of American Medical Colleges.

Sorcinelli MD: *Creating the future of faculty development: learning from the past, understanding the present,* Bolton, MA, 2006, Anker Publishing.

Steinert Y, Mann K, Centeno A, et al: A systematic review of faculty development initiatives designed to improve teaching effectiveness in medical education: BEME Guide No. 8, *Med Teach* 28(6):497–526, 2006.

Triesman U: *Lessons learned from FIPSE projects II: University of California, Berkeley, CA, The Professional Development Program,* Washington, DC, 1993, Office of Postsecondary Education.

Uijtdehaage S, Vermillion M, et al: 'Reflective practice' as a tool for programme evolution, *Med Educ* 41:1094–1095, 2007a.

Uijtdehaage S, Vermillion M, et al: Starting a pipeline program for disadvantaged students: do faculty and students value the same objectives? *American Educational Research Association (AERA) Annual Meeting,* 2007b, Chicago, eScholarship Repository.

Walling A, Chinn KC: A web-based orientation for new faculty members, *Acad Med* 77:460, 2002.

Watson RT, Romell LJ: Mission-based budgeting: removing a graveyard, *Acad Med* 74:627–640, 1999.

WFME: *Basic medical education: WFME global standards for quality improvement,* Copenhagen, Denmark, 2003, World Federation for Medical Education.

Whimbey A, Lochhead J: *Problem solving & comprehension,* ed 6, Mahway, NJ, 1999, Lawrence Erlbaum Associates.

Wilkerson L, Irby DM: Strategies for improving teaching practices: a comprehensive approach to faculty development, *Acad Med* 73:387–396, 1998.

Wilkerson L, Anderson WA: Hilliard Jason, MD, EdD: a medical student turned educator, *Adv Health Sci Educ Theory Pract* 9(4):325–335, 2004.

Wimmers PF, Schmidt HG, Splinter TA: Influence of clerkship experiences on clinical competence, *Med Educ* 40:450–458, 2006.

Further reading

Faculty development

Wilkerson L, Irby DM: Strategies for improving teaching practices: a comprehensive approach to faculty development, *Acad Med* 73:387–396, 1998.

Provides a framework for planning a faculty development programme.

Professional and Organisational Development Network: a faculty development organisation, largely focussed on classroom teaching in the university. Includes useful links and resources for faculty development programming [Online]. Available from http://www.podnetwork.org/. Accessed December, 2009.

November 2006 issue of Academic Medicine, *81 (11).*

This issue contains a series of articles on developing and evaluating longitudinal faculty development fellowships.

Student development

Quirk M: *How to learn and teach in medical schools: a learner centered approach,* Springfield, IL, 1996, Charles Thomas Publisher.

Provides a good overview of issues in the design and delivery of medical education. UT Learning Centre [Online]. Available from http://www.utexas.edu/student/utlc. Accessed December, 2009.

Provides an overview of the University of Texas Learning Center, a successful student development programme for university-level students. Includes handouts for student learning skills.

Whimbey A, Lochhead J: *Problem solving & comprehension,* ed 6, Mahway, NJ, 1999, Lawrence Erlbaum Associates.

Provides strategies useful for a student development programme, including an assessment tool for test-taking habits.

Glossary

Adult learning; see also andragogy
Describes a set of principles, originally described by Knowles in 1984, that differentiate how adult learners differ from children. They include the experience the adult has accumulated, motivation, and self-direction, and the interest in solving problems that are relevant to their everyday lives.

Andragogy; see also adult learning
An educational concept developed by Knowles, which asserts that education of adults needs to take account of their specific ways of learning, which differ from those of children. Child-orientated education is described by the more commonly used term 'pedagogy'.

Approaches to learning; see also deep learning and surface learning
These describe how students approach learning tasks. *Surface* and *deep* learning represent two different approaches. A surface approach is characterised by accepting new facts and ideas uncritically and attempting to store them as isolated, unconnected, items (rote learning). Deep learning is characterised by examining new facts and ideas critically, tying them into existing cognitive structures, and making numerous links between ideas.

Assessment The process of gathering and discussing information from multiple and diverse sources in order to develop a deep understanding of what students know and can do as the result of their educational experiences; the process culminates when assessment results are used to improve subsequent learning.

Assessment; formal That which occurs intentionally when someone comes to a view about someone's (possibly that person's own) learning, irrespective of what use (formative or summative) is to be made of that assessment.

Assessment; formative Assessment designed to help individuals develop by giving them information on their performance, usually in a non-judgemental and low-stakes environment (has no consequences in terms of the learner's progress). Often termed 'assessment for learning' or simply feedback.

Assessment; informal That which occurs naturally and often unrecognised when someone, somehow, comes to a view about someone's (possibly that person's own) learning, irrespective of what use (formative or summative) is to be made of that assessment.

Autonomy; see also conditional autonomy and principled autonomy The ability to live one's own life, according to one's own motives and reason.

Behaviourism Focuses on overt behaviour and the measurement of that behaviour. The assumptions of behavioural theorists about the nature of learning focus on the role of an individual's environment in both stimulating and shaping behaviour. What happens within individuals is of less interest as it is unobservable. From a behaviourist perspective, learning equates to changes in behavioural responses to environmental stimuli. Behaviourism is based on a causal and mechanistic model of human learning.

Codified knowledge Academic knowledge in the form of textbooks, protocols, records, manuals, etc.

Cognitive dissonance
A psychological concept developed by Festinger, which describes a state of inconsistency or disequilibrium when an individual perceives a situation, experience, or thought that is incompatible with their existing cognitive structures. The existence of cognitive dissonance motivates individuals to seek equilibrium by either avoiding a situation that caused it or, more positively, by seeking to understand the nature of the conflict and achieving resolution. Cognitive dissonance is an important concept in Constructivist and Experiential Learning theories.

Cognitive load A body of theory in cognitive psychology, which considers designs for learning as having three aspects: intrinsic (what is to be learnt); germane (how it is to be learnt); and extraneous (any other aspect not intrinsic or germane).

Cognitive scaffolding Teachers' use of structures to reduce their learners' cognitive load when acquiring subject matter.

Cognitivism Focuses on perception, memory, and meaning. The various cognitive perspectives share two important assumptions that: (a) the memory system is an active processor of information and (b) knowledge plays an important role in learning. Learning is seen as reorganising experience to increase meaning.

Competency The ability to handle a complex professional task by integrating the relevant cognitive, psychomotor, and affective skills.

Complexity theory This theory concerns the interactivity of elements in open systems, where the magnitude of effects cannot be predicted in a linear fashion from the magnitude of the elements relative to each other.

Constructivism A theory of knowledge (epistemology) whose philosophical roots can be traced back to Kant and whose psychological assumptions can be traced back to Piaget. It holds that the reality humans perceive is constructed by their social, historical, and individual contexts such that there can be no absolute shared truth. In an educational context, constructivism can be seen as a process whereby learners actively construct understandings based on their perceptions, previous experiences, and knowledge of the world. They assimilate new ideas and information by linking them to existing ideas and information. That is in contrast to a view of learning as having knowledge transmitted by a teacher. Constructivism is not a specific pedagogy, but today it underlies many approaches to learning. In small groups, those include ascertaining prior knowledge, challenging misconceptions, promoting active learning, and encouraging learners to take responsibility for their learning.

Consultant Registered and licensed specialist physician (UK).

Context The circumstances in which a task is undertaken; can be subdivided into a physical and a social context.

Contextualising learning Locating procedural skills training (or any other competence) in the context in which learners will eventually be expected to perform the skill. This is likely to include psychological, social, and physical representations of the working environment.

CoP (Community of practice) Cognitive anthropologists Jean Lave and Etienne Wenger used this term to describe a group of people who share an interest, a craft, and/or a profession. In Lave and Wenger's terms, members of a CoP are in pursuit of a shared enterprise. It is in the process of participating in that group that the members learn from each other and develop themselves personally and professionally. A CoP can be defined as an informal network that supports professional practitioners in their efforts to develop shared understandings and engage mutually in work-relevant knowledge building.

Curriculum (without a pronoun) That which underpins any learning and may be seen in the actions of teachers and learners *in situ*.

Curriculum in action The education actually being provided.

Curriculum, intended Curriculum on paper; the formal educational programme devised for an educational context.

Deep learning; see also approaches to learning A term first developed by Marton and Säljö, which refers to a learning strategy adopted by learners when they are able to interact with learning resources and teachers. In this environment, which is often a small group teaching session, learners attempt to understand material by questioning and challenging, and elaborate their understanding by application and problem solving.

Learners have an opportunity to see how their knowledge fits into an overarching framework and the bigger picture. The opposite of 'surface' learning.

Epistemology The theory or science of the method or grounds of knowledge.

Evaluation The process of assessing the strengths and weaknesses of educational programmes, policies, and organisations to improve their effectiveness. In North America, this also applies to the personnel, so learners may be 'evaluated' rather than 'assessed'. The information is often used to support quality improvement.

Experienced curriculum What students actually experience or learn at an educational site.

Experiential Learning Theory It derives from the work of David Kolb and builds on prior theories of Lewin, Piaget, Jung, and others. It asserts that learning is a process whereby knowledge is created through the transformation of experience. Raw experience is subjected to reflection, which constructs conceptual understanding and leads on to potential action. Experiential Learning Theory underpins professional development frameworks, the use of reflective portfolios, and the measurement of 'learning styles'.

Feedback Technically, it is the use of output from a process to modulate or modify the activity of the process. In educational terms, it is giving learners information about their performance to help them improve their knowledge, skills, or attitudes. Feedback is a fundamental component of formative assessment and assessment for learning.

Foundation Doctor or Foundation Trainee The Foundation Programme is a two-year postgraduate training programme designed to bridge the gap between medical school and specialty training; in the UK it is an important, formal part of the lifelong learning continuum.

GMC (General Medical Council)
Oversees the licensing of physicians in the UK. The purpose of the GMC "is to protect, promote, and maintain the health and safety of the public by ensuring proper standards in the practice of medicine."

Implicit learning The acquisition of knowledge independently of conscious attempts to learn and in the absence of explicit knowledge about what was learnt.

Informal education/learning
Learning that results from unplanned activities within an educational programme and/or daily life activities related to work, family, or leisure. It is not structured in terms of learning objectives or teaching. Informal learning may be intentional but in most cases it occurs incidentally.

Intern Historical name for a first-year postgraduate trainee in the US medical education system. An intern has an MD degree but not a license to practise unsupervised care. This term has been largely replaced with resident, with the year of training indicated by postgraduate year 1 (PGY1). The term is roughly equivalent with the European term 'foundation trainee'.

Learning A social, cognitive, and emotional process that is an integral and inseparable aspect of social practice.

Learning environment The material and social context wherein learners 'learn' (learning should be understood here as 'acquiring knowledge' as well as 'participating in practice'), which influences learners' behaviour, emotions, and practical competences.

Learning outcomes Statements defining what learners should be able to do at the end of a learning experience. They are often categorised into knowledge, skills, and attitudes and can be used to make a constructively aligned top-down curriculum.

Learning strategies These are the ways individual learners choose to achieve their goals. They may include using diagrams, taking notes, practicing skills, creating concept maps, and teaching each other.

Lifelong learning An ongoing process, through which individuals acquire the knowledge, skills, and values they will need through their life.

Maslow's hierarchy of needs A conceptual framework developed by Maslow which proposes that, in order to achieve optimal personal growth and learning ('self-actualisation'), layers of psychological and biological pre-conditions must be met. So, for example, basic physical and safety needs have to be fulfilled before one can go to 'higher-level' needs and eventually reach self-actualisation. It implies that physical surroundings matter and therefore has practical utility in ensuring that, for example, physical conditions for small group teaching and learning are adequate.

Medical (education) workplace
Any place where patients, learners, and practitioners come together for the conjoint purpose of providing/receiving medical care and learning.

Metacognition The process of thinking about how one thinks and learns. It is a reflective activity frequently used to encourage learners to identify the optimum conditions for their own learning. It can be initiated via a variety of psychometric tests, for example, Kolb's or Honey and Mumford. Refers to people's abilities to predict their performances on various tasks and monitor their current level of mastery and understanding.

Minute paper An exercise, which is often used at the end of educational sessions, to inform teachers whether students are achieving intended learning outcomes. Students are asked to reflect briefly and identify for the teacher and themselves where they are having difficulty, their major learning point(s) from the session, or a question that remains unanswered. It is useful for evaluation purposes.

Motivation; extrinsic Motivation to perform a behaviour arising from forces external to the behaviour itself such as persuasion or threats from others, material rewards, or internalisation of societal norms.

Motivation; intrinsic Motivation to perform a behaviour arising from its inherently satisfying nature.

PBL (Problem-based learning)
A small group teaching technique in which groups of learners and a facilitator engage with work-related problems and scenarios to identify their learning needs and objectives, followed by self-directed learning, and receiving feedback and arriving at conclusions within the group. It is widely used in medical education and education for other professions.

Pedagogy A body of theory and practice involved in educating young and/or junior individuals by their elders.

Portfolio A collection of information and artefacts pertaining to a learner and reflecting either 'all' or 'the best' of them for one or more educational purposes. There are very many approaches to portfolios and, as such, the specificity of the term is becoming increasingly ill-defined. A portfolio may be digital or paper-based and content may be prescribed or left to students' discretion. Despite variations in content and format, portfolios basically contain evidence about work done, feedback received, and progress made. Additionally, portfolios may stimulate reflection because collecting evidence for inclusion in a portfolio requires looking back and analysing what one has accomplished. Very often, written reflections and plans for improving competence are included.

Postgraduate trainee, see resident.

Practical theories of learning and teaching These are based on individuals' experiences, the combination of their formal and informal knowledge, and their values and beliefs. Practical theories strongly determine educational practice.

Practice Includes both clinical and non-clinical health-related work such as diagnosis, treatment, surveillance, health communications, management, and sanitation engineering.

Professionalism A concept associated with the education, training, attitudes, and ethical practices of a group of workers or practitioners. It includes a regulated educational and training system that has specific standards that are monitored and maintained. It has an ethical framework concerned with good working practices between practitioners and their clients. The work of Schön emphasises that professionalism is characterised by a variety of reflective practices that practitioners engage in to maintain their skills.

Quality improvement; see Total Quality Management An approach that is based on a manufacturing philosophy and set of methods for reducing time from customer order to product delivery, costing less, taking less space, and improving quality. Common forms of QI activities include Continuous Quality Improvement and Total Quality Management.

Reflection; reflective learning Letting future behaviour be guided by a systematic and critical analysis of past actions and their consequences or, as Eva and Regher describe it, "a conscious and deliberate reinvestment of mental energy aimed at exploring and elaborating one's understanding of the problem one has faced (or is facing) rather than aimed at simply trying to solve it." Reflective learning is the process of learning from experience through systematic reflection, returning to experience in order to re-evaluate it and glean learning that may affect one's predispositions and action in the future.

Registrar; see resident

Reliability The consistency and reproducibility of a measurement, or the degree to which an instrument, under the same condition with the same subjects, would produce an identical outcome. In the context of assessment, it is a measure of the ability of a test to differentiate reproducibly between test subjects. It is defined as the subject variability divided by the sum of subject variability and measurement error and lies between 0 and 1. Various forms include test–retest reliability and inter-rater reliability.

Resident (Registrar, post-graduate trainee); see also specialist trainee, intern, Foundation Doctor Medical school graduates undergo practice-based specialist training to be approved in their specific specialty. Resident is the common term in use in the US and, increasingly, internationally. Specialist trainee (formerly specialist registrar) is the term used in the UK. Both are post-graduate trainees.

Review; see also scoping review Literature reviews are collections of previously conducted research or evaluation studies. Reviews may be exploratory, narrative, critical, or systematic.

Scaffolding The introduction and subsequent removal of support and guidance to a learner proportionate to and in reaction to their developing mastery of a subject.

Schema building A cognitive model of understanding as a series of discrete clusters of interlinked knowledge. Learning is about adapting existing schemas and creating new ones.

Scoping review; see also review An exploratory type of review that aims to undertake a broad scope of a particular field before more extensive review work can be undertaken.

Self-actualisation A psychological concept, particularly associated with Maslow and Rogers, which asserts that all individuals wish to become the best person they can be by fulfilling all their potential; to 'become everything that one is capable of becoming'.

Self-directed learning Refers to an ongoing process through which individuals identify their learning needs, identify means to meet them, engage in relevant learning activities, and evaluate their progress and achievement in meeting their needs.

Self-efficacy From social cognitive theory, an individual's perception of their ability to perform a particular task to a desired level. Varies according to the situation and in the light of feedback from the social environment. An important influence on the goals that learners set and on their motivation to achieve.

Self-regulated learning Learners are involved in diagnosing their own learning needs, formulating goals, identifying resources, implementing appropriate strategies and activities, and self-assessing, and reflecting on both the process and outcomes of their learning. These skills are developed over time and supported by both teachers and resources in the learning environment. Self-regulated learning involves four phases: planning (identifying needs and articulating goals), learning (understanding expectations and identifying effective strategies), assessing (self-monitoring one's progress toward goals and synthesising with external feedback), and adjusting (reflecting on assessment and making necessary changes). Also involved are psychological attributes such as self-efficacy and motivation, personal choices in planning and effort, and judgements of the success of personal action.

Simulation Consensual pretence and illusion in support of training or assessment, typically through using some device, person, or environment. It should be more accurately termed 'dissimulation' as the intent is not to truly deceive.

Social cognitive theory; see also self-efficacy A theory of motivation, learning, and behaviour, which emphasises the reciprocal dynamic relationship between thoughts, actions, and society on behaviour. According to this theory, learning occurs through interaction with others and the environment. It emphasises the importance of cognition in mediating learning and function. It asserts that a significant amount of learning is associated with observing the behaviour of others in a process of vicarious experience. Self-efficacy is an important component of this theory. A major exponent is Albert Bandura.

Socio-cultural Current conceptualisations of socio-cultural theory draw heavily on the work of Vygotsky. A key feature of this emergent view of human development is that higher-order functions develop out of social interaction. Social relationships and culturally constructed artefacts – including language and tools – mediate learning and there is a two-way relationship between culture and individual learning. People learn meanings through activities that take place within individual, social, and institutional relationships.

SP (Simulated patient) An actor who is trained to portray a patient in a clinical simulation and to provide feedback to a learner.

Specialist trainee In the UK medical education system, it refers specifically to a practitioner being trained for a specialty who has completed two years as a 'Foundation Doctor'.

Student centred An educational concept that emphasises that learning should start from the needs and requirements of learners and that teachers should act more as facilitators of learning.

Summative assessment Coming to a view of someone's learning for the purpose of regulating the progression of that person and/or for some form of certification.

Surface learning; see also deep learning A concept, first developed by Marton and Säljö, which refers to a learning strategy adopted by learners when confronted by large quantities of information taught in passive and largely didactic learning environments. In such environments, learners adopt a minimalist approach, rote learn factual information, and focus on specific exam requirements at the expense of overarching understanding and the bigger picture. The opposite of 'deep learning'.

Syllabus The content of a curriculum.

Tacit knowledge Knowledge (factual or procedural) that is learnt and/or applied almost unconsciously.

Tacit learning; see also implicit learning The acquisition of knowledge independently of conscious attempts to learn, and without knowing exactly what has been learnt.

Teacher-centred An educational concept that emphasises that learning should be initiated by the prescriptions of teachers who decide what will be taught and by what methods.

Total Quality Management; see also quality improvement A culture within an organisation that is aimed at continuous improvement of educational quality.

Transferable skills Skills developed by engaging in an activity or experience that can be subsequently used in a different environment. For example, the skills of interpersonal communication that are developed during problem-based learning sessions can be used in professional conversations and patient interactions. Sometimes termed 'process' or 'generic' skills.

Validity An expression of how far the scores generated by an assessment tool make it possible to draw accurate inferences about the domain of interest; while various taxonomies exist, the concept of validity has traditionally included content validity (Does the test content correspond to the domain to be measured?), criterion validity (Do the test results correlate with results of other measures of the same domain, either concurrently or predictively?), construct validity (Do the test results accurately reflect expectations based upon underlying theory relevant to the construct being measured?), and face validity (Does it feel right?). In the context of assessment, validity is the strength of inferences which can be drawn from the outcomes (Has an assessment effectively measured what it was intended to measure?)

ZPD (Zone of proximal development) A concept developed by Vygotsky, which asserts that there is a cognitive state (the ZPD) in which learners can be helped to achieve higher levels of understanding by means of the action of others. For example, learners can be helped through the ZPD by teachers providing appropriate stimuli and intellectual scaffolding.

Index

Note: Page numbers followed by "*f*" indicate figures, "*t*" indicate tables, and "*b*" indicate boxes.